VETERINARY MEDICINE

Veterinary Medicine

A Guide to Historical Sources

PAMELA HUNTER
Freelance Archivist

Routledge
Taylor & Francis Group
LONDON AND NEW YORK

First published 2004 by Ashgate Publishing

Published 2016 by Routledge
2 Park Square, Milton Park, Abingdon, Oxon OX14 4RN
52 Vanderbilt Avenue, New York, NY 10017

Routledge is an imprint of the Taylor & Francis Group, an informa business

British Library Cataloguing in Publication Data
Hunter, Pamela
Veterinary medicine : a guide to historical sources. –
(Studies in British business archives)
1. Veterinary medicine – History – Sources – Bibliography
I. Title
016.6'3608909

Library of Congress Cataloging-in-Publication Data
Hunter, Pamela, 1967-
Veterinary medicine : a guide to historical sources / Pamela Hunter.
p. cm. – (Studies in British business archives)
Includes bibliographical references and indexes.
ISBN 0-7546-4053-1 (alk. paper)
1. Veterinary medicine–Great Britain–Sources. I. Title. II. Series.

SF610.8.H86 2003
636.089'0941–dc22

2003063713

ISBN 13: 978-0-7546-4053-0 (hbk)

Contents

Foreword

Never before have animals attracted so much attention from politicians, economists, academics, scientists, health experts, environmentalists, ethicists and the public at large. Whether as products for consumption or companionship, for military or humane practical application, for hunting or for sport, and whether in zoos, abattoirs, research stations or pits for mass disposal, animals and their relations to humans have become headline news. In one way or another, moreover, almost all of these areas of concern implicate biomedical conceptions and medical professional interventions. For this reason, among others, the history of veterinary medicine opens a window on more than merely a hitherto largely neglected branch of medicine. And it does more than supply a means to illuminate a wide variety of issues around knowledge production, professional practice and training, the development of state science, the trade in animal products and national and international agreements and regulations. It also provides a means to reflect on much of what is crucial to contemporary society, economy, politics and culture.

Veterinary Medicine: a guide to historical sources is therefore as timely as it is invaluable. The enormous range of archival material it surveys renders it a unique resource that will be of incalculable benefit to historians for generations to come. Along with its companion electronic database (compiled by the Business Archives Council on behalf of the Wellcome Trust between 1999 and 2001), the *Guide* now provides the essential starting point for documenting the long history and professionalisation of veterinary medicine. It will be found indispensable for studying the vicissitudes of both public and private practice in this area of medicine, for enquiry into the responses to animal epidemics and disease, for understanding the manufacture and marketing of veterinary products and, not least, for analysing the many different kinds of animal-human interactions that have existed among and between farmers, trade associations, pet keepers, zoo keepers, local authorities, scientists, government agencies and commissions, charities, the armed forces and animal welfarists among myriad others.

To the Business Archives Council and the Wellcome Trust we are indebted for the *Guide's* production. For gathering all the data, writing the entries and assembling them with consummate skill, Pamela Hunter, above all, deserves hearty congratulations. No labours are more prized than these.

Roger Cooter

Acknowledgements

The preparation of this *Guide* would have been impossible without the co-operation of the veterinary profession. The Royal College of Veterinary Surgeons took an active interest in the project from the outset and did everything in its power to ensure its success. In particular I would like to thank Tom Roper and the staff of the RCVS Library who have been unfailingly kind and helpful. They gave me unlimited access to their resources, checked details on numerous veterinary practices and veterinary surgeons and suggested several new lines of enquiry.

I also owe a huge debt to all those veterinary surgeons who took time out of their exceedingly busy lives to provide me with details of the records they hold. Many were kind enough to show me round their place of work and these visits were always both informative and hugely enjoyable. Although a number of retired veterinary surgeons were no doubt surprised to find me on their doorstep after little or no warning, they too were never anything other than welcoming and the information they provided gave me a valuable insight into the development of their profession over the last 60 years. Many of the practice histories rely heavily on their memories. I would also like to thank both Robert Mares, who introduced me to the archives of the Royal Army Veterinary Corps and provided a wealth of information on the history of veterinary medicine within the armed services, and Derek Lyons, who alerted me to sources for a number of Britain's leading zoos.

Archivists and librarians based at record offices, specialist repositories, veterinary colleges and research establishments across the country have been immensely helpful. I am aware that they have spent considerable amounts of time compiling lists and checking entries for me and I am grateful to them all.

I thank the Business Archives Council for its support. I am also indebted to Alison Turton and Lesley Richmond, editors of the *Studies in British Business Archives* series, who have given me much needed guidance from the start. A big thank you is also due to Professor Derek Oddy who has been unfailingly encouraging and supportive (with Merlot when necessary) throughout.

I would of course be deluding myself if I thought that I had produced a volume that was entirely free of errors. I hope, however, that they are few in number and minor in nature and take full responsibility for them all.

Pamela Hunter

Veterinary medicine: a brief history

Although the fortunes of man and beast have been bound together since early times, the evolution of veterinary medicine in Britain, both as a science and as a profession, has taken place only within the last two hundred years or so. The gradual progression from practitioner to professional, from doctoring to science, was dependent on a myriad of social, economic, political and scientific changes, all of which were necessary to drive progress forward and shape its path.

EARLY ANIMAL MEDICINE

Prior to the development of veterinary medicine both as a profession and as a science, the owner of a sick animal had few options open to him. Either he could attempt to treat the animal himself or he could call upon the services of those who made their living from animal medicine – cow leeches, horse doctors, farriers and their like. Since few of these practitioners offered much in the way of knowledge or skill, however, high mortality rates were an accepted fact of life. Many people came to regard the outbreaks of contagious disease that periodically devastated both the animal and human populations as divine punishment for the sins of man, while the truly desperate even turned to spells, charms and astrology in an effort to limit their losses.

Given their economic and social importance, it was natural that most care and attention in early times was centred on horses. It was out of concern for the poor standards of care which so many horses were being subjected to that the Mayor of London was prompted in 1356 to call upon all farriers within a seven mile radius of the City of London to form a fellowship to regulate their trade more effectively. Out of this appeal emerged the Worshipful Company of Farriers, which was granted its charter in 1674 and raised to livery company status in 1692. At first the company proposed that only its members should be allowed to practise within the City boundary, and that anyone wishing to become a member should first serve a seven year apprenticeship. This ambitious scheme soon proved impossible to enforce, however, and the company instead had to be content with a more general role, encouraging education and prosecuting wrongdoers. The compulsory registration of farriers was only achieved in 1975.[1]

Although initially concerned only with shoeing, farriers gradually widened their skills to include a number of procedures such as firing, bleeding, castrating and tail docking. Bleeding was widely regarded as a cure for all ills, whilst firing – the placing of hot irons on the skin in order to deflect pain and inflammation from their original location – persisted until well into the twentieth century. Many farriers and horse doctors also developed their own herbal dressings, ointments and powders, and by the eighteenth century were routinely applying these to cattle and even the occasional sheep or pig, as well as to horses.

PRESSURE FOR CHANGE

The eighteenth century saw a vast surge in the demand for fit and healthy horses, which in turn stimulated the need for highly skilled practitioners. The army's insatiable appetite for horses was fuelled by the numerous wars that Britain became embroiled in during the course of the century. Additionally, there was also a growing reliance on horses for both power and transport. The rapidly expanding coal, textile and iron industries all required horses to power their new machinery and transport the finished goods to and from markets, ports and canals across the country. The turnpike road system, first introduced during the seventeenth century, boomed, with 498 Turnpike Acts being passed between 1720 and 1770. By 1770, turnpike trusts were administering over 5000 miles of road, an increase of over 1500 miles in just twenty years.[2] Improved roads led in turn to a growth in the volume of traffic, particularly passenger traffic. Thirty stagecoaches were travelling along the Birmingham to London road each day by 1763, compared to only one in 1740.[3] As a result, large numbers of farriers began setting themselves up in business close to the stables and coaching inns that were springing up all over the country.

Further opportunities were created by the burgeoning interest in horseracing. Previously the preserve of royalty, its appeal broadened considerably during the eighteenth century as racetracks were set up in towns across the country. The Jockey Club was formed in 1752 to regulate the sport, while the latter part of the century saw the establishment of several classic races, notably the St Leger in 1778, the Oaks in 1779, the Derby in 1780 and the 2000 Guineas in 1807.[4] Racing became big business, and with money, pride and reputations all at stake, breeding assumed a new importance. James Weatherby's *General Stud Book*, first published in 1791, quickly became the benchmark by which all racehorses were measured, for only those who could trace their lineage back to horses listed in the *General Stud Book* could legitimately be called thoroughbreds.[5]

At the same time, hunting, particularly foxhunting, was becoming increasingly popular. The emergence of hunting clubs meant that anyone who could afford the yearly subscription was able to take an active part in the sport, thus opening it up to a much wider number of people than had hitherto been possible. Many of the most famous hunts, such as the Pytchley, Belvoir and Quorn, were established during the 1770s. The nature of hunting changed too. With the drastic reduction in open land brought about by the Enclosure Acts, it became necessary to breed horses that were not only fast but also strong enough to cope with jumping large numbers of fences, walls and rails over a sustained period of time.[6]

Demand for a higher standard of livestock medicine also increased during the eighteenth century, prompted in no small part by changes to the agricultural system. Over the previous 150 years, a range of agricultural improvements including the enclosure of land, large-scale drainage schemes and crop rotation had been introduced and developed, all of which had considerable benefits for the livestock farmer. Improved pasture led to better quality hay, which, linked with the spread of root crops such as turnips, made it possible for farmers to raise nutritional standards and thus preserve more of their livestock through the winter months. This in turn stimulated an interest in selective breeding and a number of new breeds subsequently emerged – in cattle, sheep, pigs, poultry and horses.

At the same time, farmers were coming under increasing pressure to raise productivity. Falling death rates and rising birth rates signalled a rapid growth in the size of the human population – from about 6.25 million in 1700 to 10.5 million by 1800. Demand for food was, therefore, increasing.[7] Britain was also becoming more urban. A quarter of England's population lived in towns of 5000 people or more by 1800, compared to only thirteen per cent a hundred years earlier. By the middle of the nineteenth century, more people would be living in towns than in the countryside.[8] The demand for higher productivity, therefore, had to be met by fewer and fewer people.

As the quality and value of livestock increased, farmers, breeders and industrialists all became more anxious about protecting their animals against disease. Outbreaks of cattle plague (rinderpest) in 1714 and 1745 had resulted in the loss of over half a million cattle, while a strangles epidemic in 1752 had paralysed a number of collieries in Staffordshire and Wales.[9] In strong contrast to the advances made in agriculture and industry, however, and despite a general growth in scientific awareness during the eighteenth century, including a gradual development of the three disciplines of comparative medicine – physiology, histology and pathology – that would eventually form the basis for a scientific approach to disease, veterinary science remained primitive. Eventually it became clear that the only way to meet the demand for a more scientific approach to animal medicine was to provide specialised training at veterinary colleges.

THE FIRST VETERINARY COLLEGES

The first veterinary college had been established at Lyon, France, in 1762 by Claude Bourgelat, director of the local Academy for Equitation.[10] Over the next twenty years, Bourgelat's example was followed by others at Alfort in France, Turin in Italy, Copenhagen in Denmark, Vienna in Austria, Dresden and Gottingen in Germany and Budapest in Hungary. Britain, though, lagged far behind the rest of Europe. Early attempts to form specialist colleges in England, notably in 1758 and 1766, had been restricted to equine medicine and had come to nothing.

Impetus for Britain's first veterinary college came initially from the Odiham Agricultural Society. Founded in Hampshire in 1783, it was one of many such societies formed around that time to encourage the widespread adoption of improved agricultural methods. At a meeting in 1785, the Society passed a motion stating 'that Farriery, as commonly practised, is conducted without principle of science and greatly to the injury to the noblest and most useful of our animals. That the improvement of Farriery established on a study of the Anatomy, diseases and cure of cattle particularly Horses, Cows and Sheep, will be an essential benefit to Agriculture and will greatly improve some of the most important branches of national commerce, such as Wool and Leather'.[11]

Within three years the Society had raised enough money to send two boys to the veterinary college at Alfort in France. However, a chance meeting in 1789 between Granville Penn, a Society member, and a French veterinarian called Charles Benôit Vial de St Bel led to an altogether more ambitious scheme. St Bel had for some time been trying unsuccessfully to attract support for his plan to open a veterinary college in England, based on a three-year course offering full training and education on the anatomy, physiology and diseases of all domesticated animals. After some discussion, the Society began to explore the possibility of opening a veterinary college in London. A Committee was formed in the city in November 1790 which during the following February adopted the title 'The Veterinary College, London'. From this time, though, the Odiham Agricultural Society ceased to play an active role in the college, choosing to concentrate on local issues once more. Long term interest in the Society was not sustained and it ceased to meet after 1796.

The proposed veterinary college attracted a number of distinguished subscribers, including the Prince of Wales, the Earl of Pembroke, who had done much to improve the lot of the cavalry horse, and Sir Charles

Bunbury, a notable name in horseracing circles and a former Jockey Club steward. Included in the list of honourable members were Sir Joseph Banks, President of the Royal Society, and the physicians Sir George Baker and John Hunter. Following St Bel's appointment as Professor and the selection of suitable premises near St Pancras Church, the Veterinary College, London, opened its doors in January 1792. From an initial intake of four residential students, the college by the end of the year had fourteen residential students and a number of non-residential students.[12]

Almost immediately, however, the new college ran into difficulties. St Bel, very much the driving force behind the venture, died in 1793, casting grave doubts over its future. The main difficulty was deciding on a suitable successor. At that time there was only one English veterinary graduate, William Moorcroft, who had qualified from the Lyon Veterinary College in 1791. Moorcroft, though, had little desire to leave his lucrative equine practice on London's Oxford Street. Eventually, in 1794, a compromise was reached whereby Moorcroft was appointed joint Professor with a human surgeon called Edward Coleman. Within a matter of weeks, however, Moorcroft had returned to his practice, leaving Coleman in sole charge.

Although Coleman had had little experience of animal medicine he remained Professor and Principal of the Veterinary College, London, until his death in 1839. During his long reign he made no attempt to implement St Bel's vision of a three-year course with its wide-ranging curriculum. Instead, Coleman concentrated almost exclusively on equine medicine. In 1796, following his appointment as Principal Veterinary Surgeon to the Cavalry and Veterinary Surgeon to the Board of Ordinance (Artillery), it was agreed that a veterinary surgeon should be attached to each regiment of the cavalry. The army further agreed to defray the costs of up to six men per year at the veterinary college. But when some within the army baulked at the thought of having to wait three years for qualified veterinary surgeons, especially as men were urgently needed for the war against France, Coleman offered instead to train medical men in just three months. Since a shorter course meant more students, which in turn led to more fees, both Coleman and the college governors were naturally reluctant to discontinue the practice once the army's needs had been met. Inevitably, therefore, the college was soon attracting a poor standard of entrant and turning out graduates with only the most rudimentary training

By the 1820s, the state of affairs at the Veterinary College, London, (or the Royal Veterinary College, London, as it was known from 1826), was a source of considerable dismay and disappointment to many of those who had initially welcomed its establishment. And with the introduction of two new veterinary journals in 1828 – *The Farrier and Naturalist* (later *The Hippiatrist*) and *The Veterinarian* – this disquiet could be effectively voiced for the first time. Although *The Hippiatrist* ceased publication after only two years, *The Veterinarian* continued to appear monthly until 1902, offering veterinarians, many of whom worked alone, the chance to share ideas and opinions for the first time. During its lifetime the journal contributed much to the advancement of the profession, publishing accounts of interesting cases and new treatments as well as highlighting issues affecting the profession. Crucially, its editors from the outset used their position to campaign for the reform of the Royal Veterinary College.

A more tangible challenge to the Royal Veterinary College emerged in 1823 with the establishment of a rival college in Edinburgh. At that time it was estimated that there were no more than a dozen qualified veterinary surgeons working in Scotland, since few could afford the fare to London, the college fees or the costs incurred by living there for a protracted period. To remedy this, the Lord Provost of Edinburgh, William Arbuthnot, proposed in 1821 that the University of Edinburgh establish a Chair in Comparative Anatomy. This idea was rejected by the university, which suggested instead that a veterinary college be established with the support of the Highland Society at Edinburgh (known as the Highland and Agricultural Society of Scotland from 1834). A committee was formed under the chairmanship of Dr John Barclay of the city's medical school, which in due course recommended that a veterinary course be set up. The committee also recommended that William Dick be appointed course lecturer. Dick had initially worked alongside his father as a smith and farrier, but had also found enough time to attend Barclay's lectures on anatomy as well as others on medicine and chemistry. In 1817 he enrolled at the Veterinary College, London, and obtained his diploma the following year. Nor was Dick a stranger to teaching, having already given a series of lectures in veterinary science at Edinburgh's newly founded School of Arts.

Dick's first lecture to the Edinburgh Veterinary College was given on the 24 November 1823 at the Calton Convening Rooms. During the first session, 46 lectures, covering the diseases of horses, sheep and cattle, were given to 25 students, each of whom had paid two guineas.[13] The lectures were backed up with clinical sessions at Dick's forge in Clyde Street. For the 1825–26 session, the course was extended to three lectures a week and students were encouraged to attend additional classes at the medical school. Examinations were held at the end of each session and certificates issued by the Highland and Agricultural Society of Scotland to those that passed declaring them 'qualified to practise the veterinary art'.[14] By 1833, both student numbers and curriculum had grown to such an extent that expansion was necessary. The new facilities at Clyde Street, largely paid for by Dick himself, included a lecture room, museum, dissecting room, infirmary and forge. Clinical material was provided by Dick's private practice and by his 'pauper patients'.

Despite these developments, however, the standard of veterinary care did not improve significantly. Neither the London nor the Edinburgh colleges imposed a formal entrance requirement. Fees were low and facilities limited. Students attended for only a few months before sitting an oral examination, which in London at least was conducted solely by medical men. These factors made it impossible for either college to attract a high quality of applicant or to adequately train those men that were accepted. Moreover, unlike most continental veterinary schools, the fact that both colleges were private institutions, reliant on fees and patronage for their survival, meant that they could not be held accountable to any outside body. Ultimately, those seeking reform were forced to conclude that nothing short of incorporation would guarantee an improvement in standards.

THE EMERGENCE OF THE PROFESSION

The possibility of incorporation, initially suggested at a meeting in 1828, was by 1834 being openly called for by *The Veterinarian*. Its supporters argued that incorporation would create a recognised profession and confer upon those belonging to it a degree of status, putting them on a par with their medical counterparts. A distinction between the 'professional' and 'non-professional' would make it easier for the large numbers of quacks to be eliminated, which in turn would encourage a better quality of entrant into the profession. The creation of a chartered body was also seen as the only way of gaining control over the educational standards of the colleges. Coleman's death in 1839 had briefly raised hopes that reform at the Royal Veterinary College would at last be possible, but these were quickly dashed by the appointment of Coleman's long-time assistant, William Sewell, as his successor.

At this point the initiative was seized by Thomas Mayer, a practitioner living and working in Newcastle under Lyme. Together with his son, Thomas Walton Mayer, he drafted a memorial addressed to the Governors of the Royal Veterinary College asking them to support a charter 'to protect us from illiterate and uneducated men, and to afford us the same privileges and exemptions which other professional bodies possess'.[15] A copy of the draft was sent to every veterinarian in the country together with a plea for support. Although the memorial was rejected as unnecessary by the governors of the Royal Veterinary College, who were unwilling to consent to anything that might lead to a diminution of their power, the Mayers were undeterred. A committee was set up dedicated to achieving incorporation and a petition submitted to the Privy Council in 1841. Finally, in February 1844, after lengthy negotiations and numerous redrafts, a charter of incorporation was granted.

Under the terms of the charter, veterinary medicine was formally recognised as a profession and the Royal College of Veterinary Surgeons created as its sole co-ordinating and regulatory body, with responsibility for enhancing the profession's status and controlling standards within veterinary education. To achieve these objectives, the Royal College of Veterinary Surgeons immediately introduced its own examination, to be sat by all veterinary students on completion of their studies. Only those who passed this examination would be admitted to the Royal College of Veterinary Surgeons' register as Members of the Royal College of Veterinary Surgeons (MsRCVS) and entitled to call themselves 'veterinary surgeons'.

Almost immediately, however, these plans were thrown into confusion. Both colleges had been signatories to the petition but neither had believed in its ultimate success. When the charter was duly granted, therefore, the governors of the Royal Veterinary College, London, and William Dick in Edinburgh were horrified, realising that their monopoly powers would be effectively at an end. The governors of the Royal Veterinary College lost no time in petitioning the Home Secretary, claiming that the charter infringed their privileges. This was followed by a second petition in 1845 requesting that the college be awarded a separate charter.[16] Although both petitions failed, relations between the Royal Veterinary College and the Royal College of Veterinary Surgeons remained strained for several years. Only with the election of William Sewell to the presidency of the Royal College of Veterinary Surgeons in 1852 was the breach finally healed.

The rift with William Dick proved much more damaging. At the first meeting of the newly created Royal College of Veterinary Surgeons, Dick 'protested that … several clauses had been introduced and others omitted in the Charter without his knowledge or consent'.[17] His anger was increased when the visiting Royal College of Veterinary Surgeons' examiners criticised the standard of the Edinburgh Veterinary College examinations. Standards were in all likelihood low. In common with his London counterparts, Dick held his examinations publicly in a local tavern. Students were asked a few undemanding questions to which they replied orally. Written and practical examinations were unheard of. The college, however, had been at the centre of Dick's life for over twenty years, and any criticism, no matter how mild, was bound to be taken personally. Finally, in 1848, following several years of complaint and resentment, Dick formally ended his college's affiliation with the Royal College of Veterinary Surgeons. Edinburgh graduates were once again awarded the Highland and Agricultural Society of Scotland's certificate and, in the absence of any legislation to back up the terms of its charter, the Royal College of Veterinary Surgeons found itself powerless to prevent this.

Other limitations were also becoming clear. One of the main aims of incorporation had been the creation of a recognised profession, one that would provide its members with the same status and privileges enjoyed by those of other professions, particularly the medical profession. Yet a survey carried out by the Royal College of Veterinary Surgeons in 1862–63 showed that while there were 1018 qualified veterinary surgeons in practice, there were also 1244 unqualified people calling themselves veterinary surgeons and another 1189 providing treatment for animals under various other titles.[18] Furthermore, census returns for 1861 show that some 6774 people described themselves as providers of veterinary services in England and Wales, suggesting that the qualified practitioners were outnumbered by as much as six to one.[19] The Royal College of Veterinary Surgeons was therefore forced to face the unwelcome fact that it was unable to prevent anyone, whether they were qualified or not, from calling themselves a veterinary surgeon and charging whatever fees they chose. Moreover, it lacked the power even to discipline or expel from its membership those men it felt to be guilty of 'base and dishonorable practices'.[20]

The large numbers of quacks in practice proved to be one of the biggest stumbling blocks in the veterinary surgeon's quest for improved status. Farmers with sick animals generally turned in the first instance to unqualified practitioners. All too often, the veterinary surgeon found that he was being called in to cases only as a last resort, usually when it was too late for him to be of any practical use. This then placed him in an impossible situation. If he treated the animal and it died he was blamed. If by some chance the animal recovered, the quack would then claim that the recovery was due to his treatment, rather than that of the veterinary surgeon. More significantly, owners of animals generally had little faith in the skill or knowledge of any practitioner, qualified or not. And as long as the veterinary surgeon was perceived as being no more able than his unqualified counterpart, there was little chance of the profession being able to raise its status or attract well-educated men into its ranks.

The obvious remedy was to improve the standard of veterinary education. But here again the Royal College of Veterinary Surgeons had only limited powers. While it could and did compel both colleges to increase the length of their courses to two years, it was unable to impose the other reforms necessary for raising standards – higher entry requirements, improved clinical training, a wider curriculum and the ending of examination by medical rather than veterinary men. Changes such as these could only be achieved with the co-operation of the colleges themselves, which at that time was not exactly forthcoming. Even if the colleges had been agreeable, however, it is doubtful whether such wide-sweeping changes could have been implemented, since they would have required large sums of money, impossible for private institutions to raise, and levels of scientific knowledge which at that time eluded even the most advanced scientists and teachers. Eventually the Royal College of Veterinary Surgeons was forced to concede that without legislation little could be done to improve either the profession's status or its competency.

Fundamental changes in the British way of life, meanwhile, were making the need for a competent, organised veterinary profession more pressing than ever. Rising affluence had brought about a substantial increase in the demand for meat, putting farmers under pressure to raise productivity levels once again. This demand was met partly by a surge in imports, facilitated by the relaxation of restrictions governing the importation of live animals for food purposes in 1842, followed by the introduction of free trade in 1846. As a result, large numbers of live animals began arriving from the continent at ports all over Britain. Since the demise of the first Board of Agriculture in 1822, however, there was little structure in place for monitoring livestock, making it easy for infected animals to enter the country. Once ashore they could be transported via the rapidly expanding rail network to markets and pastures throughout Britain. Conditions at markets, never very satisfactory, deteriorated further as increased numbers of animals were slaughtered and processed with no attempt to separate the healthy from the diseased. Before long several contagious diseases were being officially noted for the first time including foot-and-mouth disease (1838), pleuro-pneumonia (1841) and sheep pox (1847).

As concern about public health increased, many began to question the safety of the food being produced and consumed. The government did little, however, to allay these fears. An Act passed in 1848 giving port authorities the power to inspect and destroy animals was never implemented, while the Nuisances Removal Act of 1855, allowing local authorities to employ inspectors, had only a limited effect. A lack of scientific knowledge amongst veterinary surgeons, amply demonstrated by William Sewell, Principal of the Royal Veterinary College, who reported to the Royal Agricultural Society of England that pleuro-pneumonia was caused by 'a strange convulsion of nature, some extraordinary extrication of mephitic vapours from the bowels of the earth'[21] also prevented the introduction of significant improvements. Alarmed by these developments, and at the apparent inability of either the emergent veterinary profession or the government to deal effectively with them, the Royal Agricultural Society of England in 1842 endowed a Chair in Cattle Pathology at the Royal Veterinary College, London.

Social changes also played their part. More and more people were spending their entire lives in towns and cities, totally removed from any day-to-day contact with the animal world. In spite of, or perhaps because of this, there developed a widespread fascination with the natural world, fuelled in part by the publication of Charles Darwin's theories. Botany, zoology, ornithology and butterfly collecting all became popular hobbies and a number of zoological gardens were established, including those at London (1828) and Bristol (1835).[22] This interest, coinciding as it did with a rise in disposable income and leisure time, also led to unprecedented numbers of animals being kept as pets. Dogs, cats, birds, rabbits and even monkeys were all popular choices and inevitably led to an interest in breeding and showing. The first dog show was held at Newcastle upon Tyne in 1857, and was followed in 1863 by the establishment of the Kennel Club, while the first cat show took place at the Crystal Palace, London, in 1871.[23]

With more animals being kept as pets, the demand for small animal veterinary care increased. *The Veterinarian* published its first article on diseases of cats in 1841, and by 1850 was reporting that 'many practitioners' were restricting their practice to canine medicine.[24] Although it is unlikely that 'many practitioners' were treating pets exclusively at this time, the trend had been established and would continue to grow over the next 150 years. By this time, too, a number of scientific developments were enabling veterinary surgeons to diagnose and treat small animals more effectively. The risks attached to surgery, for example, were greatly reduced by the introduction of improved needles and suturing materials and by the development of anaesthetics such as ether and chloroform. The latter's usefulness was first demonstrated on humans by James Simpson in 1847, and he later went on to test its effectiveness on domestic animals. Other major advances included the introduction of hypodermic syringes, enabling medication to be more accurately administered, particularly vital in the treatment of small animals, and thermometers, first demonstrated by John Gamgee in 1865 and George Armatage of the Glasgow Veterinary College in 1869.[25]

As human attitudes towards animals shifted, society became less tolerant of animal cruelty. Between 1800 and 1835 no fewer than eleven Bills were introduced into the House of Commons.[26] Although most failed the Cruelty to Animals Act, outlawing animal baiting, entered the statute book in 1822 and a number of animal welfare charities were founded in its wake, notably the Society for the Prevention of Cruelty to Animals in 1824 and the Scottish Society for the Prevention of Cruelty to Animals in 1839. The former was responsible for 149 convictions for animal cruelty in its first year alone[27], whilst the latter worked hard to improve conditions for the working horse, installing drinking troughs along highways and carrying out formal inspections of pit ponies and Highland coaching horses. Within a few years both Societies were able to report a marked improvement in the health and condition of working horses and a corresponding rise in the number of unhealthy horses being sent to the slaughterhouse.[28]

It was against this background that the Royal College of Veterinary Surgeons in 1863 began its quest for statutory recognition. A Veterinary Medicine Bill was drafted which its supporters hoped would give veterinary surgeons a monopoly similar to that granted to the medical profession by the Medical Act of 1858. With such powers, the Royal College of Veterinary Surgeons would finally be able to prevent the unqualified from practising as veterinary surgeons and raise both the educational and professional standards of its members. Only then would the profession be in a position to exploit the potential of the new opportunities being created by the developments in veterinary science.

One of the main drawbacks, however, was the continued rift with the Edinburgh Veterinary College. Many in Scotland believed that if the Veterinary Medicine Bill became law, all those holding the Scottish diploma who were not also members of the Royal College of Veterinary Surgeons – about 250 men in total – would be ineligible to practise in England. This climate of suspicion was heightened by the inability of some to grasp that the Royal College of Veterinary Surgeons and the Royal Veterinary College were two entirely separate bodies, a misapprehension exacerbated by the fact that at that time the Council of each was dominated by the same men. It was feared that the Royal Veterinary College was in effect trying to take over the Edinburgh Veterinary College.[29]

Others, however, were all too aware of the harm that could result if the dispute between Dick's college and the Royal College of Veterinary Surgeons remained unresolved. The position of the former had been severely weakened by the establishment of two new veterinary colleges in Scotland, the first of which had been opened in 1858 by John Gamgee. Gamgee had initially arrived in Edinburgh in 1856 as William Dick's assistant. Frustrated by the poor facilities and low educational standards, however, it was not long before he was engaged in a series of violent disputes with his employer. After only a year, Gamgee left the Edinburgh Veterinary College and opened the New Edinburgh Veterinary College shortly afterwards, in direct opposition to his former employer. Significantly, in 1859 the New Edinburgh Veterinary College was awarded the royal sign manual, enabling its students to sit the Royal College of Veterinary Surgeons' membership examination. Despite this, and Gamgee's advanced teaching methods and ideas, the New Edinburgh Veterinary College struggled to survive in Edinburgh. In 1865 Gamgee made the decision to move to London where the college re-opened as the Albert Veterinary College . Once again, though, it failed to flourish and closed completely three years later.

Meanwhile, another college had opened at Glasgow in 1862. Its Principal, James McCall, had begun giving informal lectures at his practice in Hope Street, Glasgow, shortly after his graduation from the Edinburgh Veterinary College in 1859. Formal classes were instituted following the practice's move to Parliamentary Road in 1862 and the first three students qualified in 1865. Like Gamgee before him, McCall also successfully applied for the royal sign manual, and shortly afterwards the college moved to new premises in Buccleuch Street, which remained its home for the next century.

The establishment of two new colleges in Scotland strengthened the Royal College of Veterinary Surgeon's position considerably, while that of the Edinburgh Veterinary College was seriously undermined. Additionally, the granting of sign manuals to both Gamgee's and McCall's colleges made it clear that the Royal College of Veterinary Surgeons rather than the veterinary colleges was the profession's ruling body. If the Veterinary Medicine Bill were to succeed, therefore, the Edinburgh Veterinary College's position would become untenable, since it would be unable to offer its graduates a valid qualification. Dick, however, remained unmoved. Even a memorial signed by over seventy of his own graduates in 1865 requesting that he re-enter negotiations with the Royal College of Veterinary Surgeons failed to elicit any response.

Ultimately, however, it was another event, which, although initially serving only to expose the profession's deficiencies and ignorance, ultimately allowed it to move forward and develop.

THE CATTLE PLAGUE OF 1865

In the summer of 1865, James Beart Simonds of the Royal Veterinary College was called out to a dairy in Islington, London, where large numbers of cattle were dying. Within a few days he had diagnosed cattle plague, the first recorded outbreak in Britain for nearly a century. Simonds recommended drastic measures to bring the outbreak under control – the restriction of animal movement, the slaughter of both infected and contact beasts and the payment of compensation to those farmers and dairymen whose stock had been slaughtered. With the exception of John Gamgee, however, this advice found little favour. Such drastic action was vigorously opposed by the cattle trade, and the government, true to its *laissez-faire* beliefs, was reluctant to interfere. Instead attempts were made to treat infected animals, despite the absence of any known cure. Critically, little was done to restrict the movement of livestock, nor was there any attempt to separate imported animals from domestically reared livestock. The disease was therefore able to spread across the country unchecked, killing an estimated 400,000 animals.[30]

Only in early 1866 was the government, bowing largely to pressure from the Royal Agricultural Society of England (whose advisor Simonds was), persuaded to intervene. Many of Simonds's original recommendations were embodied in the Cattle Plague Prevention Act, which was rushed through parliament in February 1866. To oversee the eradication programme and supervise the work of inspectors, a temporary Veterinary Department was set up within the Privy Council, the body traditionally responsible for gathering statistics relating to outbreaks of disease and with the necessary powers to impose Orders relating to the importation, movement and slaughter of diseased animals.

Once these measures were in place, the effects were soon felt. The number of new cases fell from 18,000 a week in February 1866 to just eight per week by the end of the year, although it was 1867 before the country was declared entirely free of the disease.[31] Several factors made progress slower than it might otherwise have been. Firstly, because cattle plague had been unknown for so long, veterinary surgeons, practitioners and cattle owners were all equally unfamiliar with the symptoms and therefore slow to diagnose it. Secondly, administration of the eradication programme was left to local authorities who were entrusted to hire inspectors and report those breaking the law. Some took their duties seriously and were rigorous in their application of the law, but others were much more half-hearted and a few did nothing at all. Finally, too few inspectors were employed and there were serious question marks over the ability of many of those that were.

The economic effects of the cattle plague were enormous. Many had invested large sums of money and long periods of time building up quality herds, only to see them wiped out in a matter of days. Others, who relied on cattle for their living, were similarly affected. James McCall, Principal of the Glasgow Veterinary College and veterinary advisor to the City of Glasgow, estimated that cattle plague cost the city's dairymen £8978 during 1865–66. More crucially, however, McCall's figures also revealed that other diseases were in fact even more costly, since in the same year pleuro-pneumonia had accounted for losses of £54,672 and other fevers a further £14,335.[32] Such crippling losses emphasised to landowners, farmers and traders alike the dangers posed to their livelihoods by disease. But few trusted the ability of the veterinary surgeon, their attitude being summed up by the medical officer for

Hackney, Dr Tripe, who noted that London cow keepers 'believe that veterinary surgeons have not studied the diseases of cows and consequently will not employ surgeons'.[33]

Since radical changes were clearly needed if disease was to be tackled effectively, and it was acknowledged that these changes could only be brought about if the Royal College of Veterinary Surgeons was given more power, support for the Veterinary Medicine Bill became more widespread. But in 1866, after two readings in the House of Commons, the Bill was abandoned. H A Bruce, spokesman for the Privy Council, advised the Royal College of Veterinary Surgeons that too few of its members were deemed knowledgeable enough to merit the privileges of professionalism.

THE DEVELOPMENT OF THE PROFESSION

The failure of the Veterinary Medicine Bill made veterinary surgeons aware that there was still much to do before they could be regarded as professionals. Over the next fifteen years, therefore, a number of measures were introduced which aimed to unify veterinary surgeons, improve their competency and raise their profile. One of the most important was the establishment of provincial associations. The first, founded in Manchester in 1851, attracted only twelve members and was disbanded shortly afterwards. But the precedent had been set, and the West of Scotland Veterinary Medical Association, established in Glasgow in 1858, was quickly followed by a rash of others in Hampshire and Lancashire in 1862, Yorkshire and the North of England in 1863, Liverpool in 1864, Central Scotland and the West of England in 1865 and the Midland Counties in 1866. Membership of each varied between twenty and fifty and meetings were generally held every three months.[34] By giving members the chance to discuss cases and ideas with each other and to hear papers on the latest scientific breakthroughs, the meetings were an effective means of improving the general practitioner's knowledge in the diagnosis and treatment of disease.

Another important step was the organisation of the first Veterinary Congress, held in London in 1867. Recognising that the majority of veterinary surgeons lived in professional solitude with few opportunities for contact with colleagues, the Congress's organisers aimed to give participants the chance to meet and talk with fellow professionals and to foster feelings of unity amongst them.

Significant steps were also taken to improve the education system. The Royal Veterinary College in 1864 introduced a matriculation test, which required all potential students to prove that they possessed basic numeracy and literacy skills. In 1870 entrance examinations were made compulsory at all the veterinary colleges. This was followed in 1872 by the introduction of practical examinations and in 1876 by an extension of the course length to three years. Longer courses meant that more subjects could be taught and to a greater degree of depth. They also forced the colleges to expand their facilities. At the Royal Veterinary College, for example, a new dissecting room was opened in 1863, followed by an enclosure for the slaughter and post-mortem examination of hospital patients. By 1867 the college also boasted several new loose boxes, a chemistry laboratory, a lecture theatre and a new museum.[35]

The Edinburgh Veterinary College, too, underwent a series of changes, prompted largely by the death of William Dick in 1866. Under the terms of Dick's will, the Edinburgh Veterinary College was bequeathed to the city and a trust set up to fund it, the Lord Provost, Magistrates and Council of the City of Edinburgh all being nominated trustees. The following year, William Williams of Bradford, West Yorkshire, was appointed Principal and the college's future seemed assured. But in 1873, after a series of disputes, Williams resigned and, like Gamgee before him, went on to found his own rival college, the New Veterinary College, Edinburgh. Unlike Gamgee, though, Williams crucially succeeded in taking with him all but nine of the students, as well as the entire teaching staff and the college library, leaving the future of the Edinburgh Veterinary College in grave doubt. Only with the appointment of Thomas Walley in 1875 could the Edinburgh Veterinary College, or Royal (Dick) Veterinary College as it was renamed, once again look forward to a period of sustained growth. By 1904, following the removal of Williams' college to Liverpool, it had once again become the only veterinary college in Edinburgh.

At the same time, a number of important breakthroughs were being made that would later have enormous implications for the future of veterinary science. In 1876, Robert Koch successfully proved that anthrax, a highly infectious disease transmissible to humans, was caused by a bacterium. Koch's findings were backed up by the work of Louis Pasteur and led in turn to a whole host of new discoveries, culminating with the isolation of the tuberculosis bacillus by Koch in 1882. Immunology, bacteriology and microbiology signalled the future of medical and veterinary science and would eventually dispel forever the myth that contagious disease was spread by spontaneous generation.

Veterinary surgeons were also benefiting from increased government involvement. Politicians and officials could not help but be aware that the more active role adopted by their French counterparts in the setting up and running of veterinary colleges, as well as the encouragement of scientific research and the preparation of comprehensive measures designed to control outbreaks of contagious disease had resulted in the loss of only fifty to sixty beasts during the cattle plague of 1865.[36] By contrast, the little regulation that existed in Britain was mostly restricted to local by-laws and concerned solely with the seizure and destruction of unsound meat which, with the exception of Smithfield Market, London, did not apply to live animals. And as both veterinary education and research were reliant on private funding, the progress of each fell well behind the rest of Europe. It was clear, therefore, that the government would henceforth have to play a more prominent role in the management of animal health.

The temporary Veterinary Department set up within the Privy Council in October 1865 had been replaced the following April by a Cattle Plague Department, again within the Privy Council and again intended to be only a temporary body to administer the Cattle Plague Prevention Act 1866. But with the passing of the Contagious Diseases (Animals) Act in 1869 the Department's scope widened considerably, since the Act included measures aimed at dealing not only with cattle plague but also with a host of other diseases, including pleuro-pneumonia, sheep pox, foot-and-mouth, sheep scab and glanders. Under the terms of the Act, local authorities were to notify the Privy Council of any outbreaks of these 'scheduled' diseases. They were also permitted to slaughter contact as well as infected animals, although the Act fell short of compelling them to do so. Additional powers were passed to the Department by the introduction of the first Transit Order in 1870 which limited the number of ports through which animals could pass and forced the improvement of slaughter and quarantine facilities.

From a hastily assembled temporary body, therefore, the Veterinary Department rapidly developed into a permanent fixture. By 1871 it employed two senior veterinary officers and 18 full time veterinary port inspectors, while local authorities were employing 1450 inspectors, of which 372 were veterinary surgeons.[37] The Department was producing annual reports and an annual *Return of Proceedings* with details of disease outbreaks, imports and exports and compensation costs. The creation of a permanent department and the steady increase of its duties in turn boosted demand for professionally qualified veterinary surgeons, since large numbers of inspectors were required to implement the new legislation.

THE VETERINARY SURGEONS ACT OF 1881

By the mid 1870s, the Royal College of Veterinary Surgeons had seen enough progress to encourage it to try once again for legislative backing.

Hopes that a second Veterinary Medicine Bill would be more favourably looked upon were given a substantial boost by the granting in 1876 of a supplemental charter that allowed the Royal College of Veterinary Surgeons to elect Fellows as well as Honorary and Foreign Associates. The charter also compelled the Royal College of Veterinary Surgeons to keep a register of members, although it had in reality been publishing an annual register since the 1860s. More significantly, the college was granted the power to remove from the register the names of those veterinary surgeons it deemed to be incompetent or discredited.

Only one obstacle seemed to now lie between the Royal College of Veterinary Surgeons and the legislation it had fought so long for, namely the long-running dispute with the Edinburgh Veterinary College. In a move towards finally resolving the impasse the President of the Royal College of Veterinary Surgeons, Frederick Fitzwygram, proposed in 1878 that holders of the Highland and Agricultural Society of Scotland certificate be awarded the MRCVS diploma after sitting an examination and paying a fee. Although this proposal was rejected by the Highland and Agricultural Society of Scotland, lengthy negotiations produced a compromise, confirmed in a second supplementary charter in 1879, by which Highland and Agricultural Society of Scotland certificate holders were deemed eligible for membership of the Royal College of Veterinary Surgeons without sitting an examination. In return for this concession, the Highland and Agricultural Society of Scotland agreed to stop issuing certificates after 1881.

The way was now clear for legislation and in 1881 George Fleming, Principal Veterinary Surgeon to the Forces and the newly elected President of the Royal College of Veterinary Surgeons, made the Act his clear goal. Crucial support was offered by the Royal Society for the Prevention of Cruelty to Animals, which recognised that if the title 'veterinary surgeon' was applied only to qualified men it would be much easier for members of the public to avoid quacks. The Society's President agreed to introduce the Veterinary Surgeons Bill into the House of Lords while Earl Spencer, at that time Lord President of the Privy Council, took on overall responsibility for steering the Bill through Parliament. Eventually, in August 1881, the Veterinary Surgeons Act finally entered the statute book.

First and foremost, the Act confirmed both the charter of 1844 and the supplemental charters of 1876 and 1879. From that time onwards it was illegal for anyone who was not a member of the Royal College of Veterinary Surgeons to call himself a veterinary surgeon or to practise as such. There was also an awareness, however, that suddenly restricting the provision of all animal care to MRCVS diploma holders would deprive many honest and experienced people of their livelihood and create distress and hardship for both them and their families. The Act therefore made provision for the Royal College of Veterinary Surgeons to maintain a register of existing practitioners, all of whom had to have been practising since at least 1876. Further clauses allowed for the registration of the holders of colonial or foreign qualifications and the prosecution of anyone deemed to be breaching the Act, whether they were members of the college or not.

1881–1914

The year 1881 also saw the emergence of what was to become the veterinary profession's official trade association. At the first British National Veterinary Congress, held in London in July that year, veterinary surgeons from across the country, as well as from the army and the colonies, gathered to discuss a range of scientific and professional matters. During the meeting, one George Banham introduced a pamphlet entitled *Suggestions for the Formation of a British National Veterinary Association* and a resolution was passed stating that 'A British National Veterinary Association would be advantageous to the veterinary profession. A committee shall be formed to consider the subject and frame rules for its guidance'.[38] The National Veterinary Association was duly formed in 1882, with George Fleming elected as its first President. The new Association, however, had no direct links with the various provincial associations that had been forming since the 1850s. Instead, the National Veterinary Association was a non-territorial association, open to any veterinary surgeon on payment of half a guinea, and met 'in different parts of the kingdom, from time to time … under the management of a local provincial committee'.[39]

The state veterinary service continued to evolve during the 1880s and 1890s. In 1883, the Veterinary Department of the Privy Council was enlarged and renamed the Agricultural Department of the Privy Council. Five years later a departmental committee looking at pleuro-pneumonia and tuberculosis in livestock recommended that the administration of the Contagious Diseases (Animals) Acts be concentrated in a single department. This in turn led to the Board of Agriculture Act of 1889 and the establishment of a Board of Agriculture, incorporating the Agricultural Department of the Privy Council. In 1894, a separate Animals Division was formed and two years later the veterinary staff was constituted separately as a Veterinary Department. These measures, together with the introduction of the Contagious Diseases (Animals) Act 1894 which largely replaced the numerous Contagious Diseases (Animals) Acts that had preceded it, gave the Board wide-ranging powers with regard to the handling of animal diseases, the benefits of which were soon felt. An outbreak of foot-and-mouth disease in 1892 was quickly stamped out and Britain was declared free of pleuro-pneumonia in 1898.

The government also accepted that the level of scientific research would have to increase significantly if disease was to be combatted effectively. In 1893, therefore, following an outbreak of swine fever, the Board of Agriculture set up a diagnostic laboratory service in one of its rooms. By the time the laboratory moved to Alperton Lodge, Wembley, in 1908, it was carrying out research into a number of diseases including bovine contagious abortion, scrapie and Johne's disease.

Continued concern over public health, focussing particularly on the safety of meat, further enhanced the role of the veterinary surgeon. As far back as the 1860s John Gamgee had carried out an inquiry on behalf of the Privy Council, which concluded that up to a quarter of all meat consumed in the 1850s and 1860s was derived from diseased animals.[40] But Gamgee's recommendations, which included the inspection of all ports and markets by veterinary inspectors, were not acted upon at the time. Change was strongly resisted by livestock dealers, farmers and salesmen, who all feared that they would be put out of business. Besides there were nowhere near enough trained veterinary surgeons to cover every port, market and slaughterhouse in the country.

An additional stumbling block was the large number of private slaughterhouses that operated in Britain at that time. Instead of a small number of large centralised slaughterhouses which could be effectively monitored, most areas relied on a host of small privately run abattoirs, making comprehensive inspection impossible. Birmingham in 1889, for example, had over 300 private slaughterhouses, yet only two inspectors.[41] The Public Health Act of 1875 gave local authorities the power to open public slaughterhouses, which would have made the systematic inspection of meat and hygiene facilities easier to arrange. But most were unwilling to alter the *status quo*. And while such a system operated it was impossible to ensure that any meat being sold was safe to eat. Farmers suspecting disease in one of their animals would send it to the slaughterhouse as quickly as possible, before its value fell. Once at the abattoir, any visibly diseased parts could be cut away and the remainder dressed before being sent on to market. Even if diseased meat did pass through the hands of an inspector, it was by no means certain that it would be detected or condemned. The inspectors were usually butchers, policemen or ex-soldiers, men with little or no scientific training. Moreover, they judged purely on sight, which made the presence of diseases such as pleuro-pneumonia impossible to detect.

By the late nineteenth century, however, the meat industry was undergoing considerable change. The development of refrigeration from the 1870s, followed by freezing techniques in the 1880s, led to a ten-fold increase in the importation of chilled and frozen beef between the 1870s and 1890s, mainly from North and South America.[42] At the same time, new legislation aimed at disease control introduced in 1892 saw imports of European livestock fall to a trickle. Concerns about disease, though, remained. In particular, there was a strong debate over the possible links between animal and human tuberculosis. Although it had no formal responsibility for the disease until 1914, the Board of Agriculture set up a series of Royal Commissions, which reported in 1895, 1898 and 1911. The findings of the final commission concluded that milk from infected cows posed a considerable risk to humans, particularly children. A similar risk was acknowledged to be posed by the consumption of meat, although it was thought to be much less acute.[43]

With the advance of science and the increasing demands being made on veterinary surgeons by the expansion of public health services, the veterinary colleges came under renewed pressure to produce better educated and competently trained men. As a result, the length of their courses was increased to four years in 1894 and to five years in 1932. Separate written and oral examinations were introduced in 1894 and the curriculum expanded. By the 1920s, students were required to master anatomy, physiology, pathology, materia medica, surgery, hygiene, zoology, chemistry, physics and botany. The colleges also began to develop their own research interests. Professor McCall of the Glasgow Veterinary College, for example, carried out experiments in cattle plague and tuberculosis during the 1880s and 1890s, while John McFadyean, Principal of the Royal Veterinary College from 1894, founded the *Journal of Comparative Pathology and Therapeutics*[44] in 1888 and carried out his own research into a number of diseases.

1914–1939

Veterinary surgeons played a prominent role in the First World War, organising remounts and providing first aid for wounded horses and dogs before removing them to one of the eighteen veterinary field hospitals. Between 1914 and 1918, 1668 veterinary officers and 41,755 men served with the Army Veterinary Corps. Such large numbers of men were necessary since there were over a million animals on active duty across the various fronts at any one time. In all, some 2,562,549 animals were treated by the veterinary hospitals, three-quarters of which were returned to active duty.[45] In 1918, in recognition of the work carried out by the Army Veterinary Corps during the previous four years, it was granted the title of Royal Army Veterinary Corps.

Shortly after the First World War came to an end, the National Veterinary Association was dissolved and replaced by a new association. Discontent at the Association's shortcomings had been growing for some time. Charnock Bradley of the Royal (Dick) Veterinary College voiced the thoughts of many when in 1909 he called for the establishment of a single national veterinary association, incorporating all the existing regional associations. A nationally co-ordinated body, it was argued, would be better equipped to take an active role in shaping the profession and to tackle the various political, social and scientific issues that affected the veterinary surgeon but which lay for the most part outside the remit of the Royal College of Veterinary Surgeons. This led in 1919 to the establishment of the National Veterinary Medical Association (known as the British Veterinary Association from 1952). The following year, the Association took over responsibility for the professional journal, *The Veterinary Record*, founded in 1888 by the veterinary surgeon and writer William Hunting.

It was during the inter-war period too that women officially entered the veterinary profession for the first time. The first of these, Aleen Cust, had graduated from the New Veterinary College, Edinburgh, in 1900 but, following the Royal College of Veterinary Surgeon's refusal to accept her as a member, had spent the years before the First World War practising in Ireland. Although the Sex Disqualification (Removal) Act of 1919 compelled the professions to register women, it was 1922 before Aleen Cust was finally registered as a veterinary surgeon by the Royal College of Veterinary Surgeons. By 1934, thirty one women were registered members of the Royal College of Veterinary Surgeons and their numbers continued to grow until by the late 1990s more women than men were entering the profession.

The First World War led to a major expansion in the activities of the Board of Agriculture's diagnostic laboratory. Supplies of vaccine normally imported from the continent had been cut off by the war, so the laboratory was used to help make up the shortfall. Following the award of a government grant in 1914, which allowed for the purchase and development of a 40 acre site at Weybridge, Surrey, the Central Veterinary Laboratory was opened in 1917, complete with five laboratories, numerous outbuildings and a swine fever anti-serum production unit. Six veterinary officers were seconded from the Board of Agriculture to work on a range of diseases including rabies and foot-and-mouth. Further expansion during the 1930s saw the building of three new blocks – for the production of tuberculin and brucellosis vaccine and the diagnosis of and research into poultry diseases.

The Agriculture Act of 1937 heralded a major re-organisation of the government's veterinary services. In the year following the Act, the

Diseases of Animals Branch within the Ministry of Agriculture and Fisheries, created in 1919, was replaced by the Animal Health Division which brought together all the various veterinary services to form a nationally co-ordinated service of veterinary inspectors. Under the new scheme, the country was divided into twenty two areas and sub-divided into seventy eight divisions, each with its own divisional inspector.[46] The issue of research was also examined. By this time, largely due to a series of government grants and scholarships, the amount of veterinary research had greatly increased, although the Loveday Report of 1938 still called for additional funds to be made available. But progress was hampered by a lack of co-ordination. The Agricultural Research Council, established in 1931, had gone some way towards addressing the problem, but its influence over veterinary research was limited. The first veterinary surgeon was not appointed to the Council until 1936. In contrast, the Agriculture Act directly led to the establishment of a number of distinct research departments at the Central Veterinary Laboratory, covering bacteriology, biochemistry, parasitology, pathology and poultry diseases, and to the establishment of a second laboratory at Lasswade, Midlothian, to monitor the health of poultry in Scotland.

Although the horse had played a prominent role in the First World War, its importance in post-war Britain declined as both transport and machinery became increasingly mechanised. This decline, however, was slow. In 1939, there were still 550,000 horses on the nation's farms, outnumbering tractors by over ten to one.[47] It was clear, nevertheless, that veterinary surgeons could no longer rely so heavily upon equine work and that new areas of expertise would have to be developed.

Public health was one potential growth area, with many local authorities appointing full time veterinary inspectors for the first time during the post-war period. Concerns over tuberculosis persisted and responsibility for the disease was formally passed to the Board of Agriculture in 1914. Although pasteurisation, introduced in 1922, had a dramatic effect on the disease, by 1934 there were still some 2500 human deaths from bovine tuberculosis each year.[48] In a major effort to eradicate the disease from the national herd, the Ministry of Agriculture and Fisheries in 1935 introduced the Tuberculosis (Attested Herds) Scheme, involving veterinary surgeons up and down the country in the routine inspection of herds and dairies. The scheme was so successful that by 1960, every herd in Britain was declared attested.[49]

Another growth area was small animal medicine. The vogue for keeping small animals as pets, which had grown rapidly during the mid nineteenth century, showed no signs of abating. Consequently, although livestock and horses continued to dominate the caseloads of most practices down to the 1950s, many during the 1920s and 1930s began to treat an increasing number of pets, particularly cats and dogs. Simultaneously, a growing number of practices dedicated exclusively to the treatment of small animals were being set up in towns and cities across the country. This demand for small animal medicine in turn stimulated a number of scientific and technical advances that allowed veterinary surgeons to offer more effective diagnosis and treatment. A major breakthrough came in 1928, with the introduction of a canine distemper vaccine, pioneered by Patrick Laidlaw and George W Dunkin.[50]

THE SECOND WORLD WAR AND BEYOND

In marked contrast to the First World War, the overall need for animals during the Second World War was relatively small. Pack animals were required to overcome the difficult terrain in Burma and Italy, while dogs were used in far greater numbers than hitherto – as guards, messengers, casualty and arms detectors, trackers and infantry patrollers. Most veterinary surgeons, though, were concerned with ensuring the safety of the troops' food and water supplies.

The war did, however, serve to emphasise the fact that in spite of all the scientific advances made during the previous half-century, animal disease still accounted for huge agricultural losses. At a time when food supplies had became more precious than ever, each new outbreak of disease put an additional strain on the economy. Attempts to increase government funding for research projects were halted by the war, but some in the veterinary profession were unwilling to wait. In 1940 the National Veterinary Medical Association launched a survey of livestock diseases, with the intention of setting up a scheme which would then target a number of diseases in a concentrated effort. Four conditions were ultimately selected – brucellosis, mastitis, Johne's disease and infertility. Meanwhile, the Veterinary Educational Trust (later the Animal Health Trust), formed in 1942, had begun its own programme of research aimed at increasing the overall knowledge of animal disease and reducing mortality rates.

The second Loveday Report, published in 1944, re-emphasised the need for research and reiterated the recommendations made in its first report of 1938. Radical changes to the veterinary education system were outlined. The report proposed that not only should the four existing veterinary colleges – London, Edinburgh, Glasgow and Liverpool – be retained, but that two new colleges, at Bristol and Cambridge, should be created, both with an emphasis on research. Other proposals included the raising of teaching salaries and the setting up of field stations to improve students' practical skills. Additionally, the report also recommended that all six colleges be incorporated into universities.

It was this last point that caused a considerable degree of consternation at the Royal College of Veterinary Surgeons. Although it would remain the profession's governing body, with the power to inspect teaching facilities and examinations, under the proposed changes the college would no longer be able to set its own examinations. Instead it would be expected to accept the degrees awarded by the universities as sufficient qualification for MRCVS status. This led to fears that the one-portal system of entry to the profession, achieved only after a long period of struggle, would be lost, and that a variation in the standard of competency amongst veterinary surgeons would result. Only after lengthy negotiations did the Royal College of Veterinary Surgeons finally agree to the report's recommendations. For the veterinary colleges, on the other hand, incorporation into the university system had undoubted advantages, not least the benefit of closer links with medical and other scientists. The research interests of all the colleges were expanded from this time. Glasgow, for example, became increasingly involved in parasitic disease research, while Cambridge developed a number of comparative medicine research programmes.

Following an additional recommendation made by the Loveday Committee, the Chancellor Committee was set up in 1944 to re-examine the issue of unqualified practitioners. This new committee, which reported the following year, recommended that no unqualified or unregistered person should be allowed to practise as a veterinary surgeon. Like the architects behind the Veterinary Surgeons Act of 1881, however, it recognised that this would cause considerable anguish and suffering amongst those who were unqualified but had been working for some considerable time and had acquired a fair degree of competency. It therefore recommended that a supplementary register be created, made up of those who had been in practice for at least seven out of the previous ten years. Those listed on the supplementary register would not be allowed to call themselves 'veterinary surgeons' but would instead be designated 'veterinary practitioners'. They would be limited as to the types of procedure that they would be allowed to carry out and subject to the same Royal College of Veterinary Surgeons controls as registered members. The recommendations made by the Loveday and Chancellor Committees went on to form the basis of the Veterinary Surgeons Act of 1948, which was generally welcomed by veterinary surgeons, although most had hoped that unqualified persons would be excluded from practising altogether. This, however, was not achieved until the Veterinary Surgeons Act of 1966.

With the passing of the 1948 Act, the Royal College of Veterinary Surgeon's role changed significantly. Although still the profession's governing body, the fact that it could no longer set examinations reduced its role in education to one of supervision. The Veterinary Surgeons Act of 1966, however, strengthened its regulatory role, additional powers being granted which related to temporary registration and disciplinary proceedings. To carry out these functions more effectively, the Royal College of Veterinary Surgeons Council in 1966 set up a Preliminary Investigation Committee. The following year a new charter was granted, which, amongst other things, allowed the Royal College of Veterinary Surgeons to award diplomas and certificates to those training as veterinary nurses, signalling the increased role that it would come to play in the provision of continuing professional development. Both Act and charter were subsequently revised in 1980 to allow holders of approved European Economic Community veterinary qualifications to become members of the Royal College of Veterinary Surgeons.

The biggest single development of the post-war period, however, was undoubtedly the pharmaceutical revolution that swept the medical world. Until the 1930s, veterinary medication had remained relatively unaltered since medieval times. Prescriptions were made up individually, often by apothecaries or chemists, composed largely of herbal ingredients and administered in the form of balls, capsules, drenches, creams or dips. From about 1925 this system began to give way to one of pre-prepared and pre-packaged products, which were sold directly to the veterinary surgeon by the manufacturer.[51] The emergence during the 1930s and 1940s of numerous anthelmintics, antibiotics and vaccines as well as the development of procedures such as artificial insemination and chemotherapy heralded a period of rapid advancement. Suddenly a whole range of bacterial infections, including mastitis and septicemia, could be controlled more effectively. Pharmaceutical companies were quick to see the possibilities and in the immediate post-war years set up veterinary departments to conduct research and market new products. Most were initially aimed at the agricultural market and included products like *Saffelin*, introduced by Glaxo in 1955 to immunise sheep against pulpy kidney disease, and *Dictol*, an oral vaccine to combat lungworm in cattle launched by Allen & Hanburys Ltd in 1959. Later an increasing number of products offered treatments for diseases in dogs and cats, reflecting the growth in demand for small animal medicine.

Additional research was carried out by a number of independent centres including the Moredun Research Institute, established at Gilmerton, Edinburgh, in 1920, and the Roslin Institute, established in Edinburgh in 1945. The Royal Army Veterinary Corps Laboratory based at Aldershot, Hampshire, also played an important role in research.

Established in 1938 to replace the Royal Army Veterinary School, it carried out a number of tasks during the Second World War, testing new treatments, producing vaccines and supplying blood and serum to the Royal Army Medical Corps. During the post-war period, the laboratory continued its research into the effects of nuclear, bacteriological and chemical warfare on animals. Increased reliance by the army on dogs also stimulated new research into canine diseases such as haemolytic streptococci, distemper, leptospirosis and filariasis.

By the end of the twentieth century, many scientists were increasingly turning their attention towards preventative medicine. The development of major new scientific fields, such as molecular biology and quantitative genetics led to a number of breakthroughs, which in turn opened up new possibilities for disease eradication. The Roslin Institute, a recognised centre for the study of genomics, developed a number of livestock genome mapping databases, while the Animal Health Trust played a leading role in the development of genome linkage maps for both the dog and the horse. These in turn enabled scientists to develop DNA tests for inherited diseases such as progressive retinal atrophy in setters and severe combined immunodeficiency disease in Arabian horses, diseases which could then be bred out, often within a couple of generations.

Small animal medicine, or companion animal medicine as it later became known, developed rapidly from the 1950s onwards. New practices sprang up in urban centres around the country, while existing practices added consulting and treatment rooms specifically for small animal patients. This growth was reflected by the establishment in 1957 of the British Small Animal Veterinary Association 'to protect, foster and promote the cultural, scientific and professional interests of veterinary surgeons and practitioners engaged in small animal practice, teaching and research'.[52]

By the 1990s, however, practices had entered a period of significant change. Traditional small practices, run by just one or two veterinary surgeons, were being replaced by group practices employing large numbers of professional and auxiliary staff spread over several locations. This in turn made it possible for practices both to update their equipment and facilities more regularly and to offer a wider range of additional services, such as on-site laboratories. Since increasing numbers of veterinary surgeons were also choosing to specialise in particular areas of medicine, a large practice was often better placed to offer expert help in one or more fields, for example, dentistry, orthopaedics, cardiology or oncology.

Veterinary surgeons also continued to play an important role in public health. Although private slaughterhouses were closed between

1939 and 1945, many re-opened during the 1950s, making full and detailed inspections impossible once more. Finally, in 1968, it became illegal for any meat to leave an abattoir without first undergoing a post-mortem examination. The Fresh Meat Regulations, introduced after Britain's entry into the European Economic Community in the 1970s, raised standards still higher. Abattoirs were expected to provide laboratories, which in turn would make specific analyses available to veterinary inspectors. In the latter part of the twentieth century, particular efforts were made to control and eliminate a number of new diseases affecting public health, including salmonella, bovine spongiform encephalopathy and Escherichia coli.

These numerous scientific advances, legislative changes and public health issues ensured that the government's role, too, was extended in the post-war period. By the time the Ministry of Agriculture and Fisheries was renamed the Ministry of Agriculture, Fisheries and Food in 1955 the Animal Health Division had been divided into two organisations. The Inspectorate (re-designated Veterinary Field Services in 1963) was responsible for the prevention, control and eradication of animal diseases, while the Veterinary Investigation Service provided a routine diagnostic service for veterinary surgeons, employing 1500 full time staff and a further 1700 on an *ad hoc* basis. Extensive re-organisation during the 1980s and early 1990s resulted in the formation of six distinct animal health divisions: a Meat Hygiene Division; an Animal Health (Disease Control) Division, which dealt with all notifiable diseases except salmonella and bovine spongiform encephalopathy; an Animal Health (International Trade) Division, concerned with the import and export of live animals and genetic material including that relating to artificial insemination and embryo transfer; an Animal Welfare Division, with responsibility for animal health on farms, at markets and in transit; an Animal Health (Zoonoses) Division, for the control of salmonella in poultry and an Animal Health Resource Management Division, giving administrative support to the other Divisions. In addition, there was a new Animal Health and Welfare Section with responsibility for animal health schemes, particularly bovine spongiform encephalopathy, tuberculosis and brucellosis, and the importation of domestic animals.

Further changes were introduced in 2001 following a serious outbreak of foot-and-mouth disease, which resulted in the slaughter of over four million animals. In June of that year the Ministry of Agriculture, Fisheries and Food was replaced by the Department for the Environment, Food and Rural Affairs.

CONCLUSION

The changes that have occurred over the past three centuries have ensured that the veterinary surgeon of today is a very different creature from his counterpart of the past. Out of a network of individuals, lacking formal qualifications and reliant for the most part on centuries old remedies and treatments, there has emerged a recognised profession composed of highly educated men and women, all of whom are able to call upon a vast reserve of scientific knowledge to aid them in the diagnosis and treatment of disease. They have also played their part in all aspects of British life – in science and research, leisure and education, public health, the development of the colonies and warfare. It is clear, too, that veterinary medicine will continue to evolve. Already the future for many veterinary surgeons lies not in the stable or surgery but in the laboratory as the emphasis increasingly shifts from treatment to prevention. Now, at the beginning of the twenty first century, it can truly be claimed that 'science' has indeed replaced 'art'.

REFERENCES

[1] L B Prince, *The Farrier and his Craft: the history of the Worshipful Company of Farriers* (London, 1980), 1–3

[2] R Porter, *English Society in the Eighteenth Century* (London, 1990), 192

[3] Ibid, 193

[4] R H Dunlop and D J Williams, *Veterinary Medicine: an illustrated history* (USA, 1996), 480

[5] Ibid, 481

[6] Ibid, 486

[7] E J Evans, *The Forging of the Modern State: early industrial Britain 1783-1870* (London, 1983), 111

[8] Ibid, 101

[9] J Lane, 'Farriers in Georgian England', A R Michell, (ed) *The Advancement of Veterinary Science*, vol 3, 1993, 109

[10] R H Dunlop and D J Williams, op cit, 344

[11] Ibid

[12] I Pattison, *The British Veterinary Profession 1791-1948* (London, 1983), 4

[13] O C Bradley, *The History of the Edinburgh Veterinary College* (Edinburgh, 1923), 21

[14] Ibid, 25

[15] I Pattison, op cit, 18

[16] *The Veterinarian*, vol 17, no 202, Oct 1844, 605–616

[17] *The Veterinarian*, vol 17, no 196, April 1844, 184
[18] I Pattison, op cit, 62
[19] J R Fisher, 'Not Quite a Profession: the aspirations of veterinary surgeons in England in the mid nineteenth century', *Historical Research* 66 (1993), 293
[20] *The Veterinarian*, vol 40, no 464, June 1867, 486
[21] G E Mingay, (ed) *The Agrarian History of England and Wales*, vol 6 (Cambridge, 1981), 360
[22] R Porter, 'Animals, Medicine and Society: Historical Perspectives', K Arnold, R Porter, L Wilkinson (eds), *Animal Doctor: birds and beasts in medical history* (London, 1994), 5
[23] E W Jaquet, *The Kennel Club: a history and record of its work* (London, 1905), 3
[24] Dunlop and Wilson, op cit, 646
[25] Ibid, 648
[26] R Porter, op cit, 6
[27] Royal Society for the Prevention of Cruelty to Animals, annual report 1825
[28] 'A Short Historical Account of the Growth and Work of the Society Since its Inception in 1839', *SSPCA Annual Report* 1938, 1–23 [Scottish Society for the Prevention of Cruelty to Animals]
[29] *The Veterinarian*, vol 40, no 474, June 1867, 457–458
[30] Dunlop and Williams, op cit, 377
[31] I Pattison, op cit, 61
[32] *The Veterinarian*, vol 40, no 471, March 1867, 214
[33] J R Fisher, op cit, 286
[34] *The Veterinarian*, vol 40, no 472, June 1867, 526–527
[35] E Cotchin, *The Royal Veterinary College, London: a bicentenary history* (Buckingham, 1990), 79–80
[36] *The Veterinarian*, vol 40, no 474, June 1867, 493
[37] J W R Pearce, L P Pugh, J Ritchie (eds) *Animal Health: a centenary 1865–1965* (London, 1965), 35
[38] I Pattison, op cit, 95
[39] Ibid, 95
[40] R Perren, *The Meat Trade in Britain 1840–1914* (London, 1978), 65
[41] Ibid, 89
[42] D Taylor, 'The Importance of Cattle Enterprises in British Agriculture 1815–1930', *Veterinary History,* no 5, summer 1975, 23
[43] R Perren, op cit, 134
[44] W Weipers, 'The Development of Veterinary Education in the West of Scotland', *Veterinary History,* no 7, summer 1976, 9–19
[45] Dunlop and Wilson, op cit, 473
[46] Pearce et al, op cit, 109

[47] Dunlop and Wilson, op cit, 545

[48] A McDiarmid, 'The History of Bovine TB', *Veterinary History*, no 3, summer 1974

[49] Ibid

[50] Dunlop and Wilson, op cit, 607

[51] J M Kirkness, *A History of the Animal Health Register* (London, c1982), 7–8

[52] British Small Animal Veterinary Association, minutes and constitution, 1957

Veterinary records: their nature and uses

The archives relating to veterinary medicine and the veterinary profession are derived from a wide variety of sources – practices, professional associations, companies, colleges, government agencies, charities, zoos and the armed services. The following essay describes the types of records created by each and assesses their research value for historians.

EARLY RECORDS

Since horses have played an invaluable part in British life from earliest times, it is perhaps inevitable that most early documentation relates almost exclusively to their care. Some of the earliest surviving records refer in particular to the welfare of the monarch's horses. Horses were an essential part of royal life, transporting the court from palace to palace throughout the year as well as carrying armies into battle. Recognising their importance, kings such as John, Edward III and Henry VIII went to great lengths to improve the nation's stock, importing stallions from overseas and setting up their own studs. An idea of the amount of money being spent on horses and their upkeep can be found by looking at the Royal Household accounts, as well as at occasional accounts elsewhere.

Concern about the quality of care being given to horses was apparent from early times. As far back as 1356, the Mayor of London was calling upon all farriers within a seven mile radius of the city to form themselves into a fellowship, which would enable them to regulate their trade more effectively. Out of this emerged the Worshipful Company of Farriers, granted a charter in 1674 and raised to livery company status in 1692. Most of the records covering the company's early history perished in the Great Fire of London (1666), but later records provide a wealth of useful information. Registers of Freemen (1709–1864) and apprentice bindings (1619–1862), for example, give details of individual members, while minute books (1718–1862) record the quarterly meetings held by the court, made up of the Master, three Wardens and between ten and twenty assistants. These latter volumes chart the company's struggle to regulate its trade and improve standards of care. It is interesting to note, too, that while virtually all the Freemen listed in 1800 described themselves as 'farriers', by the time the Royal College of Veterinary Surgeons was awarded its charter in 1844 the vast majority were listed as 'veterinary surgeons'.

Information relating to individual farriers can be gleaned from a number of sources including apprenticeship indentures, partnership agreements, employment contracts, property deeds, wills and census returns. An apprenticeship usually lasted seven years, during which time the apprentice lived and worked with his master. No wages were paid, but the apprentice was expected to pay a premium to cover the cost of his training and board. Following the imposition of tax on all apprenticeship premiums from 1710, formally written indentures became more prevalent. Unfortunately, since farriery tended to be a family-orientated trade, there are fewer indentures then might perhaps be expected. Those that do exist, however, provide valuable details regarding training, conditions of service and the cost of premiums.

Deeds relating to property give the names of the parties involved as well as the location and size of the property being sold or leased. Additionally they provide financial details, recording sums due and the terms of payment. Wills, particularly those with inventories attached, can also yield information relating to property and finances, and as such are a useful way of gauging the financial and social status of the testator. Individuals may well also be mentioned in land tax returns, Quarter Sessions, overseers' accounts and voters' lists, although with the general absence of detailed indexing, they would be difficult to find. Printed sources, too, including trade directories, post office books and local newspapers should not be forgotten.

Records relating to other practitioners, such as cow leeches and horse doctors are limited. The most common, found in record offices, libraries and museums across the country, are examples of the cures or remedies they prescribed, and cover all manner of ailments. The list of ingredients for the various powders, balls, drenches, purges, salves and ointments, together with the instructions for their use, give us a (sometimes rather hair-raising) insight into the ideas and treatments that prevailed at a particular time. Many originated in medieval times and persisted relatively unchanged until well into the twentieth century, although the expansion of trade in the nineteenth century gave access to a much wider range of ingredients. The truly desperate, for whom all else had failed, turned to charms and spells, a number of which have also survived.

Of course, for every such document that has survived, many others must have been created that have not. A greater number still would never have been committed to paper at all, but passed from father to son, from master to apprentice, by word of mouth. Additionally, most surviving documents are isolated examples, yielding little information about either prescriber or client.

Since most remedies were ineffectual and their ingredients well known and easily available, people were accustomed to treating their animals themselves. Thus remedies can be found, scattered amongst culinary and still room recipes, in the notebooks kept by housekeepers, farmers' wives and householders. And with the development of printing came treatises, large numbers of which were published over the centuries, each one encouraging its readers to become their own animal doctor. Needless to say, the standards of these works varied considerably. The artist George Stubbs produced a series of accurate anatomical drawings, based on his own dissections, which were used to illustrate *The Anatomy of the Horse*, published in 1766. These proved to be far superior to those contained in most rival publications and set the standard for others to follow. While the advice proffered by some was sound, many others were woefully wide of the mark, and, since most writers were content to plagiarise or borrow ideas rather than formulate their own, there were far fewer new ideas being put forward than might otherwise have been the case.

A more accurate gauge of progress can be found in the patents held by the British Library's Science and Technology Service. Patents, granted by the government via the Patent Office, allow inventors the right for a period of up to twenty years to 'full power, sole privilege and authority...[to] make, use, exercise and vend' their product. Although patents cannot be granted for scientific discoveries or surgical treatments, new equipment and medicinal preparations are patentable. Relevant patents, dating from the eighteenth century onwards, relate to horseshoes and shoeing techniques, as well as to new or improved veterinary instruments including mouth openers, fetters, anaesthesia inhaling devices and castrating appliances. Various remedies and preparations have also been patented, for example Thomas Johnson's 'preparation for staining horses and other animals so as to make them match in colour' (1774) or *Major's Celebrated British Remedy*, guaranteed 'to remove spavins, ringbones, curbs, splints and other unnatural ossifications and humours from horses' (1852).

British patents are listed on CDRom, which is searchable by keyword, or can be traced via the *Name Index to Complete Specifications* which lists all patent applications year by year from 1617 alphabetically by the name of the company or individual making the application. As well as the name of the inventor, each entry will contain the patent number, the date of application and a brief description of the invention.

The patent specification gives the name, address and occupation of the patentee, followed by a detailed description of their invention. One for a medicinal cure, therefore, will list the ingredients and describe the preparation method, while that for a mechanical device will outline each stage of the manufacturing process. Sometimes drawings or plans are attached. All successful patents have to be enrolled in the Court of

Chancery within a set period of about four to six months and a note will be added to the specification where relevant, giving the date of enrolment.

The owners and managers of estates frequently called upon the services of farriers and/or veterinary surgeons, and the frequency and costs of these visits are duly recorded in ledgers and account books. A number of stud books have also survived, showing the species and breeds of animals being kept by an individual estate, useful for monitoring the progress of breeding programmes, the introduction of new breeds and the impact of disease. A search through estate collections will also yield miscellaneous bills, receipts, prescriptions and certificates of soundness which give clues about the range of animals being treated, the variety of procedures performed – bleeding, firing, castrating, docking, etc – and the fees charged. Such papers are at present somewhat difficult to locate, since they are seldom listed separately or mentioned in indexes. Instead they are generally bundled together with other papers under general headings such as 'bills and receipts' or 'factor's papers'. But the introduction of computerised cataloguing to many record offices means that in time such records will be more easily accessible.

VETERINARY PRACTICES

The earliest practices grew out of or alongside blacksmiths' forges and the first qualified veterinary surgeons were often farriers themselves or hailed from a farriering family. Many would have returned to the family business after qualification. Census returns – first gathered in 1821 but only with enough detail to be truly helpful from 1841 – are useful for establishing whether or not a practice was part of or close to a forge and for demonstrating these family connections. They also indicate where the practice was sited. Until the mid nineteenth century, the most favourable position was generally not in the centre of town, but on one of the roads leading in or out of town, enabling the practice to take full advantage of the business being generated by coaching inns and post-horse stables. The arrival of the railways led to a decline in long-distance coach travel, but in no way diminished a practice's business. Indeed, far from reducing the number of horse-drawn vehicles, railways actually increased them, since goods and people still had to be conveyed to and from stations and markets. Even the railway companies themselves kept horses to collect and deliver goods. Additional trade was generated by the large numbers of sheep and cattle that were being transported by rail then driven into nearby towns and markets.

By 2000, there were over 2200 veterinary practices and 940 branches in the United Kingdom, ranging from the single-handed to group practices employing a large number of professional and auxiliary staff spread over several surgeries. While some practices specialise in small animal, large animal or equine practice others are described as mixed. Most small animal practices are affiliated to the British Small Animal Veterinary Association (established in 1957) while those with an interest in equine medicine can apply for membership of the British Equine Veterinary Association (established in c1976). The title 'veterinary hospital' is restricted to those practices that meet certain standards relating to equipment, facilities and staffing – for example, the provision of twenty four hour nursing care and in house laboratory facilities – laid down by the Royal College of Veterinary Surgeons. Hospital status is granted only after an independent inspection and is valid for four years. Some practices will indicate a particular interest in areas such as exotic species, wild animals or game birds. A small number offer only secondary referral services, seeing cases referred to them by other practices. Non-clinical practices do not treat living animals but undertake pathological, legal and food hygiene work.

Most practices have relatively few surviving records. This can be attributed to several factors: the small size of many practices, the frequency with which they changed hands, a trend during the 1980s and 1990s to relocate and a general lack of awareness amongst veterinary surgeons that their records would be of interest to historians.

Until the late twentieth century, most practices were small concerns, often run by one or two veterinary surgeons in partnership. Some employed full time assistants while others just took on extra help for short periods, for example during the lambing season. Such small operations were unlikely to create many records initially. However, as a practice grew, the number and variety of records increased. The employment of a full time assistant required that a formal contract be drawn up, setting out the duties required of him or her and the wages he or she would be paid, together with any extra allowances, such as accommodation or a car. The establishment of branch surgeries necessitated the keeping of separate patient, accounting and property records. If the business flourished, it was not uncommon for the assistant to become a partner, resulting in new agreements which, in addition to giving the name, address and capital contribution of each partner, would also record the partnership's commencement date and the terms of any additional agreements made. Over time some practices grew into sizeable concerns, spread over several premises and employing a number of partners, assistants and auxiliary staff. This in turn led in some cases to minutes of partners' or practice meetings and correspondence files.

Practices can also change hands frequently, effectively becoming new businesses each time. The sale of a practice generally heralds a clear out, during which all records not required by the new owners are removed and destroyed. Additionally, the 1980s and 1990s saw many practices relocate to new purpose built premises, due partly to a trend amongst retiring owners to liquidate their assets by selling the (often substantial) practice building and partly to enable practices to provide improved facilities and house an increasing variety of modern equipment. In this way, many records that had lain undisturbed in attics and outhouses for decades were rediscovered and destroyed.

It should also be borne in mind that much of the information which gives the best insight into the everyday life of a veterinary practice was never written down at all, but passed from generation to generation by word of mouth. Out of the reminiscences of retired veterinary surgeons and their families come tantalizing glimpses of the veterinary surgeon at work – holding kerosene-lit consultations in sheds at the bottom of the garden, dashing around the countryside on a number of different horses each day in an attempt to look both affluent and busy, of saddle bags by the door, packed ready for midnight emergency call outs, of informal small animal surgeries held at the end of a day's farm visits – separate pots on the stove boiling both instruments and dinner while operations were carried out on the table. Also largely unrecorded is the immense amount of work carried out by veterinary surgeons' wives, who acted as receptionists, secretaries, theatre nurses, book keepers, bottle-washers and dispensers.

Amongst the records created by practices, day books, balance sheets and ledgers have generally survived best. Day books are potentially of great interest to historians, both for the amount of information they contain and because they often cover a sustained period of time. Although the degree of detail varies, a good set will give the name and address of each client, the date of the consultation, the breed or species of animal seen, the diagnosis and treatment prescribed and the charge levied. Some practices kept separate day books for large and small animals. By studying this information it is possible to chart such things as the introduction of new drugs and treatments, changes in land use, the growth of small animal work and a corresponding decline in the agricultural caseload. Additionally, day books can be used to illustrate demographic changes or regional interests such as hunting.

Annual balance sheets, compulsory for public companies from 1907 and for private companies from 1929, indicate a practice's liabilities, profits and assets. Where no other financial records have survived they are often the only source of information on such subjects as loans, staff, property and equipment and are thus invaluable for charting the ebb and flow of a practice – the decline of forges, the introduction of new-fangled appliances such as motor cars and telephones, the increased use of drugs, the employment of auxiliary staff. To a lesser extent, profit and loss accounts are also useful, summarising as they do the practice's incoming and outgoing finances and listing the items to be set against them.

Ledgers likewise contain an abundance of information. Since each account is listed at the top of a page with all transactions following below, information can be gleaned on customers and suppliers as well as products and services, wages, expenses and assets. Sometimes, too, they afford us glimpses of personal or household expenses.

Occasionally other financial records, such as invoices, receipts, cash books and wages books can be found. Details relating to charging are, however, scant, particularly prior to 1971 when the introduction of value added tax necessitated the issuing of itemised bills. Until then, bills were generally sent out quarterly and merely stated the amount due 'for professional services rendered'. Even where more detailed records do exist, they have to be treated with caution, since they seldom tell the complete story. Veterinary surgeons, in common with many other professionals, were frequently paid in kind. Many would never charge the doctor or the clergyman, knowing that their services would one day be required in turn. Farmers gave whatever produce they could spare – meat, eggs or milk – while tradesmen offered their skills. It was equally common practice to charge those on low incomes only what they could afford for minor treatments so that they would not hesitate to ask for help when their animals were more seriously afflicted.

Property has always played an important role in veterinary practice, especially since veterinary surgeons often lived and traded from the same address. For many, their property was a major asset, to be sold along with the contents and goodwill on retirement. Although quantities of title deeds have survived, they are in most cases held by banks or solicitors rather than by the practices themselves. A few inventories and purchase agreements have been preserved which list the entire extent and contents of a practice at a particular date. Architectural plans and photographs amply illustrate the changes that swept the profession in the period after the Second World War. By the 1950s, forges had all but disappeared and practices were redeveloping to cater for the growth in small animal care, providing waiting rooms, consulting rooms, operating rooms and laboratories. Rapid developments in technology and science over the next fifty years rendered the traditional home visit increasingly impractical and by 2000 practices were encouraging clients to bring their animals to the surgery whenever possible.

A number of records survive which relate to the impact made at a local level of national legislation designed to control contagious disease and improve public health which emerged from 1865. Many local authorities appointed Local Veterinary Inspectors, who would examine stock at markets, dairies and ports and notify them of any outbreaks of scheduled diseases in their area. They also administered national schemes such as the Tuberculosis (Attested Herds) Scheme, first introduced in 1935. Surviving paperwork includes official instructions issued by the Ministry of Agriculture and Fisheries to Local Veterinary Inspectors, testing books and statements of returns. Practices participating in the Tuberculosis (Attested Herds) Scheme generally kept one testing book for each farm in which they detailed the dates of visits, the tests carried out and their results. Today, these books reveal much about the local farming landscape over a sustained period, making it possible to estimate the number and size of dairy herds, for example, or to chart the widespread shift during the twentieth century from Shorthorns to Holstein-Friesians.

All practices hold records relating to patients and their owners. Until the mid 1980s, when most practices transferred such records onto computer, patient records were held on card indexes, filed alphabetically by owner, one card representing each patient. At the head of each card is the owner's name and address, followed by the name, species and, if relevant, the breed of the animal. Underneath is listed the date of each consultation, together with details of all treatments given. These could be used to trace the introduction of new drugs or a shift in emphasis, from large to small animals. But such files are rarely complete, since the cards relating to patients that have died or moved are periodically removed.

Other records found at practices could include sales literature from drug and equipment companies, lists of debtors, dangerous drug records, specimen slides, x-rays, photographs of staff, buildings and patients and newspaper cuttings. Some have papers reflecting an interest in a particular area of veterinary medicine, such as exotic species, racehorses, pigeons or greyhounds. There may also be personal papers – letters, photographs, accounts, university lecture notes – relating to individuals.

Printed sources can also reveal much. Trade and post office directories can indicate how many veterinary surgeons were working in an area and the size of the population they covered, while local newspapers will publish obituaries, advertisements and notices regarding changes of ownership or address. The trade press is another rich source of information. Two publications were launched in 1828. *The Farrier and Naturalist*, later *The Hippiatrist*, appeared monthly until 1830 while *The Veterinarian*, also a monthly journal, continued until 1902. These were followed by the *Edinburgh Veterinary Review*, founded and edited by John Gamgee and produced monthly from 1858 to 1864, *The British Veterinary Journal*, produced monthly since 1875 and *The Veterinary Record*, a weekly publication which first appeared in 1888 and has been owned by the British Veterinary Association since 1920. The latter are generally bound into indexed volumes and contain an invaluable amount of detail relating to local and national association meetings, scientific developments, legal and political issues affecting the profession and personal news regarding individuals.

COMPANIES

Until the mid twentieth century, most veterinary prescriptions were dispensed by local chemists and druggists in the form of balls, capsules, drenches, creams and dips. Additionally, chemists sold a limited range of pre-prepared products, for example *Cooper's Sheep Dipping Powder*, developed during the 1840s by William Cooper. Prescription books show what was made up for whom and when, while the buying and selling of pre-prepared products is recorded in ledgers. Some chemists maintained separate animal and human prescription books, while others recorded all prescriptions in a single series of volumes. These books gradually decrease in number from around 1925 as individually dispensed medicines gave way to pre-prepared and packaged products which manufacturers sold directly to veterinary surgeons.

The larger pharmaceutical and surgical instrument companies produce large quantities of records covering all aspects of their work. Corporate records, for example minutes and papers of directors' meetings, board meeting papers, annual reports, memoranda and articles of association, define a company's constitution and the rules by which it is to be governed, specify its aims and track its day to day administration. For the historian they are useful for explaining how and why particular decisions were made regarding policy, strategy and development. This in turn makes it possible to chart the development of, for example, animal health departments or production units, including the appointment of staff, the equipping of laboratories and the development of individual research programmes.

Accounting records can include ledgers, profit and loss accounts, balance sheets, statements of accounts, financial forecasts, budget sheets, and cash books. Private ledgers, sometimes with a lock and key attached, contain financial details intended to be seen only by a company's directors, for example details of the salaries paid to directors and senior managers. Sales and purchase ledgers show the name of each customer or supplier, the goods sold or bought and the amount paid. Profit and loss accounts illustrate to the owners or directors the difference between a company's costs and its earnings, while balance sheets list both its assets, for example the value of unsold stock or outstanding debts, and its liabilities, such as shareholder's funds and reserves. All these records can be used to show how a company is performing at a given date, while financial forecasts and budgets are useful for gauging a company's expectations for its future performance and development.

Research and development papers are a vital part of any business wishing to progress and stay ahead of its competitors. The records created by a research and development department, including reports and laboratory books, will reflect the progress of research programmes, the subsequent development of new products and the refinement of existing ones. Details of unsuccessful experiments are also useful, since they give a valuable insight into scientific thinking and knowledge at a particular time and show the paths explored before success was attained.

Sales and marketing records, including advertisements, price lists, catalogues, leaflets, press releases, brochures and representatives' sales records, will describe, and sometimes illustrate, products for both existing and potential customers. They are therefore a valuable source of detailed information relating both to the launch of new products and to the success or otherwise of existing ones. Similar information can also be found in internal publications such as staff magazines and news sheets and on corporate films and videos.

Records relating to individual members of staff can be limited. Wage books, often the only personnel records to have been kept by a company during the nineteenth and early twentieth centuries, list each employee by name but rarely give any personal details. Some do, however, show the amounts paid and the hours worked. More detailed information regarding individual employees can be found on staff record cards, although these are likely to have been created and retained only by companies with a number of workers. Staff record cards give the staff member's name, address, job title and salary. Promotions, re-gradings and disciplinary actions are also noted, all with their relevant dates. Sometimes information regarding an individual's family is also included. Occasionally, too, there are records relating to pensions, training, health and safety issues or social activities.

The number of property records a company holds necessarily depends on its size. Leases and agreements give information on when and where a company expanded. Valuations, generally generated prior to a merger, share issue or rating appeal, or to accompany a balance sheet, describe a specific premises in some detail, while inventories list, describe and value all the fixtures and fittings, thereby affording a glimpse of a factory or laboratory at a certain date. The expansion of a company into new or extended premises can also be charted by the examination of architectural drawings, correspondence files, accounts, photographs and commemorative brochures.

Information relating to a number of dissolved companies, including the Albert Veterinary College Ltd and the Veterinary Medicine Company

Ltd, as well as for several bankrupted practices can be found amongst the National Archives' series of records received from the Board of Trade and Companies House. The latter records information about dissolved companies registered under the Companies Acts within England and Wales while separate offices in Edinburgh and Dublin hold similar records for Scottish and Northern Irish Companies. Included within the files will be (where relevant) company formation documents, memoranda and articles of association, a statement of nominal share capital, a register of directors, annual share capital and debenture and shareholder returns, annual balance sheets and liquidation documents.

ROYAL COLLEGE OF VETERINARY SURGEONS

The Royal College of Veterinary Surgeons was established by royal charter in 1844. The charter, and the supplementary charters that followed, set out the college's aims and show the development of its powers and responsibilities. The college's Council is responsible for making key decisions relating to the regulation of the profession. Minute books show how these decisions were reached and cover a wide range of issues, including the co-ordination of the Member of the Royal College of Veterinary Surgeons (MRCVS) examinations, the status of foreign nationals wishing to practise in the United Kingdom, visitations to veterinary schools, disciplinary hearings and investigations of unregistered veterinary surgeons. Additionally, as the college developed, a number of committees were established, each with its own area of responsibility, for example examinations, registrations, finance or disciplinary matters, and each creating their own minute books. There were also, from time to time, sub-committees or special committees, formed to examine particular issues. These included the Indian Veterinary Service Special Committee (1923–26), the Indian and Egyptian Sub-Committee (1945–47) and the Sub-Committee on the Publication of the Loveday Report (1938, 1945–46).

The Secretary was involved in every aspect of the college's work, and this is reflected in his outgoing letter books, dating back to 1862. Their contents cover a wide range of issues, from MRCVS applications from India and Burma to petrol rationing during the First World War, from the appointment of examiners to the correct fees payable for expert witnesses, from the maintenance of buildings to the appearance of veterinary surgeons in advertising literature.

The post of Registrar, created in 1848, was usually held concurrently with that of Secretary. The Registrar was primarily responsible for maintaining the alphabetical card index of members, created around 1844 and continued until about 1960. Each card gives a member's name, place and date of graduation and the date on which they died or terminated their membership. Some cards also give dates of birth or ages at death. Additionally, all changes of addresses were noted, making the index an invaluable resource for anyone looking at the history of a particular practice or individual. It was on the card index that that the annual *Register of Members*, first published in 1852, was based. From 1881 to 1948 the *Register of Members* also included a list of existing practitioners, composed of unqualified veterinary practitioners who had been in practice since at least 1876. This latter list was replaced between 1948 and 1966 by a supplementary register of practitioners who had been working consistently for seven out of the ten years preceding 1948.

Since 1991 the Royal College of Veterinary Surgeons has also published an annual *Directory of Practices* which, as well as listing both veterinary surgeons and practices, also indicates whether a practice is small animal, large animal, mixed, equine, referral or non-clinical. Unlike the *Register of Members*, however, the *Directory of Practices* is not a complete list of all practising veterinary surgeons since participation is voluntary.

Until 1948, the Royal College of Veterinary Surgeons set an examination, to be sat by anyone wishing to legally practise as a veterinary surgeon and be admitted as a Member of the Royal College of Veterinary Surgeons. The MRCVS examination papers give an insight into the educational standards expected of veterinary surgeons by the College. They also show the type of animals and diseases a qualified veterinary surgeon was expected to come across during his working life. Examination records chart the progress of each student through university and the MRCVS examination, while registers of school qualifications give an indication of the academic standard required for admittance to veterinary college. Other records relate to the awarding of prizes to outstanding students and include lists of both prize winners and of those nominated.

PROFESSIONAL ASSOCIATIONS

Information on the work of the British Veterinary Association can be found in its weekly official journal, *The Veterinary Record*. Summaries of the Association's meetings are included, together with copies of talks given. *The Veterinary Record* also prints news of Presidential and Council elections and important notices. Additionally, the thirty two territorial divisions and twenty specialist divisions affiliated to the British Veterinary Association produce their own records. A series of minute books make it possible to construct the history of an individual association and to examine the opinions of individual veterinary surgeons on the major issues affecting their profession, for example the implementation of the Veterinary Surgeons Acts of 1881, 1948 and 1966, or the impact of new schemes such as Pet Passports. Local or specialist issues are also addressed, both in the minute books and in the supporting paperwork – lectures, reports and circulars. Papers submitted to the Veterinary Public Health Association, for example, include reports on salaries and fees for meat inspectors or drug residues in food analyses. Information on an Association's members can be gleaned from lists of members and officers, subscription registers and attendance books.

LOCAL AND NATIONAL GOVERNMENT

A variety of records have been preserved which make it possible to examine government involvement in the provision of veterinary services at both local and national level. The earliest official records relating to animal health at a local level are generally to be found within Quarter Sessions' papers and in the committees established in the wake of the Cattle Plague Prevention Act of 1866. The outbreak of cattle plague in 1865, the first for over a century, led to a rash of paperwork: minutes of committee meetings, returns, inspectors' reports, notices, suggested cures and details of compensation schemes. A series of Contagious Diseases (Animals) Acts introduced from 1867, together with an increased concern for public health, gradually led to the appointment of more inspectors and the establishment of new and permanent committees to oversee their work. By the 1920s, most county or city councils had appointed Chief Veterinary Officers. Their annual reports include an outline of the tasks carried out during the previous year, statistics relating to outbreaks of contagious disease, inspection reports for slaughterhouses, dairies, piggeries and ports and any changes in staff. Details of individual establishments, however, tend to appear only when there were grounds for an unsatisfactory report.

The development of a national veterinary service similarly grew out of the cattle plague of 1865. A temporary Veterinary Department, established within the Privy Council in October that same year, developed over time to become the present day Animal Health Division of the Department for the Environment, Food and Rural Affairs. This progress is recorded within the official files, made up of minutes, reports, memoranda and correspondence. Some files relate to particular issues such as meat inspection, quarantine procedures, the import and export of live animals, artificial insemination or the administration of health schemes for diseases such as tuberculosis or bovine spongiform encephalopathy. Others are concerned with the establishment and development of government run research institutes and laboratories, which provide diagnostic services for veterinary surgeons and farmers or carry out specialist research, for example on poultry diseases or genetics. Through the laboratory books, reports and correspondence files generated by these various institutes, it is possible to track the elimination or control of individual diseases such as rabies, swine fever or foot-and-mouth. Additionally, there are files relating to ministry staff at all levels, covering appointments, salaries, promotions, postings and pensions.

ARMY

Records reflecting the wide-ranging role played by the veterinary surgeon in army life date back to the time of the Napoleonic Wars (1793–1815). Warrants and regulations give details on the development of the Royal Army Veterinary Corps from its beginnings as the Army Veterinary Service down to the present day, while statistical reports show the numbers of men and animals serving at a particular time together with their costs. There are also lists of the equipment issued to and used by veterinary surgeons and farriers. Official records relating to individuals include lists of officers, commissions and service records. Further information can be gleaned from an individual's private papers – certificates, commissions, memoirs, obituaries, letters, photographs and diaries. Private diaries offer valuable glimpses into the day to day work of the army veterinary surgeon. Additionally they can shed light on such matters as the purchase and condition of remounts, the transportation of animals or the organisation of field hospitals.

Other records reflect the role played by army veterinary surgeons in research. Registers of experiments, reports, laboratory books and research notes cover a range of subjects including animal behaviour, nutrition and the effects of gas on horses, while animal records cards give details of individual animals, mostly horses, mules, dogs, camels and elephants. Listed on each card is the name, breed and age of an animal as well as a general physical description. All vaccinations and treatments are noted and the animal's ultimate fate. There are also a number of animal registers, which account for the animals acquired by the Corps at various times. These note the name and breed of each animal and the duties it was assigned to, together with the name and address of the donors, ranging from private individuals to animal shelters or companies such as breweries or the co-operative movement. An evaluation of a range of these records would also make a more accurate examination of a broader range of subjects possible, including the development of Dog Training Units in England and overseas or the decline in the numbers of farriers retained by the army.

VETERINARY COLLEGES

Veterinary education and training is offered by six universities. The oldest, the Royal Veterinary College, London, dates back to 1791 while the most recent, those at Cambridge and Bristol, were established in 1949. Minute books detailing the regular meetings of senate, faculty, governors and numerous committees provide information on all aspects of each college's history and development. Through them it is possible to look at a college's place within the university system, its day to day administration and the development of its courses. In addition, there are files that shed light on issues such as University Grants Committee or Royal College of Veterinary Surgeons visitations, staff appointments, funding, merger or closure plans and restructuring.

Matriculation records give details of individual students: their name, date of birth, father's name, address and school. Some also include details of school certificates, although this information is more often kept in separate registers. Examination registers detail each student's record while at university, indicating which exams they sat and when, the marks given and whether they passed or failed. While this kind of information is useful to genealogists or biographers tracing the career of an individual, it can also be used to examine a wider range of issues including student selection – the growing emphasis on science-based school certificates, for example, or the male/female student ratio, or the geographical and social areas that students were drawn from. Additionally, there are graduation lists, showing who graduated and when, and lists of prize winners.

Examination papers give an insight into what veterinary students were being taught and the types of diagnostic and treatment procedures they would be expected to perform. There are also numerous student notebooks dating from the nineteenth and twentieth centuries, making it possible to compare curriculum and teaching methods in different schools at different times. Changes in curriculum can also be used to reflect wider changes within the profession and in society generally. As science has developed, some of the diseases highlighted in early examination papers and notebooks have been eradicated, while for others the procedures being taught today would not have been known even a few decades ago. It is possible too, to chart long term changes, such as the rise of small animal medicine.

Other papers illustrate the development of teaching facilities. In the early nineteenth century, clinical teaching was generally carried out at forges using animals provided by the lecturers' private practices and by local slaughterhouses. Veterinary colleges later developed and maintained their own forges and clinics, for which a number of ledgers have survived. By the 1940s, city dairies and stables, previously valuable sources of patients for students to practise on, had virtually disappeared and the veterinary colleges were engulfed by suburban growth. This forced them to develop field stations in nearby country areas where students would be able to experience large animal practice and instigate research. Committee minutes, funding applications, architectural plans and photographs all give an insight into the development of these teaching facilities and the development of research interests. University records, however, particularly those relating to individual students, are generally closed to researchers for up to seventy five years.

CHARITIES

Records created by charities include annual reports, board or council minutes, committee minutes and associated papers. From these it is possible to outline the aims and development of an individual charity, and provide explanations for both the major and minor decisions made. Annual reports are a particularly useful starting point, since they highlight the important issues that arose over the previous year, provide a summary of accounts, list members, benefactors and new branches and pin-point the aims for the year ahead. Additionally, charity archives are often rich in publicity material: leaflets, brochures, press cuttings, magazines, photographs and the like, all of which can be used to chart changes in, say, fundraising techniques or educational programmes.

Overall, the records created by charities, as well as providing information on the history of a particular charity, can be used to examine more widespread social and economic changes. Most of the animal charities that emerged during the nineteenth century did so out of widespread concern for the plight of the working horse. As the numbers of horses on the streets diminished, however, and conditions for those that remained improved, the emphasis began to shift towards concern for the welfare of the increasing number of dogs and cats being kept as pets. It is even possible to chart changes in ethical attitudes, for example the move by many charities from the routine destruction of unwanted animals to a policy of re-homing.

ZOOS

Information on the structure and administration of a zoo can be traced through extant annual reports, committee papers and accounts. From these same papers, it is possible to glean some facts about the provision of veterinary care – for example, the names of veterinary surgeons employed and the fees or salaries paid to them. A more detailed view of the veterinary surgeon's role can be found both in the annual reports submitted to the zoo's council and in occasional more specific reports regarding a particular animal or group of animals. Most zoos have retained a number of records relating to individual animals or groups of the same species including case history cards and post-mortem reports. Case history cards give the species of the animal, its age, date of birth or arrival and its subsequent medical history. Often the date of death or removal is also noted. Post-mortem reports give detailed notes on the examination of deceased animals and the veterinary surgeon's conclusions as to the cause of death. Other useful documents include daily occurrence books, in which a day by day log of the happenings at the zoo are recorded, and registers of births, deaths, arrivals and departures. Since the emphasis during the twentieth century has shifted from preservation to conservation, notebooks and papers relating to research programmes can also be found. And, since publicity is an important part of any zoo's survival, large numbers of photographs, press releases and brochures have also been produced through the years.

CONCLUSION

A large quantity of records have survived which relate to the history of animal health care in the United Kingdom, particularly over the last two hundred years. Their contents ensure that they will be invaluable to anyone wishing to study either the history of animal health or the development of the veterinary profession. But the range of records found and the breadth of information contained within them makes them of great potential interest to many others, including social and economic historians, business historians, local historians, agricultural historians and genealogists.

BIBLIOGRAPHY

J Lane, 'Local Sources for the Study of Veterinary History', *Veterinary History*, no 1, (summer 1973)

J Lane, 'Farriers in Georgian England', in A R Mitchell (ed) *History of the Healing Professions: parallels between veterinary and medical history*, vol 3 (private publication 1993)

J Orbell, *A Guide to Tracing the History of a Business* (Aldershot, 1997)

I Pattison, *The British Veterinary Profession 1791–1948* (London, 1984)

L B Prince, *The Farrier and His Craft: the history of the Worshipful Company of Farriers* (London, 1980)

F M L Thompson, *Victorian England: the horse drawn society, an inaugural lecture* (London, 1970)

C G Trew, *The Horse Through the Ages* (London, 1953)

A Turton (ed), *Managing Business Archives* (Oxford, 1991)

Select bibliography

JOURNALS

Edinburgh Veterinary Review (monthly 1858–64)
Farrier and Naturalist, later *Hippiatrist* (monthly 1828–30)
Veterinary History Journal (twice yearly 1962–)
The Veterinarian (monthly 1828–1902)
The Veterinary Journal, later *The British Veterinary Journal* (monthly 1875–)
The Veterinary Record (weekly 1888–)

GENERAL

Anon, *A History of Johnson's Veterinary Products* (unpublished typescript, 1996)

Anon, 'The Weybridge Veterinary Laboratory During the Second World War', *Veterinary History*, 8, 1995

Anon, *Swann-Morton: sixty years of achievement 1932–1992* (private publication, 1992)

Anon, *The Royal Veterinary College, London 1791–1991* (London, 1991)

Anon, *Maria Dickin: the story of Maria Dickin, founder of the PDSA and pioneer in the field of animal welfare* [People's Dispensary for Sick Animals] (private publication, 1990s)

Anon, *Early Days of the Lancashire Veterinary Association* (private publication, c1980s)

Anon, *An Account of the Veterinary College from its Institution in 1791* [Royal Veterinary College, London] (London, 1973)

Anon, 'Central Veterinary Laboratory Weybridge, Golden Jubilee 1917–67', *State Veterinary Service*, 22, 1967

Anon, 'The Veterinary Laboratory, Lasswade', *State Veterinary Service*, 22, 1967

Anon, 'The Central Veterinary Laboratory, Weybridge 1917–67', *The Veterinary Record*, 1967

Anon, *The PDSA in Wartime: an account of the national humane work of the PDSA 1939–1945* [People's Dispensary for Sick Animals] (private publication, 1940s)

Anon, *The Royal Veterinary College and Hospital* (London, 1937)

Anon, 'A Century-Old Chesterfield Business' [A Greaves & Son Ltd], *Chemist and Druggist*, 124, 1936

Anon, 'Dr Griffith Evans, the Profession's Centenarian', *The Veterinary Record*, 1935

Anon, *The Work of the PDSA in Pictures* [People's Dispensary for Sick Animals] (private publication, 1930s)

K Arnold (ed), *Animal Doctor: birds and beasts in medical history* (Wellcome Institute, 1994)

T Ashbourne, *Shipley & Son* (unpublished typescript, 1989)

L Auchterlonie, *Sixty Years Back: some light-hearted reminiscences of a Royal 'Dick' Veterinary College graduate* (unpublished typescript, 1868)

L J Blenkinsop and J W Rainey, *History of the Great War Based on Official Documents: veterinary services* (London, 1925)

E Boden and J MacArthur Clark, *Challenges for Change: RCVS Charter 150 Symposium* (London, 1994)

O C Bradley, *History of the Edinburgh Veterinary College* (Edinburgh, 1923)

A Brown, *Who Cares for Animals: 150 years of the RSPCA* [Royal Society for the Prevention of Cruelty to Animals] (London, 1974)

R D B Carlisle, *A Century of Caring: the Upjohn story* (USA, 1987)

D Chapman-Huston and E C Cripps, *Through a City Archway: the story of Allen & Hanburys 1715–1954* (London, 1954)

H Chick, M Hume, M Macfarlane, *War on Disease: a history of the Lister Institute* (London, 1971)

J Clabby, *The History of the Royal Army Veterinary Corps 1919–1961* (London, 1963)

W Clapperton, *Clapperton's Royal Agricultural Salisbury Handbook, Containing a Concise History of the Royal Agricultural Society of England* (Salisbury, 1857)

J Clewlow, 'The Mayers of Newcastle under Lyme and their Place in the Emerging Veterinary Profession' *Veterinary History*, vol 9, no 1, 1996

J Clewlow, *The Mayers of Newcastle under Lyme: their contribution to the emerging veterinary profession* (unpublished thesis, Keele, 1995)

G W Cooke (ed), *Agricultural Research 1931–1981: a history of the Agricultural Research Council and a review of developments in agricultural science during the last fifty years* (London, 1981)

E Cotchin, *The Royal Veterinary College, London: a bicentenary history* (Buckingham, 1990)

F A E Crew, 'The Genealogy of the Poultry Research Centre, Edinburgh', *British Poultry Science*, 12, 1971

T R Currie, 'Griffith Evans: The Discoverer of the Trypanosome', *Medical Life*, May 1931

M Dickin, *The Cry of the Animal* [People's Dispensary for Sick Animals] (private publication, c1940)

M Dickin, *Can Animals Suffer?* (private publication, c1940)

C Dobell, 'D'Arcy Wentworth Thompson', *Obituary Notices of Fellows of the Royal Society*, 6, 1948–49

A J Duggan, 'Bruce and the African Trypanosomes', *American Journal of Tropical Medicine and Hygiene*, September 1977

G Evans, 'Autobiographical Memoir', *Annals of Tropical Medicine and Parasitology*, 12, 1918

R H Dunlop and D J Williams, *Veterinary Medicine: an illustrated history* (USA, 1996)

J R Fisher, 'Not Quite a Profession: the aspirations of veterinary surgeons in England in the mid nineteenth century', *Historical Research*, 66, 1993

S Foreman, *Loaves and Fishes: an illustrated history of the Ministry of Agriculture, Fisheries and Food 1889–1989* (London, 1989)

C W Forward, *Under the Blue Cross: a story of two horses in the war, etc* (London, 1915)

C Gaskell, 'University of Liverpool Faculty of Veterinary Science', *The Veterinary Record*, vol 141, no 9, 30 August 1997

N C R Goddard, *Harvests of Change: the Royal Agricultural Society of England 1838–1988* (private publication, 1988)

M Gotelee (ed), *A Record of the Past History of the Town, Park, Manor, Hundred and Castle of Odiham* (private publication, 1932)

L Hall and N Morgan, 'Illustrations from the Wellcome Institute Library: the archive of the Lister Institute of Preventative Medicine', *Medical History*, 30, April 1986

A Ingram, *The Country Animal Doctor* (Aylesbury, 1979)

L Jeffcott, 'Department of Clinical Veterinary Medicine, University of Cambridge', *The Veterinary Record*, vol 141, no 9, 30 Aug 1997

T Kelly, *For Advancement of Learning: the University of Liverpool 1881–1981* (Liverpool, 1981)

J M Kirkness, *A History of the Animal Health Register* (private publication, 1982)

R D Locke, 'The Origins of Benevolence in the Veterinary Profession', *The Veterinary Record*, 27 Sep 1997

G Macdonald, *In Pursuit of Excellence: one hundred years Wellcome 1880–1980* (London, 1980)

M McKeen, *A Brief History of Roslin Institute* (private publication, 1999)

G Mackenzie, *History of the Lasswade Veterinary Laboratory* (private publication, 1999)

J Mantle, *Pfizer at Sandwich: the story of Pfizer Ltd* (London, 1994)

Ministry of Agriculture, *Sixty Years Veterinary Investigation Service 1922–82* (HMSO, 1982)
A R Michell (ed), *The Advancement of Veterinary Science: the bicentenary symposium series*, vol 3 (Wallingford, 1993)
G E Mingay (ed), *The Agrarian History of England and Wales 1750–1850*, vol 6 (Cambridge, 1989)
F Montague, *Let the Good Work Go On* [People's Dispensary for Sick Animals] (London, 1947)
W Moorcroft and G Trebeck, *Travels in the Himalayan Provinces of Hindustan and the Panjab; in Ladakh and Kashmire; in Peshawar, Kabul, Kundaz and Bokhara ... 1819–25* (London, 1841)
P J T Morris and C A Russell, *Archives of the British Chemical Industry 1750–1914: a handlist* (Faringdon, 1988)
A W Moss, *Valiant Crusade: the history of the RSPCA* [Royal Society for the Prevention of Cruelty to Animals] (London, 1961)
A W Moss and E Kirby, *Animals Were There: a record of the work of the RSPCA during the war of 1939–1945* [Royal Society for the Prevention of Cruelty to Animals] (London, 1947)
R Onslow, *A History of the Animal Health Trust* (private publication, 1992)
I Pattison, *The British Veterinary Profession 1791–1948* (London, 1984)
I Pattison, *John McFadyean: a great British veterinarian* (London, 1981)
I Pattison, 'A History of the Veterinary Research Club 1924–74', *The Veterinary Record*, vol 94, no 6, 9 Feb 1974
J W R Pearce, L P Pugh, J Ritchie (eds), *Animal Health: a centenary 1865–1965* (London, 1965)
R Perren, *The Meat Trade in Britain 1840–1914* (London, 1978)
V Porter, *Tales of the Old Country Vets* (Newton Abbott, 1995)
L B Prince, *The Farrier and his Craft: the history of the Worshipful Company of Farriers* (London, 1980)
L P Pugh, *From Farriery to Veterinary Medicine 1785–1795* (Cambridge, 1962)
A Ramsay, *History of the Highland and Agricultural Society of Scotland* (Edinburgh and London, 1879)
H V Roberts, 'The Eighteenth Century Pharmacy at 60 High Street, Tenterden, Kent', *Pharmaceutical Historian*, Oct 1998
L C F Robson, *The Farriers of London: being an account of the Worshipful Company of Farriers as described in the records of the company* (Leeds, 1949)
L Rogers, *Happy Toil: fifty five years of tropical medicine* (London, 1950)
G A L Sarton, 'D'Arcy Wentworth Thompson 1860–1948', *Isis*, 4, 1950

J A Scott Watson, *The History of the Royal Agricultural Society of England 1839–1939* (London, 1939)

M Sewell, 'The Royal (Dick) School of Veterinary Studies', *The Veterinary Record*, vol 141, no 9, 30 Aug 1997

J B Simonds, *The Foundation of the Royal Veterinary College with Biographical Sketches of St Bel, Edward Coleman, William Sewell and Charles Spooner* (London, 1987)

C Smith, *The Blue Cross at War 1914–18 and 1939–43* (private publication, 1990)

D F Smith, 'The Agricultural Research Association: the development fund and the origins of the Rowett Research Institute', *Agricultural History Review*, 46, 1998

D F Smith, 'The Early Institutional and Scientific Development of the Rowett Research Institute', A Adam, D Smith, F Watson (eds) *To the Greit Support and Advancement of Helth: papers on the history of medicine in Aberdeen, arising from a conference held during the quincentenary year of Aberdeen University* (Aberdeen, 1996)

F Smith, *The Early History of Veterinary Literature* (London, reprinted 1976 from various earlier sources)

F Smith, *A History of the Royal Army Veterinary Corps 1796–1919* (London, 1927)

F Smith, *A Veterinary History of the War in South Africa 1899–1902* (London, 1919)

C Stone, *Salute to the National Animal Guard* [People's Dispensary for Sick Animals] (private publication, 1945)

C Stone, *The People's Dispensary for Sick Animals* (private publication, 1930s)

J Swabe, *Animals, Disease and Human Society* (London, 1999)

J A Symon, *Scottish Farming Past and Present* (Edinburgh and London, 1958)

R D'Arcy Thompson, *The Remarkable Gamgees: a story of achievement* (Edinburgh, 1974)

R D'Arcy Thompson, *D'Arcy Wentworth Thompson: the scholar naturalist 1860–1948* (London, 1958)

C Turner, *Gold on the Green: fifty years at Greenford* [Glaxo] (private publication, 1985)

G Tweedale, *At the Sign of the Plough: Allen & Hanburys and the British pharmaceutical industry 1715–1990* (London, 1990)

R P Warin, 'Medicine and Bristol Zoo', *Bristol Medico-Chirurgical Journal*, Jul/Oct 1982

J W Warner, *An Animal Hospital for Merseyside* (unpublished typescript, 1949)

J Webster, 'University of Bristol School of Veterinary Science', *The Veterinary Record*, vol 141, no 9, 30 Aug 1997

W Weipers, 'Centenary of the Foundation of the Glasgow Veterinary College', *The Veterinary Record*, vol 75, no 3, 19 Jan 1963

R G White, *The Origin and Early History of ABGRO* [Animal Breeding and Genetics Research Organisation] (unpublished manuscript, 1965)

A Wilson, *A History of the Yorkshire Veterinary Society 1863–1980* (Yorkshire, 1980)

G Wilson, 'The Brown Animal Sanatory Institution', *Journal of Hygiene*, 82, 1979

J E Wilson, 'An Account of Development at Eskgrove 1938–61', *State Veterinary Service*, 17, 1962

J Winnifrith, *Ministry of Agriculture, Fisheries and Food* (London, 1962)

N Wright, 'University of Glasgow Veterinary School', *The Veterinary Record*, vol 141, no 9, 30 Aug 1997

User's guide: arrangement of the book

The principal function of this guide is to indicate the surviving historical records relating to veterinary medicine and the veterinary profession in England, Scotland, Wales, Northern Ireland, the Channel Islands and the Isle of Man. Included are practices, professional associations, companies, veterinary schools, government agencies, the armed services, zoos, charities and research institutes as well as records created by individual veterinary surgeons and scientists. Additionally, the guide lists records relating to the veterinary surgeon's predecessors – cow leeches, horse doctors and farriers. As this is the first comprehensive survey of historical records relating to the provision of animal health care in the United Kingdom, most of the records contained within the guide, particularly those held by practices, have been listed for the first time. A number of relevant records held at record offices, libraries and museums have also been included.

ENTRIES

Entries are listed in thematic sections and within these alphabetically by name. Each entry comprises: the name of a practice, organisation or individual; the last or current trading address; a brief history; a list of relevant bibliographical references; and details of the surviving records and the location(s) at which they are kept. Minor archive collections have been grouped together by location and organised geographically in the guide to minor collections.

Name

The name of the practice, company, organisation, or individual is, in virtually all cases, the current trading name or the last known name under which they operated. Previous names, where known, are usually referred to in the history section and are also included in the extensive name index at the back of the book. Most long-established veterinary practices, however, have undergone numerous name changes as partners have come and gone and in some cases it has proved impossible to establish the full list of trading names.

Location

The location is the last known address at which a practice, company or organisation operated or, for those still trading, their present address. For those records held by individuals, the addresses given are for the known location of the records at the time of the survey.

History

A brief history of each practice, organisation or individual is provided. These histories are not definitive but outline the origins and development of each practice, organisation or individual. For most organisations and individuals the history is based on published information. Few practices, however, have published histories. Their histories, therefore, are based largely on oral accounts given by present or retired partners, together with information derived from the Royal College of Veterinary Surgeon's card index of members (maintained until around 1960), *Registers of Members* (first published in 1852, annually from the 1860s), local newspaper and trade publication obituaries and census returns.

Bibliography

The publications section lists historical books, leaflets and articles relating to the practice, organisation or individual. The publications cited in the text are included within a bibliography that also lists some important general works.

Records

The records section for each entry is headed by the address for the location of the records in December 2000, whether they are held by a practice or organisation, in private ownership or are deposited in a public repository. As far as possible, the Business Archives Council will keep a record of subsequent changes in the location of records. Changes in the address of many publicly funded record offices can be discovered by referring to the Royal Commission on Historical Manuscripts' *Record Repositories in Great Britain* (HMSO, 11th ed 1998), Janet Foster and Julia Shepherd, *British Archives* (London, 4th ed. 2001) and ARCHON on the Historical Manuscripts Commission's website at http://www.hmc.gov.uk For changes in the addresses of trading practices researchers are referred to *The Directory of Veterinary Practices*, published annually by the Royal College of Veterinary Surgeons. In many entries, records are shown at two or more locations. These locations are numbered Records (1), Records (2), and so on.

Complete consistency has not proved possible in record descriptions as information has not been made available in a standard format. The diversity of lists received from record offices, both in format and terminology, has made it difficult to standardise the record summaries or arrange them consistently in any other way. Reference numbers are placed next to the records they refer to whenever possible. Otherwise they can be found at the end of each list.

ACCESS TO RECORDS

Users of the *Guide* should be aware that the co-operation of all practices, organisations, individuals and record offices in providing details of records does not imply that access to records will be granted. Access to privately held records is at the discretion of the body or individual holding or owning the records and can only be granted when records are not deemed to be confidential and when facilities exist to accommodate researchers. Some publicly and privately held records, particularly those relating to named individuals, have closure periods of between 30 and 100 years imposed upon them. Researchers wishing access to any records should therefore write in the first instance to the address indicated in the relevant records section, explaining their research interests in full and making their enquiry as specific as possible. Instant access to archives is not always possible and particular conditions of access may exist, such as the provision of a letter of introduction and a request for the record holder to be able to review research based on information taken from archives prior to publication.

Where records have been publicly deposited, researchers should write to the chief archivist of the repository named in the relevant records section. Some records in public repositories are governed by conditions of access – such as particular closure periods for certain series of records – applied at the request of the depositor. Others are stored in off-site facilities and require a minimum period of notice to allow them to be retrieved. Researchers, therefore, should contact the appropriate repository in advance of any visit.

USEFUL ADDRESSES

Business Archives Council, enquiries in the first instance to Edwin Green, Group Archivist HSBC Holdings plc, Level 36, 8 Canada Square, London E14 5HQ; website: http://www.archives.gla.ac.uk/bac/

National Register of Archives, Royal Commission on Historical Manuscripts, Ruskin Avenue, Kew, Richmond TW9 4DU, email: nra@hmc.gov.uk; website: http://www.hmc.gov.uk

National Register of Archives (Scotland), National Archives of Scotland, HM General Register House, Edinburgh EH1 3YY
Tel: 0131 535 1314; fax: 0131 557 9569; e-mail: nra@nas.gov.uk; website: http://www.nas.gov.uk

Access to Archives, National Archives, Ruskin Avenue, Kew, Richmond TW9 4DU
http://www.a2a.pro.gov.uk

Royal College of Veterinary Surgeons, Wellcome Library, Belgravia House, 62–64 Horseferry Road, London SW1P 2AF
Tel: 020 7202 0721; e-mail: archives@rcvs.org.uk; website: http://www.rcvs.org.uk

British Veterinary Association, 7 Mansfield Street, London W1M 0AT
Tel: 020 7636 6541; fax: 020 7436 2970; e-mail: bvahq@bva.co.uk; website: http://www.bva.co.uk

ABBREVIATIONS

b	born
c	circa
cent	century
Co	company
d	died
est	established
incl	including
Ltd	Limited
misc	miscellaneous
nd	no date
p	photocopy
plc	public limited company
re	relating to
vol(s)	volume(s)
[w]	wanting – ie the record series is incomplete

List of records of practices

AARDVARK CLINIC
London

History: This small animal practice was bought in 1980 by David Dickenson.

Records: Aardvark Clinic, 151 Putney Bridge Road, London SW15 2NZ

Balance sheets 1981–; ledgers 1970–78, 1981–; day books 1981–; cash books 1981–; general accounts 1981–; receipts 1981–; invoices 1970–78, 1981–; papers re lease 1981–; client records 1981–; booster reminders, etc 1981–; photographs 1981–; notes re practice history 1981–.

ABADARE VETERINARY CLINIC
Newick, East Sussex

History: This single-handed small animal practice was established in 1987.

Records: Abadare Veterinary Clinic, 26 High Street, Newick BN8 4LQ

Balance sheets/profit and loss accounts 1987–; day books 1987–; ledgers 1987–; cash books 1987–; client records 1987–; photographs 1987–; architectural plans 1986–; x-ray monitor reports 1987–.

ABBEY LODGE VETERINARY SURGERY
Herne Bay, Kent

History: This small animal and equine practice was established in 1984 by Diana Stark.

Records: Abbey Lodge Veterinary Surgery, 118 Sea Street, Herne Bay CT6 8QZ

Balance sheets/profit and loss accounts 1984–; day books 1984–; cash books 1984–; client records 1984–.

ABBEY VETERINARY CENTRE
Abergavenny, Monmouthshire

History: This mixed practice was established in c1900. Over the years it has changed its name several times, the last four partnerships being W A Williams & Partners, D W Owen & Partners, W D Jones & Partners and Abbey Veterinary Centre. By 2000, the practice was spread over four premises and employed thirteen veterinary surgeons.

Records: Abbey Veterinary Centre, The Surgery, St Arvans Chambers, Abergavenny NP7 5PR

Partnership agreements 20th cent; client records 20th cent.

ABBEY VETERINARY CENTRE
Shrewsbury, Shropshire

History: This mixed practice was established in 1929.

Records: Abbey Veterinary Centre, 16 Holywell Street, Abbey Foregate, Shrewsbury SY2 5DB

Day books 1954–56.

ABBEY VETERINARY SERVICES
Newton Abbott, Devon

History: This histopathology laboratory was established in 1985.

Records: Abbey Veterinary Services, 39 Queen Street, Newton Abbott TQ12 2BE

Day books 1985–; client records and pathology interpretations 1985–.

ABBOTT, DRAPER & FRASER MsRCVS
Bodmin, Cornwall

History: This practice was established in 1942.

Records: Abbott, Draper & Fraser MsRCVS, The Veterinary Surgery, Harleigh Road, Bodmin PL31 1AQ

Partnership agreements 1990; balance sheets/profit and loss accounts 1990–; day books 1981–; client records 1980s–.

ABERLOUR VETERINARY CENTRE
Aberlour, Moray

History: This mixed practice was established in 1976. Previously known as Shanks & McLean MsRCVS, it has traded as Aberlour Veterinary Centre since 2000.

Records: Aberlour Veterinary Centre, Rinnachat, Aberlour AB38 9NR

Day books 1989–; ledgers 1989–; cash books 1989–; receipts 1989–; client records 1987–; architectural plans 1991–; practice magazines/leaflets 1979–.

AIREDALE VETERINARY GROUP
Keighley, West Yorkshire

History: This mixed practice was originally established in Haworth, West Yorkshire, in c1950 before moving to Keighley in c1980. It traded as Watson & Burrows until 1994.

Records: Airedale Veterinary Group, 21 Devonshire Street, Keighley BD21 2BH

Partnership agreements 1963; practice magazines/leaflets c1971–.

ALBERT COTTAGE VETERINARY CLINIC
Saltash, Cornwall

History: This mixed practice was established as Rees & Sharpe in the late 1960s and sold in 1988.

Records: Albert Cottage Veterinary Clinic, 66 Liskeard Road, Saltash PL12 4HG

Partnership agreements 1990; balance sheets/profit and loss accounts 1988–; day books 1988–; ledgers 1988–; cash books 1988–; client records 1988–.

ALLPETS VETERINARY CLINIC
West Wickham, Greater London

History: This small animal practice was established in c1960. It previously traded under the name of Pingram, Smith & Ward.

Records: Allpets Veterinary Clinic, 35 Addington Road, West Wickham BR4 9BN

Client records 1980–.

ALN VETERINARY GROUP
Alnwick, Northumberland

History: This practice was established at Wagonway Road, Alnwick, in 1899. Branch surgeries were opened in c1960 and in 1996. Although predominantly a large animal practice in the early days, sixty per cent of the work by 2000 was small animal. A large animal facility was opened in 1989 and in 1999 a neighbouring two-person mixed practice was purchased following the owner's retirement.

Records: Aln Veterinary Group, Veterinary Surgery, Wagonway Road, Alnwick NE66 1QQ

Partnership agreements c1971, 1980; balance sheets/profit and loss accounts 1982–; day books 1947–48, 1980– [w]; ledger 1948; client records (small animal) 1981–; architectural plans 1899, 1970, 1980, 1992; bill for building of veterinary surgeon's house and surgery 1899.

AMOS & PENNY MsRCVS
Falmouth, Cornwall

History: This equine and small animal practice was established in 1980.

Records: Amos & Penny MsRCVS, 1 Marine Crescent, Falmouth TR11 4BS

Balance sheets/profit and loss accounts 1980–; architectural plans c1994.

ANCHORAGE VETERINARY HOSPITAL

Acle, Norfolk

History: This mixed practice was established in 1920 at Ivy House, Acle, Norfolk, and run for many years by John Barr, who had graduated from the Edinburgh Veterinary College in 1885. Following Barr's death in 1940, the practice was sold to Oscar Vernon Gunning (1886–1974), an American who had qualified in Ohio in 1910 before coming to Britain with the Canadian Army Veterinary Corps during the First World War. On his arrival in Acle, Gunning, who had gained his MRCVS after a year's study at the Royal Veterinary College, London, in 1919, moved the practice from Ivy House to The Limes. He stayed at the practice until his death in 1974. The following year the practice relocated to South Walsham Road. It was about this time too that hospital status was first awarded to the practice.

Records: Anchorage Veterinary Hospital, South Walsham Road, Acle NR13 3EA

Day books 1977–; client records 1968–; cattle testing records 1974–77; price lists for treatment of small animals 1988, 1991; drug price list 1988; plans and papers re hospital extension 1996–97.

S ANGUS MRCVS

Ramsey, Isle of Man

History: This mixed practice was established by S Angus in 1966 and branches opened in 1972 and 1988. By 2000 there were three veterinary surgeons and nine auxiliary staff working across the three surgeries. Although initially 80 per cent of the work was large animal and 20 per cent small animal, the emphasis by 1999 had shifted to 25 per cent large animal, 65 per cent small animal and 10 per cent equine.

Records: S Angus MRCVS, The Surgery, Tower Road, Ramsey IM8 2EA

Minutes 1966–; balance sheets/profit and loss accounts 1966–; day books 1966–; client records 1966–; photographs 1966–; architectural plans 1966–; practice magazines/leaflets 1966–.

ANICARE VETERINARY GROUP
Worthing, West Sussex

History: This small animal practice was established in 1983 by Margaret Cass. John Sheridan took over the following year and stayed until 1986 at which time the practice was acquired by N J Blackwell.

Records: Anicare Veterinary Group, Unit B Limbrick Corner, Palatine Road, Worthing BN12 6JJ

Balance sheets/profit and loss accounts 1986–; day books 1996–; client records 1988–.

ANIMAL MEDICAL CENTRE REFERRAL SERVICES
Chorlton cum Hardy, Greater Manchester

History: This referral practice was established in 1990 by P Boydell and R Pike.

Records: Animal Medical Centre Referral Services, 511 Wilbraham Road, Chorlton cum Hardy M21 0UB

Balance sheets/profit and loss accounts 1990–; day books 1990–; client records 1990–; photographs 1990–; architectural plans 1990s.

ANIMED VETERINARY HOSPITAL
Wickham, Hampshire

History: This mixed practice was established in 1942 when George Begg was appointed by the Ministry of Agriculture and Fisheries to practise in the area. Begg's practice was extensive, as the shortage of veterinary surgeons during the Second World War meant that those available had to cover large areas. In 1954 Begg sold the practice to R D Locke and W B Cartmell. After Locke left in 1956 Cartmell continued to develop the practice and in 1962 opened the Wickham Laboratory. Although initially intended to process samples generated by the practice, the laboratory rapidly expanded and before long was offering a contract analytical service in microbiology, chemistry, toxicology and virology. The practice premises was rebuilt following a fire in 1971 and officially re-opened in 1976. Hospital status was granted at about the same time. By 2000 there were twelve veterinary surgeons at the practice, providing mainly small animal and equine care as well as a farm animal consultancy, whilst the Wickham Laboratory employs some fifty people across various disciplines.

Records (1): Animed Ltd, Winchester Road, Wickham PO17 5EU

Large animal ledgers 1942–58; small animal ledgers 1944–58; accounts book showing monies received/spent by each surgery in the group 1970–76; purchase ledger 1966–75.

Records (2): Hull University, Brynmor Jones Library, Cottingham Road, Hull HU6 7RX

Legal documents re alleged defamation of Animed Ltd by members of British Union of Anti-Vivisectionists and the South East Animal Liberation League 1984–89.

ANRICH VETERINARY HOSPITAL

Wigan, Greater Manchester

History: This small animal practice was established on Bolton Road, Ashton in Makerfield, Wigan, by Enid Holden (née Moody) in 1967, before moving to Wigan Road, Hindley, in 1971. Richard Weston acquired the practice in 1981 and renamed it Anrich. Branches were opened in Bolton Road, Ashton in Makerfield, in 1982, Ormskirk Road, Pemberton, in 1983 and High Street, Standish, in 1985, although those at Ashton in Makerfield and Standish were closed again in 1988. Hospital status was granted to the surgery at Hindley in 1988. In 1996, the surgeries at Hindley and Pemberton were closed and the practice moved to purpose built premises on Caroline Street, Wigan. At the same time the practice also opened its own pet superstore, Peoples Pets, the first vet-owned superstore in Britain. Although competition from rival superstores forced the closure of Peoples Pets in 1997, a smaller store called Pets by Vets was opened in 1998. The following year, the hospital's facilities were expanded, notably including the first hydrotherapy pool for small animals, useful for speeding the recovery of orthopaedic cases. The next phase of development is scheduled to include an education centre with two lecture theatres complete with viewing gallery and close circuit television for the viewing of operations. From September 2001, the centre, in partnership with Wigan & Leigh College, offered training to veterinary nurses.

Records: Anrich Veterinary Hospital, Caroline Street, Wigan WN3 4EL

Balance sheets/profit and loss accounts 1981–; client records 1984–; architectural plans 1980s; practice magazines/leaflets 1981–.

ANVIL VETERINARY CLINIC

Horsham, West Sussex

History: This practice was established by Alistair MacVicar in Holmbury St Mary, Surrey, in 1989. Originally a small animal and equine practice, by 1998 it was exclusively equine, with four veterinary surgeons employed at a new site in Copsale, West Sussex, which offered full surgical facilities and extensive in-patient stabling.

Records: Anvil Veterinary Clinic, Tuckmans, Bar Lane, Horsham RH13 7DL

Balance sheets/profit and loss accounts 1989–; ledgers 1989–; day books 1989–; cash books 1989–; general accounts 1989–; receipts 1989–; invoices 1989–; papers re assistant contracts 1989–; client records 1989–; receipts 1989–; prescription books 1989–; reports, incl laboratory reports 1990s; general letters 1990s; advertising material, press cuttings, etc 1990s; architectural plans 1990s; photographs 1990s.

ARCHWAY VETERINARY SURGERY

Highworth, Swindon

History: This equine and small animal practice was established in 1982 by S E and S V Wolfensohn. A branch was set up at 30 Devizes Road, Wroughton, Swindon, in 1990.

Records: Archway Veterinary Surgery, 21 High Street, Highworth, Swindon SN6 7AG

Balance sheets/profit and loss accounts 1982–; ledgers 1982–; client records 1982–; photographs 1982–; practice magazines/leaflets 1982–.

ARK VETERINARY PRACTICE
Stratford upon Avon, Warwickshire

History: This mixed practice was established in 1992 by Julian Marcus. An assistant was taken on later that same year and a second one in 1993. In 1997 Marcus formed a partnership with R E Lindsay. During the same year, a neighbouring practice, Greyswood Veterinary Centre, The Ridgeway, which had been purchased in 1996, ceased trading and its business was transferred to the Ark.

Records: Ark Veterinary Practice, 352–354 Birmingham Road, Stratford upon Avon CV37 0RE

Partnership agreement 1997; minutes of practice meetings 1992–; balance sheets 1992–; ledgers 1992–; day books 1992–; cash books 1992–; general accounts 1992–; receipts 1992–; invoices 1992–; client records 1992–; prescription books 1992–; press cuttings 1992–; architectural plans re extension 1997; staff registers 1992–; salary books 1992–; general correspondence 1992–; photographs 1992–.

JOHN ARMSTRONG VETERINARY CLINIC
Dudley, West Midlands

History: This practice was established in c1967 by K E Morton as a branch of his long-established practice at 98 Bridgnorth Road, Wollaston.

Records: John Armstrong Veterinary Clinic, 38 Broad Street, Kingswinford, Dudley DY6 9LP

Balance sheets 1990–; day books 1996–; cash books 1996–.

ASHDALE VETERINARY CLINIC
Harrogate, North Yorkshire

History: This small animal practice was established in 1988 by R D Partridge.

Records: Ashdale Veterinary Clinic, Pet Health Centre, 58 Otley Road, Harrogate HG2 0DP

Minutes 1988–; balance sheets/profit and loss accounts 1988–; day books 1988–; ledgers 1988–; cash books 1988–; client records 1988–; photographs 1988–; architectural plans 1988–.

ASHGROVE VETERINARY CENTRE

Aberdeen

History: George Watson Argo (1916–73) graduated from the Royal (Dick) Veterinary College, Edinburgh, in 1938 and was appointed assistant to William Hepburn (1875–1942), 74 Ship Row, Aberdeen, the following year. In 1940, Argo started a new practice at 34 Ashgrove Road, Aberdeen, moving to Lilybank, Ashgrove Road, the following year and to 10 Belmont Road in 1953. Hugh Kay joined Argo in 1962, followed by Cameron Weir in 1968. The practice by then was trading as Argo & Kay. Weir later went on to set up his own practice in Bieldside, Aberdeen, but Kay remained at Belmont Road until his retirement in 1990, at which time the practice was sold to J N Hopkins. For a time there were two branch practices in Kingsgate and Bridge of Don. Although the practice was principally large animal in its early years, its caseload since c1984 has been exclusively small animal.

Records: Ashgrove Veterinary Centre, 10 Belmont Road, Aberdeen AB25 3SR

Balance sheets 1990–; ledgers 1990–; day books 1990–; cash books 1990–; general accounts 1990–; receipts 1990–; invoices 1990; legal papers re purchase of practice 1990; client records 1980–; title deeds, nd; architectural plans 1996–97; general correspondence 1990–.

ASHLEIGH VETERINARY CLINIC

Knaresborough, North Yorkshire

History: This small animal practice was established in 1983 by N M Bryan.

Records: Ashleigh Veterinary Clinic, 61 Wetherby Road, Knaresborough HG5 8LH

Day books 1983–; cash books 1983–; client records 1983–; x-rays 1983–; consent forms 1983–.

ASHWORTH VETERINARY GROUP
Crieff, Perth & Kinross

History: This practice was established in 1903 at Union Terrace, Crieff, by William Watt, who had graduated in 1881 from the Glasgow Veterinary College. Watt died in 1933 and the practice was sold the following year to John Drummond Ferguson, who had graduated from the Glasgow Veterinary College in 1921 and had acted as Watt's assistant since 1927. Around the time of Ferguson's death in 1956 the practice was sold to a Mr Ashworth. Ashworth entered into a partnership with Mr Rodger in 1979 and the practice then traded as Ashworth & Rodger until 1991, after which it was known as Ashworth & Taylor until 1998 when it became the Ashworth Veterinary Group. Although always a mixed practice, the caseload has shifted over the years from 90 per cent large animal and 10 per cent small animal to 65 small animal, 25 per cent large animal and 10 per cent equine.

Records: Ashworth Veterinary Group, The Veterinary Centre, Union Terrace, Crieff PH7 4DE

Partnership agreements 1979–; balance sheets 1980–; ledgers 1990–; client records 1986–; architectural plans 1980–.

ASPINALL, AULD & CLARKSON MsRCVS
Abbeydale, Gloucestershire

History: This mixed practice was established in 1988.

Records: Aspinall, Auld & Clarkson MsRCVS, 20 Glevum Way, Abbeydale, Gloucester GL4 9BL

Partnership agreements 1988–; balance sheets/profit and loss accounts 1988–; day books 1988–; ledgers 1988–; cash books 1988–; architectural plans 1988–; practice magazines/leaflets 1988–.

ASTONLEE VETERINARY SURGERY
Newport Pagnell, Milton Keynes

History: This mixed practice was established in 1986 by Paul R Manning.

'Investor in People Award for Newport Pagnell Practice', *Veterinary Times*, June 1997.

Records: Astonlee Veterinary Surgery, 68 Tickford Street, Newport Pagnell MK16 9BH

Minutes for practice meetings 1990–; balance sheets 1986–; ledgers 1986–; day books 1986–; cash books 1986–; general accounts 1986–; receipts 1990–; papers re bad debt collection 1986–; clinical records 1986–; press cuttings 1986–; title deeds 1986; architectural plans 1986–; employment record cards 1986–; photographs 1986–; notes re practice history 1986–.

ATKINSON & BURGESS MsRCVS
Bideford, Devon

History: This practice was established in c1958 by D Rabbich. W I Atkinson became a partner in 1969 after which the practice traded as Rabbich & Atkinson. Following Rabbich's retirement in 1982 a new partnership was formed between W I Atkinson and K V Burgess. The practice moved to Witten Lodge in 1981.

Records: Atkinson & Burgess MsRCVS, Witten Lodge, Heywood Road, Northam, Bideford EX39 3QB

Partnership agreements 1969, 1982; balance sheets 1982–; ledgers 1982–; day books 1982–; cash books 1982–; general accounts 1982–; receipts 1982–; invoices 1982–; client records (small animal) 1985–.

G AUSTIN MRCVS
Ivybridge, Devon

History: This mixed practice was established in 1983.

Records: G Austin MRCVS, Kerswill House, Cornwood, Ivybridge PL21 9HT

Papers re practice purchase and sales of branches 1983–; balance sheets/profit and loss accounts 1983–; client records 1983–.

AVENUE VETERINARY CLINIC
Lewes, East Sussex

History: This small animal practice was established in 1951 by Miss L A Breeze along with a branch surgery at Seaford. In 1982 the practice was sold to M Westnedge. The following year surgeries at Peacehaven and Newhaven were added to the group. A partnership established between Westnedge and S C Speak in 1989 was dissolved in 2000, while a new Seaford branch was opened in Brooklyn Road in 1996.

Records: Avenue Veterinary Clinic, The Avenue, Kingston, Lewes BN7 3LJ

Partnership agreements 1989; balance sheets/profit and loss accounts 1982–; ledgers 1982–; cash books 1982–; client records 1951– [w]; architectural plans 1982–; practice magazines/leaflets 1972–.

AVENUE VETERINARY SURGERY
Redcar, Redcar & Cleveland

History: In 1988 Clive Teare bought out a branch surgery on High Street, Marske by the Sea, Redcar & Cleveland, from the Beck Veterinary Practice based at Whitby, North Yorkshire. Later that same year Teare purchased two branches of the Rosslyn Veterinary Hospital in Queen Street, Redcar, and High Street, Marske. The latter was closed after the refurbishment of the former Beck Veterinary Surgery. The premises at 2 Park Avenue, Redcar, purchased in December 1987, opened as the Avenue Veterinary Surgery in August 1988 and the surgery on Queen Street was closed shortly afterwards. In 1989, the surgery on Marske High Street was sold to Teare's assistant, James Haddow, and the income generated by the sale used to extend the premises on Park Avenue. In 1999, 4 Park Avenue was acquired, allowing the practice to expand further.

Records: Avenue Veterinary Surgery, 2 Park Avenue, Redcar TS10 3JZ

Balance sheets 1988–; ledgers 1988–; day books 1988–; cash books 1988–; general accounts 1988–; receipts 1988–; invoices 1988–; legal papers re planning, etc 1988–; client records 1988–; architectural plans 1989; salary books 1988–; general correspondence re practice 1988–; photographs 1988–.

AVON LODGE VETERINARY GROUP
Salisbury, Wiltshire

History: This mixed practice was established in 1949.

Records: Avon Lodge Veterinary Group, 21 Stratford Road, Salisbury SP1 3JN

Day book 1950; partnership agreements, minutes, receipts, photographs, architectural plans 20th cent.

AVONVALE VETERINARY GROUP
Warwick, Warwickshire

History: This surgery was established in 1984 as a branch of the Avonvale Veterinary Group.

Records: Avonvale Veterinary Group, 27 Cape Road, Warwick CV34 4JP

Partnership agreements 1984–; minutes 1984–; balance sheets/profit and loss accounts 1984–; day books 1984–; ledgers 1984–; cash books 1984–; client records 1984–; photographs 1980s–; architectural plans 1984–; practice magazines/leaflets 1984–.

AYRES VETERINARY HOSPITAL
North Shields, Tyne & Wear

History: This small animal practice was established in 1975.

Records: Ayres Veterinary Hospital, 19–21 Ayres Terrace, North Shields NE29 0HL

Balance sheets/profit and loss accounts 1975–; cash books 1975–; client records 1975–.

BAILEY & MATHEWSON MsRCVS
Bexhill on Sea, East Sussex

History: This mixed practice was established prior to 1969. There is a branch surgery at 103 De La Warr Road, Bexhill on Sea.

Records: Bailey & Mathewson MsRCVS, Green Leaves Veterinary Centre, 119 Little Common Road, Bexhill on Sea TN39 4JB

Balance sheets/profit and loss accounts 1969–.

J A BAILLIE MRCVS
Carluke, South Lanarkshire

History: This mixed practice was established by J A Baillie in c1984. A partnership was formed between J A Baillie and A J Main in 1992 and in 1998 a neighbouring practice was bought over. By 2000 thc practice employed eight veterinary surgeons.

Records: J A Baillie MRCVS, Hillend Farm, Crossford, Carluke ML8 5QN

Balance sheets/profit and loss accounts 1984–; day books 1984–; ledgers 1984–; cash books 1984–; client records 1984–.

E BARBOUR-HILL MRCVS
Bangor, Gwynedd

History: This equine and small animal practice was established in 1982.

Records: E Barbour-Hill MRCVS, Tan-y-Coed, High Street, Bangor LL57 1PX

Balance sheets/profit and loss accounts 1982–; day books 1982–; ledgers 1982–; cash books 1982–; architectural plans 1982–.

BARD VETERINARY GROUP
Dumfries, Dumfries & Galloway

History: Bard Veterinary Group was established in 1989 following the amalgamation of Allison, Murchie & Dickson of Dumfries and a single-handed practice established by Roger A Lever in Dalbeattie in 1979. Since then, the latter has been run as a branch surgery. The partners in the new group were Hugh Dickson, Roger A Lever and Alan S Marshall, Messrs Allison and Murchie having retired. Peter Lean joined the partnership in 1997. The Group remains a mixed practice.

Records: Bard Veterinary Group, Renwick Bank, 15 Catherine Street, Dumfries DG1 1JF

Partnership agreements 1989, 1997; balance sheets/profit and loss accounts 1990–; day books 1989–; ledgers 1989–; cash books 1989–; receipts 1989–; client records 1989–; architectural plans 1990, 1999.

BARN LODGE VETERINARY HOSPITAL & EQUINE CLINIC
Ormskirk, Lancashire

History: This small animal and equine practice was established in 1904.

Records: Barn Lodge Veterinary Hospital & Equine Clinic, 54a Southport Road, Ormskirk L39 1LX

Day books 1904–; ledgers 1904–; cash books 1904–; client records 1904–; horse valuations 1904–.

BARR & MACMILLAN MsRCVS
Mauchline, East Ayrshire

History: This mixed practice was established in 1954 as a branch surgery in Kilmarnock, East Ayrshire. In 1957 it was sold to George Barr who ran the practice from his home for a time before moving into purpose built premises in 1966. By 2000 there were four veterinary surgeons based at the practice. Originally the caseload was 95 per cent large animal but by 2000 it had become 50 per cent large animal and 50 per cent small animal.

Records: Barr & MacMillan MsRCVS, 16 Kilmarnock Road, Mauchline KA5 5DE

Partnership agreements 1982–; balance sheets/profit and loss accounts 1958–; day books 1957–58; architectural plans 1960s–.

BARRINGTON LODGE VETERINARY LODGE
Altrincham, Greater Manchester

History: This practice was established in 1963 by a Mr Monahon. After eighteen months Monahon sold the practice to W Gill, who in turn sold it to A F Weipers in 1973. Miss V Innes became a partner in 1998.

Records: Barrington Lodge Veterinary Lodge, 31 Barrington Road, Altrincham WA14 1HZ

Balance sheets/profit and loss accounts 1973–; day books 1973–; cash books 1973–; photographs 1973–.

A BARTHOLOMEW MRCVS
Oxford, Oxfordshire

History: This mixed practice moved from Cowley Place to Iffley Road, Oxford, during the 1940s. It was owned by a Mr Heather until the mid 1970s and since then has traded as Sheriffs & Denley, Sheriffs & Kyle, Sheriffs, Kyle & Bartholomew and A Bartholomew. A branch surgery was opened at Roman Road, Wheatley, Oxfordshire, in 1984.

Records: A Bartholomew MRCVS, 35 Iffley Road, Oxford OX4 1EA

Partnership agreements 1983–; balance sheets/profit and loss accounts 1987–; day books 1987–; ledgers 1987–; recipes 1950s; procedures, nd; price list, nd.

BARTON VETERINARY HOSPITAL
Canterbury, Kent

History: This practice was established at The Paddock, Chantry Lane, Canterbury, Kent, in 1890 by William Henry Crowhurst (1832–1919). Crowhurst, who had graduated from the Royal Veterinary College,

London, in 1856, remained at the practice until his death in 1919. In addition to serving the local farms, the practice for many years held a contract from Canterbury Corporation that required it to inspect the cattle market, held every Saturday, and the Corporation's horses. During the First World War the Royal Army Service Corps billeted horses at the practice's stables. In 1921 the practice was taken over by James George Cattell (c1883–1964), who had graduated from the Royal (Dick) Veterinary College, Edinburgh, in 1904 and served for many years in the Indian Veterinary Service. By this time the practice was based in Upper Chantry Lane, but in 1928 it moved to purpose built premises at 34 New Dover Road. George Peyton joined the practice in 1946 and took over following Cattell's retirement in 1947. In 1956 Peyton entered into partnership with two of his assistants, Norman Fowler and Derek Evans. The practice was extended and developed and in 1967 achieved hospital status. Peyton retired in 1967 and in 1970 Sidney Foster and Richard Wickham became partners. They were joined in 1987 by Dermot Stewart and Robert Thomas. In 1999 the practice was incorporated with CVS (UK) Ltd as investors.

Records: Barton Veterinary Hospital, 34 New Dover Road, Canterbury CT1 3DT

Ledgers 1956–68; appointment book 1965–66; accounts re large animals 1985–91; till book 1987–90; cash analysis books 1985–90; cash receipts 1985–86; surgery credits 1985–89; bank statements, etc 1968–80; misc rough accounts 1970s; cash books 1981–89; tax returns 1967–72, 1975–76, 1980–84; wages book (veterinary staff) 1967–75; wages book (non-professional staff) 1968–81; staff records (non-professional staff) 1960–72; correspondence, etc re veterinary posts 1976, 1984–86; correspondence re staff 1973–85; x-ray record books 1963–88; tuberculin testing records 1960s–80s; dangerous drugs register 1985–88; ophthalmic case book 1982; electrocardiogram records 1982–83; plans for building of Barton House 1926; photographs of staff, presentations, etc 1970s–; copies of photographs, certificates, etc re William Crowhurst; price lists, recipes, etc 19th–20th cent compiled for centenary display 1990; student notebooks, Bristol 1974.

A J BARTRAM & PARTNERS
Pontefract, West Yorkshire

History: This small animal and equine practice was purchased from Ashton House Veterinary Centre, Wakefield, in 1982 by Alan John

Bartram. R F Coppack joined as an assistant in 1990 and was made a partner in 1992. In 1990 a branch surgery was opened at 58 Northgate, Pontefract. A N Patrick joined the practice in 1995 and became a partner in 1998. In 1999 60 Northgate, Pontefract, was acquired.

Records: A J Bartram & Partners, 28A Minsthorpe Lane, South Elmsall, Pontefract WF9 2NY

Balance sheets 1982–; ledgers 1982–; general accounts 1982–; invoices 1982–; legal papers re purchase of practice 1982.

J BASSETT
Wadhurst, East Sussex

History: The firm of J Bassett, established at Wadhurst, East Sussex, in the late nineteenth century, traded as coach builders and painters, wheelwrights, farriers and blacksmiths. Their forge at Durgates, Wadhurst, finally closed after Rodney John Bassett (1908–92) retired in 1988.

Records: East Sussex Record Office, The Maltings, Castle Precincts, Lewes BN7 1YT

Customer account books 1893–1943, 1960–73, 1975–83; draft customer account books 1947, 1980–84; income and expenditure account books 1933–82, 1986–88; profit and loss accounts/balance sheets 1955, 1964, 1977–82; debts owed 1958–c1963; orders 1968; general register of young people employed under the Factory and Workshop Act 1901, 1901–10; accident book 1948–66; press cuttings re firm c1930, 1964, 1967, 1972–73, 1975, 1988; list of customers sending Christmas greetings c1980; office stationery c1880–1960; photographs: family members 1918–c1960, forge c1940s, 1960s; misc family papers 20th cent. [Ref: AMS 6439]

BEACON VETERINARY CENTRE
Aspatria, Cumbria

History: This mixed practice is believed to have been established in c1860 by Henry Thompson (c1837–c1920). Thompson graduated from the Edinburgh Veterinary College in 1860 and was known to be living and practising in Aspatria shortly afterwards. According to the 1891 census, Thompson was living at Brandraw House, Aspatria, along with his student assistant Thomas David Hughes. In addition to his practice, Thompson was actively involved in the setting up of a local agricultural course and was also one of the original directors of the Aspatria Farmers Agricultural Co-operative, established in 1898. Partners in more recent years have included Tom Wolf to 1982, James Buchanan 1968–90 and Martin Lord 1990 to date.

Records: Beacon Veterinary Centre, Station Road, Aspatria, Carlisle CA5 2AL

Day books 1988–89; ledger 1972.

BEGG & PARTNERS
Strathaven, South Lanarkshire

History: This largely agricultural practice is believed to have been established by Hugh Begg. Begg graduated from the Glasgow Veterinary College in 1923 and moved to Wellbrae House, Strathaven, in 1925 or 1926. He was followed into the practice by his two sons, Hugh and James, and by William (Bill) Whiteford. In 2000 the partners were T Caldwell and J Gilbert. The practice moved to purpose built premises in 1971.

Records: Begg & Partners, 40 Stonehouse Road, Strathaven ML10 6LF

Recipes 20th cent; photographs 20th cent.

BELGRAVIA HOUSE VETERINARY SURGERY
Linton, Cambridgeshire

History: This mixed practice was established in 1985 by David Urwin.

Records: Belgravia House Veterinary Surgery, 139 High Street, Linton CB1 6JT

Balance sheets/profit and loss accounts 1985–; day books 1985–; ledgers 1985–; client records 1985–.

BELL EQUINE VETERINARY CLINIC
Maidstone, Kent

History: This equine practice was established in 1989.

Records: Bell Equine Veterinary Clinic, Mereworth, Maidstone ME18 5GS

Partnership agreements 1989–; minutes 1989–; balance sheets/profit and loss accounts 1989–; day books 1989–; ledgers 1989–; cash books 1989–; client records 1989–; photographs 1989–; architectural plans 1989–.

BEVIN, BUTLER & DRUMMOND
Market Harborough, Leicestershire

History: This mixed practice is believed to have been established by a Mr Eaton. His son George Eaton (1901–67) qualified from the Royal Veterinary College, London, in 1922 and settled at Eastgates, Hallaton, Leicestershire, immediately afterwards. During the 1950s branches were established at Uppingham, Market Harborough and Corby. Following George Eaton's retirement in 1965 the practice was sold to David Heatley and John Bayliss, but their partnership was dissolved just two years later, with Heatley taking the Market Harborough and Corby branches and Bayliss the Uppingham branch. The surgery at Hallaton was closed in 1966. Heatley ran the Market Harborough surgery primarily as a large animal practice, with most of the small animal work being carried out at Corby until its sale in 1975. In c1976 a partnership was formed between Heatley and T R Bevin, who had worked at the practice as an assistant between 1966 and 1971 and again from 1974 to 1976, and the two men traded as Heatley & Bevin. Heatley retired in 1984 and Bevin entered into a new partnership with David Butler in 1986. Two years later, they were joined by Gavin Drummond. Between 1970 and 2000 the practice's caseload shifted from 90 per cent farm animal to 85 per cent small animal. The Market Harborough surgery was expanded in 1988 and branches were opened at Kibworth and Rothwell in 1990 and 1994 respectively.

Records: Bevin, Butler & Drummond, 124 Northampton Road, Market Harborough LE16 9HF

Partnership agreements 1975, 1982, 1987; diaries (Rothwell) 1996, (Kibworth) 1996; booking up sheets 1977, 1979–80; day books 1975, 1977–82; invoices: outgoing 1977–82, 1984, equine 1994, farm 1978,

1992–; expenditure ledgers 1970s, purchase ledgers 1977, 1984–85, 1988–; farm accounts ledgers 1970s, 1982–84, 1992, 1994; farm accounts 1985, 1988–91; small animal accounts 1983–84, 1986, 1988–92; purchase day books 1982–86, 1988–94; bank cash book 1976–84; cheques banked 1976–84; surgery cash books 1982–84, 1989–93; summary of surgery cash 1985, 1989–92, 1994; cheques and cash received 1988–95; cash and cheques received (Kibworth) 1990–92; surgery cash book (Kibworth) 1990–95; summary of surgery cash (Kibworth) 1990–92, 1994–95; drugs invoices 1984; sundry accounts 1971–83; stock take totals 1991; stock and equipment valuation 1988; client records 1970s–; record of operations performed 1985; record of drugs dispensed 1986; tuberculin testing notebooks 1962–c1984; Local Veterinary Inspector claim forms 1977–78, 1981–82; agreement for alterations at 2 and 2A Wellington Street, Leicester [w] 1965; plan of proposed alterations to surgery 1985; architectural plans re conversion work 1988; photographs re conversion work 1988; student notes 1970s.

BICESTER VETERINARY CENTRE
Bicester, Oxfordshire

History: This practice was established by William John Carless (1896–1978), who graduated from the Royal Veterinary College, London, in 1921. After brief spells in Worcester and Hatfield, Hertfordshire, Carless came to Wendlebury, Bicester, in 1927. He was joined in c1928 by Joseph Glyne Salt (1901–59), who had graduated from Liverpool in 1926, after which the practice traded as Carless & Salt. Following Salt's death 1959 a new partnership was formed between Carless and a Mr Niven, which lasted until 1962. The practice was then sold to William Morrison Milne. In 1975 a new partnership was formed between Milne, Dias do Nascimento and P R Ferens. Dias left in 1978 and the practice traded as Milne & Ferens until 1981. In 1981, Ferens purchased the practice outright and traded alone for three months before entering into partnership with Robert Cumming. Fiona Cornish joined the partnership in 1993 and the practice then traded as Ferens, Cumming & Cornish until 2000 when J P Williams became a partner. It was at this time that the practice became known as the Bicester Veterinary Centre.

Records: Bicester Veterinary Centre, Victoria Road, Bicester OX6 7PJ

Balance sheets 1938, 1948, 1950, 1952–56, 1959, 1975–.

BILTON VETERINARY CENTRE
Rugby, Warwickshire

History: This mixed practice was bought in 1950 by Thomas Richard Furber (1914–76), a 1940 graduate of the Liverpool Veterinary College. A partnership was later formed between Furber and F Lloyd-Griffiths, which R M Furber joined in 1965. A new surgery was built in 1967 and twice extended during the 1980s and 1990s. A branch was opened at 26 Regent Place, Rugby, in 1995. By 2000 the practice was composed of four partners and four assistants.

Records: Bilton Veterinary Centre, 259 Bilton Road, Rugby CV22 7EQ

Balance sheets/profit and loss accounts 1950–; architectural plans 1966–.

BISHOP HENDRY & EDWARDS MsRCVS
Newport, Telford & Wrekin

History: This mixed practice was established in the 1960s.

Records: Bishop Hendry & Edwards MsRCVS, 11 High Street, Newport TF10 7AR

Cash books 1960s–.

T M & J A BLACK MsRCVS
Dunoon, Argyll & Bute

History: The partnership of T M & J A Black was established in Dunoon in 1975, although T M Black had been practising in the area since 1947. It has remained a mixed practice and moved to its present site in 1978.

Records: T M & J A Black MsRCVS, The Veterinary Centre, 119 George Street, Dunoon PA23 8JX

Balance sheets/profit and loss accounts 1975– [w]; day books 1975– [w]; ledgers 1975– [w]; cash books 1975– [w]; client records 1975– [w]; architectural plans, nd.

BLYTHWOOD VETERINARY CLINIC
London

History: This small animal practice was established in Pinner in 1979.

Records: Blythwood Veterinary Clinic, 500 Uxbridge Road, Pinner HA5 4SL

Balance sheets/profit and loss accounts 1979–; day books 1979–; ledgers 1979–; cash books 1979–; client records 1979–; photographs 1979–; architectural plans 1979–; practice magazines/leaflets 1979–.

BOWBRIDGE VETERINARY GROUP
Stroud, Gloucestershire

History: This mixed practice was established in 1968.

Records: Bowbridge Veterinary Group, Butterow Hill, Stroud GL5 2LA

Partnership agreements 1975–; balance sheets/profit and loss accounts 1975–; architectural plans 1975–.

J L BOWEN MRCVS
Tenby, Pembrokeshire

History: This practice developed out of one established in Narberth, Pembrokeshire, by P Davies and J W Bowen. D I Bowen, J W Bowen's brother, joined the partnership on his return from Burma in 1948 and opened a branch in Tenby. At the same time, J W Bowen opened another branch in St Clears, Carmarthenshire (now Michell & Morgan). After the partnership was dissolved in 1950, D I Bowen traded on his own from Bredon, Warren Street, Tenby, before moving to Marsh Farm, Tenby, in 1954. The practice remained single-handed until the early 1970s, when it became a two-man practice. J L Bowen joined his father in 1979 and took over in 1985.

Records: J L Bowen MRCVS, Marsh Farm, Tenby SA70 8DU

Day books 1950–.

BREDY VETERINARY CENTRE
Bridport, Dorset

History: This mixed practice was formed by the amalgamation in 1985 of two Dorset practices – A G White, who had worked from 26 West Allington, Bridport, and R J G Smith of Prout Bridge, Beaminster.

Records: Bredy Veterinary Centre, Sea Road North, Bridport DT6 4RR
Partnership agreements 1985–; balance sheets/profit and loss accounts 1985–; day books 1985–; ledgers 1985–; cash books 1985–; client records 1985–; photographs 1985–; architectural plans 1985–.

J BROOK MRCVS
Bishops Itchington, Warwickshire

History: This practice was established in 1850. Captain John Scott (d 1962), who graduated from the Glasgow Veterinary College in 1911, was known to be practising at High Street, Nuneaton, from 1912, before moving to the Veterinary Infirmary, 7 Clarendon Avenue, Leamington Spa, in 1922. In 1946, Scott entered into a partnership with G B Brook. After Scott left in 1947 or 1948, Brook continued at the practice until 1971. J V Murphy BVSc MRCVS was made a partner in 1984. In 1990 the practice was split up. John M Brook took the equine side of the practice to Spring Paddocks, while the livestock and small animal practice remained with J V Murphy in Clarendon Street, Leamington Spa, along with the branches in Barford (est 1980) and Kineton (est 1987).

Records: J Brook MRCVS, Spring Paddocks, Bishops Itchington CV47 2QX

Partnership agreements 1984–; balance sheets/profit and loss accounts 1980–; day books 1990–; ledgers 1990–; cash books 1990–; receipts 1990–; client records 1990–; scans/x-rays 1990; photographs 1980–; practice magazines/leaflets 1995–.

BROOK VETERINARY CLINIC
Enniskillen, Co Fermanagh

History: This small animal practice was established by Maeve Lunny in 1985. Originally based at 4 Willoughby Place, Enniskillen, it moved to Rossorry Church Road in 1992.

Records: Brook Veterinary Clinic, Rossorry Church Road, Enniskillen BT74 7HB

Balance sheets/profit and loss accounts 1985–; client records 1985–; architectural plans 1985–.

BROOKEND VETERINARY SURGERY
Witham, Essex

History: This small animal practice, established in 1983 by Niall Murphy, was acquired by the Waters Partnership in 1987. Three years later the Waters Partnership split up and the Witham surgery was sold to Alison Ewbank.

Records: Brookend Veterinary Surgery, 49 Braintree Road, Witham CM8 2DD

Balance sheets/profit and loss accounts 1990–; ledgers 1990–; architectural plans 1987.

D BROWN MRCVS
Mansfield, Nottinghamshire

History: This practice was established in 1945 as a branch surgery by Hector Stewart Cockburn (d 1968), a native of Eastwood, Glasgow, who had graduated from the Royal Veterinary College, London, in 1914. By 2000 the practice's caseload was predominantly small animal.

Records: D Brown MRCVS, 25 St John's Place, Mansfield NG18 5NS

Balance sheets 1968–; cash books 1993–; receipts 1993–: invoices 1993–; clinical cards and ledgers 1972–; title deeds c1880–; photographs c1960s–90s.

BROWN & PADDON MsRCVS
Wisbech, Cambridgeshire

History: This practice was established at 4 South Brink, Wisbech, in 1859 by Robert Knowles, who had qualified from the Royal Veterinary College, London, that same year. Knowles was joined in 1888 by his son,

Robert William Knowles, who also qualified from the Royal Veterinary College, London, winning the class prize for therapeutics. Robert Knowles senior died in 1895 after which the practice was continued by his son with the help of various temporary assistants. In 1906 the practice moved to 6 South Brink, Wisbech, and in 1912 acquired its first motor car. R W Knowles' three children were all involved in the practice. His daughter Minnie acted as dispenser from the time she left school in 1916 until her marriage in 1920, while his two sons, John William (Jack) and Thomas (Tom), both attended the Royal Veterinary College, London. Jack qualified in 1917 and joined the Army Veterinary Corps as a Lieutenant, although he returned to the practice after demobilisation in 1919. Tom entered the Royal Veterinary College, London, in 1914, but left the following year to join the armed services. He too served until 1919, then worked briefly at the practice before returning to his studies, qualifying in 1922. Following R W Knowles's death in 1924, his two sons took over the practice as equal partners, trading as Knowles & Knowles. They were ably assisted by Mr Richardson, who initially acted as yardman from c1924, but went on to become a veterinary practitioner and the practice caretaker. Richardson remained at the practice until his retirement in 1983. Jack Knowles retired in 1949 leaving Tom to run the practice alone, with the help of various assistants, until 1959 when his son, Robert, who had graduated from the Royal Veterinary College, London, in 1957, was given a share of the practice. In 1960, John Machin, who had joined the practice as an assistant in 1949, became the third partner. After Tom Knowles died in 1964 the practice traded as Knowles & Machin until 1976, when Robert Knowles sold his share to Christopher John Brown. The practice then traded as Machin & Brown until John Machin retired in 1984. A new partnership was formed the following year between Christopher Brown and Nigel Paddon. The practice moved to purpose built premises on Elm Low Road, Wisbech, in 1987.

Records: Brown & Paddon MsRCVS, 214 Elm Low Road, Wisbech PE14 0DF

Notebook incl R W Knowles' student notes on cattle pathology, monthly takings 1889–1963, diary of events in family and practice life 1889–1988, prescriptions and remedies 19th cent; paper on 'Vegetable Micro-Organisms' given by R W Knowles 1888; profit and loss account 1917; invoice 1959; valuation of practice 1959; summary of profits 1959; assistants' contracts: Richard Herbert Oddy 1908, John Parry 1912, Wilfred Flanagan 1913, George A Sangster 1914; partnership agreements 1946, 1949, 1959; insurance papers for practice, staff, etc 1953–54, 1960–61; insurance schedule 1966–67; labels for medicines 20th cent; circular letter from R W Knowles re state of practice 1908; letter from National Veterinary Medical Association re advice on drawing up partnership agreement 1948; certificates: MRCVS 1859, 1888, 1922, Royal Veterinary College, London, Bachelor of Veterinary Medicine 1958; photographs of partners, etc 19th–20th cent; slides: pathological 1940s, bacteriological 1940s, preparation of canine distemper vaccine 1950s.

BROWN, SIMPSON & STOBO MsRCVS
Hawick, Scottish Borders

History: This mixed practice was established in c1966 and moved to its present location in 1973.

Records: Brown, Simpson & Stobo MsRCVS, 10 Drumlanrig Square, Hawick TD9 0AS

Partnership agreements 1966–; client records 1966–.

J A BURGESS MRCVS
Tunbridge Wells, Kent

History: This small animal practice was established by J A Burgess in 1987.

Records: J A Burgess MRCVS, The Veterinary Surgery, 20 Ashley Gardens, Rusthall, Tunbridge Wells TN4 8TU

Balance sheets/profit and loss accounts 1987–; day books 1987–; client records 1987–.

BURGHLEY VETERINARY CENTRE
Stamford, Lincolnshire

History: This practice is believed to have been established in c1850 by a Mr Whatten. He was succeeded by F W L Gooch and Frederick Leeds Gooch (d 1941), the latter of whom graduated from the Royal Veterinary College, London, in 1880.

Records: Burghley Veterinary Centre, St Leonards Street, Stamford PE9 2HU

Valuation papers 1882; client records 1965–.

I C R BUTT MRCVS
Loanhead, Midlothian

History: This mixed practice was established by I C R Butt in 1982 and moved to Fountain Place, Loanhead, in 1988.

Records: I C R Butt MRCVS, 44 Fountain Place, Loanhead EH20 9DU

Balance sheets/profit and loss accounts 1982–; day books 1982–; ledgers 1982–; cash books 1982–; client records 1982–; photographs 1982–; architectural plans 1982–.

BYRE VETERINARY SURGERY
Werrington, Peterborough

History: This small animal practice was established in 1990.

Records: Byre Veterinary Surgery, Unit 19, Papyrus Road, Werrington, Peterborough PE4 5BH

Minutes 1990–; balance sheets/profit and loss accounts 1990–; day books 1990–; ledgers 1990–; cash books 1990–; client records 1990–; architectural plans 1990–.

BYRON VETERINARY CLINIC
Nottingham, Nottinghamshire

History: This practice was established during the nineteenth century. It was based firstly at Musters Road, West Bridgford, Nottinghamshire, then St James Street, Nottingham, before moving to Nuthall Road, Nottingham, in 1992. Originally an equine and farm animal practice, it now sees mainly small animals. Previous partners have included Absalom, Percy Maurice Evershed (d 1967) who qualified from the Royal Veterinary College, London, in 1897, Symthe to 1948, John Steward from 1948 to 1980 and Butler from 1965 to 1970.

Records: Byron Veterinary Clinic, 497 Nuthall Road, Nottingham NG8 5DG

Balance sheets/profit and loss accounts 1975–; day books 1977–; client records 1988–; architectural plans 1992.

CALDER & FERGUSON MsRCVS
Forfar, Angus

History: This mixed practice was established in the early twentieth century.

Records: Calder & Ferguson MsRCVS, 225 East High Street, Forfar DD8 2HL

Partnership agreements 1988; balance sheets/profit and loss accounts 1988–; day books 1985–; ledgers 1985–; cash books 1988–; receipts 1940–; client records 1992–; architectural plans 1988.

CALWETON VETERINARY CENTRE
Callington, Cornwall

History: This mixed practice was established at Pannier Market, Callington, in 1928 by 'Old Man Drew'. The practice's name changed several times over the years, being successively Drew & Bunker, Bunker & Partners, Bunker & Brown, Brown & Partners, Brown & Helme and Calweton Veterinary Group. It moved to new premises in 1995.

Records: Calweton Veterinary Centre, 79 Tavistock Road, Callington PL17 7DQ

Partnership agreements 1995–; balance sheets/profit and loss accounts c1984–; day books c1945– [w]; ledgers c1945– [w]; receipts 1930– [w]; client records 1980–.

CAMBRIAN VETERINARY CENTRE
Tywyn, Gwynedd

History: This practice was established by G M Jenkins in 1969. It became a two-man practice with the opening of a branch surgery in nearby Machynlleth in 1984. Following the sale of the large animal side of the practice in 1999, the centre was able to concentrate on the provision of small animal and equine care.

Records: Cambrian Veterinary Centre, Llwynteg, Bryncrug, Tywyn LL36 9NU

Cash books 1969–; large animal invoices 1969–; small animal invoices 1984–; small animal client records 1984–; title deeds, nd; photographs 1969–.

CAMERON & GREIG MsRCVS
Milnathort, Perth & Kinross

History: This mixed practice was established in 1920.

Records: Cameron & Greig MsRCVS, Ardmohr, Stirling Road, Milnathort KY13 7XG

Partnership agreements, nd; balance sheets/profit and loss accounts 20th cent; day books 1990s; ledgers 1990s; cash books 1990s; client records 1990s.

CASTLE VETERINARY GROUP
Launceston, Cornwall

History: This mixed practice dates back to c1866.

Records: Castle Veterinary Group, The Surgery, Pennygillam Way, Launceston PL15 7ED

Day books 1909–; recipes, nd; client records 1980–.

CASTLE VETERINARY SURGEONS
Barnard Castle, Co Durham

History: This practice was established in c1940. Over the years the practice has grown from a four-vet mixed practice to a fourteen-vet practice spread across three divisions. Moves were made to larger premises in 1975, 1982 and 1997 and a branch surgery was set up in 1982.

Records: Castle Veterinary Surgeons, Montalbo Road, Barnard Castle DL12 8ED

Partnership agreements 1982–; minutes c1980–; balance sheets/profit and loss accounts 1980–; day books 1980–; ledgers 1980–; client records 1990–; architectural plans 1982–.

CASTLE VETERINARY SURGERY
Reading

History: This practice was established during the nineteenth century. Previous partners have included Kirkwood, Kohn, Miekle, Barber and Edgar. The practice moved from Queens Road to Tilehurst Road in 1971. The large animal side of the practice was sold c1975.

Records: Castle Veterinary Surgery, 1 Tilehurst Road, Reading RG1 7TW

Balance sheets/profit and loss accounts 1953–; bad debt ledger 1913; recipes for large animal medicaments early 1900s; client records 1963– [w].

CASTLE VIEW VETERINARY HOSPITAL
Wakefield, West Yorkshire

History: This mixed practice was established in 1982 by F J Marshall. In 2000 the goodwill was sold to CVS (UK) Ltd and the former partners retained as employees.

Records: Castle View Veterinary Hospital, Belle Isle Health Park, Wakefield WF1 5PN

Partnership agreements 1980s–; balance sheets 1983–; cash books 1983–; receipts 1985–; invoices 1985–; client records 1991–; architectural plans 1982, 1997; photographs 1997.

CHALKS ROAD VETERINARY CLINIC
St George, Bristol

History: This small animal practice was established in 1984.

Records: Chalks Road Veterinary Clinic, 31 Lyndale Road, St George, Bristol BS5 7AA

Day books 1984–; ledgers 1984–; cash books 1984–; architectural plans 1984.

CHAMINGS & CARMAN MsRCVS

Malvern, Worcestershire

History: This mainly small animal practice was established in Worcester Road, Malvern, by R J Chamings in 1985.

Records: Chamings & Carman MsRCVS, 38 Worcester Road, Malvern WR14 4AA

Balance sheets/profit and loss accounts 1985–; day books 1985–; ledgers 1985–; cash books 1985–; photographs 1985–.

CHAPELFIELD VETERINARY PARTNERSHIP

Norwich, Norfolk

History: This practice was believed to have been established by Garwood George Whincop (d 1908), who graduated from the Royal Veterinary College, London, in 1867. After a brief stay in Lowestoft, Suffolk, Whincop came to 46 Thorpe Hamlet, Norwich, in c1869. In 1886 or 1887 Whincop was joined by John Pollock (c1855–1909), who had qualified from the Glasgow Veterinary College in 1877 and spent some time practising in Lanarkshire before coming to Norfolk. Shortly afterwards, branches were opened at Oxford Place, Prince of Wales Road and Dereham Road. The Oxford Place branch later became the centre of the practice. In addition to his practice, Pollock acted as veterinary surgeon to Norwich Corporation and gave lectures on farriery under a scheme run by Norfolk County Council. He also invented several instruments for use in veterinary medicine. Following Pollock's death in 1909, the practice was acquired by Harry P Standley (d 1944), who had been practising in Wymondham, Norfolk, since his graduation from the Royal Veterinary College, London, in 1895. Standley was later joined by his son, also called Harry (c1902–49), who graduated from the Royal Veterinary College, London, in 1923, after which the practice traded as Harry P Standley & Son. Following the death of Harry Standley junior the practice was sold to John McLintock. In 1962 the practice moved to a purpose built facility on Chapelfield Road, where it traded as McLintock & Partners. Following McLintock's retirement in c1980 the practice's name was changed to the Chapelfield Veterinary Partnership. Over the years, branches were established at Wymondham, Long Stratton and Costessey.

Obituary of Harry Standley, *The Veterinary Record*, 13 Feb 1909; obituary of John Pollock, *The Veterinary Record*, 30 April 1949.

Records: Chapelfield Veterinary Partnership, McLintock House, 21 Chapelfield Road, Norwich NR2 1RR

Ledgers 1957–77; visits book 1956–59; general accounts book incl bad debts, drawings, etc 1957–62; cash books 1958–64; expenditure book 1956–59; bills issued 1911, 1967; Christmas bonus book 1910–91; photographs of staff c1960s, c1990.

CHARLTON PARK VETERINARY GROUP

Keynsham, Bristol

History: Charlton Park Veterinary Group, established in 1984 by a husband and wife team, was sold in 1988. It was originally a small animal and equine practice, but the equine goodwill was sold in 1997.

Records: Charlton Park Veterinary Group, 52 Charlton Park, Keynsham, Bristol BS31 2ND

Partnership agreements 1988–97; balance sheets 1998–; ledgers 1998–; day books 1998–; cash books 1998–; general accounts 1998–; receipts 1998–; invoices 1998–; client records 1984–; salary books 1988–.

CHARTER VETERINARY SURGEONS

Newcastle under Lyme, Staffordshire

History: This practice was established in Newcastle under Lyme in 1812 by Thomas Mayer. Mayer was later joined by his sons, Thomas Walton Mayer and John Smith Mayer. All three men lobbied hard during the 1830s to improve the standard of veterinary education and were largely responsible for organising the petition that led to the granting of a charter to the Royal College of Veterinary Surgeons in 1844. Although Thomas Walton Mayer left the practice in 1855 to fight in the Crimean War, his brother remained until his death in 1863, after which the practice was sold to William Henry Llewellyn. In 1870, the practice changed hands once again, passing this time to R Cadwallader Trigger, a future president of the Royal College of Veterinary Surgeons (1896). His nephew, William Trigger, qualified in 1904 and the two men traded together until the senior man's death in 1927. William Trigger continued to practise until his own death in 1961, after which the business was acquired by Frank Sims, who had already established his own practice at Congleton, Cheshire, in 1958. The Newcastle under Lyme practice became a branch of this business along with other surgeries at Biddulph, Smallthorne and Butt Lane, Staffordshire. After John Clewlow was made a partner in 1970 the business was renamed Sims & Partners. In 1994, following Sims' retirement, the practice was renamed Charter Veterinary Surgeons, in recognition of the 150th anniversary of the granting of the charter to the Royal College of Veterinary Surgeons.

J Clewlow, 'The Mayers of Newcastle under Lyme and their Place in the Emerging Veterinary Profession', *Veterinary History*, New Series, vol 9, no 1, 1996; J Clewlow, 'The Mayers of Newcastle under Lyme: Their Contribution to the Emerging Veterinary Profession' (MPhil, Keele, 1995).

Records: in private ownership of Mr J Clewlow, Ferndale, 5 Grange Road, Biddulph, Stoke on Trent ST8 7SB

Account rendered by Thomas Mayer 1811; press cuttings, architectural drawings and photographs re renovation of Newcastle under Lyme veterinary surgery and house 1982–83; correspondence re history of Newcastle under Lyme house and buildings 1983–84; history of Mayer family, nd.

M K CHRISTIAN MRCVS
Kelsall, Cheshire

History: This small animal and equine practice was established in 1979 by M K Christian.

Records: M K Christian MRCVS, The Firs, Dog Lane, Kelsall CW6 0RP

Balance sheets 1979–; ledgers 1979–; day books 1979–; cash books 1979–; general accounts 1979–; receipts 1979–; invoices 1979–; client record cards 1979–; architectural plans for a new surgical unit 1986.

CLAREMONT VETERINARY GROUP
Bexhill on Sea, East Sussex

History: This small animal practice was established by Stephen White in 1979.

Records: Claremont Veterinary Group, 44 Sidley Street, Bexhill on Sea TN39 5BQ

Balance sheets/profit and loss accounts 1979–; client records 1979–; photographs 1979–; architectural plans 1979–.

CLARENDON STREET VETERINARY PRACTICE
Cambridge, Cambridgeshire

History: This small animal practice, established in 1955 by a Mr Flemming, was sold to Clive Jordan in 1970.

Records: Clarendon Street Veterinary Practice, 28 Clarendon Street, Cambridge CB1 1JX

Balance sheets 1970–; ledgers 1993–; day books 1993–; cash books 1993–; general accounts 1993–; receipts 1993–; invoices 1993–; architectural plans, nd.

CLARK & SCOTT MsRCVS
Gateshead, Tyne & Wear

History: This practice was established in 1963 by H M Clark. Colin Mills became a partner in 1968, followed by W R Clark in 1980. H M Clark retired in 1984 while Dr A Henfrey joined the partnership in 1995. Originally a mixed practice, it became exclusively small animal in 1981. Hospital status was awarded in 1971 and branch surgeries established at Whickham in 1973 and Washington in 1981.

Records: Clark & Scott MsRCVS, Sheriffs Highway Veterinary Hospital, 94 Sheriff's Highway, Gateshead NE9 5SD

Partnership agreements 1963–; balance sheets/profit and loss accounts 1976–; day books 1992–; ledgers 1973–; cash books 1973–; client records 1992–; architectural plans 1963–.

CLARKE & HAMILTON MsRCVS
St Helier, Jersey

History: This small animal practice was established in 1973 by J H W Clarke and Mrs A Hamilton.

Records: Clarke & Hamilton MsRCVS, Veterinary Surgery, 19 Oxford Road, St Helier JE2 4LJ

Day books 1973–; cash books 1973–; client records 1973–; architectural plans 1973–.

CLAYTON & COX MsRCVS
Newent, Gloucestershire

History: This practice is believed to date back to the early nineteenth century. In 1900 it was bought by William James Boyd, who had graduated from the Royal Veterinary College, London, a short time before. Boyd based his practice first at Hillfields, Kempley, before moving to Church Street, Newent, in 1931.

Records: Clayton & Cox MsRCVS, Millpark Veterinary Centre, Newent GL18 1AZ

Partnership agreement 1981; balance sheets 1974–; ledger 1946; day books 1970–; cash books, general accounts, invoices, client records, prescription books, architectural plans, photographs 20th cent.

CLIFTON LODGE VETERINARY GROUP
Hartlepool

History: This mixed practice was established in the 1950s.

Records: Clifton Lodge Veterinary Group, 24 Stockton Road, Hartlepool TS25 1RL

Partnership agreements 1983; minutes 1983– [w]; balance sheets/profit and loss accounts 1983–; day books 1983–; ledgers 1983–; cash books 1983–; client records 1960s–; x-rays 1983–; architectural plans 1985–.

CLINIGAU CEFFYLAU FYRNWY EQUINE CLINICS '93
Llanymynech, Powys

History: This equine practice has grown steadily since its establishment by Rh ap Rh Owen in 1978. By 1999 there were six veterinary surgeons based at the practice.

Records: Clinigau Ceffylau Fyrnwy Equine Clinics '93, Llanymynech SY22 6LG

Partnership agreement 1993; balance sheets 1978–; ledgers 1978–; day books 1978–; general accounts 1978–; receipts 1978–; invoices 1978–; client records 1978–; salary books 1978–; photographs 1978–; general correspondence re practice 1978–.

COCKBURN VETERINARY GROUP
Coalville, Leicestershire

History: This mixed practice was established in 1918.

Records: Cockburn Veterinary Group, 100 London Road, Coalville LE67 3JD

Partnership agreements 1966–; balance sheets/profit and loss accounts 1968–; ledgers 1970–; cash books 1990–; recipes 1960s; architectural plans 1972–.

THOMAS A COE
Bury St Edmunds, Suffolk

History: Thomas A Coe may have worked for a time with Walter Brown Coe [his father?], a veterinary surgeon based at 107 Rigsbygate Street, Bury St Edmunds. By 1922 Thomas was a partner in Coe & Hudson, veterinary surgeons and canine specialists, and by 1941 the practice was trading as Thomas A Coe, Canine Surgery.

Records: Suffolk Record Office, Bury St Edmunds Branch, 77 Raingate Street, Bury St Edmunds IP33 2AR

Day books 1919–50; account books 1922–51; correspondence, insurance documents, photographs, dog show catalogues and other printed material, misc papers 20th cent. [Ref: HC 554]

WALTER BROWN COE
Bury St Edmunds, Suffolk

History: Walter Brown Coe (c1848–1921) qualified from the Royal Veterinary College, London, in 1868 and was known to be working in Bury St Edmunds from c1875, probably alongside Walter Coe [his father?], himself an Royal Veterinary College, London, graduate in 1836.

Records: Suffolk Record Office, Bury St Edmunds Branch, 77 Raingate Street, Bury St Edmunds IP33 2AR

Ledgers 1890–1908; day books 1913–14, 1917–19; letterbooks 1912–15; zoology notebook, Royal Veterinary College, London, nd; zoology rough notebook, nd; book re Thorpe Morieux Hall 1843–1914. [Ref: HC 514]

J H C COLDICOTT MRCVS
Tewkesbury, Gloucestershire

History: This mixed practice was established in 1974.

Records: J H C Coldicott MRCVS, 55 Barton Street, Tewkesbury GL20 5PX

Balance sheets/profit and loss accounts 1974–; ledgers 1974–; client records 1974–.

COLEBROOK VETERINARY SURGERY
Solihull, West Midlands

History: This small animal practice was established in 1985 by Dr J H Marston.

Records: Colebrook Veterinary Surgery, 61 Colebrook Road, Shirley, Solihull B90 2JZ

Balance sheets/profit and loss accounts 1986–; day books 1985–; client records 1985–; x-ray records 1985–; scientific data re early years of embryo transfers in primates, nd; safety records re University of Birmingham outbreak of smallpox 1978.

F COLEMAN MRCVS
Orby, Lincolnshire

History: This small animal practice was established in 1984 by a retired veterinary surgeon from Skegness, Mr Kortien, who worked from his home in Sausthorpe, Lincolnshire, until his sudden death later that same year. The practice was then acquired by Robert Greenwell and Sheila Cunningham and moved to Orby, Lincolnshire, before being sold to F Coleman in 1986.

Records: F Coleman MRCVS, Ranby House, Marsh Road, Orby, Skegness PE24 5HY

Balance sheets/profit and loss accounts 1986–; day books 1986–; ledgers 1986–; cash books 1986–; client records 1986–; architectural plans 1993.

COLES & COLES MsRCVS
Hay on Wye, Powys

History: This mixed practice was established in c1948 by A L Hughes and run from his home in Cusop, Herefordshire. It was acquired by D J G Coles and R M Coles in 1984 and, with the exception of part of the equine practice, moved to new premises in Hay on Wye shortly afterwards.

Records: Coles & Coles MsRCVS, Lamb House, 17 Newport Street, Hay on Wye HR3 5BG

Balance sheets/profit and loss accounts 1984–; day books 1984–; client records 1987–.

COMPANION VETERINARY CLINIC
Newark on Trent, Nottinghamshire

History: This small animal practice was established in 1982 as a branch surgery to the Broughton Veterinary Centre, Brant Broughton,

Nottinghamshire. It was sold to P S Dowie in 1989 and renamed the Companion Veterinary Clinic.

Records: Companion Veterinary Clinic, 9 Bullpit Road, Balderton, Newark on Trent NG24 3PT

Balance sheets/profit and loss accounts 1989–; day books 1989–; architectural plans re structural changes 1992–95.

COOMARA VETERINARY PRACTICE

Carlisle, Cumbria

History: This practice was established in 1964 by Mark Wharton. In 1971 Wharton entered into a partnership with Mr Earp. Following Wharton's retirement in 1989, a new partnership was formed between Earp and Graham Brooks.

Records: Coomara Veterinary Practice, Coomara, Carleton, Carlisle CA4 0BU

Partnership agreement 1989; practice minute book 1989–; balance sheets 1989–; farm animal ledger 1980–98: client records c1985–; press cuttings 1990s.

P R COOPER MRCVS

Hastings, East Sussex

History: This mixed practice was established in 1979. A branch surgery was opened at 309 The Ridge, Hastings, in 1982.

Records: P R Cooper MRCVS, 5 Victoria Avenue, Ore, Hastings TN35 5BY

Balance sheets/profit and loss accounts 1979–; ledgers 1979– [w]; cash books 1979–; client records 1979– [w]; architectural plans 1983–.

COOPER, JINMAN & PARTNERS
Hereford, Herefordshire

History: This practice is believed to date back to the nineteenth century. From the 1950s it was based in Victoria Street, Hereford, before moving to Ryeland Street in 1979.

Records: Cooper, Jinman & Partners, The Laurels Veterinary Centre, 4 Ryeland Street, Hereford HR4 0LA

Partnership agreements 1950–; balance sheets 1950–; day books 1950–; recipe books 1900s; prescription books 1900s; promotional material 1980–.

COPTHORNE VETERINARY CENTRE
Shrewsbury, Shropshire

History: This small animal practice was established in 1980.

Records: Copthorne Veterinary Centre, 114 Copthorne Road, Shrewsbury SY3 8NA

Balance sheets/profit and loss accounts 1980–; ledgers 1980–; cash books 1980–; architectural plans 1980s–.

COUTTS & SHACKLETON MsRCVS
Biggleswade, Bedfordshire

History: This small animal practice was established in 1967.

Records: Coutts & Shackleton MsRCVS, Veterinary Surgery, 15 Shortmead Street, Biggleswade SG18 0AT

Partnership agreements 1967–; minutes 1967–; ledgers 1967–; cash books 1987–; client records 1967–; photographs 1997–; architectural plans 1967–.

M G COWGILL & S J PEMBLE MsRCVS
Lytham, Lancashire

History: This mixed practice was established by J R Rigby in 1908. Rigby studied at the New Veterinary College, Edinburgh, and at Liverpool, qualifying in 1907. He remained at the practice until selling out to Roger B Hornby in 1949. Hornby in turn sold the practice to B D W Hardy in 1965. A J Smith and M G Cowgill acquired the practice, based by this time at 2 Albert Street, Lytham, in 1970.

Records: Department of Special Collections and Archives, Sydney Jones Library, University of Liverpool, PO Box 123, Liverpool L69 3DA

Practice diary 1909; day book 1909–22; case book 1935–48; student notebooks: Rigby early 1900s, D Jenkins Thomas 1900, A B Howe early 20th cent, unidentified student early 20th cent; diplomas 1907, nd; MRCVS certificate 1907; veterinary instrument catalogues and associated publications from Arnold & Sons, etc 1885–1951, nd. [Ref: D. 492]

ROBERT J CRANE MRCVS
Heavitree, Devon

History: This small animal practice was established by Robert J Crane in 1989.

Records: Robert J Crane MRCVS, The Veterinary Surgery, 64–66 Fore Street, Heavitree, Exeter EX1 2RR

Balance sheets/profit and loss accounts 1989–; day books 1989–; ledgers 1989–; cash books 1989–; client records 1989–; architectural plans 1990s; practice magazines/leaflets 1989–.

CRANMORE VETERINARY CENTRE
Childer Thornton, Cheshire

History: This practice was established in a former coaching house at 104 Chester Road, Childer Thornton, by Neil McKechnie Barron. A native of Turriff, Aberdeenshire, Barron (c1841–1903) graduated from the Edinburgh Veterinary College in 1873 and came to Childer Thornton in c1876, where, in addition to his practice he also acted as Local Veterinary Inspector for the Wirral Division of Chester County. After his death the practice passed to his son, William Knight Barron (1876–1957), who had graduated from Edinburgh earlier that year. William Knight Barron continued to run the practice until the outbreak of war in 1914 when he left to join the Army Veterinary Corps. After the war ended, he failed to return to Cheshire, choosing instead to practise in Haverfordwest, Pembrokeshire, at that time an important centre for heavy horse breeding. The practice in Childer Thornton was sold to Edmund Francis Wood in 1920, and sold again in 1950 to Cecil Twizell. Twizell was succeeded by Coles & Lowe in 1978, who in turn sold out to G C Skerritt in 1994. Although originally an agricultural practice, by 1978 it had become exclusively small animal and referral, specialising in neurology and avian medicine. A branch surgery, Church Farm Veterinary Clinic, was established at Neston Road, Willaston, in 1993.

Records: Cranmore Veterinary Centre, 140 Chester Road, Childer Thornton CH66 1QN

Architectural plans re refurbishment of practice 20th cent; photographs of building c1910.

CRESCENT VETERINARY CENTRE
Tewkesbury, Gloucestershire

History: This mixed practice was established in 1990.

Records: Crescent Veterinary Centre, 31 Church Street, Tewkesbury GL20 5PD

Balance sheets/profit and loss accounts 1990–; day books 1990–; ledgers 1990–; cash books 1990–; client records 1990–; photographs 1990–; architectural plans 1990–.

CROFT HOUSE VETERINARY CLINIC
Batley, West Yorkshire

History: Mrs C M Oakes joined this small animal practice in 1988 and became the sole owner in 1991.

Records: Croft House Veterinary Clinic, 378 Soothill Lane, Batley WF17 6EU

Day books 1988–; cash books 1988–; client records 1988–.

CROMLYN HOUSE VETERINARY CLINIC
Hillsborough, Co Down

History: This equine and small animal practice was established in 1984 by C J Heffron and L E Heffron.

Records: Cromlyn House Veterinary Clinic, 2 Main Street, Hillsborough BT26 6AE

Balance sheets/profit and loss accounts 1984–; ledgers 1984–; cash books 1984–; client records 1984–; architectural plans 1984–.

J R F CROUCH MRCVS
Leigh, Dorset

History: This equine practice was established in 1987.

Records: J R F Crouch MRCVS, Willow Tree Farm, Leigh DT9 6HJ

Balance sheets/profit and loss accounts 1993–; day books 1994–; ledgers 1994–; cash books 1993–; receipts 1965–; photographs 1989.

DAVID CUFFE & ASSOCIATES
London

History: This mixed practice was established by David Cuffe in 1990.

Records: David Cuffe & Associates, 348 South Lambeth Road, Stockwell, London SW8 1UQ

Balance sheets/profit and loss accounts 1990–; day books 1990–; accounts 1990–; architectural plans 1990s; practice magazines/leaflets 1990s.

DACRE HOUSE VETERINARY CLINIC
Tunbridge Wells, Kent

History: This small animal practice was established in 1986.

Records: Dacre House Veterinary Clinic, 91 Powdermill Lane, Southborough, Tunbridge Wells TN4 9ED

Balance sheets/profit and loss accounts 1986–; day books 1986–; ledgers 1986–; cash books 1986–; client records 1986–; architectural plans 1986–.

PETER DALTON'S GAME CONSULTANCY
Salisbury, Wiltshire

History: This practice, specialising in the care of game birds, was established in 1982.

Records: in private ownership of John Robert Dalton, 32 Gravel Close, Downton, Salisbury SP5 3JQ

Balance sheets/profit and loss accounts 1986–; day books 1982–; photographs 1982–; day books re Salisbury Poultry Laboratories Ltd 1968–72.

DAMSON HOUSE VETERINARY CLINIC
Solihull, West Midlands

History: This small animal practice was established in 1989 by David More and acquired by Heidi and Ian Strong in 1990.

Records: Damson House Veterinary Clinic, 82 Damson Lane, Solihull B92 9JP

Balance sheets/profit and loss accounts 1990–; day books 1990–; ledgers 1990–; client records 1990–.

DARLEY HOUSE VETERINARY SURGERY
Farnworth, Greater Manchester

History: This small animal practice was established in 1963.

Records: Darley House Veterinary Surgery, 19–25 Peel Street, Farnworth, Bolton BL4 8AA

Day book 1970; cash book 1970; mortgage deeds 1852–.

DAVEY & DAVEY MsRCVS
Whittlesford, Cambridgeshire

History: This practice was established in 1983 by Paul W Davey. C A Davey joined in 1985 and by 1999 there were four veterinary surgeons at the practice, seeing mainly small animals.

Records: Davey & Davey MsRCVS, The Veterinary Surgery, 39 Station Road, Whittlesford CB2 4NL

Partnership agreement 1985; balance sheets/profit and loss accounts 1983–; day books 1983–; ledgers 1983–; cash books 1983–; client records 1983–.

DAVIES, JOHNSON & STALEY MsRCVS
Woodplumpton, Lancashire

History: This mixed practice was established in 1932.

Records: Davies, Johnson & Staley MsRCVS, The Veterinary Surgery, Woodplumpton Road, Woodplumpton, Preston PR4 0TA

Partnership agreements 1978–; balance sheets/profit and loss accounts 1980–; day books 1971–; ledgers 1971–; cash books 1971–; client records 1985–; photographs 1978–; architectural plans 1970–80; practice magazines/leaflets 1980–.

DAVIES & ROUTLEDGE MsRCVS
Royston, Hertfordshire

History: This mixed practice was established in Newmarket Road, Royston, in 1939, since when there have been just three partners: Ronald Percival Webber, J C Davies and J K Routledge.

Records: Davies & Routledge MsRCVS, Coed-y-Brain, Valley Rise, Newmarket Road, Royston SG8 7HD

Ledger 1939–40.

DAVISON VETERINARY SURGEONS
Nottingham, Nottinghamshire

History: This mixed practice was established at 63–65 Ilkeston Road, Nottingham, in 1933 by Lindsay Alexander Auchtolonie, a graduate in 1911 from the Royal (Dick) Veterinary College, Edinburgh. After the practice was sold to F L Davison in 1947 there were a number of different partnerships, including Davison & Denholm, Davison & Taylor, F L & J L Davison, J L & J E B Davison, J C & J E B Davison & W Butler, J L & J E B Davison. Additional branches have been established at 81 South Road, West Bridgford, Nottingham, and at 101 Nottingham Road, Keyworth, Nottingham.

Records: Nottinghamshire Archives, County House, Castle Meadow Road, Nottingham NG2 1AG

Treatment books and financial records 1935–91. [Ref: Acc 5876]

DERW VETERINARY SURGEONS
Builth Wells, Powys

History: This mixed practice was established in c1950 by J N M Hills. W A Jones became a partner in 1957, after which the practice traded as Hills & Jones. C J M Hills, the son of J N M Hills, joined the partnership in c1976. Following the retirement of Hills senior in 1983, D J England was made a partner and the practice became known as Hills, Jones & England. Hills left in 1986 and the practice then traded as Jones & England until Jones' retirement in 1996, after which England became the sole owner. It was at this time that the practice's name was changed to Derw Veterinary Surgeons.

Records: Derw Veterinary Surgeons, Garth Road, Builth Wells LD2 3NL

Balance sheets/profit and loss accounts 1980–; day books 1982–; ledgers 1955–; client records 1982–; architectural plans 1950s.

T A DOLLAR & SONS
London

History: Thomas Aitken Dollar (1833–1909) studied at the Edinburgh Veterinary College and was awarded the Highland and Agricultural Society's certificate in 1851. He then worked as an assistant to Cuthbert Simpson in Manchester before moving to London to set up his own equine practice at 56 New Bond Street. The practice flourished, so much so that by the time Dollar died in 1909 it was considered to be one of the largest in London. Dollar himself, though, still found time to be involved in the wider issues surrounding veterinary medicine. He was an examiner for the Highland and Agricultural Society's certificate and did much to persuade the Royal College of Veterinary Surgeons to recognise the qualification. In 1880 he served as Vice President of the Royal College of Veterinary Surgeons. Some time after 1861, Dollar was joined by his brother, Peter Salmon Dollar (1836–1912), but after only a brief stay Peter Dollar left to take up an appointment as Chief Veterinary Surgeon at East & Co. During the 1880s, Thomas Dollar's two sons, William Watt Dollar (1860–1938) and John Archibald Watt Dollar (1866–1947), entered the practice which was renamed T A Dollar & Sons. During the 1890s, the stables and surgery at 56 New Bond Street were extensively rebuilt. John Archibald Watt Dollar spent much time travelling abroad and took every opportunity to visit veterinary colleges. He was credited with introducing the first equine operating table, designed by himself, to Britain. Between 1897 and 1899 he served as President of the Central Veterinary Society, representing the Royal College of Veterinary Surgeons at various international conferences. Additionally, he was Warden of the Worshipful Company of Farriers from 1900 to 1903 and President of the Royal College of Veterinary Surgeons in 1904–05. He and his brother continued to work together at their practice, which moved to Baker Street in 1919, until their retirement in 1926, at which time the practice was sold to a Mr Tay.

Records (1): in private ownership of Mrs J Dollar, 53 St Ann Place, Salisbury SP1 2SU

Mortgage indenture for 56 New Bond Street 1881; architectural plan of 56 New Bond Street and veterinary surgery (p) c1888; Corporation of City of London city lands committee, certificate of approval for rebuilding stabling and premises at 56 New Bond Street 1889; John Mowlem & Co, builders: agreement 1890, estimate for building works 1891, receipts for payment received from T A Dollar 1890–91, correspondence re dispute 1891; Musgrave & Co Ltd, receipts for fittings supplied 1890; letters from Robert Walker, architect and surveyor, to T A Dollar re formal approval of building plans 1891; John Archibald Watt Dollar: bound memoirs 1866–1948, photograph as President of Royal College of Veterinary Surgeons c1904–05, obituaries 1947–48, chronology of life compiled by his son A T J Dollar, nd, booklet, *A Surgical Operating Table for the Horse*, providing details of his invention 1900; Thomas Aitken Dollar: inaugural address to Royal (Dick) Veterinary College 1894, photograph as Upper Warden of Worshipful Company of Farriers c1903, obituary (p) 1909; Peter Salmon Dollar, obituary (p) 1916; William Watt Dollar: albums of family photographs c1920s–30s, obituaries 1938; *Dollar's Veterinary Surgery* and other publications, nd; photographs of 56 New Bond Street, nd.

Records (2): Edinburgh Room, Edinburgh Central Library, George IV Bridge, Edinburgh EH1 1EG

Thomas Aitken Dollar, inaugural address to Royal (Dick) Veterinary College 1894. [Ref: YSF 779]

R A DONCASTER MRCVS

Ipswich, Suffolk

History: This practice was established by M B Lingwood at 27 St Helens Street, Ipswich, in 1966, before moving to 49 Christchurch Street in 1972. After Lingwood's death in 1980 the practice was acquired by R A Doncaster.

Records: R A Doncaster MRCVS, 49 Christchurch Street, Ipswich IP4 2DF

Balance sheets/profit and loss accounts 1963–; day books 1963–; ledgers 1963–; cash books 1963–; receipts 1963–; client records 1963–; architectural plans 1963–.

RAOUL DOWDING

Gainsborough, Lincolnshire

History: This practice was established in 1924 by Rowland Swaby. In addition to his regular duties, Swaby was for over sixty years the veterinary attendant at the Lincolnshire County Show. The practice was sold to James Hart in 1965, but sold again only three years later, to James Harte. Harte in turn sold the practice to Daniel Bardsley in 1984. In 1999 the practice was acquired by Raoul Dowding.

Records: Raoul Dowding, 8 Morton Terrace, Gainsborough DN21 2RF

Balance sheets 1984–; ledgers 1984–; day books 1984–.

DRYFE VETERINARY GROUP
Lockerbie, Dumfries & Galloway

History: This mixed practice was established during the 1930s. Partners have included Pearson & Findlay until the 1960s, D S Roger from the 1960s to 1989, D R Fountain from 1982 and G A Veitch from 1991.

Records: Dryfe Veterinary Group, 34 Townhead Street, Lockerbie DG11 2AE

Day books 1978–; ledgers 1989– [w]; client records 1986–.

DUNLUCE VETERINARY CLINIC
Bushmills, Co Antrim

History: This single-handed mixed practice was established in 1985.

Records: Dunluce Veterinary Clinic, 53 Ballytober Road, Bushmills BT57 8UU
Day books 1985–; ledgers 1985–; cash books 1985–; client records 1985–; practice magazines/leaflets 1985.

J DUNTON MRCVS
Fordingbridge, Hampshire

History: This practice was established in 1985 by J Dunton.

Records: J Dunton MRCVS, The Beeches, Fordingbridge Road, Alderholt, Fordingbridge SP6 3BE

Balance sheets/profit and loss accounts 1985–; day books 1985–; ledgers 1985–; cash books 1985–.

DURTNELL VETERINARY CENTRE

Leeds, West Yorkshire

History: This small animal practice was established in 1978 by Richard Durtnell.

Records: Durtnell Veterinary Centre, 260–262 Tong Road, Armley, Leeds LS12 3BG

Balance sheets 1988–; cash books 1988–; land registry documents (copies) 1979–80, 1988, 1993; client records 1994–; salary books 1988–.

EARLSWOOD VETERINARY HOSPITAL

Belfast, Co Down

History: This practice was established at 56–58 Chichester Street, Belfast, in 1890 by Samuel R Thompson. Thompson was later joined by his two sons, Jim (1921) and Alex (1926). Although originally a heavy horse and livestock practice, Alex Thompson built up the small animal caseload while Jim significantly extended the thoroughbred and leisure horse side of the practice. Jim's son Desmond joined the practice in 1961 and in 1967 the practice moved to 193 Belmont Road, Belfast. Hospital status was granted in 1970, after which time the practice traded as the Earlswood Veterinary Hospital. A new partner, Ian Miller, joined in 1976. The practice has been exclusively small animal from 1985.

Records: Earlswood Veterinary Hospital, 193 Belmont Road, Belfast BT4 2AE

Partnership agreement 1976.

EDWARDS & GLAS MsRCVS

Langport, Somerset

History: This mixed practice was established in 1940 at North Street, Langport, and moved to Bow Street in 1975.

Records: Edwards & Glas MsRCVS, Regency House, Bow Street, Langport TA10 9PS

Day books 1940–; ledgers 1940–; receipts 1940–.

STEPHEN P ELWOOD
Boston, Lincolnshire

History: This practice was established by David Eckford in 1974. After a period of partnership, Stephen Elwood took over in 1991. Although the practice is mainly small animal, Elwood has a special interest in orthopaedics and cases are frequently referred from other practices in the area. By 2000 there were four veterinary surgeons and eight support staff based at the practice.

Records: Stephen P Elwood MRCVS, 36 Boston Road, Kirton, Boston PE20 1DS

Partnership agreements 1991; day books 1974–; ledgers 1990–; cash books 1990–; client records 1974–; architectural plans 1989; diaries 1974– [w].

EQUIPET VETERINARY CENTRE AND HOSPITAL
Kirkcaldy, Fife

History: This small animal practice was acquired in 1990 by Miss R I Denton and R W Gray.

Records: Equipet Veterinary Centre and Hospital, 24 Nicol Street, Kirkcaldy KY1 1NY

Balance sheets/profit and loss accounts 1990–; cash books 1990–; receipts 1990–; client records 1980s–.

C C EVANS MRCVS
Fort William, Highland

History: This practice was established in 1947.

Records: C C Evans MRCVS, Callart Cottage, Victoria Road, Fort William PH33 6BJ

Balance sheets/profit and loss accounts 1947–; day books 1947–; ledgers 1947–; cash books 1947–; client records 1947–; architectural plans 20th cent; practice magazines/leaflets 20th cent.

EWING & GIDLOW MsRCVS
Wooler, Northumberland

History: This cattle and sheep practice was run for many years at Strathmore, 18 Ryecroft Way, Wooler, by William Malcolm Lyons, a graduate of the New Veterinary College, Edinburgh. Initially based in Ayrshire, Lyons came to Wooler in 1886 or 1887, possibly to take over from John Carr (graduated New Veterinary College, Edinburgh, 1879) who died in 1887. Lyons' nephew, Hugh Bain, who graduated from the Royal (Dick) Veterinary College, Edinburgh, in 1927, came to Wooler in 1931 or 1932 and is thought to have taken over the practice around the time of his uncle's death in 1933. In 1955, Bain entered into partnership with Thomas J Dunn and their practice traded as Bain & Dunn until John Ewing joined the partnership in 1970, after which the practice briefly traded as Bain, Dunn & Ewing before changing to Dunn & Ewing in 1971. A new partnership formed in 1987 between Ewing and Stephen K Lomax traded as Ewing & Lomax until they were joined by Mrs J R Gidlow in 1994, after which the practice was known as Ewing, Lomax & Gidlow until 1996 when it became Ewing & Gidlow.

Records: Ewing & Gidlow MsRCVS, The Veterinary Surgery, 29 Ryecroft Way, Wooler NE71 6DY

Partnership agreements 1987–; balance sheets/profit and loss accounts 1969–; day books 1987–; cash books 1987–; recipes 1919–28.

EXETER STREET VETERINARY SURGERY
Salisbury, Wiltshire

History: This single-handed small animal practice was established in 1982 by T N St John.

Records: Exeter Street Veterinary Surgery, 123 Exeter Street, Salisbury SP1 2SG

Balance sheets/profit and loss accounts 1982–; day books 1982–; client records 1982–; photographs 1982–.

FERGUSON & BONNIWELL MsRCVS
Oban, Argyll & Bute

History: This practice is believed to have been established by John MacDougal (1854–1947) who qualified from the Glasgow Veterinary College in 1879 and arrived in Oban that same year. Following his retirement in 1936 the practice was bought by Dugall Sinclair Brown (b 1898), a graduate in 1924 from the Glasgow Veterinary College. In 1957 Brown sold the practice to Donald A Bremner. Bremner entered into partnership with H K MacLachlan in c1960, then with Donald A Ferguson in 1973, the latter of which was dissolved in 1982. In 1986 Ferguson formed a new partnership with Max A Bonniwell. The practice was originally agricultural but has evolved into a mixed practice. There have been about three changes in address, the most recent of which was in 1976.

Records: Ferguson & Bonniwell MsRCVS, The Veterinary Surgery, 14 Tweedale Street, Oban PA34 5DD

Partnership agreement 1973; balance sheets/profit and loss accounts 1973–; day books 1971–; client records 1982–.

FIRS VETERINARY SURGERY
Bath, Bath & North East Somerset

History: This small animal and equine practice was established in 1972.

Records: Firs Veterinary Surgery, 21 The Firs, Combe Down, Bath BA2 5ED

Balance sheets/profit and loss accounts 1972–; day books 1972–; ledgers 1972–; cash books 1972–; client records 1980–; photographs 1970s–; practice magazines/leaflets 1970s–.

FIRTH VETERINARY CENTRE
Annan, Dumfries & Galloway

History: Alfred James Milligan (c1869–1943) graduated from the Glasgow Veterinary College in 1890 and is believed to have set up this mixed practice at 5 Ednam Street, Annan, in 1920. In 1939 he entered into partnership with a Mr Hector. Hector continued the practice after

Milligan's death in 1943 and in 1949 formed a new partnership with a Mr Burns. J W Gilliland became a partner in 1975, G A Baxter in 1986 and P Armstrong in 1991.

Records: Firth Veterinary Centre, 3–5 Ednam Street, Annan DG12 6EF

Partnership agreements 1978–; balance sheets/profit and loss accounts 1978–; ledgers 1978–; cash books 1978–; client records 1978–.

W J FORD & SONS
Mildenhall, Suffolk

History: W J Ford & Sons are listed as blacksmiths at West Row, Mildenhall, in mid to late nineteenth century directories.

Records: Suffolk Record Office, Bury St Edmunds Branch, 77 Raingate Street, Bury St Edmunds IP33 2AR

Account books, rough day books 1891–1987; detailed account books recording payments for work carried out incl entries for attending to sick animals c1917–39; misc papers 18th–20th cent. [Ref: HC 556]

FOREST HOUSE VETERINARY GROUP
Windsor, Windsor & Maidenhead

History: The origins of the Forest House Veterinary Group can be traced back to two nineteenth century practices. Henry Allnutt (1828–1904), a native of High Wycombe, Buckinghamshire, qualified from the Royal Veterinary College, London, in 1855 and set up his practice in Thames Street, Windsor, in 1862. That same year he was appointed surgeon in charge of the stables at the Royal Gardens and later assumed control of the equine establishments at the Royal Farms and Dairy. In 1875 Allnutt was appointed veterinary surgeon to Queen Victoria at Windsor Castle. Robert Craig Tennant (c1865–1936) qualified from the Royal Veterinary College, London, in 1888 and joined Allnutt the following year. Following Allnutt's retirement in 1899, Tennant took over both the practice and the royal appointments. Meanwhile, another practice had been established at Gordon House, Peascod Street, Windsor, by George Simpson (b c1812). Like Allnutt and Tennant, Simpson was a landowner of some substance as well as a veterinary surgeon. His son, Henry Lunnon Simpson (1842–1900), was made a partner in 1861. Henry Simpson took an active role in the running of the Royal College of Veterinary Surgeons, serving on the Council between 1882 and 1890. He was elected Vice President in 1881 and President in 1887. Also in 1887, Henry Simpson was elected Mayor of Windsor and given the arduous task of overseeing the town's celebrations to mark Queen Victoria's Golden Jubilee. His efforts earned him a knighthood. His son, Henry G Simpson, joined him in the practice after graduating from Glasgow Veterinary College in 1896. The two practices were eventually combined in 1906 when Henry G Simpson sold out to Tennant. In 1913 Tennant moved the entire practice to William Street. After his retirement in 1935, the practice was taken over by Edmond Paterson who stayed until 1954. Edmund Bowditch joined in 1947, retiring in 1978. Philip Ayrton Grime came to the practice in 1950 and remained until his retirement in 1992. Two further veterinary surgeons were taken into partnership in 1962; John Taylor, who emigrated to Canada in 1966, and Ian Guthrie, who bought out the Slough branch (est 1964) in 1973. Anthony Hilbery joined the practice in 1968, Jeremy Ridgway in 1978 and Martin Watson in 1990. All later went on to become partners. In 1973 the practice moved to Clewer Hill Road, Windsor. Two branch practices were established at Egham, Surrey, in c1964 and Ascot in c1985. Over the years the practice has enjoyed a varied clientele. In common with many practices, there was until the early 1950s a forge attached to the practice with stabling for twenty eight horses, the latter used predominately by military men based at the local garrison. Today, equine care still forms part of the practice's activities. Veterinary services are provided at the Royal Windsor and Ascot racecourses and a representative from the practice has sat on the committee of the Royal Windsor Horse Show since its foundation as a war-time fundraiser in 1943. Veterinary services were also provided at Slough (1950–85) and Reading (1950–65) Greyhound Stadiums. In addition, the practice was involved in the treatment of animals at Windsor Safari Park from 1973 until its closure in c1994 and at the two circuses that wintered in the area each year.

Records (1): Forest House Veterinary Group, 28 Clewer Hill Road, Windsor SL4 4BS

Accounts ledgers 1943–46, 1960–65; Robert Craig Tennant's private account book 1917–21.

Records (2): in private ownership of Mr Philip Ayrton Grime, Woodland Manor, St Leonards Hill, Windsor SL4 4AT

Partnership agreement between Henry Allnutt and Robert Craig Tennant 1899; proposed terms of partnership between E S Paterson and [-], nd; profit and loss sheets for Bell Farm, belonging to Robert Craig Tennant 1901–13, 1918, 1921–32; profit and loss sheets for the Thames Street practice 1901–13, 1918, 1921–32, 1936–38, 1941; inventory of veterinary surgery and farrier's stable occasioned by the sale of the practice from Simpson to Tennant 1906; misc price lists, advertisements, catalogues for drugs and equipment 1930s; occasional letters re practice 1930s, 1960s; plan for small animal surgery c1952.

FOREST VETERINARY CENTRE
Nottingham, Nottinghamshire

History: This practice was established in 1963 by Andrew Kettles and traded for many years under his name before changing to Kettles & Crowther. After Kettle's retirement the practice became known as the Forest Veterinary Centre. Originally a mixed practice, it is now entirely small animal.

Records: Forest Veterinary Centre, 12 Gregory Boulevard, Hyson Green, Nottingham NG7 6BG

Partnership agreements, nd; balance sheets/profit and loss accounts 1963–; ledgers 1963–; cash books 1963–; receipts 1963–; photographs 1963–; architectural plans 1963–.

FOREST VETERINARY CLINIC
Mansfield, Nottinghamshire

History: This practice dates back to the nineteenth century, although popular myth has it that the original building was constructed in 1792 for a farrier.

Records: Forest Veterinary Clinic, 5 Terrace Road, Mansfield NG18 2BP

Papers re transfer of ownership 1885–.

FOREST VETERINARY CLINIC
Pontypridd, Rhondda Cynon Taff

History: This small animal practice was established in 1983 by G W Marshall.

Records: Forest Veterinary Clinic, 16 River Street, Treforest, Pontypridd CF37 1TD

Partnership agreements 1983–; balance sheets/profit and loss accounts 1983–; day books 1983–; ledgers 1983–; cash books 1983–; receipts 1983–; client records 1983–; photographs 1983–; practice magazines/leaflets 1983–.

FOTHERINGHAM & PARTNERS
Strichen, Aberdeenshire

History: This practice was established in c1940.

Records: Fotheringham & Partners, Buchan House Veterinary Clinic, 19–21 High Street, Strichen AB43 4SQ

Partnership agreements c1970–; balance sheets/profit and loss accounts c1970–; day books c1970–; ledgers c1970–; cash books c1970–; client records 1985–.

FOXGROVE VETERINARY CENTRE
Beckenham, Greater London

History: This small animal practice was established in The Avenue, Beckenham, by Captain Richardson and bought by Mr Hawkin in 1968. Hawkin's first partner, Jeremy David, emigrated to Sydney, Australia, in 1976 while his second partner, Ian Graham, left in 1982. Clinton Jefferies became Hawkin's third partner in 1984 and acquired the practice in 1992.

Records: Foxgrove Veterinary Centre, 8 Foxgrove Road, Beckenham BR3 2AT

Partnership agreements 1976, 1984, 1992; balance sheets/profit and loss accounts 1976–; day books 1985–; ledgers 1979–; cash books 1979–; client records 1985–.

K J FRASER MRCVS
Abingdon, Oxfordshire

History: This small animal practice was established in 1987 by K J Fraser.

Records: K J Fraser MRCVS, 37 Caldecott Road, Abingdon OX14 5EZ

Balance sheets/profit and loss accounts 1987–; day books 1987–; cash books 1987–; client records 1987–; architectural plans 1987–.

FURNISS & MORTON MsRCVS
Weston Super Mare, Somerset

History: This mixed practice was established in 1972.

Records: Furniss & Morton MsRCVS, The Veterinary Centre, Summer Lane, Worle, Weston Super Mare BS22 6BE

Day books 1985–; client records 1980– [w].

GARDEN & GILMORE MsRCVS
Standish, Greater Manchester

History: This small animal practice was established in 1985.

Records: Garden & Gilmore MsRCVS, 52 High Street, Standish WN6 0HF

Balance sheets/profit and loss accounts 1985–; day books 1985–; ledgers 1985–; cash books 1985–; client records 1985–; architectural plans 1985–.

RONALD E GARDNER & ASSOCIATES
London

History: This practice is believed to have been established at 727 High Road, Leyton Village, in the late nineteenth century by Edward Henry Scott (c1854–1914). His son, Eustace Edward Scott, who qualified from the Royal Veterinary College, London, in 1923, later took over the practice. As well as treating horses and pets, the practice was actively involved in the export of horses and 'Spratts' dogs from the local docks. A large kennels was attached to the yard for this purpose. Sometime during the 1920s Scott was joined by Mr Leat, a veterinary practitioner. Difficulties, however, arose after Scott's death in 1964. New regulations, and the terms of the Spratts' contract, dictated that the practice could not continue without a qualified veterinary surgeon. To overcome the difficulty, Mr Provan, a veterinary surgeon in Ware, Hertfordshire, became a named partner but took no active role in the running of the practice. This arrangement continued until Leat's death in 1972 left Provan with two practices. A manager was appointed to run the Leyton practice but could not prevent it from failing the following year. In 1974 the practice was acquired by Ronald Gardner. Gardner at first intended to run the practice from his home, but was unable to get the necessary planning permission. Instead he bought an empty premises on Leyton High Road from one of his clients, George Wise of G Wise Motors.

Records: Ronald E Gardner & Associates, 655 High Road, Leyton, London E10 6RA

Ledgers 1974–; day books 1974–; cash books 1974–; general accounts 1974–; receipts 1974–; invoices 1974–; legal papers re purchase of practice 1974; advertising and promotional material c1975; press cuttings c1985; architectural plans 1970s; staff registers c1975–; salary books c1975–; pension papers c1975–; magazines c1975–; photographs 20th cent.

GARRETT & FREEMAN MsRCVS
Braintree, Essex

History: This mixed practice, established in 1982 by A B Farrow and S N Bayer, traded as Farrow & Bayer until 1987 when it became Farrow, Bayer & Garrett. Between 1995 and 1997 the practice was known as Farrow, Bayer, Garrett & Freeman, then Bayer, Garrett & Freeman from 1997 to 1998, followed by Garrett & Freeman from 1998. A branch practice was established at 35 Church Street, Coggeshall, in 1990.

Records: Garrett & Freeman MsRCVS, 64 Coggeshall Road, Braintree CM7 9BY

Partnership agreements 1988–; balance sheets/profit and loss accounts 1987–; architectural plans 1982–.

GARSTON VETERINARY GROUP

Frome, Somerset

History: Sydney James (1831–1907), graduated from the Royal Veterinary College, London, in 1853 and set up his business in North Parade, Frome, some time afterwards. In addition to his practice, James was for many years Honorary Veterinary Surgeon for the Frome Agricultural Society and a Local Veterinary Inspector under the Contagious Diseases (Animals) Acts for the Frome Division. His son, William Henry James, qualified from the Royal Veterinary College, London, in 1891 and held several assistantships before joining his father at Frome. Following his father's death in 1907, William James continued to practise until 1911 when he sold up and left for British Columbia, Canada. On 1 June 1911, following his qualification from the Royal Veterinary College, London, and with financial backing from his father, William Kingdom Stephens (d 1955) became the practice's new owner. He lived at the top of North Parade, close to his predecessor, and practised from a small lock up premises in the old Frome Market Yard before purchasing Garston House in 1919. Stephens practised single-handedly, with the help of various locums, until his two sons were able to join him. Trevor Kingdom Stephens (1915–91) graduated from the Royal Veterinary College, London, in 1937, winning both the coveted Williams memorial prize and the first Fitzwygram prize. He went on to complete a post-graduate degree before joining the practice in 1938. Arthur Douglas Stephens (b 1918) qualified in 1939 and joined the Royal Air Force in 1942, only returning to Frome at the end of the war. The two brothers then ran the practice until their retirements in 1980 and 1981. In 1954 they added an extension to improve the small animal facilities. Further expansion followed with the purchase of the adjacent property, 1 Portway, in 1966 and V C Ward's Warminster practice in 1982. By 2000 there were fourteen veterinary surgeons at Garston House, providing small animal, agricultural and equine care. Since 1965, the practice has provided veterinary services to Longleat Safari Park.

Records: Garston Veterinary Group, Garston House, Frome BA11 1PZ

Partnership agreements, agreements of service 1937–; day books 1911–12, 1935–37, 1958–62 (surgery), 1960–62 (visits); message books 1955, 1958, 1961; appointment diaries 1981–; duty rota diaries 1948, 1950, 1960, 1989–; profit and loss account 1913–14; record of weekly takings 1920–52; cash books 1936–43, 1945–63; cash receipt book 1974–84; private expenses book 1940–54; ledger c1957–62; petrol and car repairs ledger 1955–65; extracts from ledgers showing expenses, bad debts, turnover of each veterinary surgeon, etc 1938–54; wages book 1961–65; list of fees c1970s; recipe books 1918, nd; misc bottles 1930s; laboratory book 1938–39; pathology slides, nd; tuberculin testing books 1946–47; papers re tuberculin testing 1958–61; notebooks of clinical records for cow herds: Haycroft Farm, Warminster 1942, 1951, Lower West Barn Farm 1940; notebook of insurance policies taken out by various named farmers 1933; proposal form for foaling policy taken out by Wilfred Farrier, Knoll Farm, nd; deeds re Garston House c1600–; plans for various alterations and refurbishments at Garston House 20th cent; William K Stephens' visiting cards c1910–11; scrapbooks re practice c1920–60s; Trevor Stephens' student notebooks: obstetrics, parasitology, surgery III, histology 1934, 1937, nd; Arthur Stephens' student notebooks: biology I, biology/embryology I and II, animal husbandry I with feeding notes, chemistry, physics, parasitology, medicine, anatomy 1936–37, nd; certificates: William K Stephens' Royal Veterinary College, London, pathology & bacteriology 1911, Trevor Stephens MRCVS 1937, Fitzwygram prize 1937, Williams memorial prize 1937, Arthur Stephens MRCVS 1940; photographs: Royal Veterinary College, London, association football team 1907–08, Royal Veterinary College, London, v Royal Veterinary College, Ireland rugby teams 1935, Royal Veterinary College, London, rugby club 1937–38, Garston House, staff, patients, etc c1950–; Ministry of War transport notice re non-issue of vehicle licences c1940.

GIBBONS & SPRINZ MsRCVS
Thame, Oxfordshire

History: This practice was established in 1950.

Records: Gibbons & Sprinz MsRCVS, The Veterinary Hospital, 23 Wellington Street, Thame OX9 3BW

Partnership agreements 1950–; minutes 1950–; balance sheets/profit and loss accounts 1950–; day books 1950–; architectural plans 1950–; practice magazines/leaflets, nd.

D A GILLON MRCVS
Letchworth, Hertfordshire

History: This practice was established in c1956 by Esther Denham. Over the next few years Mrs Denham established a chain of practices before entering into partnership with Jim Evans, a former president of the British Small Animal Veterinary Association. The Letchworth and Stevenage practices were later bought out by Evans and John Cartwright while the rest of the group gradually split up into individual practices during the 1960s and 1970s. After Jim Evans left in 1964, John Cartwright formed a new partnership with David Green and Chris Hislop. This partnership was dissolved in 1984 and replaced in 1986 by one between Donald Gillon and Chris Hislop. Following Hislop's retirement in 1999, Donald Gillon continued to run the practice under his own name.

Records: D A Gillon MRCVS, The Veterinary Centre, Norton Way North, Letchworth SG6 1BS

Partnership agreements 1984–; balance sheets/profit and loss accounts 1984–; architectural plans 1980–.

GLEDHILL, ALLISON & PEARSON MsRCVS
Cromer and Holt, Norfolk

History: This practice was established in Cromer, Norfolk, in 1930 by Norman Pollock, before moving to West Runton, Norfolk, in c1939. Pollock ran the practice with the help of various assistants until 1959, when he entered into partnership with Kenneth Gledhill, who had arrived at the practice as an assistant the previous year. In 1960 Gledhill set up a branch in Holt while Pollock continued to practise in West Runton. Pollock sold his remaining share in the practice to Gledhill in 1963 but continued to work part time until 1966. Gledhill then ran the practice single-handedly for a time, with various temporary assistants, opening a branch in Cromer in c1967. In 1972 the Holt practice was moved to new premises. That same year, David Allison joined the practice as an assistant and set up a branch in Sheringham, Norfolk, before becoming a partner in 1974. Another branch was opened in Wells, Norfolk, in c1982 and the partnership became three-way in 1984 with the inclusion of Bridget Pearson. Gledhill retired in 1988 and in 1990 the practice was split up, Allison taking the small animal Sheringham surgery and Pearson the predominantly large animal surgery at Holt, although the latter now also caters largely for small animals.

Records: in private ownership of Mr K C Gledhill, 8 Town Close, Holt NR25 6JN

Day book 1963–71; income and expenditure accounts 1959–88.

GLENBRAE VETERINARY CLINIC
Bearsden, East Dunbartonshire

History: This mixed practice was established in 1990 by Mrs W E McGrandles.

Records: Glenbrae Veterinary Clinic, 11–12 Baljaffray Shopping Precinct, Bearsden, Glasgow G61 4RN

Balance sheets/profit and loss accounts 1990–; day books 1990–; ledgers 1990–; cash books 1990–; client records 1990–.

M A GORDON MRCVS
London

History: This practice, established by Madeleine Shepherd and her husband in 1932, was acquired by M A Gordon in 1967. An ophthalmology referral service was started in 1978 and the range of services gradually expanded to include orthopaedics, homeopathy, soft tissue surgery, dermatology, ultrasonography and dentistry.

Records: M A Gordon MRCVS, 35 Alexander Street, Bayswater, London W2 5NU

Balance sheets/profit and loss accounts 1968–; ledgers 1986–.

GRAHAMS ROAD VETERINARY CLINIC
Falkirk

History: This mixed practice was established at James Street, Falkirk, in 1919 by Captain Henry Fairburn Downie who had qualified from the Royal (Dick) Veterinary College, Edinburgh, the previous year. In 1922 Downie moved his practice to 91 Grahams Road. T B Newlands became a partner in 1946 and continued the practice following Downie's death in 1966. In 1990 Newlands retired, selling his share of the partnership to R J Scott. D G Reed became a partner in 1995. The practice moved to 53 Grahams Road in 1960.

Records: Grahams Road Veterinary Clinic, 53 Grahams Road, Falkirk FK2 7DJ

Day books 1967– [w]; ledgers 1967– [w]; cash books 1967– [w].

GRANT, NORRIE & ALMOND MsRCVS
Masham, North Yorkshire

History: This mixed practice was established in 1900.

Records: Grant, Norrie & Almond MsRCVS, Oaklands, Park Street, Masham HG4 4HN

Partnership agreements 1979; balance sheets/profit and loss accounts 1980–; day books 1980–; ledgers 1980–; cash books 1980–.

LORNA GRAY VETERINARY CENTRE
Uddingston, South Lanarkshire

History: This small animal practice was established by Lorna Gray on Main Street, Uddingston, in 1984, before moving to Bellshill Road in 1994.

Records: Lorna Gray Veterinary Centre, 80 Bellshill Road, Uddingston G71 6NR

Balance sheets/profit and loss accounts 1984–; day books 1984–; client records 1984–; architectural plans 1984–.

GRAZELY VETERINARY CENTRE
Farnborough, Hampshire

History: This small animal practice was established in 1973 by G G Beadle and initially based at 26A Guildford Road West, Farnborough, before moving to 12 Guildford Road West in 1977. Two branches, Castle Veterinary Centre, Farnborough, and Wellesley Veterinary Centre, Frimley, Surrey, were established, although the latter was sold in 1997.

Records: Grazely Veterinary Centre, 12 Guildford Road West, Farnborough GU14 6PU

Balance sheets/profit and loss accounts 1973–; diaries 1973–; ledgers 1973–; cash books 1973–; photographs 1973–; architectural plans 1973–.

GROVE LODGE VETERINARY GROUP
Worthing, West Sussex

History: This small animal practice was established in 1948.

Records: Grove Lodge Veterinary Group, Upper Brighton Road, Worthing BN14 9DL

Partnership agreements 1948–; day books 1990–; client records 1990–; architectural plans 1990s.

GROVE VETERINARY CENTRE
Ballymena, Co Antrim

History: This mixed practice was established in 1970.

Records: Grove Veterinary Centre, 17 Grove Road, Ballymena BT43 6UB

Partnership agreements 1970–; balance sheets/profit and loss accounts 1970–; day books 1970–; ledgers 1970–; cash books 1970–; client records 1970–; architectural plans 1970–; practice magazines/leaflets 1970–; x-rays 1970–.

HALL COURT VETERINARY GROUP
Sheffield, South Yorkshire

History: This mixed practice was established in 1900.

Records: Hall Court Veterinary Group, 1 St Leonard's Close, Dinnington, Sheffield S31 7RL

Partnership agreements c1979– [w]; balance sheets/profit and loss accounts 1992–; day books 1992–; ledgers 1992–; cash books 1992–; client records 1992–; architectural plans c1970–.

HAMPDEN VETERINARY HOSPITAL
Aylesbury, Buckinghamshire

History: This practice was established in c1935.

Records: Hampden Veterinary Hospital, 49 Cambridge Street, Aylesbury HP20 1RP

Partnership agreements c1970–; minutes c1980–; balance sheets/profit and loss accounts 1985–; architectural plans c1965–.

R HANDS MRCVS
Coventry, West Midlands

History: This small animal practice was established by R Hands in 1969.

Records: R Hands MRCVS, 255 Broad Lane, Coventry CV5 7AQ

Partnership agreements 1969–; balance sheets/profit and loss accounts 1969–; day books 1969–; receipts 1969–; photographs 1969–.

C J & P M HANSON MsRCVS
Altrincham, Greater Manchester

History: This small animal practice was established in 1982 by C J and P M Hanson.

Records: C J & P M Hanson MsRCVS, 40 Barrington Road, Altrincham WA14 1HJ

Balance sheets/profit and loss accounts 1982–; ledgers 1982–; cash books 1982–.

S F HARVEY MRCVS
Tewkesbury, Gloucestershire

History: The goodwill to this mixed practice was sold to Simon Harvey by E T A White of The Mythe, Tewkesbury, in 1978. Harvey initially based his practice at 29 Barton Street, Tewkesbury, before moving to Folly Gardens in 1983.

Records: S F Harvey MRCVS, 1 Folly Gardens, Tewkesbury GL20 5QP

Appointment books 1990–95; booking diaries 1987–91; day books 1985–92; outgoing invoices (duplicates) 1978–94; purchase invoices 1978–79,

1988–90; large animal bills 1978–94; small animal accounts 1988–90; small animal bills 1993; cash books 1980–90; petty cash books 1978–80, 1987–90; payment ledgers 1984–86; value added tax books 1980–88; list of debtors 1988; drug order books 1991–96; patient record cards 1980s–; vaccine record cards 1980s–; hospitalisation sheets c1991; laboratory reports 1985–94; wages books 1986–94; papers, accounts, etc re provision of People's Dispensary for Sick Animals care 1992–93; Local Veterinary Inspector claim forms for fees 1980–87; Local Veterinary Inspector's reports 1987–92; Ministry of Agriculture, Fisheries and Food circulars re procedures for Local Veterinary Inspectors, brucellosis, tuberculosis, etc 1980s; receipts re building work 1978–80; certificates: Frederick Harvey MRCVS 1885 and fellowship 1891, Henry Harvey MRCVS 1931.

HARWELL VETERINARY CENTRE
Peverell, Plymouth

History: This single-handed small animal practice was established in 1970 by Edmund H Shillabeer at 4 Wesley Villas (later known as 94 Hyde Park Road), Peverell. In c1979, 96 Hyde Park Road was purchased and the practice extended across the two properties. A branch surgery was established at 4 Haye Road South, Elburton, Plymouth, in 1971. After part of the latter was demolished in 1989 the practice introduced a mobile surgery, which was in use until 1997. Additional branches were opened at 56 Maker Road, Torpoint, Cornwall, in 1972, and 44 Ryder Road, Stoke, Plymouth, in 1998.

Records: Harwell Veterinary Centre, 94–96 Hyde Park Road, Peverell, Plymouth PL3 4RE

Day books/diaries 1970–; cash books 1970–; petty cash books 1977–85; practice bank account ledgers 1970–82; receipts 1970–73; diaries from employment at other practices 1965–69.

HAYDON VETERINARY GROUP
Bridport, Dorset

History: This practice was established in 1980 by George Dickinson.

Records: Haydon Veterinary Group, Corbin Way, Bridport DT6 3UX

Papers re partnership breakup 1980; client records 1950–; receipt books 1975–; prescription books 1990–; photographs taken during service in Royal Army Veterinary Corps 1940–46.

HAYES & BORRAJO MsRCVS
Leicester, Leicestershire

History: This practice was established in 1980 by Ian McDonald. A partnership formed with M J Hayes in 1982 lasted until McDonald's retirement in 1984. In 1991 a new partnership was formed between M J Hayes and John Borrajo. Originally a mixed practice, it became exclusively small animal from c1985. A branch surgery was later opened at 84 Sibson Road, Birstall, Leicester.

Records: Hayes & Borrajo MsRCVS, 192 Uppingham Road, Leicester LE5 0QG

Partnership agreements 1982, 1984, 1991; balance sheets 1987–; client records 1986–; architectural plans re Birstall extension 1996; photographs of Birstall surgery prior to extension, nd; salary books 1980–.

HEATH VETERINARY GROUP
Cardiff

History: This practice was established by John George Wright (1897–1971) who graduated from the Royal Veterinary College, London, in 1923 and later went on to become Professor of Surgery and Principal of Liverpool University Veterinary College. Wright was initially based at 5 Dumfries Place, Cardiff, before moving to 1 Fitzalan Place, Cardiff, in 1925 or 1926. Later the surgery moved again, to Newport Road, Cardiff. In 1959 Lewis Jessop took over the practice and traded from his home on Whitchurch Road, Cardiff. Jessop decided early on to specialise in small animal medicine and built up a large practice which eventually took over the whole house, forcing his family to move out. On Jessop's retirement in 1987, the practice was sold to Marina Crockford and Chris Troughton. Later, a large extension was added, housing a new operating theatre and hospital wards. Two branch surgeries, in Cyncoed, Cardiff, and Rhiwbina, Cardiff, opened in 1994.

Records: Heath Veterinary Group, 326 Whitchurch Road, Cardiff CF4 3NG

Balance sheets/profit and loss accounts 1987–; client records 1989–.

J R HEGARTY MRCVS
Bournemouth, Dorset

History: This small animal practice was established in 1985.

Records: J R Hegarty MRCVS, 5 Stokewood Road, Bournemouth BH3 7NL

Balance sheets/profit and loss accounts 1985–; day books 1985–; ledgers 1985–; cash books 1985–; receipts 1985–; client records 1985–; architectural plans 1985–.

HEY AND GREENWOOD MsRCVS
Rufford, Lancashire

History: This practice was established in 1920 by Captain William Drummond Allan (1866–1939), at Beech House, Rufford. After his death, the practice was sold to Thomas Edmund Hey, who had been running his own practice in Leyland, Lancashire, since 1936.

Records: Hey and Greenwood MsRCVS, 9 Holly Lane, Rufford, Ormskirk L40 1SH

Day books 1942, 1946–48, 1957, nd; day/cash book 1964; visit diaries 1953, 1955, 1959–62; cash books 1944–63 [w]; ledgers 1944–55; invoice book 1958; expenditure book, nd; misc letters re drugs, tuberculin testing, purchase of motor car 1947–48; Ministry of Agriculture and Fisheries guidelines on coupon free buying of protective clothing 1940s; student notebooks: biochemistry, anatomy, physiology, shoeing, veterinary hygiene, systematic surgery & obstetrics 1931–34; notes on protozoology, nd; *The Veterinarian* 1838–40, 1842.

HIGHFIELD VETERINARY SURGERY
Broxbourne, Hertfordshire

History: This small animal practice was established in 1982 at White Stubbs Lane, Broxbourne, Hertfordshire, by R H Lockyer. It moved to Highfield Stables, White Stubbs Lane, in 1990. A branch surgery was opened at 62 Longfield Lane, Flamstead End, Cheshunt, Hertfordshire, in 1986.

Records: Highfield Veterinary Surgery, Highfield Stables, White Stubbs Lane, Broxbourne EN10 7QA

Accounts 1983–; architectural plans for new surgery c1990.

A T M & C W HILL MsRCVS
London

History: This small animal practice was bought from a non-qualified veterinary practitioner in c1971 and moved to its present location in 1976.

Records: A T M & C W Hill MsRCVS, 178 Park Road, Crouch End, London N8 8JT

Day books early 1970s–; accounts early 1970s–.

C H O L HODGES MRCVS
Sherborne, Dorset

History: This small animal practice was established by C H O L Hodges in 1988.

Records: C H O L Hodges MRCVS, Dymor, Sandford Orcas Road, Sherborne DT9 4RW

Balance sheets/profit and loss accounts 1988–; day books 1988–; ledgers 1988–; cash books 1988–; client records 1988–; laboratory reports 1988–.

E J HODGKINSON MRCVS
Leek, Staffordshire

History: This practice has been trading since at least 1910.

Records: Moorland Veterinary Centre, St Lukes House, Vicarage Road, Leek ST13 6AS

Ledgers 1910–56.

GEORGE HOLTHAM
Gloucester, Gloucestershire

History: George Holtham (1845–1927) graduated from the Royal Veterinary College, London, in 1870 and established a practice in Gloucester some time after. He retired in 1923.

Records: Gloucestershire Record Office, Clarence Row, Alvin Street, Gloucester GL1 3DW

Ledger of clients' accounts 1901–24; Gloucestershire Old Spot Pig Society herd books 1915–24 [w]; photographs of 124 Westgate Street and other properties c1900. [Ref: D2648]

HOPE & DAVIES MsRCVS
New Malden, Greater London

History: This small animal practice was established in 1971 by H P Hope. In 1979 Hope entered into partnership with John Davies. By 2000 there were five veterinary surgeons based at the practice.

Records: Hope & Davies MsRCVS, 14 Burlington Road, New Malden KT3 4NY

Partnership agreements 1979; balance sheets/profit and loss accounts 1971–; client records 1980–; architectural plans 1980–; practice magazines/leaflets 1994–.

HORSEPOND VETERINARY CENTRE
South Molton, Devon

History: This practice was established in c1940.

Records: Horsepond Veterinary Centre, Horsepond Meadow, South Molton EX36 4EJ

Day books 1970–; ledgers 1970–; cash books 1970–; recipes 1960; architectural plans 1983.

P M HOUGHTON MRCVS
Oakham, Rutland

History: This practice was established in c1980. It was sold in 1992 after which it moved to new premises. A branch surgery was opened in 1993.

Records: P M Houghton MRCVS, 12a Ayston Road, Uppingham, Oakham LE15 9RL

Ledgers 1980s–; cash books 1980s–; client records 1980s–.

HOWE & STARNES MsRCVS
Uckfield, East Sussex

History: This mixed practice was established at Fairfield House, Uckfield, in 1953 by D E Gunner and P B Clarke, although there had been a practice on the same site previously. K J Grainger joined the practice in 1956, staying until 1984. Gunner left in 1968 and was replaced by Miss C M Howe. A F Starnes joined in 1980, L K Gatward in 1984 and P S Blowey in 1994. P B Clarke left in 1993.

Records: Howe & Starnes MsRCVS, Fairfield House, Uckfield TN22 5DG

Partnership agreements 1982–; balance sheets/profit and loss accounts 1970–; day books 1970–; ledgers 1980–; receipts 1955–; client records 1980–; photographs 1970–.

HUBBARD & WILLIAMS MsRCVS
Caernarfon, Gwynedd

History: This mixed practice was established by G P Davies in c1965 and acquired by G E and N T Hubbard in 1978. Dewi Williams became a partner in 1986. The practice moved twice, in 1986 and 1997.

Records: Hubbard & Williams MsRCVS, Cibyn Veterinary Clinic, Llanberis Road, Caernarfon LL55 2BD

Partnership agreements 1986–; minutes 1986–; day books 1975–; client records 1974–; practice magazines/leaflets 1986–.

A J HUTCHESON MRCVS
Longridge, Lancashire

History: This mixed practice was established in 1960 by J D Scrambler. Based initially at Ashfield, Inglewhite Road, Longridge, it moved to Preston Road in 1988. Following Scrambler's retirement in 1990, the practice was sold to A J Hutcheson.

Records: A J Hutcheson MRCVS, 54 Preston Road, Longridge, Preston PR3 3AY

Partnership agreements 1978–; balance sheets/profit and loss accounts 1975–; ledgers 1975–; cash books 1975–; client records 1990–; architectural plans 1989.

HUTCHISON, DUNLOP & BAIRD MsRCVS
Wetherby, West Yorkshire

History: John Sanderson (b c1819) was known to be practising as a veterinary surgeon in Castle Street, Spofforth, North Yorkshire, in 1857. His son, Joseph William Sanderson (1844–1912), graduated from the Royal Veterinary College, London, in 1867 and the 1871 census shows the two men living and practising together in Castle Street, Spofforth, next door to a forge run by George Bailey. Joseph Sanderson moved to North Street, Wetherby, in c1893 and was succeeded by George Wilkie Davidson (d 1945) who qualified from the Royal (Dick) Veterinary College, Edinburgh, in 1904 and was known to be practising at Swan House, Wetherby, by 1920. Shortly before his death Davidson was approached by Joseph Powley (qualified Edinburgh 1904) who wished to buy the practice on behalf of his son, George Seaton Powley, at that time a partner in Tyreman & Withers, Harrogate, North Yorkshire. Powley's turnover for his first month in Wetherby was reputed to be £30, and the practice grew steadily, boosted by the presence in those days of up to 200 racehorses in the town. Working alongside Powley was his father, who also acted as a Local Veterinary Inspector for the Ministry of Agriculture and Fisheries, another veterinary surgeon and a yardman who helped administer the anaesthetics. During the 1950s the surgery at Harrogate was sold to Richard and Judith Beckett, while the Wetherby practice was moved to a converted cow shed on Hallfield Lane in 1955. J L H Cuthbertson joined as an assistant in 1956 and became a partner in 1963, after which the practice traded under the name of Powley & Cuthbertson. John Hutchison came to the practice as an assistant in 1976 and was made a partner in 1982, after which the practice traded as Powley, Cuthbertson & Hutchison. Following Powley's retirement in 1986 the practice became known as Cuthertson & Hutchison. Gordon Dunlop started at the practice in 1989 and was joined a year later by John Baird. In 1993, Cuthbertson retired and the partnership of Hutchison, Dunlop & Baird was formed.

Records: Hutchison, Dunlop & Baird MsRCVS, The Veterinary Surgery, Hallfield Lane, Wetherby LS22 6JU

Day books 1954–55, 1957–nd; ledgers 1948–50; small animal ledger 1961; dog accounts list 1962; receipted invoices for incoming goods and services 1949–50, 1954–55; Ministry of Agriculture, Fisheries and Food defence training of the veterinary surgeon professional short course, joining instructions, course instructions, etc 1964; drugs register (blank), nd; headed notepaper for Powley & Cuthbertson, nd; student notebooks: G S Powley, anatomy, surgery, histology, medicine, entomology, biochemistry, nd, John Hutchison, medicine, clinical pathology, surgery 1974, radiology 1975, A R Withers, physiology class B, nd.

P H JANAWAY MRCVS
Didmarton, Gloucestershire

History: This equine practice was established in 1970 by P H Janaway.

Records: P H Janaway MRCVS, Buryhill House, Didmarton GL9 1DX

Balance sheets/profit and loss accounts 1970–; client records 1970–.

J P JARVIS MRCVS
Evesham, Worcestershire

History: This small animal practice was purchased in 1977 by J P Jarvis.

Records: J P Jarvis MRCVS, Veterinary Surgery, Northwick House, Coopers Lane, Evesham WR11 6BY

Balance sheets/profit and loss accounts 1977–; day books 1982–; cash books 1982–; client records 1982–.

JOHNSON, DANIELS & PARTNERS
Watford, Hertfordshire

History: This mixed practice was established in the late nineteenth century.

Records: Johnson, Daniels & Partners, Park Veterinary Centre, 256 Cassiobury Drive, Watford WD1 3AP

Partnership agreements 1974; balance sheets/profit and loss accounts 1980s–; day books 1970s–; ledgers 1960s–; cash books 1970s–; receipts 1970s–; client records 1970s–; architectural plans 1970s.

ALAN K JONES MRCVS
Crawley, West Sussex

History: This practice was established by Alan K Jones in 1985.

Records: Alan K Jones MRCVS, The Cottage, Turners Hill Road, Worth, Crawley RH10 4LY

Partnership agreements 1985–; day books 1985–.

S P KAVANAGH MRCVS
Sittingbourne, Kent

History: This mixed practice was established in 1978 by S P Kavanagh.

Records: S P Kavanagh MRCVS, The Veterinary Surgery, Dover Street, Sittingbourne ME10 3EH

Ledgers 1978–; cash books 1978–; receipts 1978–; architectural plans 1978–.

KEARNS & REA VETERINARY SURGEONS
Tewkesbury, Gloucestershire

History: This practice was established by L G Harries of Upton upon Severn, Worcestershire. Following Harries's death in 1986, the practice was run by his daughter, L A Harries, until 1989 when it was sold to Kearns and Rea.

Records: Kearns & Rea Veterinary Surgeons, Three Counties Equine Hospital, Stratford Bridge, Ripple, Tewkesbury GL20 6HE

Partnership agreements 1989–; balance sheets 1989–; ledgers 1989–; day books 1989–; cash books 1989–; general accounts 1989–; receipts 1989–; invoices 1989–; legal papers 1989–; client records 1989–; recipe books 1989–; title deeds, nd; architectural plans, nd; staff registers 1989–; salary books 1989–; pension papers 1989–; magazines 1989–; photographs 1989–; general correspondence re practice 1989–.

KINGDOM VETERINARY CLINIC

Glenrothes, Fife

History: This practice was established by Major Bryant in the 1960s and later sold to R J Low. R F Waterston joined as a partner in 1970 after which the practice traded as Low & Waterston until 1975 when Low left to join another practice. In 1985 Waterston formed a new partnership with W A Wooton. The practice moved to North Street, Glenrothes, in 1989, since when it has traded as the Kingdom Veterinary Clinic.

Records: Kingdom Veterinary Clinic, North Street, Glenrothes KY7 5NA

Day books 1975–; cash books 1975–; photographs, mainly of staff 1975–; architectural plans for original surgery 1960s.

DONALD KINGSNORTH & ASSOCIATES

Chobham, Surrey

History: This mixed practice was established by R Y Christie in 1975 and sold to Donald Kingsnorth in 1992.

Records: Donald Kingsnorth & Associates, Cedar Cottage, 2 Brimshot Lane, Chobham GU24 8RN

Balance sheets/profit and loss accounts 1975–; day books 1975–; ledgers 1975–; cash books 1975–; client records 1975–.

KINGSTON VETERINARY GROUP
Sherborne, Dorset

History: This practice was established at Kingston House, Long Street, Sherborne, by Charles Hedworth Golledge (c1859–1929), who graduated from the Royal Veterinary College, London, in 1879. After short periods in Wiltshire and Somerset, Golledge came to Sherborne in 1885 or 1886 and rapidly became a familiar sight in the area, dashing about the countryside on horseback in an effort to look busy. Following the outbreak of the First World War, Golledge joined up, leaving the practice in the hands of his son, Lionel St Bel Golledge (d 1960), who was at the time still a student at the Royal Veterinary College, London. After completing his studies in 1919, Lionel Golledge returned to Sherborne and entered into practice with his father and his brother Hedley. Hedley Charles Davys Golledge (1889–1942) had qualified in 1910 and was made a Fellow of the Royal College of Veterinary Surgeons in 1917. He did not remain at Sherborne for long, however, becoming a Board of Agriculture Assistant Inspector before moving to Silchester House, Yeovil, Somerset, from where he ran a mixed practice. Lionel Golledge, in addition to his duties at Kingston House, sat on the Council of the Royal College of Veterinary Surgeons and acted as official veterinary surgeon at both Wincanton and Taunton racecourses. In 1947 he entered into partnership with Robert Brown (d 1978) and in 1949 they opened a branch surgery at Grove Dene, Preston Road, Yeovil. This surgery was moved to a purpose built clinic at The Forum, Abbey Manor Park, Yeovil, in 1990. Other partners at the practice have included G L Barker (1956–92), H L Trump (1960–83), K R C Ferguson (1967–94), M J Coleman (1979–), J M Wilde (1980–84), P N Atkinson (1985–), A F Lees (1989–) and K M Jones (1994–). Since the 1960s the practice has changed its name several times, becoming Brown, Barker, Trump & Ferguson in 1967, then Barker & Partners from 1981 and finally the Kingston Veterinary Group in 1994. An equine hospital, established at Rimpton, Somerset, in 1972 by G L Barker, was moved to Long Burton, Somerset, in 1994. By 1999 there were ten veterinary surgeons providing treatment for both small and large animals at surgeries in Sherborne, Yeovil, Long Burton and Milborne Port in Somerset. The practice also continues to provide veterinary services to both Taunton and Wincanton racecourses.

Records: Kingston Veterinary Group, Kingston House, Long Street, Sherborne DT9 3DB

Day books 1933–60; cash books 1923–55; account sheets c1923–45; visits book 1946–47; message books 1978–95; bill for professional services rendered 1948; telegram asking veterinary surgeon to attend 1924; misc letters, drug advertisements, etc c1955; list of price amendments c1955; drug list, nd; map of Blackmoor Vale hunt country with an advertisement for H J Everitt, dispensing, veterinary and photographic chemist, nd; misc unidentified photographs c1900.

J E KNEEN MRCVS
Arbroath, Angus

History: This practice was established in c1910 by Alexander S Wallace (1852–1922), who had graduated from the Royal (Dick) Veterinary College, Edinburgh, in 1889. After Wallace's death the practice was sold to Archibald Linton Robertson (d 1972) who had graduated from the Glasgow Veterinary College in 1918. Robertson based his practice at 40 Hill Street, Arbroath, before moving to 16 Hill Place in 1926 then to 30 Wellbank in 1930. John Kneen became a partner in 1957 and sole owner in 1965. A branch was opened in Carnoustie, Angus, in c1978. The practice was sold following Kneen's retirement in 1997.

Records: in private ownership of Mr J E Kneen, Hill House, Arbroath DD11 1AH

Large animal day books 1968–71, 1974–75, 1982–84; small animal day book 1968–72; accounts 1965–97; dangerous drug record c1955–97; patient record cards 1980s–90s.

A V KRASNO MRCVS
Basingstoke, Hampshire

History: This equine and small animal practice was established by A V Krasno in 1982.

Records: A V Krasno MRCVS, Veterinary Surgery, 16 The Street, Old Basing, Basingstoke RG24 0BN

Partnership agreements 1980s–; balance sheets/profit and loss accounts 1982–; day books 1982–; ledgers 1982–; cash books 1982–; client records 1982–; architectural plans 1980s–.

KYNANCE VETERINARY CLINIC
London

History: This practice was established in a converted stable in Mayfair by Keith Butt in 1962. It grew rapidly over the next decade and handled a wide variety of cases, including horses, monkeys, snakes and big cats as well as dogs, cats and birds. Peter Arbeid became a partner in 1966 and Woodthorpe Veterinary Surgery, Putney, established in 1959, was purchased in 1985. Since 1979 the practice has been linked to the Elizabeth Street Emergency Service. By 2000 there were four partners at the clinic.

Country Life, Nov 1997, Snowdon's Country Life.

Records: Kynance Veterinary Clinic, 8 Kynance Mews, London SW7 4QP

Partnership agreement 1996; balance sheets 1962–; photographs, nd.

KYNOCH & PARTNERS
Crowthorne, Bracknell Forest

History: This small animal practice, established in 1987, is part of a group of practices set up in Berkshire, Hampshire and Surrey by Ian Kynoch from 1971. In addition to the regular practice, the Pine Grove surgery also offers a referral service.

Records: Kynoch & Partners, Pine Grove Veterinary Clinic, 51 Dukes Ride, Crowthorne RG45 6NE

Partnership agreements 1998–; minutes 1994–; balance sheets/profit and loss accounts 1987–; day books 1987–; ledgers 1987–; cash books 1987–; receipts 1987–; client records 1987–; architectural plans 1997; x-rays, laboratory and referral reports 1988–.

LANSDOWN VETERINARY SURGEONS
Stroud, Gloucestershire

History: This practice was established in 1950 and offers small animal care as well as an avian and exotic referral service. There are branch surgeries at Oldmarket Place, Nailsworth, and Middle Hill Farm, Chalford Hill, Stroud.

Records: Lansdown Veterinary Surgeons, Clockhouse Veterinary Hospital, Wallbridge, Stroud GL5 3JD

Partnership agreements 1985–; minutes 1990–; balance sheets/profit and loss accounts 1980–; day books 1992–; ledgers 1992–; cash books 1992–; client records 1992–; architectural plans 1987–; practice magazines/leaflets 1995–.

HENRY LAWRENCE AND PHILIP GREEN

Brentwood, Essex

History: Philip Green (d c1889) graduated from the Royal Veterinary College, London, in 1832. Henry Lawrence (c1844–1904) also trained at the Royal Veterinary College, London, graduating in 1863.

Records: Essex Record Office, Southend Branch, Central Library, Victoria Avenue, Southend on Sea SS2 6EX. Not all records are stored on-site. Researchers are therefore advised to contact the office in advance of any visit.

Memorandum of agreement 1880. [Ref: D/DGs B303]

ALISON P LEE VETERINARY SURGERY

Carnforth, Lancashire

History: This mixed practice was established in 1984.

Records: Alison P Lee Veterinary Surgery, 2 Queen Street, off Lancaster Road, Carnforth LA5 9EB

Balance sheets/profit and loss accounts 1984–; day books 1984–; ledgers 1984–; cash books 1984–; receipts 1984–; client records 1984–; photographs 1984–; architectural plans 1984–; practice magazines/leaflets 1984–.

LEWIS-JONES & ASSOCIATES
Honiton, Devon

History: This mixed practice was established in 1980.

Records: Lewis-Jones & Associates, 5 High Street, Honiton EX14 1PR

Partnership agreements 1980–; client records 1980–; photographs 1980–; practice magazines/leaflets 1980–; farm reports 1980–; papers re feed, prescriptions, etc 1980–.

LLOYD FAMILY
Tyberton, Herefordshire

History: Successive generations of the Lloyd family were blacksmiths, farriers and horse doctors in Tyberton from at least 1870 to 1960.

Records: Herefordshire Record Office, The Old Barracks, Harold Street, Hereford HR1 2QX

Ledgers 1865–1959 [w]; day books 1919–24; account books: receipts and payments 1918–26, cash payments 1907–11, carrier's business 1895–1914; customer accounts 1924–38; notebook containing farriery recipes 1882; *The Modern System of Farriery* incl handwritten list of oils for cuts and bruises 1864; pocket books 1863, 1886; school exercise books 1896, 1942. [Ref: AF100/1–28, 30]

LOCKE & SON
Manchester, Greater Manchester

History: Samuel Locke (1846–1910) graduated from the Glasgow Veterinary College in 1869 and shortly afterwards became an assistant at Thomas Taylor's practice based at 98 Grosvenor Street, Manchester. Locke later went on to acquire the business. In 1891 he was elected Honorary Secretary of the National Veterinary Benevolent & Mutual Defence Society. Locke's son, George Harry Locke (1875–1960) graduated from the New Edinburgh Veterinary College in 1896 and joined his father shortly afterwards. Both men served as President of the Royal College of Veterinary Surgeons, Samuel from 1909 to 1910 and Harry from 1934 to 1935. Harry was also Honorary Secretary of the Victoria Veterinary Benevolent Fund until 1913. In 1923 Harry's son,

Richard Conway Locke (1902–67), graduated from the Royal Veterinary College, London, and joined the family practice, which by that time was trading as Locke & Son. Richard Conway Locke was appointed Veterinary Officer to the Veterinary and Milk Control Department of Manchester Corporation in 1934 and by the late 1940s the practice had ceased trading. Richard Conway's son, Richard David Locke, qualified from Liverpool University's Veterinary College in 1950 and after a brief period in practice worked for the Ministry of Agriculture, Fisheries and Food. He too acted as Honorary Secretary of the Veterinary Benevolent Fund, between 1990 and 1995.

Records (1): in private ownership of Mr R D Locke, 4 Rathmore Road, Cambridge CB1 7AD

G H Locke's address as president of the Royal College of Veterinary Surgeons to George V on 25th anniversary of his accession 1935; correspondence: G H Locke to S Locke while with Remount Service during Boer War 1902, W E Harwood, solicitor to G H Locke re Grosvenor Street premises 1923, practice employees to R C Locke wishing him luck in his final examinations 1923, R D Locke with Royal College of Veterinary Surgeons 1950; certificates: R C Locke, Diploma in Veterinary State Medicine, Victoria University of Manchester 1925, R D Locke, Bachelor of Veterinary Science, University of Liverpool 1950, R D Locke, Diploma in Veterinary State Medicine, University of Edinburgh 1961; photographs: S Locke, G H Locke, R C Locke and R D Locke, nd, surgery premises c1906, G H Locke in remount service 1914–17, misc college and family, nd.

Records (2): Manchester Central Library, Local Studies Unit, St Peter's Square, Manchester M2 5PD

Bills issued by Thomas Taylor 1867, 1869–70. [Ref: M35/9/62/13–17]

LODGE VETERINARY CENTRE

Birmingham, West Midlands

History: This small animal practice was established during the 1950s. In 1998, following the introduction of a new partner, it changed its trading name from Harrington Lodge to the Lodge Veterinary Centre. A branch surgery was established in Coleshill, Birmingham, during the late 1980s.

Records: Lodge Veterinary Centre, 64 Coleshill Road, Hodge Hill, Birmingham B36 8AB

Balance sheets/profit and loss accounts 1980s–; day books 1980s–; ledgers 1980s–; cash books 1980s–; client records 1980s–; architectural plans c1970s.

WILLIAM LOTHIAN SENIOR AND WILLIAM LOTHIAN JUNIOR

Duns, Scottish Borders

History: William Lothian senior qualified in 1844 and afterwards practised as a veterinary surgeon in North Street, Duns. His son, also William Lothian (c1864–1940), qualified in 1884 and later took over his father's practice, moving it to 20 Newtown Street, Duns. Both men acted as Local Veterinary Inspectors for the area and William Lothian junior also wrote extensively on veterinary matters. On his retirement in 1939, the practice was sold to a Mr Milne.

Records: Archivist, Edinburgh University Library, George Square, Edinburgh EH8 9LJ

William Lothian senior: certificates of attendance at lectures, testimonials 1842–44, veterinary college certificate 1844, MRCVS certificate 1844, inspection returns re cattle plague 1866, sheep scab 1872–74, foot-and-mouth disease 1869–74, accounts submitted for services and travelling expenses as inspector of cattle for Duns 1865–66, returns in accordance with the 1878 Contagious Diseases (Animals) Act 1879, notebooks 1850, 1883, letters incl some addressed to his son 1873, 1879–1916, veterinary certificates re visits to clients 1871, 1880, nd, recipe for mud fever cure, nd, misc recipes and notes 1860, nd, annotated copy of Royal College of Veterinary Surgeons' annual report 1881, circular advertising publication of *The Principles and Practice of Bovine Medicine and Surgery* and other works 1881, price list for Burgoyne, Burbridge, Cyriax & Farries, wholesale druggists & manufacturing chemists 1881, receipts for veterinary instruments bought from Arnold & Sons 1878–79; William Lothian junior: certificates issued by New Veterinary College, Edinburgh, stating that he had acted as a dispenser, clinical dresser and visitor 1884, card requesting attendance at Royal College of Veterinary Surgeons examination 1884, notification of dates, etc for preliminary examination at Royal (Dick) Veterinary College 1902, letter and recommendation 1892, nd, inspection returns re anthrax 1892–1910, notes of method of examination for bacillus tuberculosis c1913, recipes and costs for preparations from Harkness, Beaumont & Co Ltd, wholesale manufacturers of pharmaceutical products, Edinburgh, 1940, photograph of delegates to National Veterinary Medical Association annual congress, Aberdeen, 1924, obituary 1940, illustrations of dissected horse showing development of teeth and internal structure, nd.

H J LOVELESS MRCVS
Clacton on Sea, Essex

History: Harry John Loveless (1900–75), a native of Diss, Norfolk, graduated from the Royal Veterinary College, London, in 1921 and was known to be practising in Clacton on Sea from 1932. He was based initially at High View Avenue before moving to 110 Pier Avenue in 1933 and then to Norfolk House, Pier Avenue, in 1939.

Records: Essex Record Office, Colchester & North-East Essex Branch, Stanwell House, Stanwell Street, Colchester CO2 7DL

Day books 1953–57; ledgers 1939, 1945, 1955. [Ref: D/F 46]

LUCAS VETERINARY SURGERY
Longwell Green, Bristol

History: This practice was established in 1985 at 146 Bath Road, Longwell Green, Bristol, by Stephen Lucas. After Lucas's death in 1990, his widow, Susan, took over the running of the practice, which moved to Court Farm Road, Longwell Green, Bristol, in 1993.

Records: Lucas Veterinary Surgery, 1 Court Farm Road, Longwell Green, Bristol BS30 9AA

Balance sheets 1985–; ledgers 1985–; day books 1985–; cash books 1985–; general accounts 1985–; receipts 1985–; invoices 1985–; client records 1985–; recipe books 1985–; staff registers 1985–; salary books 1985–; title deeds 1985–; architectural plans 1985–; photographs 1985–99.

MACARTHUR, BARSTOW & GIBBS MsRCVS
Droitwich, Worcestershire

History: This mixed practice was established in 1956.

Records: MacArthur, Barstow & Gibbs MsRCVS, 8 Corbett Street, Droitwich WR9 7BT

Partnership agreements 1956–; minutes 1956–; balance sheets/profit and loss accounts 1956–; day books 1956–; ledgers 1956–; cash books 1956–; receipts 1956–; client records 1956–; photographs 1956–; practice magazines/leaflets 1956–.

MACKAY & TAYLOR MsRCVS
Bridgwater, Somerset

History: This mixed practice was established at The Woollands, Brent Road, Cossington, in 1976 by P H S Mackay and R H Taylor.

Records: Mackay & Taylor MsRCVS, The Woollands, Brent Road, Cossington, Bridgwater TA7 8LF

Partnership agreements 1976–; balance sheets/profit and loss accounts 1976–; day books 1970s– [w]; ledgers 1970s– [w]; cash books 1970s– [w]; receipts 1976–; client records 1970s– [w]; photographs 1976–; architectural plans 1976–.

MACQUEEN VETERINARY CENTRE
Devizes, Wiltshire

History: This practice was established in 1987 by R Geering and branches subsequently opened in Melksham and Corshaom. When the practice split up in 1990, the Devizes surgery was bought by I G and J C Macqueen. The practice moved to new premises in 2000 and now operates as a small animal clinic. About 40 per cent of its work is derived from orthopaedic referrals.

Records: Macqueen Veterinary Centre, 57 New Park Street, Devizes SN10 1DP

Balance sheets/profit and loss accounts 1987–; day books 1987–; cash books 1987–; client records 1987–; architectural plans 1987–.

F J MAGUIRE MRCVS
Withington, Greater Manchester

History: This practice has been trading since at least 1980.

Records: F J Maguire MRCVS, 331 Yew Tree Road, Withington, Manchester M20 9FP

Partnership agreements 1985–; balance sheets/profit and loss accounts 1980–; appointment books 1980–; day books 1980–; ledgers 1985–; cash books 1980–; client records 1980–; architectural plans 1985–.

MALLON VETERINARY PRACTICE
Dungannon, Co Tyrone

History: This mixed practice was established by B P Mallon in 1988.

Records: Mallon Veterinary Practice, 99 Killycolpy Road, Killywoolaghan, Dungannon BT71 5AW

Day books 1988–; cash books 1988–; receipts 1988–.

THE MALTHOUSE SURGERY
Minsterley, Shropshire

History: This mixed practice was established in c1950.

Records: The Malthouse Surgery, Minsterley, Shrewsbury SY5 0AA

Day books c1985–; ledgers c1985–; cash books c1985–; client records c1985–.

MANSFIELD COTTAGE VETERINARY SURGERY
Cheshunt, Hertfordshire

History: This small animal practice was established in 1969 by B A Mallows. It relocated in 1974 and was sold to R A Drew in 1975. By 2000 there were four veterinary surgeons based at the practice.

Records: Mansfield Cottage Veterinary Surgery, 24 Crossbrook Street, Cheshunt EN8 8JQ

Balance sheets/profit and loss accounts 1975– [w]; day books 1975– [w]; ledgers 1975– [w]; cash books 1975– [w]; client records 1975–; x-rays 1975–.

MAPLE VETERINARY SURGERY
Penketh, Warrington

History: This small animal practice was established in 1986 by Lesley Morris.

Records: Maple Veterinary Surgery, 95 Maple Crescent, Penketh, Warrington WA5 2LQ

Balance sheets 1986–; ledgers 1986–; day books 1986–; cash books 1986–; general accounts 1986–; receipts 1986–; invoices 1986–; legal papers 1986–; client records 1986–; advertising/promotional material 1986–; press cuttings 1986–; architectural plans 1980s; photographs 1986–.

MCKEATING, LEHNER & SOMERS
Bishop's Stortford, Hertfordshire

History: This practice was established in Rye Street, Bishop's Stortford, by John Square Brunskill, who graduated from the Royal Veterinary College, London, in 1878. After spending some time in High Barnet, Greater London, Brunskill came to Bishop's Stortford in 1885 or 1886. Like many practices at that time, Brunskill's was attached to a forge on the outskirts of town and derived much of its trade from passing dray and coach horses. The town's other practice, next to the Bricklayers Arms, was run by a veterinary practitioner and offered a more limited service. After Brunskill's death in 1903, his widow Alice entered into a ten-year partnership agreement with Archibald Millar (c1870–1939), who had graduated from the Glasgow Veterinary College in 1890. Under the terms of this agreement, the practice kept the name J S Brunskill and Millar was forbidden to practise anywhere within the surrounding area if he broke the agreement within the stipulated ten years. When the partnership ended in 1913, Millar stayed at Rye Street and was later joined by his two sons, Ramsay (b 1912), who qualified from the Royal Veterinary College, London, in 1934, and Alistair. The three men all lived in the house next door to their practice and always kept saddle bags in the kitchen overnight, arguing that it was often quicker to reach a farm by riding across the fields than by using a car. During the First World War the surgery premises were used by the Army Remount Corps to process some of the large numbers of horses, mules and asses being imported from the colonies to sustain the war effort. Wooden panels, used to test branding irons during that period, are still kept at the surgery. During the 1930s and 1940s, Sir Frederick Hobday regularly carried out his 'Hobday procedure' on horses with paralysed larynxes on the cobbled yard behind the surgery, while large numbers of shunting horses were driven into the yard for castration before being put to work at the local railway yard. Additionally, until the 1950s large numbers of cattle, sheep and pigs arrived each Thursday for sale at the market by Northgate End. Archibald Millar retired in 1938 and was replaced the following year by Lionel Wakley. The post-war period saw further changes as Ramsay Millar left and two new partners, Joseph Paterson and Henry Mills, arrived. Mills, who came to Bishop's Stortford after service with the Sudan Veterinary Service, left again in 1973, but Wakley and Paterson both stayed until their retirements in 1981 and 1986 respectively. Alistair Millar retired in the 1950s. F J McKeating became a partner in 1978, Robert Lehner in 1981 and Mrs Somers in 1997. During the 1980s and 1990s there was a sharp decline in the number of agricultural cases, although equine care continued to form an important part of the practice's work. The emphasis, however, has shifted from working horses to hunters, riding horses and ponies. Like many other practices, demand for small animal care has increased rapidly. In 1985, after extensive refurbishment, the practice was granted hospital status.

Records: McKeating, Lehner & Somers, The Veterinary Hospital, Rye Street, Bishop's Stortford CM23 2HA

Partnership agreement between Alice Brunskill and Archibald Millar 1903; Archibald Millar's correspondence with Field Roscoe & Co, solicitors, London, and Wm Gee and Sons, solicitors, Bishop's Stortford, re negotiations to end partnership 1913–15; balance sheets/profit and loss accounts incl lists of creditors 1904–06, 1908–12; balance sheet 1913; settlement account at dissolution of partnership 1913; lists from forge and veterinary ledgers of debtors and amounts owing 1913; list of amounts owed to sundry creditors 1913; list from branch ledger of amounts owed by sundry creditors 1913; Buntingford branch: list of expenses and sales 1910, account sheet 1911; national air raid precautions for animals committee report on casualties (copy) 1941; specification, plan and estimate for proposed new waiting room 1950; photographs: Archibald Millar and family, practice stables, etc 1900–40, hospital, facilities, equipment, patients, etc 1980s.

J R McNAUGHTON
West Bromwich, West Midlands

History: Henry James Dawes FRCVS (c1864–1931) graduated from the Royal Veterinary College, London, in 1885 and shortly afterwards established himself in practice at Camden House, High Street, West Bromwich, specialising in equine medicine. His son, Howard Winnington Dawes CBE, FRCVS (1892–1977), graduated from the Royal Veterinary College, London, in 1913, and joined his father's practice after serving as a Captain in the Army Veterinary Corps during the First World War. Howard Winnington Dawes was an authority on the horse and acted as judge and senior veterinary surgeon at numerous prestigious horse shows. He served on the Council of the Royal College of Veterinary Surgeons from 1934 to 1953, becoming Vice President in 1945, President between 1946 and 1949 and Vice President again from 1949 to 1951. He was also for a time President of the Veterinary Benevolent Fund. Despite these duties, Dawes continued to run his practice, entering into partnership with Paul Young and moving to new premises at 78 New Street, West Bromwich, in 1964. In 1965, John R McNaughton joined the practice and the business was renamed Dawes, Young & McNaughton. After Dawes retired in the mid 1970s, the practice traded as Young & McNaughton until Paul Young's death in 1981, when it was renamed J R McNaughton.

Records: J R McNaughton, 78 New Street, West Bromwich B70 7PZ

Bank account books, H J Dawes 1888–1900; receipts 1887–90, 1897; letter from District Bank Ltd re cancellation of guarantee 1951; prescription book 1928–48; loose prescriptions, nd; certificate book for examination of horses 1887–97; H W Dawes's paper to British Veterinary Association entitled 'The Relationship of Soundness and Conformation in the Horse' 1957; diaries, H J Dawes 1907–08; student notebook, H W

Dawes 1910; *The Comparative Anatomy of the Domesticated Animals*, annotated by H W Dawes 1909; press cuttings re horse disease and cases of cruelty to horses in which H J Dawes gave evidence in court, nd; letter book, H J Dawes 1900–01; correspondence: C H S Townsend, farmer, re operation on a cow 1952, British Equine Veterinary Association with H W Dawes re attendance at Congress incl copy of Congress programme 1962, nd, Royal College of Veterinary Surgeons to J R McNaughton re application for re-approval of practice as a training centre for veterinary nurses 1992; photographs: H W Dawes as President of Royal College of Veterinary Surgeons c1948, horses, horse shows, dignitaries and foot-and-mouth crisis 20th cent; National Greyhound Racing Club, rules booklets incl reference to H W Dawes as a steward and member 1952, 1966.

R MCNEILL MRCVS
Northampton, Northamptonshire

History: This small animal practice was established in 1983 by R McNeill.

Records: R McNeill MRCVS, 5 Bliss Lane, Flore, Northampton NN7 4LJ

Balance sheets/profit and loss accounts 1983–; receipts 1983–; photographs 1980s–; architectural plans 1980s.

MEADOWBANK VETERINARY CENTRE
Holywell, Flintshire

History: This practice was established in 1984 by Mrs Wyn-Jones at Moor Lane, Holway, Holywell. It closed in 1987.

Records: Meadowbank Veterinary Centre, Ty'n y Caeau, Northop, Mold CH7 6BE

Day books 1984–87.

MEADOWS VETERINARY CENTRE
Oldmeldrum, Aberdeenshire

History: This mixed practice traded as Silver & Lawson before becoming the Meadows Veterinary Centre in 1996. It moved from the Square to Station Road in 1990.

Records: Meadows Veterinary Centre, Station Road, Oldmeldrum AB51 0EZ

Client records 1988–; architectural plans 1989.

MERLIN VETERINARY GROUP
Carmarthen, Carmarthenshire

History: This large animal practice was established in c1940 and formed its first partnership in 1967. It became known as the Merlin Veterinary Group in c1972. A branch practice was opened in the mid 1970s.

Records: Merlin Veterinary Group, 4 St Catherines Street, Carmarthen SA31 1RE

Balance sheets/profit and loss accounts 1975–; day books 1992–; photographs 1967; architectural plans 1972.

MERLIN VETERINARY GROUP
Kelso, Scottish Borders

Records: Merlin Veterinary Group, Edinburgh Road, Kelso TD5 7EN

Day books 1970, 1980, 1990; photographs of former members of staff, nd.

MIDSUMMER VETERINARY GROUP
Stantonbury, Milton Keynes

History: This mixed practice was established by D J Smith in 1985.

Records: Midsummer Veterinary Group, 36 Purbeck, Stantonbury, Milton Keynes MK14 6BL

Balance sheets/profit and loss accounts 1985–; day books 1985–; ledgers 1985–; cash books 1985.

MILAN VETERINARY CLINIC
Douglas, Isle of Man

History: This practice was established in c1959. Prior to 2000 it traded as Vanderplank, Davies & Cox.

Records: Milan Veterinary Clinic, Somerset Road, Douglas IM2 5EB

Partnership agreements 1991; balance sheets/profit and loss accounts 1986–; day books 1989–; ledgers 1989–; cash books 1989–; photographs late 1980s.

MILDMAY VETERINARY CENTRE
Winchester, Hampshire

History: This mixed practice was established in 1976.

Records: Mildmay Veterinary Centre, Eastgate Street, Winchester SO23 8DZ

Balance sheets/profit and loss accounts 1976–; client records 1976–.

MILFEDDYGON BODRWNSIWN VETERINARY GROUP
Anglesey, Isle of Anglesey

History: This mixed practice was established in 1910.

Records: Milfeddygon Bodrwnsiwn Veterinary Group, Bodrwnsiwn, Rhosneigr, Anglesey LL63 5SG

Partnership agreements 1985–; balance sheets/profit and loss accounts 1985–; day books 1980–; rota plans, nd; x-rays 1980–; architectural plans 1910.

MILL HOUSE VETERINARY SURGERY AND HOSPITAL
King's Lynn, Norfolk

History: This practice was established by David and Carole Clarke in 1984. An assistant was taken on in 1986 and the practice steadily grew until by 1999 there were seven veterinary surgeons and twelve nurses working at the surgery. The practice was initially located in King St before moving to Tennyson Avenue in 1990. It has remained a small animal practice, although it did provide morbillivirus treatment for seals between 1987 and 1989.

Records: Mill House Veterinary Surgery, 20 Tennyson Avenue, King's Lynn PE30 2QG

Minutes 1986–; balance sheets 1984–; ledgers 1984–; day books 1984–; client records 1989–; press cuttings, advertisements, etc 1984–; title deeds 19th–20th cent; architectural plans 1983–84, 1989–90; salary books 1990–; photographs 1984–.

MORGAN & MCGHEE
Warwick, Warwickshire

History: This practice was established by William Stanley (d 1815), with James Rose, a descendant of a family of Warwickshire farriers, as his assistant. Following Stanley's death, the business was acquired by James Rose and traded as Rose & Stanley. During the 1850s a branch was established at Leamington Spa, Warwickshire. The Warwick practice was sold to Robert Bacon Palmer shortly after his graduation from the Royal Veterinary College, London, in 1906. Palmer traded from The Butts, Warwick, before moving to Stokesleigh, Coton End, Warwick, in 1939. After his death in 1948, the practice was sold to John McGhee and Trevor Morgan who traded as Morgan & McGhee. John McGhee died in 1983 and Trevor Morgan retired in 1987, at which time the practice was sold to Richard Lane and M J Murray.

Veterinary History, no 6, winter 1975–76.

Records (1): Shakespeare Birthplace Trust Records Office, Henley Street, Stratford upon Avon CV37 6QW

Receipted bill from William Stanley to Henry Verney for veterinary medicines 1809 [Ref: DR 98/1654/249]; James Rose, draft conveyance to

John Caleb Adkins of Milcote, gentleman, of nine leys of woodland in Alveston Pastures 1847. [Ref: DR 149/154/180]

Records (2): Warwickshire County Record Office, Priory Park, Cape Road, Warwick CV34 4JS

Settlement re marriage of James Rose and Charlotte Stanley 1820 incl a contract of James Rose as servant to Mrs Stanley 1815 [Ref: CR 556/774/1]; mortgage of a house in the Market Place, Warwick, to James Rose 1835 [Ref: CR 611/165/1]; conveyance of a cottage at Tiddington in Alveston adjoining the turnpike road, from James Rose to Thomas Vincent 1846 [Ref: CR 611/499]; deeds re execution of will of Thomas Wallis incl affidavits by James Rose 1854–55 [Ref: CR 237/360/8; CR 237/368/16; CR 237/369/37]; financial records 1950s–80s; client ledgers 1934–76; practice diaries 1957–85. [Ref: CR 2724]

MOTT CLINIC
Broadclyst, Devon

History: The Mott Clinic was established in 1970 by Dr C J Chesney. The main part of the practice was sold in 1995 but Dr Chesney continues to practise as a veterinary dermatologist.

Records: Mott Clinic, Broadclyst, Exeter EX5 3JH

Balance sheets 1970–; ledgers 1970–; day books 1970–; cash books 1970–; general accounts 1970–; receipts 1970–; invoices 1970–; client records: written records 1970–80, dermatology records 1990–; advertising and promotional leaflets 1990s; architectural plans 1976; salary books 1970– [w]; general correspondence 1970–; notes re history 1970–.

C M NEWMAN MRCVS
Denham Green, Buckinghamshire

History: This mixed practice was established in 1987 by C M Newman.

Records: C M Newman MRCVS, 20 Penn Drive, Denham Green UB9 5JP

Balance sheets/profit and loss accounts 1987–; day books 1987–; ledgers 1987–; cash books 1987–; client records 1987–.

NICOLL & WALTON MsRCVS
London

History: This small animal practice was established in c1920. Nigel Norris bought into David Roberts' practice in 1967 and stayed until his retirement in 1988. In 1998 the practice changed hands again and since then has traded as Nicoll & Walton MsRCVS.

Records: Nicoll & Walton MsRCVS, 496 Hornsey Road, Holloway, London N19 4EF

Partnership agreements 1967–; balance sheets/profit and loss accounts 1967–; day books 1967–; ledgers 1967–; cash books 1967–.

F NIND MRCVS
Currie, Edinburgh

History: This small animal practice was established in 1976.

Records: F Nind MRCVS, 5 Riccarton Mains Road, Currie EH14 5NQ

Balance sheets/profit and loss accounts 1976–; day books 1976– [w]; cash books 1976– [w]; client records 1985–; architectural plans 1976–.

NISBET & HARRIES MsRCVS
Haverfordwest, Pembrokeshire

History: Alister Nisbet graduated from the Glasgow Veterinary College in 1937 and came to Haverfordwest in 1939 or 1940. He was later joined by Griffith Michael Harries, who graduated from the Royal Veterinary College, London, in 1948.

Records: Pembrokeshire Record Office, The Castle, Haverfordwest SA61 2EF
Income and expenditure book 1952–54. [Ref: D/PR/633]

NIXON & MARSHALL MsRCVS
Buckingham, Buckinghamshire

History: This mixed practice was established in 1988.

Records: Nixon & Marshall MsRCVS, Overton, Maids Moreton, Buckingham MK18 1RE

Partnership agreements 1988–; day books 1988–; ledgers 1988–; cash books 1988–; client records 1988–; practice magazines/leaflets 1988–.

F NOBLE & J CARR MsRCVS
Teignmouth, Devon

History: This small animal practice was established in 1974.

Records: F Noble & J Carr MsRCVS, Teign View Veterinary Surgery, Maudlin Drive, Teignmouth TQ14 8RU

Partnership agreements 1997–; balance sheets/profit and loss accounts 1989–; day books 1974– [w]; ledgers 1974– [w]; cash books 1974– [w]; client records 1988–; architectural plans 1996.

OAK BECK VETERINARY CLINIC AND HOSPITAL
Harrogate, North Yorkshire

History: This practice was established by R D Partridge in 1988. In 1992 it became a two-man practice and moved to larger premises in Oak Beck Way, Harrogate. The following year the practice became the first registered veterinary hospital in North Yorkshire. Since 1994 it has also been an approved training centre under the Veterinary Nursing Scheme.

Records: Oak Beck Veterinary Clinic and Hospital, Oak Beck Way, Harrogate HG21 3HU

Minutes 1995–; balance sheets 1988–; ledgers 1988–; day books 1988–; cash books 1988–; general accounts 1988–; receipts 1988–; invoices 1988–; legal papers re bad debt collection 1988–; client records 1988–; recipe books 1988–; prescription books 1988–; advertising and promotional leaflets 1988–; press cuttings 1988–; title deeds, nd; architectural plans 1988–; photographs 1988–; staff registers 1988–; salary books 1988–; pension papers 1988–; general correspondence re practice 1988–.

OAKS VETERINARY CENTRE
Saltcoats, North Ayrshire

History: This mixed practice was established in West Kilbride, North Ayrshire, by James Donaldson (c1875–1954), who qualified from the Glasgow Veterinary College in 1897 and was known to be living in West Kilbride from 1922. He was succeeded in the mid 1950s by Edward (Ted) Holmes, who graduated from the Glasgow Veterinary College in 1940 and was known to be practising at Hillview, Cubrieshaw Street, West Kilbride, in 1952. In 1968 the practice was sold to Gilbert Kennedy. A branch was established in Largs, North Ayrshire, around the same time. The main practice relocated to a purpose built surgery behind Kennedy's house in Caledonia Road, Saltcoats, in 1972, a move largely prompted by the increasing demand for small animal treatment. Melissa Donald joined the practice in 1990 and became a partner in 1993. Following Kennedy's retirement in 1998, the practice was renamed the Oaks Veterinary Centre. It remains on the same site, although the postal address has changed from Caledonia Road to Bute Terrace.

Records: Oaks Veterinary Centre, 7 Bute Terrace, Saltcoats KA21 5BA

Ledgers 1973–80; cash books 1974–78; income/expenditure account 1973–74; summary of income/expenditure 1988–92; summary of income 1991–92; client records 1980s–; papers re Ministry of Agriculture, Fisheries and Food instructions to Local Veterinary Inspectors 1965–73.

OAKS VETERINARY SURGERY
Oldham, Greater Manchester

History: This small animal practice was established in 1982 in a former Victorian mill owner's house and extended in 1999–2000.

Records: Oaks Veterinary Surgery, 56 Manchester Road, Shaw, Oldham OL2 7DE

Balance sheets/profit and loss accounts 1982–.

OATHALL VETERINARY GROUP
Haywards Heath, West Sussex

History: This practice was established in c1904 by Henry Taylor (1870–1954). Taylor, who graduated from the New Veterinary College, Edinburgh, in 1899, based his practice first at Sunnyside, Haywards Heath, then Ormerod House, also in Haywards Heath. Kenneth Stuart, Taylor's son-in-law, took over in c1940 and was in turn succeeded by his son, A N Stuart, in c1976. Since 2000, the practice has traded as the Oathall Veterinary Group.

Records: Oathall Veterinary Group, 30 Oathall Road, Haywards Heath RH16 3EQ

Balance sheets/profit and loss accounts, day books, ledgers, cash books 20th cent; prescription book 1950s; castration records 1920s; architectural plans 1980s; Henry Taylor, certificate of fellowship 1905; Kenneth Stuart, MRCVS certificate 1934; partnership agreement re a practice at 50 Brewer Street, Soho, London 1899.

DR J A O'CONNOR MRCVS
Pembroke, Pembrokeshire

History: This practice was established in 1939 by Peter Drewett who originally came to the area as an assistant to Brychan Jeffries Rees (d 1947), an equine specialist based in Picton Road, Tenby. Until that time no veterinary surgeon had been able to make a living in Pembroke with most of the farm cases being seen by a blacksmith on horseback. The war, however, brought increased agricultural prosperity to the area and by 1945 Drewett had built up an extensive farm practice based at 89 Main Street, Pembroke. In 1955 Gerald Hudson arrived as Drewett's assistant, later buying into the practice and eventually succeeding Drewett as Principal in 1973. By this time the practice had moved to 91 Main Street. Hudson was largely responsible for the opening of two branch surgeries, at Begelly, Pembrokeshire, and 8 Bush Street, Pembroke Dock, although both were closed after Drewett's retirement in 1973. There then followed an unsettled period, with a number of assistants and partners coming and going, until John O'Connor was made a partner in 1983. Branches were opened at Great North Road, Milford Haven, Powys, in 1986 and at Streamline House, Kilgetty, Pembrokeshire, in 1996. The success of the latter reflected the increasing numbers of people retiring with their pets to the Saundersfoot and Tenby areas. By 1990 the main practice had outgrown the premises on Main Street and was moved to 13 East Back, Pembroke.

Records: Dr J A O'Connor MRCVS, 13 East Back, Pembroke SA71 4HL

Partnership agreements 1973, 1979, 1984, 1986; balance sheets 1985–; ledgers 1982–; day books 1992–; cash books 1992–; general accounts 1985–; invoices 1992–; legal papers re mortgage, lease, etc 1990; case history cards [w] 1992–; practice booklet 1993; general correspondence 1982–.

OKEFORD VETERINARY CENTRE
Okehampton, Devon

History: This mixed practice, established during the nineteenth century, moved to School Way, Okehampton, in 1981. The partners in 2000 were R C Young, P T Davies, A J Hill and R R Cunningham. In addition to the main surgery, there is a branch at Chagford, Newton Abbott.

Records: Okeford Veterinary Centre, The Veterinary Clinic, School Way, Okehampton EX20 1EU

Partnership agreements 1974–; balance sheets 1975–; ledgers 1940s; receipts 1962–; client records early 1980s–; architectural plans 1981–.

A F O'MEARA MRCVS
Ewell, Surrey

History: This small animal practice was established in c1947 by a veterinary practitioner called Naylor-Hayes. It was sold to Alistair Macrae in 1977 then to Adrian O'Meara in 1980. Branches were established at Chessington, Greater London, in 1984, Epsom Downs, Surrey, in 1985 and Banstead, Surrey, in 1995.

Records: A F O'Meara MRCVS, North Lodge, 150 Kingston Road, Ewell KT17 2ET

Balance sheets/profit and loss accounts 1980–; day books 1980–; ledgers 1980–; cash books 1980–; client records 1980–; photographs 1980–; architectural plans 1980–.

OUNDLE VETERINARY SURGERY
Oundle, Northamptonshire

History: This mixed practice was established in the early twentieth century.

Records: Oundle Veterinary Surgery, 92 South Road, Oundle, Peterborough PE8 4BP

Partnership agreements, balance sheets/profit and loss accounts, day books, architectural plans 20th cent.

C PAGE MRCVS
Cambridge, Cambridgeshire

History: This small animal practice was established in 1984 by D Shaw and sold to C Page in 1999.

Records: C Page MRCVS, 32 Arbury Road, Cambridge CB4 2JE

Balance sheets/profit and loss accounts 1984–; client records 1984–.

H L PAPWORTH MRCVS
Biggleswade, Bedfordshire

History: This mixed practice was established in 1982 by Helen Papworth and moved to Old Warden, Biggleswade, in 1998.

Records: H L Papworth MRCVS, The Shuttleworth Centre, Old Warden, Biggleswade SG18 9EA

Balance sheets 1982–; ledgers 1982–; day books 1982–; cash books 1982–; general accounts 1982–; receipts 1982–; invoices 1982–; legal papers re purchase of the original building 1982; client records 1982–; architectural plans 1980s–; salary books 1982–.

PARKSIDE VETERINARY GROUP
Dundee

History: This mixed practice was established in c1930. There are two branches in Broughty Ferry, Dundee, at 12 Lawrence Street and 58 Dalhousie Road.

Records: Parkside Veterinary Group, 61 Constitution Road, Dundee DD1 1LA

Partnership agreements 1980–; minutes 1994–; day books 1980–; ledgers 1980–; cash books 1980–; client records 1980–.

PAWS VETERINARY HEALTH CENTRE
Nuneaton, Warwickshire

History: This mixed practice was established in c1910 at 71 Princes Street, Nuneaton. There have been a number of partners through the years, including Henry Arthur Barrett (1862–1952), who graduated from the Edinburgh Veterinary College in 1884, and Walter Henry Newey (1913–75), who graduated from the Royal Veterinary College, London, in 1934. The practice has traded under several names including Barratt, Newey & Peace, Newey & Peace, Peace Windridge, Peace Windridge Smith and Peace Windridge Smith Price Henderson. It moved from Princes Street to Edward Street in 1994.

Records: Paws Veterinary Health Centre, Edward Street, Nuneaton CV11 5RP

Partnership agreements, client records, photographs, architectural plans, practice magazines/leaflets 20th cent.

PENNARD VETERINARY GROUP
Sevenoaks, Kent

History: This practice was established at Pennard House, Sevenoaks, in 1895 by D L Pugh (d 1944), five years after his graduation from the Royal Veterinary College, London. After the First World War, Pugh was joined by his son, Major Leslie Penrhys Pugh, who had graduated from the Royal Veterinary College, London, in 1917. John William Bruford (1903–75) also joined the practice following his graduation from the

Royal Veterinary College, London, in 1926. L P Pugh (d 1983) went on to have a distinguished academic career, culminating in his appointment as Professor of Veterinary Clinical Studies at Cambridge University Veterinary School. He was an active member of the Royal College of Veterinary Surgeons, serving as a Councillor between 1944 and 1965, Vice President in 1955 and 1958 and President from 1956 to 1957. The practice traded as Pugh & Bruford until 1983, after which it was known as the Pennard Veterinary Group. Originally it treated mainly large animals but the growth in demand for small animal healthcare led to a gradual shift in emphasis. While in 1972 the caseload was 60 per cent large animal and 40 per cent small animal, by 2000 95 per cent of the work was small animal. The premises have undergone considerable alteration over the years and branch surgeries were opened at Borough Green, Kent, in 1980 and Allington, Kent, in 1995. Eton Veterinary Hospital, Tonbridge, Kent, was purchased in 1998.

Records: Pennard Veterinary Group, Pennard House, 5 Eardley Road, Sevenoaks TN13 1XY

Partnership agreements 1975–; minutes 1985–; balance sheets/profit and loss accounts 1970–; ledgers 1990s–; cash books 1990s–; client records 1990s–; architectural plans 1970–; practice magazines/leaflets 1996–.

PETCARE ANIMAL CENTRE
London

History: This small animal practice was established in 1985.

Records: Petcare Animal Centre, 146 Goldhawk Road, Shepherds Bush, London W12 8HH

Balance sheets/profit and loss accounts 1985–; day books 1992–; cash books 1991–; client records 1985–; laboratory and x-ray results 1985–.

PETCARE ANIMAL CLINIC
London

History: This small animal practice was established in 1935.

Records: Petcare Animal Clinic, 113 Chiswick High Road, Chiswick, London W4 2EQ

Balance sheets/profit and loss accounts 1984–; photographs 1984–; architectural plans 1984–; practice magazines/leaflets 1984–.

D H PHILLIPS MRCVS
Aberdare, Rhondda Cynon Taff

History: This small animal practice was established in 1960.

Records: D H Phillips MRCVS, 17–18 Dean Street, Aberdare CF44 7BN

Balance sheets/profit and loss accounts 1960–; ledgers 1960–; cash books 1960–; receipts 1960–; client records 1960–; architectural plans 1960–.

PHILLIPS & OSBORN MsRCVS
Ipswich, Suffolk

History: This practice, latterly based at 139 London Road, Ipswich, was established in 1912 and closed in 1978. A branch surgery, established at 83 Queen's Road, Felixstowe, Suffolk, during the 1950s by another Ipswich practice, Castle & Leason, was acquired during the 1960s and later sold to Smith, Ryder Davies & Partners of Woodbridge, Suffolk.

Records: in private ownership of Captain R N Phillips, The Elms, Little Blakenham, Ipswich IP8 4NF

Balance sheets 1947–77; recipe books 1912–77; photographs 20th cent.

PIG DISEASE INFORMATION CENTRE
Cambridge, Cambridgeshire

History: The Pig Disease Information Centre was established as a special project at the University of Cambridge Veterinary School in 1991 following the outbreak of a serious epidemic that killed two million pigs across Europe. Gradually the Centre's remit was broadened to include a wide range of porcine diseases and welfare issues. A lack of public funding led to it becoming an independent company in 1996 and it presently operates as a non-clinical veterinary practice.

Records: Pig Disease Information Centre, 4 New Close Farm Business Park, Bar Road, Cambridge CB3 8DS

Minutes 1996–; balance sheets/profit and loss accounts 1996–; day books 1996–; ledgers 1996–; cash books 1996–; photographs 1991–; architectural plans 1996; practice magazines/leaflets 1991–; papers and publications on pig disease and welfare 1991–.

PINFOLD HOUSE VETERINARY SURGERY
Misterton, Nottinghamshire

History: This practice was originally established as a branch of a practice in Gainsborough, Lincolnshire, before being sold to R W Gibbons in 1978. Gibbons in turn sold the practice to Mrs J F Turner in 1995, at which time the name Pinfold House Veterinary Surgery was adopted. The surgery was expanded in 1976 and 1979 and again during the 1980s and 1990s.

Records: Pinfold House Veterinary Surgery, 4 Church Street, Misterton, Doncaster DN10 4AH

Balance sheets/profit and loss accounts 1978–; photographs 1978–; architectural plans 1970s–.

POLESBURN VETERINARY CENTRE
Ellon, Aberdeenshire

History: This mixed practice was established in 1960.

Records: Polesburn Veterinary Centre, Polesburn, Methlick, Ellon AB41 7DU

Partnership agreements 1982–; balance sheets/profit and loss accounts 1982–; day books 1990–; ledgers 1990–; photographs 1992–; architectural plans 1992–.

A J POOLE MRCVS
Harpenden, Hertfordshire

History: This single-handed small animal practice was established in 1992 by Alistair J Poole.

Records: A J Poole MRCVS, The Veterinary Surgery, 169 Luton Road, Harpenden AL5 3BN

Balance sheets 1992–; ledgers 1992–; day books 1992–; cash books 1992–; general accounts 1992–; receipts 1992–; invoices 1992–; client records 1992–; title deeds 1992–; staff registers 1992–; salary books 1992–.

PRIORS LEAZE VETERINARY CENTRE
Chichester, West Sussex

History: This predominantly small animal practice was established by R W Kynoch in 1983. A branch surgery was opened at Rowland's Castle, Hampshire, in 2001.

Records: Priors Leaze Veterinary Centre, Priors Leaze Lane, Nutbourne, Chichester PO18 8RH

Balance sheets/profit and loss accounts 1983–; bank statements 1983–; day books 1983–85; client records 1989–; architectural plans 1983–.

PRIORY VETERINARY SURGERY
Taunton, Somerset

History: This mixed practice was established in 1978.

Records: Priory Veterinary Surgery, 17 Canon Street, Taunton TA1 1SW

Balance sheets/profit and loss accounts 1978– [w]; day books 1978– [w]; ledgers 1978– [w]; cash books 1978– [w]; client records c1990–; photographs 1978–; architectural plans 1978–; practice diaries 1978–.

S J PRITCHETT MRCVS
Newmilns, East Ayrshire

History: This single-handed practice, seeing mainly small animals, was established in 1981 by S J Pritchett.

Records: S J Pritchett MRCVS, 6 Isles Street, Newmilns KA16 9DP

Balance sheets/profit and loss accounts 1981–; day books 1981–; ledgers 1981–; client records 1981–.

PROSPECT VETERINARY CENTRE
Sowerby Bridge, West Yorkshire

History: This small animal practice was established in 1985 by Chris and Eleanor Dale.

Records: Prospect Veterinary Centre, 1 Wakefield Road, Sowerby Bridge HX6 2AP

Balance sheets/profit and loss accounts 1990–; day books 1985–; ledgers 1985–; client records 1985–; practice magazines/leaflets 1985–.

J S PYBUS MRCVS
Hastings, East Sussex

History: This practice was established in 1943 by a veterinary surgeon from Robertsbridge, East Sussex, and passed through several owners before being acquired by J S Pybus in the 1950s. Latterly it was based at 30 Mount Pleasant Road, Hastings, until its closure following Pybus's retirement in 1998.

Records (1): J S Pybus MRCVS, 30 Mount Pleasant Road, Hastings TN34 3SH

Balance sheets/profit and loss accounts 1951–98; day books 1951, 1992–98; accounts 1951–98.

Records (2): The World of James Herriot, 23 Kirkgate, Thirsk YO7 1PL

J S Pybus, student notes on therapeutics, toxicology and materia medica II 1940.

A G RAFFERTY MRCVS
Grantown on Spey, Highland

History: This mixed practice was established by A G Rafferty in 1991.

Records: A G Rafferty MRCVS, The Veterinary Centre, Forest Road, Grantown on Spey PH26 3JJ

Balance sheets/profit and loss accounts 1991–; day books 1991–; ledgers 1991–; cash books 1991–; client records 1991–; photographs 1991–; practice magazines/leaflets 1996–.

RAINBOW EQUINE CLINIC
Malton, North Yorkshire

History: This practice was established in 1986 by R M Ordidge. An assistant was taken on in 1987 and a partner, I V Pritchard, in 1991.

Records: Rainbow Equine Clinic, Rainbow Farm, Old Malton, Malton YO17 0SG

Partnership agreement 1991; balance sheets 1986–; ledgers 1986–; day books 1986–; cash books 1986–; general accounts 1986–; receipts 1986–; invoices 1986–; case histories 1986–; recipe books 1986–; title deeds 1985; photographs 1986–; architectural plans, nd.

RAWLE & MATTHEWS
Rackenford, Devon

History: According to the 1851 census, Michael Rawle (b c1788) was practising as a 'veterinary surgeon to horses' at Chapelcourt, Rackenford. Next door was a blacksmith's shop run by Thomas Matthews (b c1788), while beyond him lived Aaron Matthews (b c1817), veterinary surgeon. Aaron's son, Frank Rawle Matthews (b c1848), was working as a veterinary practitioner by 1883.

Records: North Devon Record Office, Tuly Street, Barnstaple EX31 1EL

Accounts 1850–63. [Ref: 3058 add 4/23/1–2]

REED, BROWN & CAMERON MsRCVS
St Boswells, Scottish Borders

History: This mixed practice was established by Jim Scott in 1969 and moved to Braeheads Stables, St Boswells, in 1974. After Scott's death in

1976, the practice was sold to his assistant, John Reed. A branch surgery was opened in Jedburgh, Scottish Borders, in 1979. Nigel Brown, who had joined the practice as Reed's assistant in 1976, was made a partner in 1980, while Ewan Cameron arrived as an assistant in 1983 and became a partner in 1987. A fourth veterinary surgeon was employed as an assistant in 1990.

Records: Reed, Brown & Cameron MsRCVS, Braeheads Stables, St Boswells TD6 0AZ

Partnership agreements 1980s; balance sheets/profit and loss accounts 1974–; day books 1974–; ledgers 1974–.

REES & REEVES VETERINARY CENTRE
Warrington

History: This small animal practice was established as the Cinnamon Veterinary Centre in 1984 at 6 Cinnamon Lane, Fearnhead, Warrington. It moved to its present location in 1999 and now trades as the Rees & Reeves Veterinary Centre.

Records: Rees & Reeves Veterinary Centre, 86 Orford Avenue, Warrington WA2 7QQ

Partnership agreements 1984–; balance sheets/profit and loss accounts 1984–; day books 1984–; ledgers 1984–; cash books 1984–; client records 1984–; architectural plans 1984–.

RETFORD POULTRY PARTNERSHIP
Retford, Nottinghamshire

History: This poultry practice was established in 1992.

Records: Retford Poultry Partnership, Unit 5, Stirling Road, West Carr Industrial Estate, Retford DN22 7SN

Balance sheets/profit and loss accounts 1992–; day books 1992–; ledgers 1992–; cash books 1992–; receipts 1992–; client records 1992–; photographs 1992–; practice magazines/leaflets 1992–.

RHODES VETERINARY SURGERY
Northampton, Northamptonshire

History: This small animal practice was established by John Rhodes in 1958.

Records: Rhodes Veterinary Surgery, 95 Queens Park Parade, Northampton NN2 6LR

Partnership agreements, nd; balance sheets/profit and loss accounts 1958–; ledgers 1958–; photographs 1958–; architectural plans 1958–.

PETER ROBINS & ASSOCIATES
Cambridge, Cambridgeshire

History: This practice was established in 1955 by L M Kirkbride. In 1965, Kirkbride entered into partnership with J G Carter and they were joined by P G Robins in 1981. After Carter left in 1983 the practice traded as Kirkbride & Robins until 1988 when it was renamed Peter Robins & Associates. Originally based in King Street, Cambridge, it moved to 12 Willow Walk, Cambridge, in 1962. A branch surgery, opened on Chesterton Road, Cambridge, in 1972 became the sole surgery in 1975. In 1982 the practice moved to Hamilton Road, Cambridge. A branch surgery was established at Chivers Jam Factory Warehouse Yard, Histon, Cambridgeshire, in 1975, moving to Signal Box, Station Yard, Histon, in 1985. Originally a mixed practice, the caseload since 1995 has been exclusively small animal.

Records: Peter Robins & Associates, Midsummer Veterinary Surgery, 25 Hamilton Road, Cambridge CB4 1BP

Partnership agreements 1981–; balance sheets/profit and loss accounts 1973–; day books 1987–; ledgers 1980–; cash books 1980–; architectural plans 1981.

ROSEMULLION VETERINARY PRACTICE
Falmouth, Cornwall

History: This practice is thought to have been established by E R Smythe, who graduated from the Royal Veterinary College, London, in 1885 and was known to be in Falmouth by 1887. From the 1950s the practice traded under the name of Smythe & Turnbull, changing to Turnbull & Roberts in the 1960s, Turnbull in the 1970s and Turnbull, Wilson & Cockerham in the 1980s. It was renamed the Rosemullion Veterinary Practice in 1997.

Records: Rosemullion Veterinary Practice, The Veterinary Centre, 66 Melvill Road, Falmouth TR11 4DD

Partnership agreements 1970s–; minutes 1970s–; balance sheets/profit and loss accounts 1970s–; day books 1970s–; ledgers 1970s–; cash books 1970s–; receipts c1930–40; client records 1990–; architectural plans 1997.

ROSSLYN VETERINARY CENTRE
Linthorpe, Middlesbrough

History: This practice, established by Colin Haith in the mid 1960s, was one of the first to be given hospital status, although this status has since lapsed.

Records: Rosslyn Veterinary Centre, 1 The Crescent, Linthorpe, Middlesbrough TS5 6SD

Partnership agreements 1992–94; balance sheets 1992–; ledgers 1992–; day books 1992–; cash books 1992–; general accounts 1992–; receipts 1992–; invoices 1992–; client records 1992–; press cuttings 1994–95; title deeds 1992; architectural plans 1992–; photographs 1996.

ROWE VETERINARY GROUP
Wotton under Edge, Gloucestershire

History: This practice was established by John F W Rowe at his home in Coombe Mount, Wotton under Edge, in 1948. His wife, Ruth, acted as secretary, receptionist, nurse and book-keeper. The practice grew rapidly, its client base in the early days made up largely of livestock. Small animals were seen at the house at the end of the day. Conditions quickly became cramped, with instruments being boiled on the stovetop while small animal operations were carried out on the kitchen table. In 1951 a much needed extension was added and an assistant taken on. A branch surgery was opened next to the livestock market in Station Road, Yate, Gloucestershire, in 1970. Again, this was primarily aimed at farm animals, although a thirty minute small animal surgery was held each afternoon. A second branch opened in Pullins Green, Thornbury, Gloucestershire, in 1979 and a third at Bradley Stoke, Gloucestershire, in 1991. In 1981, shortly after the death of John Rowe, a new, purpose built veterinary hospital was opened by the Duke of Beaufort. The following year a new partnership was formed between Helen Rowe, Richard Rowe, Philip Marsh and Brian Hildick-Smith, at which time the practice assumed the name Rowe Veterinary Group. Chris Artingstall joined the partnership in 1989. By the time the practice celebrated its golden anniversary in 1998, there were a total of five partners, eight assistant veterinary surgeons, a practice manager, sixteen veterinary nurses, a laboratory technician, thirteen receptionists and two office staff working across four surgeries, providing treatment for farm animals, horses and small animals. Since 1989 the practice has also treated animals at Bristol Zoo. A new veterinary hospital was opened at Bradley Stoke in 1999.

Records: Rowe Veterinary Group, The Veterinary Hospital, Bradley Green, Wotton under Edge GL12 7PP

Day books 1948–51; ledger 1948–54; cash book 1948–54; expenditure book 1948–54; account book for drugs purchased c1974–80; notebook of prices 1970s, incl a scale of fees for veterinary treatment of prison livestock and dogs 1974–75; letters, etc re opening of veterinary hospital 1981; papers re anniversary 1998; photographs: John Rowe 1943, opening of hospital 1981, staff, surgery, equipment 1980s; practice leaflets re openings, services, etc 1970s–90s; certificates: John Rowe, MRCVS 1944, hospital status 1981; John Rowe's college notebooks on jurisprudence, hygiene & nutrition c1942; *Sport and Country Magazine* incl illustrated article on Royal Veterinary College, London's evacuation to Goring, Oxfordshire, and Streatley, West Berkshire 1943; press cuttings 1970s–90s.

RYELANDS VETERINARY CLINIC

Leominster, Herefordshire

History: This practice is thought to have been established by Walter Vernon Tuson (d 1919), a graduate in 1877 from the Royal Veterinary College, London, who was known to be practising in Leominster in 1878. Based for a time at The Tan House, 71 Bridge Street, Leominster, the practice had moved by 1895 to Westbury House, Bridge Street, and moved again in c1900 to Marsh House, Bridge Street. By 1922, John Wallace Peatt had replaced Tuson at the practice. Peatt was succeeded by his son, John, in c1937 and the practice moved to 126a South Street. Alfred Malcolm Barker joined as an assistant in 1954 and entered into partnership with John Peatt in 1961, after which the practice traded as Peatt & Barker. In 1963, the practice moved to converted stables at Ryelands Road, Leominster. John Peatt retired in 1965 and in 1967 a new partnership was formed between Barker and Brian Jones, which traded as Barker & Jones. Andrew Praill joined the partnership in 1978 after which the practice became known as Barker Jones & Praill. Following Jones's death in 1984, the practice traded as Barker & Praill until Barker's retirement in 1991, at which time it was renamed Ryelands Veterinary Clinic.

Records: in private ownership of A M Barker, Plovers, Norton, Bromyard HR7 4PJ

Partnership agreements 1968, 1978, 1988.

ST IVES VETERINARY SURGERY
St Ives, Cornwall

History: This small animal practice was established in c1981 by Shaun Halbert and sold to Stephen Putnam in 1990.

Records: St Ives Veterinary Surgery, Trenwith Lane, St Ives TR26 1DA

Balance sheets 1990–; day books 1990–; general accounts 1990–; receipts 1990–; invoices 1990–; legal papers re purchase of practice 1990; client records 1990–; practice newsletters 1990–; photographs 1990–; general correspondence 1990–.

H L L & L P SALMON MsRCVS
Cheriton Bishop, Devon

History: This mixed practice was established in 1970 and sold to H L L and L P Salmon in 1985.

Records: H L L & L P Salmon MsRCVS, Wolfgar Veterinary Surgery, Wolfgar, Cheriton Bishop, Exeter EX6 6HH

Balance sheets 1985–; ledgers 1985–; day books 1985–; cash books 1985–; general accounts 1985–; receipts 1985–; invoices 1985–; legal papers 1985–; client records 1985–; practice information leaflets 1990s; press cuttings 1985–; architectural plans, nd; photographs 1985–; staff registers 1985–; salary books 1985–; general correspondence 1985–.

SANDON VETERINARY GROUP
Edgbaston, Birmingham

Records: Sandon Veterinary Group, 373 Hagley Road, Edgbaston, Birmingham B17 8DL

Ledgers 1988–; day books 1989–; invoices 1988–; salary books 1972–.

SENLAC VETERINARY CENTRE
Battle, East Sussex

History: This practice was established in 1932 at the Old House, 89 Battle High Street, Battle, by Simon Percival Hendry (1901–59), who had graduated from the Royal (Dick) Veterinary College, Edinburgh, in 1926. William Hopkin (1922–83), who graduated from the Royal Veterinary College, London, in 1946 and came to the practice as an assistant in 1948 was made a partner in 1954. Although originally a large animal practice, the small animal caseload has been gradually developed. Norman Nuthall joined the practice in 1968 and entered into partnership with Hopkins in 1974, after which the practice traded as Hopkins & Nuthall. Following Hopkins's death the practice moved to Mount Street, Battle, and was renamed the Senlac Veterinary Centre. Peter Clark and Tim Pitman became partners in 1989, and joint partners in 1999 following Norman Nuthall's retirement. A branch surgery was opened at Robertsbridge, East Sussex, in 1993.

Records: Senlac Veterinary Centre, Mount Street, Battle TN33 0EG

Partnership agreements 1999; minutes 1990–; balance sheets/profit and loss accounts 1930s–; day books 1930s– [w]; ledgers 1930s– [w]; cash books 1930s– [w]; client records 1980s–; architectural plans 1980s–.

SHIPLEY & SON
Great Yarmouth, Norfolk

History: William Shipley (d 1877) graduated from the Royal Veterinary College, London, in 1823 and established his practice in North Walsham, Norfolk, shortly afterwards. His son, also named William Shipley (b 1833), graduated in 1856 and practised at Southtown, Great Yarmouth. He in turn was joined by his son, another William Shipley (d 1917), who qualified in 1888, after which the practice traded as Shipley & Son. In 1884 William Shipley II built a veterinary infirmary at Steam Mill Lane, Southtown, Great Yarmouth. Steam Mill Lane was renamed Southtown Road in 1913, and later changed its name once again to Bridge Street. In 1915, a fourth William Shipley, son of William Shipley III, joined the practice. His son, also William Shipley, graduated in 1952 and went on to acquire the business. He continued to practise, under the name Shipley & Son, until 1992 when the business was sold to his partners, J A Higginson and R M Livie. In 1998 they were still practising at the old veterinary infirmary, the street name having changed again to Bridgefoot, and the practice name to Haven Veterinary Surgeons.

T Ashbourne, *Shipley & Son* (unpublished typescript, Great Yarmouth, 1989).

Records: in private ownership of Mr W Shipley, Beechcroft, 28 Southtown, Great Yarmouth NR31 0DT

Invoice 1880; reference from William Shipley re Richard Hughes for post of hospital surgeon at Royal Veterinary College, London 1881; description of premises, nd; correspondence: Professor Cotchin, Royal Veterinary College, London 1984–85, Linda Warden, Royal Veterinary College, London, re research into first William Shipley 1984, Terry Ashbourne of the Great Yarmouth & District Archaeological Society re practice history 1989, Department for Culture, Media and Sport re listing of veterinary infirmary 1998; photographs of grooms, blacksmiths and veterinary helpers 1907; practice history 1989.

SHIRES VETERINARY PRACTICE
Eccleshall, Staffordshire

History: This practice was established in 1920.

Records: Shires Veterinary Practice, Stone Road, Eccleshall ST21 6DL

Partnership agreements 1976–; balance sheets/profit and loss accounts 1968–; architectural plans 1982–.

SHUTTLEWORTH VETERINARY GROUP
Rawtenstall, Lancashire

History: This practice was established in 1979 by L A Gould and relocated in 1980. It traded as Gould & Shuttleworth from 1983 to 1988, then as the Shuttleworth Veterinary Group between 1988 and 1989, Shuttleworth & Bonham from 1989 to 1995 and the Shuttleworth Veterinary Group once more from 1995. There were branch surgeries at Haslingden, Lancashire, between 1982 and 1990 and at Bacup, Lancashire, from 1986 to 1996. A third branch at Ramsbottam, Greater Manchester, established in 1983, was sold to Mr Bonham in 1995.

Records: Shuttleworth Veterinary Group, 209A Bacup Road, Rawtenstall BB4 7PA

Partnership agreement 1983; balance sheets/profit and loss accounts 1983– [w].

SINCLAIR & WIGHT
Thirsk, North Yorkshire

History: William Howard Wood (d 1944) graduated from the New Veterinary College, Edinburgh, in 1883 and initially worked in Middleton, Manchester, before arriving in Thirsk in c1890. It is possible that he worked alongside Thomas M Harrison, who graduated from the Royal Veterinary College, London, in 1847 and was known to be in Thirsk by 1854, and took over the practice entirely following Harrison's death in 1892. On his retirement in 1940, Wood sold the practice to Donald Sinclair, who had been working as an Assistant Veterinary Officer in Wakefield, West Yorkshire, since his graduation from the Royal (Dick) Veterinary College, Edinburgh, in 1933. Sinclair was joined shortly afterwards by Alf Wight (1916–95), who had graduated from the Glasgow Veterinary College in 1939. Initially a salaried partner, Wight became a full partner in 1949. Sinclair & Wight's practice covered a large area, and during the 1940s and 1950s saw mainly agricultural cases. The first in a series of assistants was employed in 1951. Sinclair also acted as the attending veterinary surgeon for Thirsk racecourse. In common with many other practices, small animal work became an increasingly important part of the practice's finances from the 1960s. Wight's son, Jim, joined the practice as an assistant in 1967 and became a salaried partner in 1976. In 1970, the first of Alf Wight's books based on life at the practice, *If Only They Could Talk*, written under the pseudonym James Herriot, was published. Its success led to a series of sequels as well as two films and the long running British Broadcasting Corporation television series *All Creatures Great and Small*. Alf Wight retired from the practice in 1989, followed by Donald Sinclair in 1991. In 1996 the practice moved from its original home at 23 Kirkgate, Thirsk, to new premises on the outskirts of the town. A museum devoted to the life of Alf Wight and the history of veterinary medicine was opened at 23 Kirkgate in 1999.

J Wight, *The Real James Herriot: the authorised biography* (London, 1999).

Records: The World of James Herriot, 23 Kirkgate, Thirsk YO7 1PL

Partnership agreement 1948; day books 1941–42, 1968–89; diaries 1987–88; ledgers c1971–73; payment books 1968–90; receipt books 1964–90; cash payment books 1982–89; receipts issued for work done c1970s–90s; invoices 1984–89; list of debtors and creditors 1976; feed prescriptions book 1987–88; drug order book 1964–72; petty cash books 1967–90; wages books 1961–90; daily cash book 1980–81; tuberculin testing records 1956–c1988; Ministry of Agriculture, Fisheries and Food instructions to Local Veterinary Inspectors re Tuberculosis (Attested Herds) Scheme 1947; Alf Wight: Royal College of Veterinary Surgeons certificate of general education 1933, diary 1934; Jim Wight: student notebooks for anatomy, histology and surgery 1960s, notes re poultry legislation 1980s; photographs, literary manuscripts, etc 1940s–90s.

SMITH & CLARE VETERINARY SURGEONS
Pontypool, Torfaen

History: This practice was established in 1989 at 71 The Highway, New Inn, Pontypool, by R V Smith. V A Clare, who had worked at the practice as a part time assistant since 1989, became a full partner in 1996. The following year the main practice moved to Fairwater Square, Fairwater, Cwmbran, leaving the Pontypool premises as a branch surgery performing only minor surgical procedures. Although the practice originally saw both small animal and equine cases, by 1999 it was exclusively small animal.

Records: Smith & Clare Veterinary Surgeons, 71 The Highway, New Inn, Pontypool NP4 0PN

Balance sheets/profit and loss accounts 1989–; client records 1989–; architectural plans 1989–.

SOUTHILL VETERINARY GROUP

Sherborne, Dorset

History: This mixed practice was established by S F More in 1982. It was sold to the Southill Veterinary Group, Wincanton, Somerset, in 1998 and relocated later that same year.

Records: Southill Veterinary Group, Bazzleways, Milborne Port, Sherborne DT9 5EH

Balance sheets/profit and loss accounts 1982–; day books 1982–; ledgers 1982–; cash books 1982–; receipts 1982–; client records 1982–; photographs 1982–.

SPARROW FAMILY

Rochford, Essex

History: In about 1870 Henry Frost Sparrow was taken into the employment of Edward Simmons, a veterinary surgeon based in Market Square, Rochford. It is thought that Sparrow went on to acquire the practice following Simmons's death in c1897. Shortly afterwards Sparrow moved to Fir Tree House, East Street, Rochford, before moving again in 1911 to purpose built premises at 19 East Street, Rochford. That same year Sparrow was joined by his son, Harry Davis Sparrow (1890–1959), who had just graduated from the Royal Veterinary College, London. Leonard Harry Sparrow (1915–66) graduated from the Royal Veterinary College, London, in 1941 and, after serving in the Royal Army Veterinary Corps during the Second World War, entered into practice with his father and grandfather.

Records: Essex Record Office, Southend Branch, Central Library, Victoria Avenue, Southend on Sea SS2 6EX. Not all documents are stored on-site. Researchers are therefore advised to contact the office in advance of any visit.

Bills, receipts, correspondence and general papers 1933, 1938–44 [w], nd; papers and correspondence of Harry Davis Sparrow 1912–48; list of existing veterinary practitioners incl entries for Sparrow family c1881; Henry Frost Sparrow's obituary 1953; photograph of Harry Davis Sparrow at work in his office c1955; family tree and notes re Sparrow family, nd. [Ref: D/DS 279, 425; TS/515]

SPIRE VETERINARY GROUP
Chesterfield, Derbyshire

History: This mixed practice was established in 1985 by I K Taylor.

Records: Spire Veterinary Group, 161–163 St Johns Road, Newbold, Chesterfield S41 8PE

Balance sheets/profit and loss accounts 1985–; day books 1985– [w]; ledgers 1985–; cash books 1985–; client records 1985– [w].

STANHOPE VETERINARY CENTRE
Strood, Medway

History: This small animal practice was acquired by the present owners in 1987.

Records: Stanhope Veterinary Centre, 29 Stanhope Road, Strood ME2 3EJ

Balance sheets/profit and loss accounts 1987–; day books 1987–; ledgers 1987–; cash books 1987–; architectural plans 1987–.

STATION ROAD VETERINARY CLINIC
Lower Weston, Bath & North East Somerset

History: This mixed practice has been trading since at least the 1970s.

Records: Station Road Veterinary Clinic, 15A–15B Station Road, Lower Weston, Bath BA1 3DX

Partnership agreements 1987; balance sheets/profit and loss accounts 1977–; architectural plans 1973; practice magazines 1990–91.

STATION VETERINARY CLINIC

Stocksfield, Northumberland

History: This small animal practice was established in 1987 by Miss C F Shield.

Records: Station Veterinary Clinic, Station Yard, Main Road, Stocksfield NE43 7HJ

Balance sheets/profit and loss accounts 1987–; day books 1987–; ledgers 1987–; cash books 1987–; client records 1987–; architectural plans 1987–; practice magazines/leaflets 1987–.

S T STEAD MRCVS

Ancomb, York

History: This small animal practice was established in 1985.

Records: S T Stead MRCVS, 2 Plantation Drive, Ancomb, York YO2 6AG

Balance sheets/profit and loss accounts 1985–; day books 1985–; ledgers 1985–; cash books 1985–; client records 1985–; photographs 1985–; architectural plans 1985–; practice magazines/leaflets 1985–.

T & R STEELE MsRCVS

Lisburn, Co Antrim

History: This practice was established in 1946. Since 1970 its caseload has been exclusively equine. The present partners, Robert and Thomas Steele, qualified in 1975 and 1993 respectively.

Records: T & R Steele MsRCVS, Beechfield, 185 Moira Road, Lisburn BT28 1JA

Day books 1946–; ledgers 1946–.

STEVENSON, LARWOOD & KENNEDY MsRCVS
Dereham, Norfolk

History: This mixed practice was established in 1960.

Records: Stevenson, Larwood & Kennedy MsRCVS, 7 Wellington Road, Dereham NR19 2BP

Day books 1960–; ledgers 1960–; receipts 1960–; architectural plans 1960–; radiographs 1960–.

STOKESLEY VETERINARY PRACTICE
Stokesley, Middlesbrough

History: This practice was established in c1900 and took the name of Stokesley Veterinary Practice following the dissolution of the Miller & Whimster partnership in 1999.

Records: Stokesley Veterinary Practice, Bridge View, Stokesley, Middlesbrough TS9 5DP

Partnership agreements 1975–99; balance sheets/profit and loss accounts 1975–; day books 1990–; ledgers 1990–; cash books 1990–; receipts 1990–; client records 1990–.

STONE LION VETERINARY CENTRE
London

History: This small animal practice dates back to c1900.

Records: Stone Lion Veterinary Centre, 41 High Street, Wimbledon, London SW19 5AV

Poison registers c1900; notes re practice history 1995.

STONEHENGE VETERINARY HOSPITAL
Salisbury, Wiltshire

History: This small animal practice was established by C Irvine-Smith in 1991.

Records: Stonehenge Veterinary Hospital, Larkhill Road, Durrington, Salisbury SP4 8DP

Photographs 1990s; architectural plans 1990s.

THE STORRAR PRACTICE

Chester, Cheshire

History: James Storrar (c1823–1906) qualified from the Edinburgh Veterinary College in 1848. After practising and farming in his native Aberdeenshire for a time he moved to Chester in 1865 and quickly built up an extensive practice based in Frodsham Street. Storrar also acted as the Local Veterinary Inspector for both the County of Cheshire and the City of Chester and as Veterinary Officer for the Earl of Chester's Yeomanry Cavalry. He became a Fellow of the Royal College of Veterinary Surgeons in 1886 and sat on the Council. His son, also called James Storrar (1858–1923), joined his father after graduating from the Glasgow Veterinary College in 1879, the two men trading as James Storrar & Son. Shortly afterwards the practice moved to premises in Newgate Street, Chester, with stables and a forge attached. The younger Storrar continued the practice from the time of his father's death until his own death in 1923, after which it passed to his two sons, another James (1893–1972), and Eric Rowe Dutton Storrar (1898–1961), who graduated from Liverpool Veterinary College in 1924 and 1926 respectively. Eric was eventually bought out by his brother in 1927. In 1938, the Newgate Street premises were sold and the business moved to Park Cottage, Duke Street, Chester. James's son, James Eric Storrar, joined him at the practice in 1952 and they traded as James Storrar & Son until the senior man's retirement in 1971, after which James Eric Storrar formed a partnership with Peter Wrather and the practice was renamed Storrar & Wrather. In 1979 James Eric Storrar's son, James Andrew Storrar, joined the practice. James Eric Storrar retired in 1990, and the practice briefly traded as Wrather & Storrar until Peter Wrather's retirement in 1992, after which it was renamed The Storrar Practice. James Andrew Storrar's son, James, graduated from Liverpool University's veterinary school in 2001.

Obituary of James Storrar, *The Veterinary Record*, vol 18, no 935, 9 June 1906.

Records (1): The Storrar Practice, Park Cottage, Duke Street, Chester CH1 1RP

Day books 1970, 1980, 1991; cash books 1952–69; payment receipts: Mr Dutton, Saighton 1896, Mr Venables, butcher, for castration of two cats 1932; letter from Walter Conway & Co, practice accountants 1923; advertisement re establishment of practice in Chester 1865; Newgate Street premises: deed of assignment and release, Eric Rowe Dutton Storrar to James Storrar 1927, mortgage agreement 1927, title deeds 1930, contract and conditions of sale 1938, correspondence with J H Dickson, Town Clerk 1930, 1937–38, correspondence with R G Williams, solicitor, re sale 1938–39; certificate of registration of business name James Storrar & Son 1927; certificates: James Storrar II, Fellowship of the Royal College of Veterinary Surgeons 1886, James Storrar II, Membership of Glasgow Veterinary Medical Society, nd, James Eric Storrar, Royal (Dick) Veterinary College, Edinburgh 1952, James Eric Storrar, MRCVS 1952, James Storrar V, Bachelor of Science, University of Saskatchewan, Canada 1978; letters: James Storrar II to James Storrar I stating that he has passed qualifying examinations 1879, R G Williams, solicitor 1927, Joseph Hankness to James Eric Storrar re his military successes during Second World War 1945; photographs: James Storrar II late 1880s, James Storrar II outside Newgate Street premises early 20th cent, James Storrar III on a horse c1930s, James Storrar III calving a cow and treating a cow for milk fever early 1950s, family friend inside Newgate Street premises c1950s, Storrar family early 20th cent; booklet giving names of Local Veterinary Inspectors including James Storrar & Son early 20th cent; observations on health of farm livestock by John Butler, nd; poems re veterinary surgeons by Edward Carter, proprietor of Collinge Pedigree Poultry Farm, Backford, near Chester.

Records (2): Cheshire and Chester Archives and Local Studies, Cheshire Record Office, Duke Street, Chester CH1 1RL

Diary and almanac containing accounts and memoranda re hire of horses, etc 1898. [Ref: CR 139]

STRACHAN, TYSON & HAMILTON MsRCVS

Newcastle upon Tyne, Tyne & Wear

History: This mixed practice was established by D Strachan in 1970. D Tyson joined in 1971 and P Hamilton in 1974.

Records: Strachan, Tyson & Hamilton MsRCVS, 36 Heaton Road, Newcastle upon Tyne NE6 1SD

Balance sheets/profit and loss accounts 1970–; day books 1970– [w].

STRAMONGATE VETERINARY CENTRE
Kendal, Cumbria

History: This practice, acquired by Ralph Rimmer in c1885, had surgeries in both Kendal and Milnthorpe, Cumbria. It has occupied its present site since 1905.

Records (1): Cumbria Record Office, County Offices, Kendal LA9 4RQ

Nominal ledger 1885; ledgers 1887–88, 1895–1901; day book 1893–96; sale book of farming stock at Yew Tree, Underbarrow, for Handley Robinson c1957; invoice from T D Carlisle, saddle maker 1906; remittance advice from Lieutenant Colonel Sandys 1895; diaries 1895, 1905; letter from F J Crossfield requesting to be taken on as a pupil 1895. [Ref: WDB 93/1–10]

Records (2): Stramongate Veterinary Centre, 52 Stramongate, Kendal LA9 4BD

Practice meetings notebook 1970–; formulary 1936.

SUMMERFIELD LODGE VETERINARY SURGERY
Tunbridge Wells, Kent

History: This small animal practice was established in 1988 by J D Hayward.

Records: Summerfield Lodge Veterinary Surgery, 24 Eridge Road, Tunbridge Wells TN4 8HJ

Balance sheets/profit and loss accounts 1988–; ledgers 1988–; cash books 1988–; client records 1988–; architectural plans 1988–.

SWANSPOOL VETERINARY CLINIC
Wellingborough, Northamptonshire

History: This practice was established at 1 London Road, Wellingborough, in c1848 by Benjamin Blunsom Aris. In 1879 Joseph

Bainbridge, who had just graduated from the Royal Veterinary College, London, was taken on as Aris's assistant. Bainbridge later married Aris's younger daughter and left to set up his own practice nearby, which traded until about 1920. Following Aris's death in c1900 the practice at London Road was sold to a Mr Parks. In 1939, Parks sold out to a Mr Dunlop, already the owner of a practice in Northampton. During the Second World War the Wellingborough practice flourished as the pressure to produce more food increased. In 1946 Dunlop sold his Northampton practice but retained the Wellingborough one. After a brief partnership with a Mr Ellis, Dunlop entered into partnership with John Edwards in 1947. In 1961, J R Bainbridge, Aris's great-grandson, joined the practice. By 1999 there were six veterinary surgeons and an auxiliary team of eight. Recent years have seen a decline in the livestock side of the practice but a corresponding growth in demand for small animal and equine care, the latter a reflection of the growing numbers of leisure and competition horses in the area. The premises, originally a house with stables and coach house nearby, have been extensively altered through the years.

Records (1): in private ownership of J R Bainbridge, Byre Cottage, Wilby, Wellingborough

B B Aris's recipe book, incl occasional letters 1879–nd; B B Aris' visiting card c1880; Mr Parks' recipe book 1940s; annual balance sheets 1965–; account book 1968–72; day books 1944–62 [w]; visits book c1950s; J Bainbridge's notebooks on horse dentition 1879, nd; printed copy of paper given by Brigadier Peatt at British Veterinary Association conference on 'Acid Firing for Sprain of the Flexer Tendons in the Horse' 1956; *Veterinary Pharmacoepia* 1874; *Mackey's Veterinary Diary and Almanac* (blank) 1899; pencil drawing of 1 London Road 19th cent; photograph of horse slaughterer [Chettle?] with horse and cart 19th cent; photographs: surgery (interior and exterior), veterinary surgeons at work, alteration works 1970–; articles of partnership 1964; draft of partnership deed 1994; assistantship agreement 1967; Joseph Bainbridge's will 1928; John Edwards's college notes on medicine and hygiene c1938; John Edwards's retirement: final accounts and related letters, list of clients who subscribed to his present 1972.

Records (2): Swanspool Veterinary Clinic, 1 London Road, Wellingborough NN8 2BT

MRCVS certificates: B B Aris 1848, J Bainbridge 1879; clinical notes 1990–; accounts 1990–; drugs supplied 1990–; message books 1990–; operations books 1990–; x-rays 1990–; plans of alterations 1972, 1990s.

TEMPLE END VETERINARY SURGEONS
High Wycombe, Buckinghamshire

History: This mixed practice was established in c1900.

Records: Temple End Veterinary Surgeons, 43 Temple End, High Wycombe HP13 5DN

Day book 1947.

DAVID M TERRY MRCVS
Hull, Kingston upon Hull

History: This practice was established at 2 Park Street, Hull, by Arthur Weighton in 1898. Weighton, who had graduated from the Edinburgh Veterinary College in 1896, ran the practice with various assistants before being joined by his son, John, following the latter's qualification in 1925. John Weighton continued the practice after his father's death in 1956. David Terry, who joined as an assistant in 1972, became a partner in 1977 and took over the practice after John Weighton's retirement in 1983. 1 Park Street was purchased in 1963. The practice was extended in 1973 and extensively remodelled in 1992. Originally a large animal practice, it is now almost exclusively small animal. A branch surgery was opened at 16–18 New Village Road, Cottingham, East Riding, in c1985.

Records: David M Terry MRCVS, 1–2 Park Street, Anlaby Road, Hull HU3 2JF

Balance sheets/profit and loss accounts 1948–54, 1956–71; cash book 1974–83, incorporating wages book 1975–97; summary account book 1974–96; statement of trust accounts prepared by the executors of Arthur Weighton 1956; David Terry's contract as assistant to John Weighton (copy) 1972; letters and plans re purchase and repairs to 1 Park Street 1963; letters, application forms and plans re proposed extension of 2 Park Street 1973; plans and papers re maintenance of surgeries and extension of 1–2 Park Street 1988–94.

THAMES WOOD VETERINARY CLINIC

Swindon

History: This small animal practice was established in 1986 by Nicholas Hartley and his wife.

Records: Thames Wood Veterinary Clinic, 62–64 Purton Road, Swindon SN2 2LZ

Balance sheets 1986–; ledgers 1986–; day books 1986–; cash books 1986–; general accounts 1986–; receipts 1986–; invoices 1986–; client records 1993–; press cuttings 1986–; photographs 1986–; salary books 1993–.

TODDBROOK VETERINARY CENTRE

Harlow, Essex

History: This practice was established in 1976. Although predominantly a large animal practice at first, its small animal facilities have been significantly increased in recent years.

Records: Toddbrook Veterinary Centre, Toddbrook House, Harberts Road, Harlow CM19 4DT

Balance sheets/profit and loss accounts 1976–; day books 1976–; ledgers 1976–; student notes, nd.

TOFT LODGE VETERINARY CENTRE

Easingwold, North Yorkshire

History: This practice was established in 1969 by R W Turnbull and N J Jackson, although Jackson became sole owner following Turnbull's retirement in 1989. The caseload was originally 70 per cent large animal and 30 per cent small animal but by 2000, when the practice changed its name to the Toft Lodge Veterinary Centre, the division was 60 large animal and 40 per cent small animal.

Records: Toft Lodge Veterinary Centre, Toft Lodge, Raskelf Road, Easingwold YO6 3LA

Client records 1970s–; architectural plans, nd.

TOWCESTER VETERINARY CENTRE
Towcester, Northamptonshire

History: This practice was established in 1905 at Carlisle House, 23 Park Street, Towcester, by David Forwell (c1876–1955). Forwell, who had graduated from the Glasgow Veterinary College in 1899 and had served in the Army Veterinary Corps during the First World War, also acted as a Local Veterinary Inspector for the Ministry of Agriculture and Fisheries. During the 1930s, as his health began to fail, Forwell was joined by Arthur William Gill (1896–1947). Gill, who graduated from the Royal (Dick) Veterinary College, Edinburgh, in 1934, gradually took over the practice, working from his home at The Mount (now Mandalay House), Daventry Road, Towcester. After Gill's death in 1947, the practice was run for two years by various locums on behalf of his widow before being sold to Alistair Andrew Lamont. In 1951, Lamont moved the practice to Chattrice House, 114 Brackley Road, Towcester. The garage was converted into a dispensary and a new surgery created at the back of the building. Mrs Lamont acted as book-keeper, receptionist and nurse. Charles Wright, who had been an assistant at the practice between 1950 and 1953, returned as a partner in 1953 after a brief time in Stafford. In 1954 the practice moved once again, this time to 57 Brackley Road, Towcester. Soon afterwards, William Blackwell's practice at Well House, Wood Burcote, Northamptonshire, was bought out, leaving Lamont & Wright as the only practice in the Towcester area. The partnership of Lamont & Wright continued until Lamont's retirement in 1980. The following year Peter Saunders and Robert Lloyd Francis joined the partnership, becoming joint partners in their own right after Wright's retirement in 1986. In 1970 a plot of land was bought on Wood Burcote Road from the estate of Lady Florence Hesketh, and a purpose built veterinary surgery constructed, complete with waiting room, reception room, dispensary, consulting room and operating room. There was further expansion in 1983 with the addition of a single storey extension, which provided further office space, recovery kennels, a preparation room and a small animal operating theatre. The site was expanded again in 1991, with the enlargement of the reception and waiting areas and the addition of four consulting rooms, reflecting the increase in small animal work. At the same time, a larger dispensary, two operating theatres, a large preparation room, a reception area, increased kennelling facilities and living accommodation for veterinary nurses were added. The facilities were increased again in 1998, resulting in a total of six consulting rooms, one of which was used mainly by a veterinary nurse for pet health counsellor work. Sue Jennings became a partner in 1994 and Helen Pope in 1995. Robert Francis died in 1996 and Andrew Hayes became a partner in 1999. By 2000 the practice caseload was 70 per cent small animal, 25 per cent large animal and 5 per cent equine.

Records: Towcester Veterinary Centre, The Veterinary Surgery, Burcote Road, Towcester NN12 6JW

Partnership agreements 1982–; large animal client records c1989–; photographs 20th cent; architectural plans c1970–; client list compiled from William Blackwell's ledger 1942–50.

TOWN & COUNTRY VETERINARY GROUP
Banchory, Aberdeenshire

History: This practice was established in 1987 with C E Wiper as its Principal. Three neighbouring practices were purchased in 1990 and another branch opened in 1997. The majority of the caseload is small animal, with some equine and large animal work.

Records: Town & Country Veterinary Group, 14a Bridge Street, Banchory AB31 5SX

Balance sheets/profit and loss accounts 1987–; day books 1987–; ledgers 1987–; cash books 1987–.

TOWNLEY, CARTER & DAVIES MsRCVS
Shaftesbury, Dorset

History: This mixed practice was probably established by Edward Langford (c1859–1949), who graduated from the Royal Veterinary College, London, in 1881 and was known to be practising at Park House, Langfords Lane, Shaftesbury, shortly afterwards. Benjamin Donald Bassett, who qualified in Dublin in 1940, came to Shaftesbury in 1946 and was living at Park House by 1948. In 1955, Bassett sold the practice to J H Cripps. R H Hiscock joined the practice in 1956, while D B Townley joined in 1964 and was made a partner in 1969. Cripps retired in 1985 and Hiscock in 1989, while A P Carter and L R Davies joined in 1981 and 1989 respectively. The practice moved to new premises at Longmead in 1979.

Records: Townley, Carter & Davies MsRCVS, Longmead Veterinary Practice, Longmead, Shaftesbury SP7 8PL

Partnership agreements 1969–; balance sheets/profit and loss accounts 1966–; day books 1974–; photographs of original surgery 1960s; architectural plans for new premises 1979.

PETER TURNBULL MRCVS
Midsomer Norton, Bath & North East Somerset

History: Peter Turnbull qualified in 1940 and shortly afterwards was appointed assistant to Mr Haydon of Midsomer Norton and Radstock. In 1943 Turnbull set up in business for himself, renting a room above the garage on the High Street, Midsomer Norton, and holding additional surgeries at nearby Radstock and Poulton. His wife, Joyce, acted as book-keeper, nurse and dispenser. An assistant was appointed in c1945 and the practice moved to Stone's Cross House, Midsomer Norton, around the same time. The branches at Radstock and Poulton were later closed but another branch was opened at Bear Flat, Wells Road, Bath, in c1955, which held surgeries every evening and on Saturdays. On his retirement in 1968, Turnbull sold the practice to his assistant, David Walker, who, in partnership with Mr Zagni, moved the practice to North Road, Midsomer Norton.

Records: Somerset Archive and Record Service, Obridge Road, Taunton TA2 7PU

Patient history cards, incl details of treatments and charges c1950–68; day books 1950–68; boarding kennels ledger 1964–67; account book 1954–57; client payments book 1966–67; outgoing receipt books 1947–55; bills/receipts for pharmaceutical products, surgical instruments, etc 1940s–68; recipe book c1940; tuberculin testing records 1950s–60s; bank statements, etc 1950s–60s; catalogues for Arnold & Sons, Hauptman and others 1940s–60s; J Wy Williams, University of Liverpool, pathology slides 1932.

TURNER, HOUSE & FLAVIN MsRCVS
Crediton, Devon

History: This practice was established at the end of the Second World War and run single-handedly by several veterinary surgeons until a partnership was formed in 1955. C B Turner bought the practice in 1961. By the time he retired in 1989 there were four veterinary surgeons at the practice, seeing mainly agricultural cases.

C B Turner, monograph re clinical research carried out whilst engaged in general practice 1957–61.

Records: In private ownership of C B Turner, Nymet Hill, Nymet Rowland, Crediton EX17 6QX

Day book 1966.

UPLANDS WAY VETERINARY GROUP

Diss, Norfolk

History: This mixed practice was established in c1942 by the forming of a partnership between Claud Horace Downe (1910–80) and William Frederick Loveless (1901–66). Prior to this, each had practised separately in the town, Loveless at Millfield House from 1933, and Downe in Denmark Street. Over the years there have been several changes in partners and a change in premises.

Records: Uplands Way Veterinary Group, Uplands Way, Diss IP22 3DF

Partnership agreements 1969–; balance sheets/profit and loss accounts 1969–; day books 1969–; ledgers 1969–; cash books 1969–.

THE VALE VETERINARY GROUP

Stourport on Severn, Worcestershire

History: John Alexander McLauchlan (d 1973) graduated from the Royal (Dick) Veterinary College, Edinburgh, in 1906 and set up his practice in the village of Clows Top, Worcestershire, shortly afterwards. After serving in the Army Veterinary Corps during the First World War, McLauchlan bought Foxall Farm, Great Witley, Worcestershire, with the help of a loan from Herbert Banks, a local auctioneer, and resumed his practice. A broken arm, however, limited McLauchlan's ability to work and the loan was called in, forcing him to sell the farm and move to Stourport on Severn. When finances improved he purchased Kingston House, Areley Kings, Stourport on Severn, along with 3.5 acres of land, 2 loose boxes and various other outbuildings. One loose box became a surgery while the other buildings were converted into boarding kennels. The surgery had no electricity or water and heating was provided by a paraffin stove. In 1947 McLauchlan sold the practice to Roger Henry Vale, who had seen practice with him as a student, and moved to Putney where he helped out at the Royal Society for the Prevention of Cruelty to Animals' clinic. After two and half years of single practice in Stourport on Severn, Vale took on his first assistant, who later became a partner. Two other partners were to join the practice, which then traded as Vale & Partners. By 1999, the practice employed five veterinary surgeons and had moved to purpose built premises.

Records: The Vale Veterinary Group, Areley Kings, Stourport on Severn DY13 0TH

Partnership agreement 1946; prescription books 1947–72; general correspondence 1947–60; video transferred from 8mm film photographed in a mixed practice 1959–60.

THE VETERINARY CENTRE
Hotwells, Bristol

History: This practice was established in 1986 by Judith Glushanok.

Records: The Veterinary Centre, 4 Merchants Road, Hotwells, Bristol BS8 4RD

Balance sheets 1986–; ledgers 1986–; day books 1986–; cash books 1986–; general accounts 1986–; invoices 1986–; client records 1986–.

VETERINARY CENTRE
Usk, Monmouthshire

History: This mixed practice was established in 1947 and moved twice, in 1955 and 1978. By 1999 there were nine veterinary surgeons employed at the centre.

Records: Veterinary Centre, Porth-y-Carne Street, Usk NP5 1RZ

Partnership agreements 1979–; day books 1960s–; architectural plans 1978–.

THE VETERINARY CLINIC
Birmingham, West Midlands

History: This small animal practice was established in 1972 and sold to Douglas Cave in 2000.

Records: The Veterinary Clinic, 749 Chester Road, Erdington, Birmingham B24 0BY

Minutes 1972–; balance sheets/profit and loss accounts 1972–; day books 1972–; ledgers 1972–; cash books 1972–; receipts 1972–; client records 1972–; architectural plans 1972–.

THE VETERINARY SURGERY
Marske by the Sea, Redcar & Cleveland

History: This equine and small animal practice was established in 1976 and sold to James Haddow in 1989.

Records: The Veterinary Surgery, 45 High Street, Marske by the Sea, Redcar TS11 6JQ

Balance sheets/profit and loss accounts 1989–; day books 1989–; client records 1976–; photographs 1988–; practice magazines/leaflets 1990s.

F J WADSWORTH VETERINARY CENTRE
Ballasalla, Isle of Man

History: In 1982 Frank J Wadsworth was asked to open a small animal surgery and hospital in the southern part of the Isle of Man, having previously run a similar practice in London for thirty seven years. He remained the surgery's Principal until his retirement in 2000.

Records: F J Wadsworth Veterinary Centre, The Sycamores, Douglas Road, Ballasalla IM9 2DN

Balance sheets 1992–; ledgers 1992–; journals 1992–; cash books 1992–; general accounts 1992–; receipts 1992–; invoices 1992–; papers re house purchase insurance 1982; papers re Veterinary Defence Society Ltd 1982–; client records 1982–; title deeds 1985; staff registers 1998–; salary books 1998; pension papers 1992; general correspondence 1982–; notes re practice history 1982–.

WAKERLEY & SPEED MsRCVS
Dronfield, Derbyshire

History: This practice was established at 1 Holborn Avenue, Dronfield, in 1973 by Mr Burley and sold to Mr and Mrs Ross two years later. In 1976 Mrs L J Ross took over the practice entirely. Julie Wakerley joined as an assistant in 1987 and became a partner in 1993. Following Mrs Ross's retirement in 2000, Wakerley entered into a new partnership with Mr Speed, after which the practice traded as Wakerley & Speed. The practice also used a converted ambulance as a mobile surgery, allowing it to offer veterinary services to a number of mining villages in the surrounding area. This service was replaced in 1999 by the opening of a branch surgery at Killamarsh, Derbyshire.

Records: Wakerley & Speed MsRCVS, 1 Holborn Avenue, Dronfield S18 2NA

Statements of accounts 1979–80, 1987–92; ledgers 1987, 1989, 1991; accounts, etc 1986–87, 1989–92; salary sheets 1986–87; photographs: building of extension 1980, animals, staff, mobile surgery, etc 1970s–; architectural plans and related papers re extension 1980.

WALKER, GLANVILL & RICHARDS
Hook Norton, Oxfordshire

History: The origins of this practice date back to nineteenth century Long Compton, Warwickshire, where generations of Walkers acted as farriers, horse doctors, castrators, tail dockers and herbalists. The choice of Long Compton was a shrewd one, marking as it did the halfway point on the main coaching route from London to Birmingham via Oxford. At one time the village boasted four coaching inns. The introduction of the railway created further traffic, since cattle and sheep bought cheaply in Wales were brought to Moreton in the Marsh station, unloaded, and driven along the toll road through Long Compton to Banbury where they were sold to the wealthier eastern side of the county. By the end of the Second World War, there were three members of the Walker family practising in the area: William James Walker (1877–1946) and his sons Joseph John (Jack) (1911–88) and Alfred William (1903–96). The two latter signed the supplementary register as veterinary practitioners in 1948. In 1949, Jack Walker moved the practice to Burmington, Warwickshire, where he continued to specialise in the treatment of horses and cattle. In 1981, Jack's son, John Alan Walker, moved the practice once again, this time to Sibford Road in Hook Norton, Oxfordshire. At first it operated from a garage as a solo practice, but grew rapidly and was granted hospital status in 1984. By 1999 there were eight veterinary surgeons at the practice, working alongside five veterinary nurses and eleven auxiliary staff, providing comprehensive small and large animal and equine care. Two branch surgeries were opened at Charlbury, Oxfordshire, and Shipston on Stour, Warwickshire.

V Porter, 'Of Farriers and Cow Doctors', *Tales of the Old Country Vets* (Newton Abbott, 1995).

Records: Walker, Glanvill & Richards, Sibford Road, Hook Norton, Banbury OX15 5JZ

Advertising card for W J Walker & Sons c1930; W J Walker's recipe book c1930; misc recipes belonging to W J Walker c1930s; itemised quarterly account from W J Walker to Mr Joe Hands of Shipston on Stour 1936; J J Walker's recipe book, being a list of cattle medicines, liniments, ointments and antiseptics c1950; Wyleys Ltd, analytical and operative chemists, Coventry: analytical report re angleberry paint 1938, catalogue of animal preparations, veterinary instruments, etc c1930s; Leonard Smith & Co (branch of A S Price & Co Ltd) veterinary chemists of Birmingham, catalogue of preparations, oils, etc 1951; transcript on calving from *A Living from the Land*, a British Broadcasting Corporation broadcast of 11 October 1956; correspondence re orders for preparations from J M Loveridge plc, manufacturing chemists, incl recipes 1980s; photographs of W J Walker, J J Walker, J A Walker, W J Walker's father, J J Walker swimming horses in the canal by Deddington, and various unidentified c1900–80.

WARBRECK VETERINARY CENTRE
Liverpool, Merseyside

History: This small animal practice, established by Ted Wescott, was sold to B G McVey in 1990.

Records: Warbreck Veterinary Centre, 11 Warbreck Road, Orrell Park, Liverpool L9 8EE

Balance sheets/profit and loss accounts 1990–; day books 1990–; ledgers 1990–; cash books 1990–; client records 1990–; architectural plans 1990–; practice magazines/leaflets 1990–.

WARREN HOUSE VETERINARY SURGERY

Rochester, Medway

History: This practice was established in 1982 by A Piercy as a single-handed small animal practice. Branches were opened in Walderslade Road, Chatham, Medway, in 1985, Christmas Lane, High Halstow, Medway, in 1993 and Lordswood, Medway, in 1995. By 2000 the practice employed ten veterinary surgeons.

Records: Warren House Veterinary Surgery, Anchor Road, Rochester ME1 2PR

Partnership agreements 1980s–; balance sheets 1982–; ledgers 1982–; day books 1982–; cash books 1982–; general accounts 1982–; receipts 1982–; client records 1982–; press cuttings 1980s–90s; title deeds, nd; architectural plans, nd; general correspondence 1982–; photographs 1980s–.

WATERLOO HOUSE VETERINARY SURGERY

Swadlincote, Derbyshire

History: This practice was established by S J McKay in 1977 and expanded rapidly to become a three-vet practice within eighteen months.

Records: Waterloo House Veterinary Surgery, 49 West Street, Swadlincote DE11 9DN

Balance sheets 1977–; ledgers 1977–; day books 1977–.

WAY & LEE MsRCVS

Lincoln, Lincolnshire

History: This practice was established at 43 Friars Lane, Lincoln, in 1893 by Charles Hartley (c1856–1915), who had qualified from the Royal Veterinary College, London, in 1883. On his arrival, Hartley greatly extended the premises by adding a large two storey stable block. Hartley's son, also Charles, graduated from the Royal Veterinary College, London, in 1907 and worked at the practice until his sudden death at an Army Remount parade in 1930. In 1933 the practice was leased by Hartley's widow to Major Arthur Norman Foster (c1882–1941), who had graduated from the Royal Veterinary College, London, in 1903. Three years later Foster's son Charles (1902–78), a 1925 graduate from the Royal (Dick) Veterinary College, Edinburgh, joined the practice. In 1965 the latter entered into partnership with Colin Sutherland (b 1940). A new partnership was formed between Sutherland and Edward Way in 1981, with Martyn Lee becoming a third partner in 1989. Following Sutherland's resignation in 1993 the partnership was renamed Way & Lee. Originally a mixed practice, it became exclusively small animal in 1999. A branch at Bassingham, Lincolnshire, was disbanded in 1985 and replaced with a branch surgery at Birchwood, Lincolnshire.

Records: Way & Lee MsRCVS, 43 Friars Lane, Lincoln LN2 5AL

Partnership agreements 1981–; balance sheets/profit and loss accounts late 1980s–; day books mid 1980s–; ledgers mid 1980s–; cash books mid 1980s–; client records early 1980s–; architectural plans mid 1980s–.

WELL ANIMAL CLINIC
London

History: This small animal practice was established in 1945 by Dr Eugen Kaufman (1894–1967), who had graduated from the Royal Veterinary College, London, in 1937. In 1963 Kaufman sold the practice to J Abraham, who entered into partnership with Bryan Down in 1981. The partnership ended in 1993.

Records: Well Animal Clinic, 292 West End Lane, Hampstead, London NW6 1LN

Partnership agreements 1981; balance sheets/profit and loss accounts 1989–; day books 1989–; ledgers 1989–; client records c1989–.

C J WELLS MRCVS
Seaford, East Sussex

History: This small animal practice was established in the mid 1960s.

Records: C J Wells MRCVS, 37 Stafford Road, Seaford BN25 1UE

Partnership agreements 1994; balance sheets/profit and loss accounts 1980s–; day books 1980s–; ledgers 1980s–; cash books 1980s–; architectural plans 1980s–.

WENDOVER HEIGHTS VETERINARY CENTRE

Aylesbury, Buckinghamshire

History: This mixed practice was established in 1965 by John Parker and moved to Tring Road in 1991. By 1999 it employed nine veterinary surgeons and a consultant.

Records: Wendover Heights Veterinary Centre, 1 Tring Road, Halton, Aylesbury HP22 5PN

Partnership agreements, minutes, balance sheets, ledgers, day books, recipe books, photographs 20th cent.

WEST FARM VETERINARY CLINIC

Cowbridge, Vale of Glamorgan

History: This practice was established in 1984 by J H H James as a single-handed mixed practice. The following year it became a two-man practice and continued to grow steadily, moving to larger premises in 1988, 1992 and 1999. By 1995 the demand for agricultural work had largely disappeared and the practice's caseload was made up of 70 per cent small animal, 25 per cent equine and 5 per cent other animals. A third veterinary surgeon joined the practice in 1999.

Records: West Farm Veterinary Clinic, North Road, Cowbridge CF71 7DF

Balance sheets 1984–; ledgers 1984–; day books 1984–; cash books 1984–; general accounts 1984–; practice brochure, nd; architectural plans 1988, 1992, 1999.

WHARFE VETERINARY GROUP
Haslemere, Surrey

History: This small animal practice was established in 1989, although the building was first used as a veterinary surgery in the late 1930s or early 1940s. In 1992 the group bought out a neighbouring practice owned by Colin Gray.

Records: Wharfe Veterinary Group, Crofts Veterinary Surgery, Petworth Road, Haslemere GU27 2HR

Partnership agreements 1982–; minutes 1992–; balance sheets/profit and loss accounts 1982–; client records c1970s–; radiographs and radiograph exposure book, nd.

P E G WHEELER MRCVS
Sudbury, Suffolk

History: This single-handed small animal practice was established in 1982 by P E G Wheeler.

Records: P E G Wheeler MRCVS, Gentrys, Little Henny, Sudbury CO10 7NG

Balance sheets/profit and loss accounts 1982–; day books 1982– [w]; financial analysis books 1990–; cash books 1990–; receipts 1990–; client records 1982–.

A J WHITE MRCVS
Penwortham, Lancashire

History: This mixed practice was established in Penwortham in 1928 and moved to 32 New Lane in 1981.

Records: A J White MRCVS, The Beeches, 32 New Lane, Penwortham, Preston PR1 9JJ

Partnership agreements 1992; day books 1981–.

WHITEFORD, RAMSAY & HERD MsRCVS
Perth, Perth & Kinross

History: This mixed practice was established in c1940 by R R Macrae. It has since traded as R R Macrae & Partners (incorporating R R Macrae, J W Taylor and J Strachan), Taylor, Whiteford & Ramsay and, most recently, as Whiteford, Ramsay & Herd.

Records: Whiteford, Ramsay & Herd MsRCVS, 26 Kinnoull Causeway, Perth PH2 8HQ

Day books 1979–; client records 1979–.

WHITEGATES VETERINARY SURGERY
Washingborough, Lincolnshire

History: This mixed practice was established in 1984.

Records: Whitegates Veterinary Surgery, 3 Main Road, Washingborough LN4 1AT

Partnership agreements 1992; balance sheets/profit and loss accounts 1984–; day books 1984–; client records 1984–.

WILDBORE VETERINARY GROUP
Worksop, Nottinghamshire

History: This practice was established in c1885 by Captain Harry Moore (d 1933). Moore, who qualified from the Royal Veterinary College, London, in 1877, ran the practice single-handedly until 1901, when he was joined by Thomas Bowett. Bowett took over the practice after Moore's retirement in 1925 and was later joined by his son, John, who became the senior partner in the early 1940s and remained at the practice until his retirement in 1964. J G S Wildbore joined the practice as a new graduate in 1945.

Records: Wildbore Veterinary Group, 5 Newcastle Street, Worksop J80 2AB

Recipe books 20th cent.

WILKINS & PARTNERS
Chard, Somerset

History: This mixed practice was established in 1902.

Records: Wilkins & Partners, Glynswood Veterinary Centre, Furnham Road, Chard TA20 1AF

Partnership agreements 20th cent; balance sheets/profit and loss accounts 1950–; day books 1950–; ledgers 1950–; client records 1950–.

WILLETT HOUSE VETERINARY SURGEONS
Staines, Surrey

History: This practice grew out of a forge established by John Willett in 1862. Willett's son, Albert, was admitted to the Royal College of Veterinary Surgeons' supplementary register as a veterinary practitioner in 1881 and later passed the practice on to his two sons, F W and A E Willett. The last Willett, Reginald Albert, retired in 1963. In 1976 the practice moved from Staines High Street to Kingston Road.

Records: Willett House Veterinary Surgeons, Willett House, 138 Kingston Road, Staines TW18 1BL

Partnership agreements, ledgers, day books, client records, title deeds, architectural plans, photographs 20th cent.

WILLOW LODGE VETERINARY CENTRE
Leatherhead, Surrey

History: This practice was established by Peter A Culpin in 1979. Originally based at 7 Corfe Close, Ashtead, Surrey, the practice moved to Willow Lodge, 173 Barnet Wood Lane, Ashtead, in 1982 and then to 291 Kingston Road, Leatherhead, in 1984. In January 2000 it was sold to the David Callaghan Partnership, a large Surrey-based veterinary group with branches in Fetcham, Woking, St Johns, Knaphill, Guildford, Shalford, East Horsley and Badshot Lea.

Records: Willow Lodge Veterinary Centre, 291 Kingston Road, Leatherhead KT22 7PJ

Client records 1991–; photographs c1980–.

M B WILSON MRCVS
London

History: This single-handed small animal practice was established in 1986 by M B Wilson.

Records: M B Wilson MRCVS, Rosemary Avenue Veterinary Clinic, Rosemary Avenue, Enfield, London EN2 0SR

Balance sheets/profit and loss accounts 1986–; ledgers 1986–; architectural plans 1986–.

SAMUEL WILSON
Liverpool, Merseyside

History: Samuel Wilson, who qualified from the Royal Veterinary College, London, in 1818, practised as a blacksmith and veterinary surgeon in Liverpool between at least 1839 and 1849. From 1845, he traded from premises in Williamson Street, Liverpool.

Records: National Museums and Galleries on Merseyside, Merseyside Maritime Museum, Albert Dock, Liverpool L3 4AQ

Bank book 1837–46; shoeing account for Joseph Mosscrop 1846; receipts and bills, nd; apprenticeship indentures: John Sefton 1839, Joseph Burrows 1844, Patrick Hardiman 1848; apprenticeship indenture between Thomas Houghton and James Hambles 1842; lease re Williamson Street 1840; memorandum granting lease of Williamson Street property to Samuel Wilson 1845; rent book 1844–48; inventory, nd; correspondence 1848–49, nd. [Ref: DX/251]

JAMIE WINSTONE MRCVS
Burton upon Trent, Staffordshire

History: This small animal practice was established in 1989.

Records: Jamie Winstone MRCVS, 30 Horninglow Road North, Horninglow, Burton upon Trent DE13 0SL

Balance sheets/profit and loss accounts 1989–; day books 1989–; ledgers 1989–; cash books 1989–; client records 1989–; practice magazines/leaflets 1989– [w].

WITHY GROVE VETERINARY CLINIC
Preston, Lancashire

History: This small animal practice was established in 1984 by M E Clarke.

Records: Withy Grove Veterinary Clinic, 39 Station Road, Bamber Bridge, Preston PR5 6QR

Balance sheets/profit and loss accounts 1990–.

WOODHORN VETERINARY CENTRE
Chichester, West Sussex

History: This farm animal and game bird practice was established in 1969 by Ian Hutchinson. Based originally at The Causeway, Arundel, West Sussex, it moved to Oving, Chichester, in 1998. A partnership was formed between Paul J Crossman and Keith Baxter in 1999, after which the practice traded as the Woodhorn Veterinary Centre.

Records: Woodhorn Veterinary Centre, Oving, Chichester PO20 9BX

Partnership agreements 1979; balance sheets/profit and loss accounts 1966–; day books 1969–.

WOODLANDS VETERINARY CLINIC
Cheltenham, Gloucestershire

History: This practice was established in 1992 by M J S Daly. G Simpson became a partner in 1998 and two full time assistants and one part time assistant were employed shortly afterwards. The practice sees mainly small animal and equine cases, although its avian and exotic work is expanding. It also offers acupuncture treatments. In 2000 the practice was named Veterinary Practice of the Year.

Records: Woodlands Veterinary Clinic, Salisbury Avenue, Cheltenham GL51 3GA

Partnership agreements 1998; balance sheets 1992–; ledgers 1992–; day books 1992–; cash books 1992–; general accounts 1992–; receipts 1992–; invoices 1992–; clinical records 1992–; title deeds 1992; salary books 1992–; pension papers 1992–; photographs 1992.

YEW TREE VETERINARY CENTRE
Cranleigh, Surrey

History: This practice was established in 1974 by Richard Hankinson. C D Culley joined as an assistant in 1995 and became a partner in 1998.

Records: Yew Tree Veterinary Centre, Horsham Road, Cranleigh GU6 8DP

Balance sheets 1974–; ledgers 1974–; receipts 1974–; invoices 1974–; legal papers re lease 1974–; client records 1974–; architectural plans, nd.

M O YOUNG MRCVS
Penicuik, Midlothian

History: This mixed practice was established in 1979.

Records: M O Young MRCVS, 16 Carnethy Avenue, Penicuik EH26 8AR

Day books 1979–; ledgers 1979–; cash books 1979–; client records 1979–; photographs 1979–; practice magazines/leaflets 1979– [w].

List of records of individuals

EMMANUEL CIPRIAN AMOROSO
London

History: Emmanuel Ciprian Amoroso, veterinary physiologist (1901–82), studied medicine at University College, Dublin, graduating in 1929 with the highest marks ever awarded to a student in the final examinations. A travelling studentship in 1930 enabled him to study in Berlin and Freiburg, after which he undertook a PhD at University College, London. In 1934, Amoroso was appointed senior assistant in charge of histology and embryology at the Royal Veterinary College, London. In 1948 he became Professor of Physiology at the University of London, then Professor of Veterinary Physiology from 1950. Between 1956 and 1963 Amoroso also acted as the Privy Council's representative to the Houghton Poultry Research Station. Following his retirement in 1968, the University of London conferred the title of Emeritus Professor upon him, while the Royal Veterinary College, London, made him a fellow. During the 1970s Amoroso held a series of visiting professorships in the US, Chile, Australia, Canada and Nairobi, and lectured extensively across the world. In addition, he was appointed Special Professor to the Department of Physiology and Environmental Studies at Nottingham University in 1973, and worked at the Institute of Animal Physiology, Cambridge. He was also elected a Fellow of the Royal Society in 1957, the Royal College of Surgeons in 1960, the Royal College of Obstetricians and Gynaecologists in 1965, the Royal College of Physicians in 1966 and the Royal College of Pathologists in 1973. Other honours included a CBE in 1969, the Trinity Cross in 1977 and honorary associateship of the Royal College of Veterinary Surgeons in 1959. In 1988, a new award for outstanding veterinary preclinical research was designated the Amoroso Award. Although his research interests included cancer and the seried veins in the giraffe's neck, Amoroso's speciality was reproductive biology, particularly the structure and function of the placenta. Publications included a chapter on placentation in the 3rd edition of Marshall's *Physiology of Reproduction* (1952), *The Physiology of the Domestic Fowl* (1965), *Protein Utilization by Poultry* (1967) and *Reproductions in the Female Mammal* (1967).

Records: Archives and Manuscripts, Wellcome Library for the History and Understanding of Medicine, 183 Euston Road, London NW1 2BE

Correspondence re: Trinidad and Tobago, honours and awards, Cayman Turtle Farm, general 1970s; lecture/address notes 1970s; misc notes, reprints 1970s; papers re Royal Society 1960s; photographs 1970s. [Ref: PP/AMO]

ROBERT STARMER AUDAS
Sudan

History: Robert Starmer Audas, veterinary surgeon (d 1965), served with the Egyptian Army Camel Corps in Sudan between 1909 and 1911 before taking up an appointment as veterinary inspector to the Sudanese government in 1912, a post he held until 1935.

Records: Archives and Special Collections, Durham University Library, Palace Green Section, Durham DH1 3RN

Memoirs of service in Sudan 1965; photograph 1962; slides, mainly of game 1920s.

WILLIAM HENRY BRADLEY
London

History: William Henry Bradley BA, DM, FRCP (1898–1975) was Resident Medical Officer at Downside School, Bath, from 1925 until the 1930s. In 1939 he joined the Ministry of Health as Medical Officer in the Epidemiology Section and went on to become Senior Medical Officer in 1946 and Principal Medical Officer in 1956. Bradley retired in 1963.

Records: Archives and Manuscripts, Wellcome Library for the History and Understanding of Medicine, 183 Euston Road, London NW1 2BE

Myxomatosis advisory committee papers 1954–57. [Ref: PP/JRH/B.66–69]

MARY BRANCKER
Tamworth, Staffordshire

History: Mary Brancker (b 1914) graduated from the Royal Veterinary College, London, in 1937. Shortly afterwards she became an assistant at Henry William (Harry) Steele-Bodger's surgery in Tamworth,

Staffordshire, and went on to become a partner in 1944. Following Steele-Bodger's death in 1952 the practice, which by then included surgeries in Lichfield, Staffordshire, and Sutton Coldfield, West Midlands, was divided between Mary Brancker and Steele-Bodger's sons Alasdair and Michael. Alasdair and Michael assumed control of the Lichfield and Tamworth surgeries respectively, while Mary took charge of the Sutton Coldfield surgery. In addition to her general practice work, Mary Brancker conducted research into poultry farming, fish breeding and fish health, and served on the advisory committee of the White Fish Authority. She was also an active member of the National Federation of Zoological Gardens of Great Britain and Ireland, and veterinary surgeon on call at her local zoo. In 1967 Brancker became the first woman to be appointed President of the British Veterinary Association. This proved to be a challenging presidency, coinciding as it did with an outbreak of foot-and-mouth disease in Britain. Mary Brancker retired from practice in 1983 but retained an active interest in veterinary medicine, carrying out research into invertebrates and acting as an inspector of zoos. She was awarded an OBE in 1969 and a CBE in 2000.

V Porter, 'Chickens, Chimps and Halibut, Mary Brancker OBE', *Tales of the Old Country Vets* (Newton Abbott, 1995).

Records: in private ownership of Miss Mary Brancker, 38 Streetly Lane, Sutton Coldfield B74 4TU

Correspondence: Nuffield Foundation re application of science to development of fish farming 1973, Emrys Jones of the Ministry of Agriculture, Fisheries and Food re organisation of fish farming trip 1973, National Federation of Zoological Gardens of Great Britain and Ireland awarding life membership 1986; Society of Veterinary Practitioners committee of veterinary education, memorandum, nd; memorandum re proposed further participation of the universities in veterinary education, nd; photographs: celebration of 50th anniversary of graduation 1987, Royal Veterinary College, London, dinner c1990s; press cuttings re foot-and-mouth crisis 1968.

DAVID BRUCE
Malta, Africa, England

History: David Bruce (1855–1931) was educated at the University of Edinburgh, graduating MB, CM in 1881. In 1883 he entered the Army Medical School and was posted to Malta the following year. There his studies into the pathological and bacteriological aspects of a fever then prevalent on the island led him to identify the organism responsible, which he called micrococcus melitensis, later renamed brucella melitensis. Bruce left Malta in 1888 and the following year was appointed Assistant Professor of Pathology at the Army Medical School, Netley, Hampshire. After five years he was posted overseas again, this time to Natal, where his investigations into a disease decimating the local animal population enabled him to identify the organism later known as Trypanosoma brucei in the bloodstream of infected animals. Although he returned to England in 1901, by 1903 Bruce was back in Africa, seconded by the War Office to continue his investigations into sleeping sickness, this time in Uganda. Bruce was able through his own research and that of others to conclude that trypanosomiasis was transmitted by the tsetse fly. Further postings followed, to Malta, Uganda and Nyasaland. During the First World War, Bruce was based at the Royal Army Medical College, where his research interests included trench fever and tetanus. David Bruce retired in 1919. Among the honours conferred upon him were Fellowship of the Royal Society in 1899, CBE in 1905, a knighthood in 1908 and KCB in 1918.

A J Duggan, 'Bruce and the African Trypanosomes', *American Journal of Tropical Medicine and Hygiene*, September 1977; B Mathews, 'A Detective of the Mystery Microbe', *Outward Bound*, August 1921.

Records: Archives and Manuscripts, Wellcome Library for the History and Understanding of Medicine, 183 Euston Road, London NW1 2BE

Experiment notebooks re research into anthrax, rabies and nagana 1893–96; reports, lectures and press cuttings re trypanosomiasis 1903–25; notes re sleeping sickness 1899–1910; announcement of Theiler's discovery of Trypanosoma theileri with note and drawing 1902; correspondence with Royal Society of Tropical Medicine and Hygiene 1906–07, 1929; correspondence with British scientists in Uganda re sleeping sickness 1903–07; photographs and reports re nagana in Zululand 1894–1903; photographs of insects and skin eruptions 1911–12; illustrations of trypanosomes 1908–13. [Ref: WTI/RST/C.5, G.18–20, G.24–37; Royal Army Medical Corps Muniment Collection]

WILLIAM ANDREW CARTWRIGHT
Whitchurch, Shropshire

History: William Andrew Cartwright MRCVS, FRCVS (1801–82) qualified from the Royal Veterinary College, London, in 1840 and afterwards practised in Whitchurch, Shropshire.

Records: Manchester Central Library, Local Studies Unit, St Peter's Square, Manchester M2 5PD

Correspondence with veterinary surgeons re professional matters, especially treatment of horses and articles for *The Veterinarian* 1822–54; will 1865; extract from baptism register 1802; notes re family history, nd. [Ref: O6/3/1–6; O6/5/1; O6/6/1]

WELDON DALRYMPLE-CHAMPNEYS
London

History: Weldon Dalrymple-Champneys, Bart (1892–1980) was educated at Oriel College, Oxford, before taking up an appointment as Assistant Medical Officer of Health at Willesden in 1927. He became Deputy Chief Medical Officer of Health in 1940, a post he held until his retirement in 1956. Dalrymple-Champneys additionally held several Presidencies at the Royal Society of Medicine, namely Epidemiology and Public Health (1943–45), Comparative Medicine (1954–55) and the History of Medicine (1957–59). He was also Vice President Emeritus at the Royal Society of Health, a Fellow of the Royal Veterinary College, London, and a member of the Animal Health Trust's Council. Particular interests included brucellosis and bovine tuberculosis, reflected by his chairmanship of the Joint Food and Agriculture Organisation and World Health Organisation Expert Panel on Brucellosis. Publications included *Undulant Fever* (1929), *Bovine TB in Man, with Special Reference to Infection by Milk* (1931), *The Supervision of Milk Pasteurising Plants* (1935), *Undulant Fever, a Neglected Problem* (1950) and *Brucella Infection and Undulant Fever in Man* (1960) as well as numerous articles for scientific journals.

Records: Archives and Manuscripts, Wellcome Library for the History and Understanding of Medicine, 183 Euston Road, London NW1 2BE

Certificate of fellowship of Royal Veterinary College, London 1973; lectures on laboratory tests in brucellosis to Laboratory Section of

American Public Health Association 1950; lecture to Royal Veterinary College, London, students 1957; presidential address to the Veterinary Hygiene Section of the Royal Society of Health's Congress 1960; papers re brucellosis 1933–56; correspondence with J T Edwards re cattle testing station, Pirbright, Surrey, nd; reports of the Joint Food and Agriculture Organisation and World Health Organisation Expert Panel on Brucellosis 1951–53; programme of fourth Inter-American Brucellosis Congress 1957; photographs of World Health Organisation Veterinary Public Health Group, Geneva 1955; leaflet and circular letter re veterinary education 1980. [Ref: GC/139/D.9–10, E.13, F.17, 24, 26, H.4/1–4, I/4–5, 9–10; PP/JRH/D.17–19]

COLIN DAVENPORT
France, India, England

History: Colin Davenport (d 1973) graduated from the Royal Veterinary College, London, in 1913 and was immediately commissioned as a Lieutenant in the Army Veterinary Corps, rising to the rank of Major by 1927. During the First World War he served in France and was based at no 8 field veterinary hospital during 1917–18 before becoming second in command at no 7 field veterinary hospital for 1918–19. He later served in India and was known to be at Mukhtesar in 1920 and Meerut in 1922. In 1924 the Royal College of Veterinary Surgeons awarded him a fellowship. In 1937 Davenport bought a practice in Christchurch, Dorset, basing himself first at Magnolia House before moving to Brockhills House, New Milton, Hampshire, in 1939.

Records: The Army Medical Services Museum, Keogh Barracks, Ash Vale, Aldershot GU12 5RQ

War diary, incl intelligence summary, reports and correspondence 1919; war diary 1923; private diaries: at no 8 field veterinary hospital 1917–18, at no 7 field veterinary hospital 1918–19; notes on bacteriology, vaccine therapy and serum therapy at Mukhtesar 1920; report on anti-rinderpest inoculation, India 1921; record of all Army Veterinary Corps officers and men who served in no 9 mobile veterinary section 1914–19; personal letters 1914–19; misc concert programmes, Christmas cards, etc 1914–19; commissions: Lieutenant 1913, Major 1927; notification of OBE 1920; speech on departure from Veterinary Club, Jhansi, India, nd. [Ref: Boxes 4, 5, 18, 21]

FITZ-PATRICK EASSIE
British Salonica, South Africa, Macedonia

History: Brigadier General Fitz-Patrick Eassie (c1859–1943), graduated from the Royal Veterinary College, London, in 1885 and entered the Army Veterinary Corps shortly afterwards. He was known to be in Dublin from 1920.

Records: The Army Medical Services Museum, Keogh Barracks, Ash Vale, Aldershot GU12 5RQ

War diary 1919; record of service 1899–1938; report on manpower in the British Salonica Force 1917; notes on horse management and lectures on horse breeding 1929; misc papers incl lecture notes 1938; plan of arrangements, nd; album of photographs, reports, press cuttings re South African War 1899–1901; photographs incl field veterinary hospitals, in Macedonia nd. [Ref: Box 6]

CHARLES ARTHUR LOVATT EVANS
London

History: Charles Arthur Lovatt Evans (1884–1968), physiologist, graduated as an external student from London University in 1910 before taking up the Sharpey scholarship at the Department of Physiology at University College, London. There he worked closely with Ernest Starling, mainly on metabolisms of the heart. At the same time Evans studied medicine at University College Hospital, qualifying in 1916. Between 1916 and 1918 he worked at the Anti-gas Department of the Royal Army Medical Corps, then, after brief spells at Leeds University and the National Institute for Medical Research, he was appointed Professor of Physiology at St Bartholomew's Medical College, London, in 1922. Later he was appointed Professor of Physiology at University College, London, where he worked closely with A V Hill. During the Second World War Evans worked at the Chemical Defence Experimental Establishment at Porton Down, Wiltshire, returning to University College, London, in 1945. On his retirement in 1949, however, he returned to Porton Down where he remained for most of the rest of his life. In addition to his work in human physiology, Evans carried out substantial research into various veterinary subjects including sweating in the horse. He was a governor of the Royal Veterinary College, London, from 1933 and served as chairman of the Royal Veterinary College's Council between 1949 and 1963. He also sat on the Medical Research Council between 1947 and 1950 and chaired the Military Personnel Research Committee from 1948 to 1953. Honours included a Fellowship of the Royal Society in 1925 and a knighthood in 1951.

Records: Archives and Manuscripts, Wellcome Library for the History and Understanding of Medicine, 183 Euston Road, London NW1 2BE

Correspondence and arrangements re Queen Elizabeth's visit to Royal Veterinary College, London 1958–59; correspondence re William Dick Memorial Lecture, Royal (Dick) Veterinary College, Edinburgh 1963–65; Jockey Club and National Hunt committee correspondence re proposed research panel on detection of drugs in racehorses 1963; Research Defence Society, committee papers and correspondence re need for animal experimentation and Cruelty to Animals Act 1876, 1963–65. [Ref: PP/CLE/A.12–13, C.2–3]

GRIFFITH EVANS
Canada, India, England, Wales

History: Griffith Evans (1835–1935), qualified from the Royal Veterinary College, London, in 1855. In 1861 he entered the Army Veterinary Service, serving with the Royal Artillery in Canada where he was awarded the Canadian General Service Medal with two bars in 1870. Alongside his official duties, Evans also found time to study medicine part time at McGill University, graduating in 1864. In 1870 he returned to Britain and was based at Ipswich, Suffolk, before being posted to India in 1877. It was in India, in 1880, that Evans discovered that surra, a disease principally found amongst horses and camels, was due to flagellated protozoa in the circulating blood. Evan's work, on what is now known as Trypanosoma evansi, is generally recognised to be the first step in the discovery of some nine or ten diseases affecting both animals and humans caused by members of the genus Trypanosoma. Evans returned to England in 1885 and, following his retirement from the army in 1890, moved to Bangor, Gwynedd, where he lectured at the University College's agricultural department for the next twenty years. His work was recognised by the awarding of several honours: the Mary Kingsley medal by the Incorporated Liverpool School of Tropical Medicine (1917), the Steel medal (1918) and an honorary Doctor of Science from the University of Wales (1918).

T R Currie, 'The Discoverer of the Trypanosome', *Medical Life*, May 1931; 'Dr Griffith Evans, the Profession's Centenarian', *The Veterinary*

Record 1935; G Evans, 'Autobiographical memoir', *Annals of Tropical Medicine and Parasitology*, vol 12, 1918.

Records: National Library of Wales, Department of Manuscripts and Records, Aberystwyth SY23 3BU

Report re surra 1880 (p) with letter from Secretary, Indian government, to Adjutant General, India, re report 1881; report by Royal Microscopical Society re nomenclature of Trypanosoma evansi, nd; report on presentation of Mary Kingsley medal to Evans c1917; correspondence re: local blacksmith's cure for eye complaint in a colt 1857, explanation of how Evans' work on pathogenesis of microbes came to be neglected 1906, experiment performed on turtle in Canada 1913, observations made when carrying out experiments on milk 1916, investigation of anthracoid diseases in India 1918, University of Wales' decision to confer honorary Doctor of Science 1918, Steel medal and honorary Doctor of Science 1919, Fred Bullock, Secretary, Royal College of Veterinary Surgeons, re Evans's status and recollections 1925, Sydney H Slocock, President, Royal College of Veterinary Surgeons, offering congratulations on reaching 70th anniversary of qualification as MRCVS 1925, general veterinary and medical matters 1907–35; programme of meeting at which paper, 'The discoverer of the trypanosome', was given 1931; photograph of presentation of scroll by Sir Frederick Hobday to Evans on behalf of Royal Veterinary College, London 1935; obituary notice 1936; signed portrait, nd; biographical notes and articles 1918–35, nd; press cuttings: medical and scientific subjects 1875–96, biographical 1918–35. [Ref: Griffith Evans collection 111/1–21, 304, 448, 467, 475, 478–79, 494, 497, 499, 519, 521–24, 530, 556, 589, 594, 599]

J T R EVANS
Sudan

History: J T R Evans graduated from the Royal Veterinary College, London, in 1928 and in 1930 joined the Sudan Veterinary Service as an Assistant Veterinary Research Officer. He was appointed Veterinary Research Officer in 1937, and transferred to Khartoum four years later. In 1944 Evans was promoted to the position of Senior Research Officer and went on to become Director of Veterinary Services in 1952, retiring in 1955. During his time in the service Evans published numerous papers and organised mass treatment campaigns against cattle plague and bovine trypanosomiasis. He was also a founder member and first president of the Sudan Veterinary Association.

Records: Archives and Special Collections, Durham University Library, Palace Green Section, Durham DH1 3RN

Reports on bovine trypanosomiasis and animal husbandry 1950–53; résumés of careers of Evans and others with Sudan Veterinary Service; personal correspondence 1980s; paper re animal resources in Sudan 1975; speech by President of Sudan Veterinary Association 1971; photographs illustrating work of Sudan veterinary officer 1952. [Ref: JTR Evans]

JOHN GAMGEE
Edinburgh and London

History: John Gamgee (1830–94) was the second son of the veterinary surgeon Joseph Gamgee, and the brother of the physician Joseph Sampson Gamgee. He initially set out to study medicine in Italy, but soon changed his mind and entered the Royal Veterinary College, London, in 1849, qualifying in 1852. The following three years were spent travelling the continent, during which time he visited a number of veterinary colleges. On his return to England in 1855, Gamgee worked briefly as a veterinary assistant in Thirsk, North Yorkshire, before succeeding John Barlow as Professor of Anatomy and Physiology at William Dick's Edinburgh Veterinary College. Within a year, however, the two men had fallen out and in 1857 Gamgee left to establish a rival college. The New Edinburgh Veterinary College, based in Drummond Street, was granted the royal sign manual in 1859, enabling its students to sit the examination for membership of the Royal College of Veterinary Surgeons and thus practise as veterinary surgeons. In 1858 Gamgee set up the *Edinburgh Veterinary Review*, a monthly publication which continued until 1864. Maintaining two veterinary colleges in Edinburgh proved impossible, however – soon the New Edinburgh Veterinary College was losing £1000 a year – and in 1865 Gamgee took the decision to transfer his college to Bayswater, London. But the Albert Veterinary College, as it became known, also failed to gain enough support and closed in 1868. Gamgee's influence and interests, however, extended beyond undergraduate education. Recognising that increased movement of animals and meat made the international control and elimination of disease more vital than ever before, he organised the first International Congress of Veterinary Surgeons in Hamburg in 1863, bringing together veterinary surgeons from across the world. During the cattle plague crisis of 1865–66, Gamgee was one of the principal witnesses called to give evidence by the Cattle Plague Commissioners and amongst the first to recommend a policy of restriction of movement and mass slaughter. He was also the first veterinary surgeon to successfully use the thermometer for clinical purposes, measuring body temperatures of animals in the incubative and clinical stages of cattle plague. His volume on *The Cattle Plague* was published in 1866. After the failure of the Albert Veterinary College, Gamgee worked for a time in North America, devoting much of his energy to the problems surrounding the transportation of frozen meat.

R D'Arcy Thompson, *The Remarkable Gamgees: a story of achievement* (Edinburgh, 1974); S A Hall, 'John Gamgee and the Edinburgh New Veterinary College', *The Veterinary Record*, vol 77, no 3, 15 July 1965.

Records (1): in private ownership of Dr David Boddington, The Down House, Bromyard HR7 4QH

Correspondence with relatives, mostly re academic activities 19th cent; pamphlets re domestic animals, nd; paintings of pathological specimens 1853; photographs, nd.

Records (2): Department of Manuscripts, British Library, 96 Euston Road, London NW1 2DG

Correspondence with John Poyntz, 5th Earl Spencer re Albert Veterinary College, treatment of horses, etc 1866–73, 1887. [Ref: Add Ms 77239]

Records (3): Wellcome Library, Royal College of Veterinary Surgeons, Belgravia House, 62–64 Horseferry Road, London SW1P 2AF

Regulations and rules for Albert Veterinary College 1865.

JOSEPH GAMGEE
Edinburgh and London

History: Joseph Gamgee (1801–95) was interested in the care of horses from an early age. In 1820 he travelled to Italy to become huntsman to Prince Petrulo A'Aqualla, visiting the Veterinary College, London, *en route*. After a year's apprenticeship with a London farrier, he entered the Veterinary College, London, in 1823, qualifying the following year. In 1825 Gamgee returned to Italy and practised as a veterinary surgeon in Naples. By 1855 he had returned to London and in 1857 became a lecturer at his son's newly established New Edinburgh Veterinary College. The college moved to London in 1865 and reopened as the Albert Veterinary College. Although it failed shortly afterwards, Gamgee continued to lecture on horse foot care and to speak out against cruelty to animals.

R D'Arcy Thompson, *The Remarkable Gamgees: a story of achievement* (Edinburgh, 1974).

Records (1): in private ownership of Dr David Boddington, The Down House, Bromyard HR7 4QH

Notebooks outlining studies at St Pancras Veterinary College 1824; notes re various European travels incl cost of travel and horses 1850–53; passports with accompanying notes 1852–55; lecture notes whilst lecturer at New Edinburgh Veterinary College 1860; Edinburgh Infirmary day book 1864–65; notes re horse shoeing and lameness early 19th cent; correspondence with relations re veterinary profession and veterinary matters 19th cent; publication re horse shoeing and lameness 1811; letters and notes re hoof ointment, nd.

Records (2): Department of Manuscripts, British Library, 96 Euston Road, London NW1 2DG

Two letters to John Poyntz, 5th Earl Spencer c1865. [Ref: Add Ms 77239]

JOSEPH SAMPSON GAMGEE
Birmingham, West Midlands

History: Joseph Sampson Gamgee (1828–86), was the eldest son of Joseph Gamgee, an eminent veterinary surgeon, and the brother of John Gamgee, founder of the New Edinburgh Veterinary College. In 1847 Joseph Sampson entered the Royal Veterinary College, London, and was awarded his diploma in 1849, after which he enrolled as a student at University College Hospital, London. Although he retained an interest in veterinary medicine, visiting a number of European veterinary colleges, writing up cases and carrying out investigations into diseased meat, Joseph Sampson Gamgee's later career, from 1857 to 1881, was in human medicine and surgery. He practised in Birmingham and was known to be an early advocate of asefisis. He was elected to the Royal College of Veterinary Surgeons' Council in 1858.

R D'Arcy Thompson, *The Remarkable Gamgees: a story of achievement* (Edinburgh, 1974); H M Kafiadia, *Sampson Gamgee: contributions to surgery* (unpublished dissertation, University of Birmingham, 2000).

Records: in private ownership of Dr David Boddington, The Down House, Bromyard HR7 4QH

Lecture notes taken whilst a student at Royal Veterinary College, London 1848–49; diary of European travels incl notes on veterinary colleges 1849; research notes on pathological anatomy and clinical surgery, with illustrations by his brother John Gamgee 1856; original manuscript of *Wounds and Fractures* 1878; pamphlets re veterinary surgery, human surgery and social history 1848–80; medico-social pamphlets, letters, account books and job references, nd; pamphlets by other authors 1850s, nd.

PERCY CYRIL CLAUDE GARNHAM
Kenya and England

History: Percy Cyril Claude Garnham (1901–94), protozoologist, graduated MRCS, LRCP MB BS (St Barts) in 1923. He then worked for the Colonial Medical Services in Kenya between 1925 and 1927 before undertaking further study which resulted in an MD from University College, London, in 1928 (with Gold Medal) and the Diplôme de Médicine Malariol in Paris in 1931. In 1947 Garnham joined the Department of Parasitology at the London School of Hygiene and Tropical Medicine, becoming head of department in 1952. In 1968 he was appointed Heath Clark lecturer at the University of London and senior research fellow at the Imperial College Field Station, Ascot. Scientific achievements included the discovery of the liver stages of the malaria parasite and the elucidation of the full life cycle, as well as the fine structure, of many species of malaria parasites. Additionally, Garnham was actively involved in the eradication of onchocerciasis from Kenya and undertook research into a number of parasitic infections, including piroplasmosis. Honours conferred upon him included Fellowship of the Royal Society in 1964.

Records: Archives and Manuscripts, Wellcome Library for the History and Understanding of Medicine, 183 Euston Road, London NW1 2BE

Research notebooks 1925–67; correspondence and papers re research 1929–79; notebooks and diaries re working trips abroad: Mauritius and East Africa 1950, Brazil 1955, Uganda 1956, British Honduras 1958, 1963, Colombia 1959; correspondence and papers re visits abroad: Uganda 1950, US and Canada 1968–70, 1972–75, Germany 1969–70; notes re Diploma in Protozoology course [1913]; correspondence with individuals and institutions 1951–79; lectures and papers: Heath Clark lecture 1968, correspondence, notes, papers, photographs 1955–70, Gaillard Festschrift, papers 1969–72; notes, etc re biographical memoir of Edward Hindle 1973–74; correspondence, drafts, reprints, notes and illustrations re dissertation on Linnaeus 1972–79; unpublished papers 1918, 1920; personal correspondence 1929–84; honours 1964, 1971; diary 1957; photographs 1938, 1947–67. [Ref: PP/PCG]

WALDO H GLANVILLE
Sudan

History: Waldo H Glanville was a veterinary inspector for the Sudanese government between 1928 and 1946, and Director of the Sudan Veterinary Service from 1946 to 1952.

Records: Archives and Special Collections, Durham University Library, Palace Green Section, Durham DH1 3RN

Letter in praise of veterinary service 1942; photograph of Glanville and graduates of Khartoum Veterinary School 1940; soldier's driving permit 1940.

HENRY GRAY
London

History: Henry Gray qualified from the Royal Veterinary College, London, in 1885 and established The London Infirmary in Earl's Court Road shortly afterwards. He also wrote extensively on veterinary matters.

Records: Wellcome Library, Royal College of Veterinary Surgeons, Belgravia House, 62–64 Horseferry Road, London SW1P 2AF

Letters to Henry Gray 1886–38, nd; letter by Gray's daughter re his papers 1951; letter to Gray's daughter from [-] 1954; photograph of The London Infirmary 19th cent.

GEORGE RICHARD GRIFFITH

Egypt and Sudan

History: George Richard Griffith (d 1920) graduated from the Royal Veterinary College, London, in 1880 and immediately enlisted in the Army Veterinary Corps. He went on active service to Egypt in 1882 and was present at the actions of El Magfar, Masameh, Kassassin and the battle of Tel-el-Kebir before returning to England in November that same year. Griffith returned to Egypt in 1884 as part of the Nile Expedition and remained there until his retirement in 1907. Seconded to the Egyptian Army in 1889 as Principal Veterinary Officer, he organised the Egyptian Army Veterinary Service, and later went on to set up the Sudan Veterinary Service . He was present at nearly every engagement up to the Battle of Omdurman in 1898 and at the re-conquest of Sudan the following year. During his long career, Griffith rose to the rank of Lieutenant Colonel, was mentioned in dispatches three times and awarded the DSO.

Records: The Army Medical Services Museum, Keogh Barracks, Ash Vale, Aldershot GU12 5RQ

Personal papers 1896–1907, 1917; warrant for award of DSO 1896; record of service compiled c1980; photographs 1897, 1907. [Ref: Box 21]

RUPERT LANCELOT LEON HART

Zambia and Uganda

History: Rupert Lancelot Leon Hart (b 1885) graduated from the Royal Veterinary College, London, in 1906 and after a short period at a practice in Devon went to North East Rhodesia as a Veterinary Officer in 1910. He was appointed Veterinary Officer for Uganda in 1914, promoted to Senior Veterinary Officer in 1920 and Acting Director of Veterinary Services in 1932.

Records: Rhodes House Library, South Parks Road, Oxford OX1 3RG

Diary of experiences in Africa, incl notes on stock inspections, cattle census and condition of animals 1910–12; history of veterinary services in North East Rhodesia 1954. [Ref: MSS.Afr.r.112; MSS.Afr.s.1390]

RICHARD HOLLIDAY
Purton, Wiltshire

Records: Barton Veterinary Hospital, 34 New Dover Road, Canterbury, Kent CT1 3DT

Notebook containing veterinary recipes and accounts 1807.

JAMES RANDAL HUTCHINSON
Manchester, Wigan and London

History: James Randal Hutchinson (c1880–1955) was Senior Assistant to the Medical Officer of Health, Manchester, between 1908 and 1910, then Medical Officer of Health for Wigan from 1910 to 1911. In 1911 he was appointed Medical Inspector to the Local Government Board, remaining there until 1919 when he took up an appointment as Medical Officer at the Ministry of Health. There he worked on a number of infectious diseases, including some that affected animals. From 1926 to 1947 he was Secretary to the Ministry of Health/Medical Research Council Committee on Vaccine. Hutchinson retired in 1947.

Records: Archives and Manuscripts, Wellcome Library for the History and Understanding of Medicine, 183 Euston Road, London NW1 2BE

Papers re: anthrax 1917–26, foot-and-mouth disease 1922–41, meat inspection, knackers' yards and animal inoculation 1922–39, psittacosis 1930–52, glanders 1939–48, trichinosis 1941–46. [Ref: PP/JRH/A.1–6, 186, 188, 196, 230–33, 261–66]

EDWARD ANEURIN LEWIS
Kenya

History: Edward Aneurin Lewis worked in the Department of Veterinary Sciences in Kenya during the 1930s and 1940s, rising to the position of Chief Field Zoologist. Much of his work centred on the eradication of trypanosomiasis and led to his appointment as Deputy Director of the East Africa Tsetse and Trypanosomiasis Research and Reclamation Organisation in 1949. He became director of the organisation in 1952 and retired in 1954.

Records: Archives and Manuscripts, Wellcome Library for the History and Understanding of Medicine, 183 Euston Road, London NW1 2BE

East Africa Tsetse and Trypanosomiasis Research and Reclamation Organisation: summary of objectives, nd, annual report 1953, draft annual reports 1952–54, officers' duties 1952, reports re cattle trypanosomiasis c1947–50, reports and papers re tsetse distribution 1951–53, reports on tsetse research programmes at Central Tsetse Research Laboratory 1948–53, report of the Ankole land utilisation sub-committee to the Uganda tsetse and trypanosomiasis advisory committee 1951, notes re experiments on cattle c1952, correspondence, proposals and grant applications re pilot schemes for land reclamation (tsetse eradication) 1945–54, notes on reclamation projects 1949–53, conference proceedings 1943, handing over notes 1951–54, review of work of West African Institute for Trypanosomiasis 1954, memoranda on anti-tsetse measures in other countries 1950–53, article on trypanosome in camels, nd, letter and notes re history of trypanosomiasis in Uganda 1919–48, 1953, list of publications 1923–53, historical notes 1948–54; Central Trypanosomiasis Research Institute: proposals for creation 1949, research programme 1953; research report of International Scientific Committee for trypanosomiasis 1952; abstracts of reports and papers on animal diseases in East Africa 1911–25; reports: tsetse control projects in Kenya 1932–47, activity experiment (with photographs) 1948, land development in Kenya 1954; notes, graphs, reports and correspondence re: different trypanosomes and different districts 1941–46, virulence of different strains of trypanosome 1940–51, observations on tsetse flies 1944–46; records of experiments 1932, 1945–46; foreword to *Bulletin of Entomological Research* re proposed establishment of committee to centralise information on African insects 1910; literature on tsetse flies and trypanosomiasis in Kenya 1903–12; records of tsetse activity 1944–46; summary of trypanosomiasis cases on farms in Machakos district 1935–37; papers re African vegetation 1923–51; copy of presidential address to Society of American Bacteriologists 1934; press cuttings re animal diseases and husbandry in East Africa 1936–45; correspondence re identification of specimens 1936–39; maps of tsetse distribution in Africa 1909–c1946. [Ref: WTI/EAL]

ANDREW LINTON
Egypt and Kenya

History: Andrew Linton of Gilmanscleugh, Selkirk, qualified as an agriculturalist in the late nineteenth century before taking up an appointment at the School of Agriculture in Cairo. He appears to have worked as Director of Agriculture on government farms in Nairobi and Naivasha in the East Africa Protectorate during the early 1900s. He also researched, wrote and corresponded about veterinary medicine and animal disease. Linton died in 1951.

Records: Scottish Borders Archive and Local History Centre, St Mary's Mill, Selkirk TD7 5EW

Highland and Agricultural Society of Scotland: diploma in agriculture 1896, second class certificate in forestry 1896, certificate of registration as free life member 1896; Royal Agricultural Society of England, first class certificate 1897; School of Agriculture, Cairo: job descriptions re professorships, nd, notice re appointment to school, nd; articles on research into animal disease 1920 for meetings of Animal Diseases Research Association 1920–21; papers on: history of Animal Diseases Research Association 1920–21, sheep tick 1938; notes for a treatise on sheep, nd; notes and ideas re animal diseases, nd; correspondence re: government farms in East Africa Protectorate 1905, laboratory of Board of Agriculture and Fisheries 1914, Brown Animal Sanatory Institution 1914, Royal Veterinary College, London 1915, braxy infected sheep 1920, criticism of Professor Gaiger's views on sheep disease 1920; notes re Linton family history, nd. [Ref: SC/S/10/6/10–12, 15; SC/S/10/9/14–16; SC/S/10/16/3–17, 20, 26, 29, 34]

JOHN MATTHEWSON

Records: Archivist, Edinburgh University Library, George Square, Edinburgh EH8 9LJ

University class cards 1833; letter certifying attendance at lectures 1834; apprenticeship indenture, Walter Halliday to John Matthewson 1846; *Small's Veterinary Tablet* c1850.

WILLIAM MOORCROFT

London and India

History: William Moorcroft (1765–1825) originally intended to follow a medical career and with this in mind studied under Dr Lyon at the Liverpool Infirmary. Following an outbreak of cattle plague in 1783, however, the local medical authority was asked to provide a student to investigate the cause of the outbreak and Moorcroft was the student selected. This awakened his interest in animal medicine and he went on to study veterinary science at Lyon Veterinary College, France, from 1790 to 1791 before setting up his own equine practice at 224 Oxford Street, London. On the death of Charles Vial de St Bel, Professor of the newly established Veterinary College, London, in 1793, Moorcroft was appointed joint Professor with Edward Coleman. After only a few weeks, however, Moorcroft left the college and returned to his equine practice, which he ran jointly with John Field (1768–1833). The practice proved highly lucrative and enjoyed the patronage of the King. In addition to his practice, Moorcroft ran a successful breeding stud for the East India Company near Romford, Essex. One of his special interests at this time was the lameness of horses. He also wrote extensively, producing such works as *An English Translation of Vallis' Experiments in Animal Electricity* (1793), *Directions for Using the Portable Horse-Medicine Chest Adopted for Service in India* (1795) and *A Cursory Account of the Various Methods of Shoeing Horses Hitherto in Use* (1800). By the early 1800s, however, Moorcroft was in financial difficulties, having lost large sums on two patents for the mechanised manufacture of horseshoes. In 1808 he was appointed veterinary surgeon to the Bengal Army and Superintendent of the East India Company's stud at Pusa near Cawnpore, India. There he introduced oat cultivation, greatly reduced disease at the breeding stud and began producing quality horses for use by the cavalry. At the same time he developed an interest in agriculture and trade and in 1811–12 travelled to Tibet to explore the possibility of trade with neighbouring countries. In 1819 Moorcroft embarked on a second expedition, having been granted permission to travel to Bukhara to purchase stallions for the East India Company's stud. Although he was given several assistants and a sepoy guard most of the expeditions' expenses were borne by Moorcroft himself. Some horses were purchased, but the expedition made slow progress, being forced into extended stops at various points *en route*. These stops, however, enabled Moorcroft to write various letters and notes on, amongst other things, agriculture. Moorcroft died on the return journey in 1825.

G Alder, *Beyond Bokhara: the life of William Moorcroft, Asian explorer and pioneer veterinary surgeon 1767–1825* (London, 1985); W Moorcroft and G Trebeck, *Travels in the Himalayan provinces of Hindustan and the Panjab; in Ladakh and Kashmir; in Peshawar, Kabul, Kunduz and Bokhara*; ... *from 1819–1825, prepared for the Press from original journals and correspondence by Horace Hayman Wilson*, (London, 1841).

Records (1): University of London Library, Senate House, Malet Street, London WC1E 7HU

Volume of notes on agriculture in Kashmir incl references to animals and animal diseases 1822–23. [Ref: MS.630]

Records (2): Oriental and India Office Collections, British Library, 96 Euston Road, London NW1 2DB

Journals 1820–25; correspondence 1812–26; accounts, bills, etc 1811–23; stud papers 1817–18; misc papers, notes, etc 1819–25, nd. [Ref: MSS Eur K307–364; J823–824]

Records (3): Science and Technology Service, British Library, 96 Euston Road, London NW1 2DB

Patents re manufacturing of horseshoes 1796, 1800. [Ref: 2104, 2398]

Records (4): National Library of Scotland, Department of Manuscripts, George IV Bridge, Edinburgh EH1 1EW

Correspondence with Gilbert Elliot Murray Kynynmound, 1st Earl of Minto, re East India Company stud and proposed appointment of an assistant veterinary surgeon 1809–13. [Ref: MS11287, 11299, 11319, 11330, 11331, 11590, 11593, 11604]

ANTHONY WILLIAM POLDEN
Sudan

History: Anthony William Polden (d 1997) served as a veterinary inspector to the Sudanese government from 1949 to 1955.

Records: Archives and Special Collections, Durham University Library, Palace Green Section, Durham DH1 3RN

Employment contract with Sudan government 1949; notes on Nuer districts c1955; memoirs entitled 'the Upper Nile from a veterinary point of view', nd; letters to his mother 1950–51; photographs of Polden, housing, servants and cattle vaccination, nd; humorous verses re hand-over of power to his successor, nd. [Ref: Anthony William Polden]

LEONARD ROGERS
India and London

History: Major General Sir Leonard Rogers (1868–1962) was educated at St Mary's Hospital Medical School, London, qualifying in 1892. The following year he entered the Indian Medical Service where he began his work on tropical diseases. After gaining his MD (1897) and MRCP (1898) in London, Rogers returned to India and was immediately seconded to the All-India Veterinary Bacteriological Laboratory at Mukhtesar. His research there led to the improved control of cattle plague by inoculation and to a better understanding of the transmission of trypanosomiasis (surra) in horses and camels. In 1900 Rogers was posted to the Bengal Civil Medical Department, Calcutta, as Deputy Sanitary Commissioner, where his work tended to concentrate on human infectious diseases, especially leprosy and amoebic dysentery. This was followed in 1906 by his appointment as Professor of Pathology at Calcutta Medical College. After retiring from the Indian Medical Service in 1921, Rogers took up a lectureship at the London School of Hygiene and Tropical Medicine, remaining there until 1937. He retained his links with India, however, notably as a member of the India Office Medical Board from 1922 and president of the same from 1928. He was also responsible for the establishment of the British Empire Leprosy Relief Association in 1923 and did much to bring about the construction of the Calcutta School of Tropical Medicine. The many honours conferred upon him included a knighthood in 1914.

Biographical Memoirs of Fellows of the Royal Society, no 9, 1963, 261–282; L Rogers, *Happy Toil: fifty five years of tropical medicine* (London, 1950).

Records: Archives and Manuscripts, Wellcome Library for the History and Understanding of Medicine, 183 Euston Road, London NW1 2BE

Clinical notebooks re cattle plague experiments in India 1899–1900; correspondence and notes: cattle plague research at the Veterinary Laboratory 1899–1902, surra research 1899–1904, 1920–21; published articles re animal disease, animal experimentation and veterinary research 1933–36. [Ref: PP/ROG/B.4, C.3/1–13, C.4/1–11, E.133, E.135–38]

L A SCRIVENS
British Salonica and Constantinople

History: L A Scrivens served as a private in the Army Veterinary Corps during the First World War, seeing service in British Salonica and Constantinople.

Records: National Army Museum, Royal Hospital Road, Chelsea, London SW3 4HT

Farewell message from Director of Veterinary Services, British Salonica 1919; pass to enter Salonica 1919; pass to enter Constantinople 1919; certificate of transfer to reserve 1920. [Ref: Acc 7611–30]

FREDERICK SMITH
England, Africa and India

History: Major General Sir Frederick Smith (1857–1929) entered the Royal Veterinary College, London, in 1873 and qualified in 1876 with prizes in physiology and cattle pathology as well as the Coleman medal for an essay on specific ophthalmia. In December 1876 he passed the army veterinary examination and was gazetted to the Royal Artillery early the following year, moving to the 12th Royal Lancers as a veterinary captain in 1880. The years 1877 to 1886 were largely spent in India, where Smith succeeded in demonstrating that the problem of sore backs amongst horses was caused by ill-fitting saddles rather than by poor riding. In 1882, along with John Henry Steel, he established the *Quarterly Journal of Veterinary Science in India*, which ran until 1889. By this time, however, Smith was back in England, having in 1886 joined the staff of the Army Veterinary School, Aldershot, as assistant instructor, before being appointed professor the following year. His publications during this time included the *Manual of Veterinary Hygiene* (1887), the *Manual of Sore Backs* (1891), which later formed part of the army's *Manual on the Care and Management of Horses*, and the *Manual of Veterinary Physiology* (1892), as well as numerous papers for professional journals. His tour of continental veterinary colleges led to the establishment at Aldershot of a Vaccine Institute in 1888. In 1892 Smith left the Army Veterinary School for the Remount Department. He was promoted to major in 1896 and lieutenant colonel in 1899, and served in the Nile Expedition of 1898 and the South African War from 1899 to 1902. At the end of the latter, Smith chose to stay in South Africa as Principal Veterinary Officer, only returning to England in 1905 when he was appointed Principal Veterinary Officer, Eastern Command, with the rank of colonel. In 1907, he was appointed Director General of the Army Veterinary Service with the rank of major general. During his three years in charge, he reorganised the system of veterinary stores, took an active role in the organisation of the veterinary service within the newly established Territorial Army and campaigned to have the veterinary service removed from the Remount Department and placed instead under the Quartermaster General. Smith retired in 1910, but was employed on home service during the First World War. After the war ended, he concentrated on writing. His publications included *The Veterinary History of the War in South Africa* (1919), *The History of the Royal Army Veterinary Corps 1796–1919* (1927) and *The History of Veterinary Literature* (4 vols, 1919–33) On his death in 1929, Smith left his estate to the Royal College of Veterinary Surgeons for the establishment of a fund for veterinary research.

Records (1): Wellcome Library, Royal College of Veterinary Surgeons, Belgravia House, 62–64 Horseferry Road, London SW1P 2AF

Correspondence with Henry Gray, MRCVS, 1912–29; letters to Frederick Bullock, secretary of Royal College of Veterinary Surgeons 1910–29; letters to Mrs Bullock and Wilfred Bullock 1919–23, 1926–28; letters from L Moule, Marne, France 1914, 1921–23; general letters to Smith, mostly re his publications 1877–1929; Bullock's correspondence with various people re Smith's books 1929–34; correspondence and papers re Smith's estate 1929, 1938–39; official papers re Army Veterinary Corps during the First World War incl conditions of service 1914–18; draft of opening of *The History of Veterinary Literature* (vol 2) with amendments; notes on his time as Director General of the Army Veterinary Corps, nd; *Queen's Regulations and Orders for the Army* (incomplete) 1883; invitation, tickets, etc to funeral of Edward VII 1910; statutes of the Most Distinguished Order of St Michael and St George 1902, 1917; statutes of the Most Honourable Order of the Bath 1904, 1925; licence to accept and wear insignia of the 4th Class of the Imperial Ottoman Order of the Medjidick 1900; royal warrants appointing Smith: Commander of the Most Distinguished Order of St Michael and St George 1901, 1903, Companion of the Order of the Bath 1905, Knight Commander of St Michael and St George 1918; commissions as veterinary surgeon, land forces 1876–77; thanks of George V for services rendered during First World War c1918; thanks of Prime Minister for services rendered during General Strike 1926; original scheme of work 1888; list of investments 1931; misc biographical notes, nd; reports: *General Report of the Army Veterinary Department in the Zulu War* 1879, *Veterinary Reports from the Nile Expeditionary Force* 1882, 1884, 1898, *Report re Cavalry equipment* 1883; *Report from 1st Class Veterinary Surgeon Anderson, Army Veterinary Department, to the Principal Veterinary Surgeon in India* 1883, *Report on the Kuram Field Force by G A Oliphant Officiating Veterinary Surgeon* 1883, *Report with Related Correspondence from F Duck, Veterinary Surgeon with the Bechuanaland Field Force* 1886, *Report on the Working of the Army Veterinary Department with the Chitral Relief Force from Veterinary Lieutenant Colonel Richard Poyser, Inspecting Veterinary Officer, to the Assistant Adjutant and Quarter Master General* 1895, *Report on the Working of the Army Veterinary Department with the Waziristan Field Force from Veterinary Major G J R Reyment, Army Veterinary Department, 3rd Brigade Waziristan Field Force, to the Deputy Assistant Adjutant General* 1895, *Report on the Working of the Army Veterinary Department with the Suakin Force* 1896, *Report on the Working of the Army Veterinary Department with the Tochi Field Force from H Thomson, Veterinary Colonel and Principal Veterinary Officer in India to the Adjutant General* 1897–98, *Report on the Working of the Army Veterinary Department with the Tirah Expeditionary Force from the Principal Veterinary Officer in India to the Adjutant General* 1897–98, *Report on the Working of the Army Veterinary Department with the Mohmand, Malakand and Buner Field Forces from H Thomson, Veterinary Colonel, Principal Veterinary Officer in India to the Adjutant General in India* 1897–98, *Report of the Working of the Army Veterinary Department with the China Expeditionary Force from Veterinary Captain E H Hazelton, Inspecting Veterinary Officer, China Field Force, to the Principal Veterinary Officer in India* 1900–01, *Extract from the Report on Demobilisation of the South African Field Force Army Veterinary Department* 1902–03, *Report from the Professor of the Army Vaccine Institute to the Principal Medical Officer, 1st Army Corps, on the Working of the Army Vaccine Institute,* with notes and photographs 1903, *Statistical and General Report of the Army Veterinary Service for 1907–09* by Frederick Smith, *Report on the Working of the Army Veterinary Department with the Bazar Valley Field Force from Major A England, Army Veterinary Corps, Senior Veterinary Officer, 1st Peshawar Division to the Principal Veterinary Officer in India* 1908, *Veterinary Report on the French operations in Morocco for the relief of Fez* 1911, *Report from Colonel James Irvine Smith, Director of Veterinary Services, Union Defence Forces, South African Veterinary Corps re the German South West African campaign, the rebellion and subsequent period* 1915–16; notes from *The Veterinarian* 1828–70; abstracts from *Proceedings of the Veterinary Medical Association* 1841–44 and from *Transactions of the Veterinary Medical Association* 1845–50; notes taken by unidentified student during chemistry classes at the

Army Veterinary School 1887–92; notes re research at Public Record Office, British Museum, Royal Veterinary College Library and elsewhere gathered by Smith for his publications incl some on regimental standing orders, cavalry inspections, Army Medical Service, Abyssinian Expeditionary Force of 1868, farriers and army shoeing 1909–10, anatomy, mobilisation, pay, formation and organisation of the Army Veterinary Corps Territorial Division c1910; misc notes on the Army Veterinary Corps c1900–10; notes re: history of Cavalry and Royal Artillery, Russian Army Veterinary Corps, Veterinary Department during Afghan War, India, Egypt, Arabia, English Antiquities, 16th cent veterinary care, ancient medicine, tuberculosis, insulin, joint disease, anthrax, veterinary hygiene, liver and spleen, vitamins, cytology, skin, anatomy and anthropology, heredity and hygiene, cancer and tumours, South African War, Royal Society 19th–20th cent; copy of War Office correspondence re Astor-Jackson case of 1914–16; numerous offprints of articles incl some by Smith; *The Early History of Veterinary Literature and its British Development* vols 1–3 (unbound); reviews of Smith's books early 20th cent; photographs: Army Veterinary School 1886, 1889, Boers mobilising at Potchefstroom 1899, South African War 1899–1902, Veterinary School at Aldershot and Smith's laboratory late 19th cent, Army Veterinary Department on the road late 19th cent, visits of Queen Victoria and Edward VII to Aldershot late 19th–early 20th cent, views of Tibet 1903–04, Canadian Army Veterinary Corps at Salisbury 1914, field ambulance Frith Hill Camp 1912, Frederick Smith 1916, nd.

Records (2): The Army Medical Services Museum, Keogh Barracks, Ash Vale, Aldershot GU12 5RQ

Licence issued (copy) 1886; certificate of licence renewal (copy) 1887; renewals of licenses (copies) 1888–91; certificate of authorisation to destroy animals if in pain, nd. [Ref: Box 21]

Records (3): Department of Manuscripts, British Library, 96 Euston Road, London NW1 2DB

Letter to E T Hutton 1890. [Ref: Add Ms 50093 f 187]

Records (4): The Library, Royal Veterinary College, Royal College Street, London NW1 0TU

Drafts, correspondence and notes re life of Napoleon Bonaparte 19th–20th cent.

HENRY WILLIAM STEELE-BODGER
Tamworth, Staffordshire

History: Henry William (Harry) Steele-Bodger (1896–1952), began working as a farrier whilst serving with the Royal Engineers during the First World War. After qualifying from the Royal (Dick) Veterinary College, Edinburgh, in 1922 he established himself in practice in Tamworth, Staffordshire. He later acquired two further practices in Sutton Coldfield, West Midlands, in the early 1930s and Lichfield, Staffordshire, in 1938. Steele-Bodger also undertook many visits to veterinary colleges overseas and wrote extensively on bovine infertility and pregnancy diagnosis. Between 1936 and 1939 he was Examiner in Animal Management for the Royal Veterinary College, London. He also served as President of the National Veterinary Medical Association from 1939 to 1941 and established the Society of Veterinary Practitioners (later the Society of Practising Veterinary Surgeons) in the mid 1930s.

Records (1): in private ownership of Miss Mary Brancker, 38 Streetly Lane, Sutton Coldfield B74 4TU

Presidential address to National Veterinary Medical Association general meeting 1941; booklet on suggested technique to be employed in bovine pregnancy diagnosis 1942; photographs of Steele-Bodger: as President of National Veterinary Medical Association c1940, at work c1940s; obituaries 1952; funeral order of service 1952; death notice, *Tamworth Herald* 1952.

Records (2): British Veterinary Association, 7 Mansfield Street, London W1M 0AT

Biographical notes, nd.

C E STUTTARD
Egypt

History: C E Stuttard enlisted as a veterinary surgeon with the 18th Mobile Section of the Army Veterinary Corps in January 1915 and served in Egypt until illness forced his evacuation in August that same year.

Records: Imperial War Museum, Lambeth Road, London SE1 6HZ

Discharge certificate from 3rd East Lancashire Brigade 1911; reply to application to join Army Veterinary Corps 1914; employer's reference 1914; diary describing experiences during service with Army Veterinary Corps 1915; correspondence with mother 1915; correspondence re hospitalisation 1915; forms re demobilisation from 13th field veterinary hospital 1915; wound label issued on evacuation through sickness 1915; race card, Alexandria Sporting Club horserace meeting 1915; press cuttings 1915–60; papers re pension application 1920; son's application for war widow's pension for his mother 1961. [Ref: 90/7/1]

D'ARCY WENTWORTH THOMPSON
Dundee and St Andrews, Fife

History: D'Arcy Wentworth Thompson (1860–1948) graduated from Edinburgh University in 1883 with a degree in natural science. The following year he was elected Professor of Biology at University College, Dundee, and stayed there until 1917 when he accepted the Chair in Natural History at United College, University of St Andrews. In addition to his natural science research, Thompson published numerous papers on a wide range of subjects including classical studies, mathematics and zoology. Among the many honours conferred upon him were a Doctor of Literature in 1912 for his *Glossary of Greek Birds* and a knighthood in 1937.

C Dobell, 'D'Arcy Wentworth Thompson', *Obituary Notices of Fellows of the Royal Society*, 6, 1948–49; G A L Sarton, 'D'Arcy Wentworth Thompson, 1860–1948', *Isis*, 4, 1950; R D'Arcy Thompson, *D'Arcy Wentworth Thompson: the scholar naturalist, 1860–1948* (London, 1958).

Records: University of St Andrews Library, North Street, St Andrews KY16 9TR

Copies of [Joseph?] Gamgee's publications 1861–83; scrapbook re Joseph Gamgee, nd; lecture notes and writings on veterinary subjects by Joseph Gamgee, nd; press cuttings and notes on veterinary subjects chiefly re horses c1863–73; correspondence, scrapbooks, notebooks, lecture notes and photographs on a variety of subjects incl some veterinary 1878–1948. [Ref: MS 9013–MS29950; MS 40500–MS48549 (et ff)]

S E W VILES
Coltishall, Norfolk

History: S E W Viles served as a non-commissioned officer with the Air Ministry Falcon Unit at RAF Coltishall, Norfolk, between 1948 and 1949. The unit carried out research into the military use of hawks and the use of falcons to keep military airfields clear of birds.

Records: Imperial War Museum, Lambeth Road, London SE1 6HZ

Falcon daily reports (p) 1948–49; correspondence re veterinary matters, publicity and falconry (p) 1948–49; press cuttings re military uses of falcons (p) 1948–49; papers re food, medicine and weight of falcons (p) 1948–49. [Ref: 80/8/1]

GRAHAM SELBY WILSON
London and Manchester

History: Graham Selby Wilson (1895–1987), was educated at King's College, London, and Charing Cross Hospital, London, qualifying in 1916. After serving as a Captain in the Army Veterinary Corps between 1916 and 1920, he was appointed Demonstrator in Bacteriology at Charing Cross Hospital, London. In 1923, Wilson moved to Manchester to take up a lectureship there and shortly afterwards began researching the hygiene and pasteurisation of milk. He was appointed Reader in Bacteriology at the London School of Hygiene and Tropical Medicine in 1927, and went on to become Professor of Bacteriology in 1930, a post he held until 1947. In 1929 Wilson was co-author, with W W C Topley, of *Principles of Bacteriology and Immunity*. During the late 1930s, he was one of the leading men behind the establishment of the Emergency Public Health Laboratory Service (EPHLS), which aimed to control epidemics brought about by the mass movement of people in wartime. In 1941, he became Director of the EPHLS and played a major role in its evolution into the Public Health Laboratory Service with some sixty local laboratories. Following his retirement in 1963 Wilson sat on the editorial board of the journal *Research in Veterinary Science* from 1964–68. He was elected a Fellow of the Royal College of Physicians in 1930, a Fellow of the Royal Society in 1978 and knighted in 1962.

Records: Archives and Manuscripts, Wellcome Library for the History and Understanding of Medicine, 183 Euston Road, London NW1 2BE

Veterinary Research Club: membership cards and club rules 1953–87, correspondence and papers 1968–86, draft of speech 1969; lectures at Royal Veterinary College, London: food poisoning 1961, 1968, 1984, epidemiology 1974–75, brucellosis and leptospiral infections, nd; editorial correspondence re *Research in Veterinary Science* 1964–71; papers re visit to Sudan to advise the Veterinary Research Administration on epidemiological problems and development of the service: journal 1976, correspondence 1976, memorandum and plans re design and structure of bacteriological laboratories 1976; correspondence re arrangements for lectures at Royal Veterinary College, London 1984–86. [Ref: PP/GSW/D.24, 30–34, 139, 141 /E.56–60, /F.51–53]

List of records of companies

ALLEN & HANBURYS LTD
Greenford, Greater London

History: The origins of Allen & Hanburys Ltd date back to 1715 and the opening of a pharmacy at Old Plough Court, Lombard Street, London, by Silvanus Bevan. Ten years later Bevan's younger brother, Timothy, was apprenticed to him. The two men went on to form a partnership in 1731, their business trading under the name Silvanus and Timothy Bevan, Apothecaries, Lombard Street. Over the next century, the company became known both for the quality of its products and the integrity of its partners, who brought their Quaker philosophy to bear on their business dealings. After Silvanus Bevan's death in 1765, the firm became known as Timothy Bevan and Sons, druggists and chemists. Timothy Bevan retired in 1775, handing over the business to the younger son of his second marriage, Joseph Gurney Bevan. Under J G Bevan the company concentrated largely on the manufacture and sale of wholesale drugs and instruments to merchants and surgeons in London and the colonies. In 1794 J G Bevan retired and sold the business to Samuel Mildred who shortly afterwards entered into partnership with one of Bevan's former clerks, William Allen, renaming the company Mildred & Allen. Allen bought Mildred out in 1797 and entered into a new partnership with Luke Howard. While Allen concentrated on the Plough Court business, Howard assumed control of the company's laboratory at Plaistow, Greater London. The two branches rapidly diverged, however, and the partnership was dissolved in 1806. Howard developed a chemical manufacturing business at Plaistow, while Allen kept control of Plough Court and specialised in the production of galenicals. Two of Allen's nephews by his second wife were brought into the firm: Daniel Bell Hanbury in 1808 and Cornelius Hanbury in 1813. Both went on to become partners in 1824. A further partner was included from 1818, John Thomas Barry, who had acted as Allen's clerk and done much to facilitate the winding down of the largely unprofitable overseas trade. All four men were influential in the establishment of the Pharmaceutical Society of Great Britain in 1841 and William Allen was elected the Society's first president. Following the retirements of Barry and Cornelius Hanbury, in 1856 and 1858 respectively, the business became known as Allen & Hanburys. Two new partners were admitted: Daniel, eldest son of Daniel Bell Hanbury, and Cornelius, son of Cornelius Hanbury. Daniel Bell Hanbury retired in 1868 and was succeeded by Cornelius Hanbury's only other surviving son, Frederick Janson Hanbury. The period between 1850 and 1920 proved to be one of rapid expansion. The dispensing and manufacturing premises at Plough Court were enlarged during the 1860s, while a factory was established at Bethnal Green, Greater London, in 1874, followed by a second retail outlet at Vere Street, Cavendish Square, London, in 1884. Additionally, during the early 1880s a small forge and workshop were set up at the Bethnal Green factory to manufacture surgical instruments. This side of the business later moved to Wigmore Street, London, to be near the medical community of Harley Street. In 1893 the company was incorporated as a limited liability company, Allen & Hanburys Ltd. This was followed in 1896 by the acquisition of a mill at Ware, Hertfordshire, for the production of malted food, pastilles and galenicals. Allen & Hanburys Ltd's most successful products during this period included cod-liver oil, malted extract, pastilles, compressed tablets and baby milk, and a number of overseas subsidiaries were established between 1902 and 1913. After the First World War, the company, by this time under the chairmanship of Frederick Janson Hanbury, established an analytical laboratory at the Bethnal Green factory and had an early success, becoming in 1923 one of the first producers of insulin. Overall, though, the period between 1920 and 1950 proved undynamic. Allen & Hanburys' major customer, the retail chemist, was disappearing as national retailing outlets such as Boots emerged, while the entrance of Glaxo into the baby milk market hit profits hard. By 1953, the production of milk products had ceased altogether. The 1950s, however, saw a growth in the company's veterinary output. Although the firm had always sold veterinary products these now assumed a greater importance. A new veterinary division was established and the marketing policy altered, enabling the veterinary surgeon, rather than the farmer, to be targeted by specially trained staff. The division's greatest success was *Dictol*, launched in 1959 as an oral vaccine to combat lungworm in cattle. Hitherto the disease had cost the farming industry thousands of animal lives a year, but a research breakthrough by scientists at Glasgow University's Veterinary Faculty meant that over 250,000 calves were being vaccinated annually by the early 1960s. By this time, however, Allen & Hanburys Ltd was no longer an independent company, having agreed to a merger with Glaxo Laboratories Ltd in 1958. Three years later, Glaxo Research Ltd was established to co-ordinate the research functions of the two companies. Dr David Jack was appointed research director at Ware and promptly carried out a restructuring of the research facilities, moving the parasitology laboratory to Glaxo at Greenford, Greater London, and setting up a new pathology department at Ware. In 1962 the research division at Ware became a separate entity charged with developing new medicines for animals and humans. Over the following decades it had particular success in developing drugs to combat respiratory diseases. All research activities were eventually concentrated at Greenford in 1979. An interest in the manufacture of surgical instruments was also retained, culminating in the incorporation of all the relevant Glaxo subsidiaries into Allen & Hanburys (Surgical Engineering Ltd) in 1963.

P Baker, 'London Origins of the Glaxo Group', *Supplement to the Pharmaceutical Journal*, 30 July 1983; D Chapman-Huston & E C Cripps, *Through a City Archway: the story of Allen & Hanburys, 1715–1954* (London, 1954); E C Cripps, *Plough Court: the story of a notable pharmacy, 1715–1927* (London, 1927); J C Hanbury, 'Early Developments in the Fine Chemical Industry: an historical survey', *Chemistry & Industry*, 1952; R L Hanbury, 'The History and Development of Allen & Hanburys Ltd, 1715–1965' (unpublished typescript, 1965); K Holland, 'Sir John Hanbury', *Pharmaceutical Journal*, 28 Nov 1992; A A Locke, *The Hanbury Family*, 2 vols (London, 1916); C S Stander, 'A History of the Pharmaceutical Industry With Particular Reference to Allen & Hanburys, 1775–1843' (unpublished thesis, London University, 1956); G Tweedale, *At the Sign of the Plough: Allen & Hanburys and the British pharmaceutical industry 1715–1990* (London, 1990); M E Weeks, 'The Chemical Contributions of William Allen', *Journal of Chemical Education*, 35, 1958.

Records (1): (Historical Records) Records Centre, Glaxo Wellcome plc, 891–995 Greenford Road, Greenford UB6 0HE

Directors' meetings, minutes and related papers 1894–; general meetings, minutes 1894–; memoranda and articles of association 1951–60; board papers 1955–78 [w]; executive committee, minutes and papers 1966–78; research and development (finance and policy) committee, minutes 1955–61; patents committee, minutes 1955–56; new products development (veterinary) committee, minutes 1954–56; new products committee, minutes 1957–61; marketing committee, minutes 1967–76; papers re merger with Glaxo Laboratories Ltd 1958; share registers 1926–35, 1941–69; dividend lists 1912–25; share valuation 1938–49; stock exchange papers 1920–62; papers and correspondence re debentures 1894–1965; share purchases 1964–66; annual reports and accounts 1921–68; accounting schedules and papers 1934–74; budget sheets 1974–76; accounts 1953–78; general ledger 1783–1804; journals: private 1948–72 [w], reserves and provisions 1956–58, exports 1965, 1970; cash books 1960–70; financial registers: assets 1970–71, 1974–75, capital 1971–72, plant 1946–70, motor 1970–73; capital control statements 1974–77;

capital expenditure papers 1968–78; investment grant applications 1966–76; papers re taxation 1921–54, 1961–75; audit papers 1940–75 [w]; papers re acquisition, nd; commercial papers, negotiations and correspondence 1953–74, nd; papers re subsidiary companies 1954–58, nd; production rationalisation papers 1964; research papers and correspondence 1940, 1949–50; licence agreements 1968; papers re surgical division 1947–49; overseas representatives' papers, nd; correspondence re: export business 1793–1823, 1925–50s, Cornelius Hanbury 19th cent, investments 1966–69, Midland Bank re overdraft facilities 1947–56; valuations of plant and equipment, Bethnal Green 1950; papers re property 1948, 1954–63; statutory form and misc papers 1957–78; papers re overseas subsidiaries 1904–08, 1931–57; historical notes and articles 1965–66, nd; private ledger no 3 c1822–43; letterbook of Joseph Gurney Bevan, nd; orders addressed to Mildred & Allen, early 19th cent; family letters, diaries, papers 18th–19th cent; notebooks of D Hanbury, nd; journal 1863; William Allen's preparation book, nd; Daniel Hanbury's notebooks 1842–78; Cornelius Hanbury's letterbook 1896–99; prescription books, nd; William Allen, letters 19th cent; trial balance 1826; laboratory notebook 1881; letters and papers of Cornelius Hanbury 1880s onwards; trust deeds, other legal documents and filing re debentures, etc 19th cent; photographs: *Dictol* production 1960s, *Vitablend* production 1960s, poultry buildings, eggs, chickens and veterinary procedures at Bury Green Farm 1960s–70s, laboratory and office at Bethnal Green, nd; catalogue of veterinary instruments and equipment 1955; unlisted records 18th–20th cent.

Allen & Hanburys (Farms) Ltd
Minutes 1956–85; register of directors' shares 1967–68.

Allen & Hanburys Research Ltd
Annual reports and accounts 1958, 1964–70.

Allied Laboratories Ltd
Directors' meetings, minutes 1937–nd; chairman's meetings, minutes 1960–64; combined register of members, directors and share ledger 1937–61; annual reports and accounts 1938–63 [w]; trading and profit and loss accounts, nd; journals: 1959–65; accounting papers 1956–65; audit papers 1965; papers re acquisition by Edinburgh Pharmaceutical Industries Ltd and Allen & Hanburys Ltd, nd; payroll papers 1963–65; statutory documents and correspondence 1957–80.

AB Insulin Ltd
Register of directors' shares 1967–69; annual reports and accounts 1963–68; ledger 1961–68; auditor's reports 1963–67; finance directors' papers 1958–69; directors' attendance book 1964–68; statutory forms 1964–78.

Eschmann Bros & Walsh Ltd
Order book 1955; catalogue of silver, plated and celluloid surgical instruments, etc 1930; catalogue of elastic gum deaf aids and veterinary instruments 1955.

Records (2): Museum of the History of Science, University of Oxford, Old Ashmolean Building, Broad Street, Oxford OX1 3AZ

Prescription books 1840–94 [w]; pharmaceutical and chemical supplies, orders and invoices 1795, 1802, nd; scrapbook of autographed prescriptions from distinguished physicians collected by Hanbury family 1790, 1822–nd. [Ref: MSS Allen & Hanburys 1–9]

Records (3): Library and Archives, Royal Botanic Gardens, Kew, Richmond TW9 3AE

Correspondence and misc reports of Daniel Hanbury, Cecil Hanbury, Frederick Janson Hanbury and Sir Thomas Hanbury re drugs and plants 19th cent. [Ref: Directors' correspondence 26, 29, 31–39, 41, 87, 109, 121, 134, 142, 146, 148, 152, 214, 218; R Melville – Drugs – Misc]

Records (4): Archives and Manuscripts Section, Wellcome Library for the History and Understanding of Medicine, 183 Euston Road, London NW1 2BE

Outgoing letter book of Daniel Hanbury to overseas correspondents 1858–60. [Ref: MS 5304]

Records (5): Museum, Royal Pharmaceutical Society of Great Britain, 1 Lambeth High Street, London SE1 7JN

Laboratory calculation book 1795–98; drug notebooks 1920–49; stock book 1810–11; price lists 1844–46; correspondence, notes and papers: William Allen 1824, 1833, Daniel Hanbury 1856–75, nd; marriage entry for Silvanus Bevan and Elizabeth Quare 1715; Allen & Hanburys & Barrys Ltd, cost price book 1824–44; page from notebook depicting chemical symbols, nd. [Ref: IRA.1996.037, 090, 230–231; IRA.1997.008–10, 021, 044, 072, 134, 117]

Records (6): Society of Friends, Library of the Religious Society of Friends, Friends House, 173–177 Euston Road, London NW1 2BJ

William Allen, diary fragments 1815. [Ref: Temp MSS 57/13]

Records (7): Rural History Centre, University of Reading, Whiteknights, PO Box 229, Reading RG6 6AG

Veterinary catalogue 1955. [Ref: TR ARN P2/B1]

ARNOLD & SONS LTD
London and Basildon, Essex

History: This company was established in Smithfield, London, in 1819 as Arnold & Sons, manufacturers of surgical instruments and equipment. It was bought by John Bell & Croyden Ltd in 1923, which in turn was bought by Savory & Moore in 1928. During the 1950s Arnold & Sons was incorporated as two limited liability companies. Arnold & Sons Veterinary Instruments Ltd, based at 54 Wigmore Street, London, was responsible for retail sales, while Arnold & Sons Basildon Ltd, based at Honywood Road, Basildon, Essex, concentrated on the manufacture of veterinary and surgical instruments.

Records (1): Rural History Centre, University of Reading, Whiteknights, PO Box 229, Reading RG6 6AG

Catalogues: Arnold & Sons (Savory & Moore Ltd) 1935, 1938–40, nd, Arnold & Sons Veterinary Instruments Ltd 1954, 1964, Arnolds Veterinary Products Ltd 1968; product leaflets, nd. [Ref: TR ADA P2/B22–25, 28–30, 32–38; TR ARN P2/A1–4; TR CXL P2/B1; TR HSE P2/B594; TR 2MRL P2/B13]

Records (2): Museum, Royal Pharmaceutical Society of Great Britain, 1 Lambeth High Street, London SE1 7JN

Catalogue of veterinary and surgical instruments 1954. [Ref: 615.46/7 (085)]

Records (3): John Bell & Croyden Ltd, 50–54 Wigmore Street, London W1H 0AU

Catalogue of surgeon's instruments 1927; photographs of shop window displays, nd.

Records (4): Mitchell Library, Arts Department, North Street, Glasgow G3 7DN

Catalogue of surgical instruments, nd. [Ref: 399457 Shelf no 5430]

THE BOOTS COMPANY PLC

Nottingham, Nottinghamshire

History: The history of The Boots Company plc can be traced back to 1849, and the opening of the British and American Botanic Establishment at 6 Goose Gate, Nottingham, by John Boot, who made and sold his own herbal remedies. From the 1880s, additional shops were opened up in Nottingham and beyond until by 1900 a total of 250 stores made up the Boots Pure Drug Company Ltd, as it had by then become known. Further expansion followed the Pharmacy Act of 1908, which allowed stores such as Boots to offer dispensing services, and the Health Insurance Act of 1911, which extended medical benefits to all working people. By 1913 Boots owned 560 stores in England, Wales and Scotland and the number continued to rise, reaching 1000 by 1933. In 1929, Boots set up an agricultural division. The Ardnamurchan Estate, Argyll, purchased in 1934, was used partly to research and develop veterinary and horticultural products, which could then be sold in Boots stores. By 1952, the company was farming 4500 acres at various locations in England and Scotland. In 1965, Boots Farm Sales Ltd was formed to sell agricultural (including veterinary) products directly to farmers. It was merged with Fisons Ltd in 1980 to form FPC Holdings Ltd and sold in 1983. Veterinary products ceased to be sold in Boots stores from about 1980.

Records: Records Centre and Company Archives, The Boots Company plc, Thane Road West, Nottingham NG90 4XY

Annual reports 1929–; product files and literature c1940–80; price lists for veterinary pharmaceutical products and instruments c1932–65; packaging designs c1930–60s; label specimen books 1945–48; statistical returns giving expense allocation for veterinary products incl a list of agricultural shows Boots advertised at 1925–60; sales review and analysis 1965, 1972; statistical returns, giving expenses for Veterinary Science Section at Thurgarton and Ardslignish, Highland 1935–60; booklet on veterinary research at Thurgarton 1950s; publications: *Veterinary and*

Agricultural Bulletin 1928–29, *Boots Products for the Veterinary Profession* 1963.

COOPER ANIMAL HEALTH LTD
Berkhamsted, Hertfordshire

History: In 1843, William Cooper (d 1885) moved to Berkhamsted, Hertfordshire, from Clunbury in Shropshire and established himself as a veterinary surgeon there. Gradually he began to manufacture and sell his own chemical sheep dip – *Cooper's Sheep Dipping Powder.* In 1852 a mill was acquired in Ravens Lane, Berkhamsted, enabling the dip to be manufactured in bulk and the product range to be expanded. During the 1870s Cooper was joined in the business by his nephews, William Farmer Cooper (d 1882), Herbert Cooper (d 1891) and Richard Powell Cooper (d 1913). In around 1883, the business was renamed William Cooper & Nephews. Richard Powell Cooper's son, Richard Ashmole Cooper, joined the company in 1898 and assumed full control after his father's death. By 1900, Coopers had developed a string of successful companies in major stock-raising countries across the world including Argentina, Africa and Australia. The Cooper Technical Bureau, formed in 1919, soon became an acknowledged world centre of expertise in the development and field use of sheep and cattle dips. First located in London, it moved to Berkhamsted in 1940. William Cooper & Nephews was incorporated as a limited liability company in 1920, and in 1925 merged with another sheep dip manufacturer, McDougall & Robertson Ltd, to form Cooper McDougall & Robertson Ltd. In 1959, Cooper McDougall & Robertson Ltd was acquired by the Wellcome Foundation Ltd, the former's emphasis on dips and dressings complementing the latter's expertise in biologicals. Each company also carried an anthelmintic range and had a common interest in the manufacture of foot-and-mouth disease vaccines. A gradual amalgamation of the two companies' research programmes was completed in 1973 with the establishment in Berkhamsted of the Wellcome Research Laboratories incorporating the Cooper Technical Bureau and the Cooper Research Station. In 1984 a new company, Coopers Animal Health Ltd, was established following the merger of the veterinary interests of the Wellcome Foundation Ltd and Imperial Chemical Industries Ltd. Coopers Animal Health Ltd was wound up in around 1990.

G Macdonald, *In Pursuit of Excellence: one hundred years Wellcome 1880–1980* (London, 1980); P J T Morris and C A Russell, *Archives of the British Chemical Industry 1750–1914: a handlist* (Oxford, 1988).

Records (1): (Historical Records) Records Centre, Glaxo Wellcome plc, 891–995 Greenford Road, Greenford UB6 0HE

Minute books and meeting papers of board and other meetings, statutory records under the Companies Acts, papers of the company secretary and other senior officers incl K J Merrifield and A L McNeilly, material re relations with external bodies and acquisition of companies, reports on overseas visits, financial records, legal agreements and related papers, papers re litigation, patents, records re research and development and manufacturing, company publications incl product literature, external publications, accounts of company history, papers re Cooper family and company employees, photographs, films 19th cent–1980s; William Cooper's notebooks 1859–80s; Cooper Technical Bureau, veterinary research and development records incl correspondence, reports, experiment results, etc 1896–1956; correspondence with War Office re supplies of veterinary products 1914–17; sheep dipping experiment tables 1918–37; complaints register c1940–47. [Ref: Acc 99/2/1–9; Acc 99/60; Acc 99/6/7, 18–22]

Records (2): Rural History Centre, University of Reading, Whiteknights, PO Box 229, Reading RG6 6AG

Leaflets, pamphlets, labels and stationery samples 1880s–1920s, nd; rival firms' advertisements, posters and leaflets 1880s–90s; press cuttings c1889–1905; company publication re agricultural depression 1896; testimonials 1908–16; posters advertising sheep dips for home and overseas markets 1913–17; articles re company history 1960, 1972; annual review 1987; company brochure c1980s; *Cooper's International News* 1987–89. [Ref: TR CMR/AC7/1; P1/B1; P2/A–B; P3/A–B1; P4/1–4; P8–9; SP1]

DAY & SON (CREWE) LTD
Crewe, Cheshire

History: Thomas Day began manufacturing animal medicines at Wantage, Oxfordshire, and Red Lion Street, London, in 1834. In 1840, the business was incorporated as a limited liability company, Thomas Day Ltd. The following year, Day was joined in the business by his brother, James Henry Day. This was a short lived affair and James Henry Day left shortly afterwards to establish his own business, H W & J H Day, in Stafford. Thomas Day continued to develop his business, concentrating on the manufacture of equine remedies for working horses across the country. In 1846 he closed down his London operation and concentrated the entire business in Wantage. Day's son, William Henry Day, became a partner in 1852 after which the business traded as Day & Son Ltd. In 1856 the company re-established itself in London, with premises at 12 Sheldon Street, Paddington, although the Wantage site continued to be active. Shortly afterwards, George Frederick Hewitt was taken into partnership and the company was renamed Day, Son & Hewitt Ltd. In 1862 it moved from Sheldon Street to 22 Dorset Street, London, and during the 1880s relocated to Hope Street, Crewe, where it was renamed Day & Son (Crewe) Ltd. Thereafter the business flourished, and was for a time the largest manufacturer of equine medicines in the country. During the 1920s, however, the demise of the working horse led to a corresponding decline in the company's fortunes that continued until the 1950s. In the 1970s Day & Son (Crewe) Ltd relocated to purpose built premises in First Avenue, Weston Road, Crewe, and expanded its product range to include veterinary preparations aimed mainly at the large animal market. However, by the early 1990s the company was again in decline and in 1994 it was sold to its managing director, Geoffrey McLaughlan, who set about turning it around and increasing its product range. It continues to trade as Day & Son (Crewe) Ltd.

Records (1): Day & Son (Crewe) Ltd, First Avenue, Weston Road, Crewe CW1 1BE

Wages books 1947–61; product formulae cards 19th cent–1950s; product formulae book 20th cent; product lists: veterinary preparations 1940s, animal medicines 1940s; price lists for veterinary preparations and sundries 1940, 1961–82, 1984; product packaging and advertising material, many with directions for use and prices 1940s; correspondence, E G Dennett to Mrs Twigg re company history 1982; company publications 1885, 1912–13, 1940s.

Records (2): Rural History Centre, University of Reading, Whiteknights, PO Box 229, Reading RG6 6AG

Day, Son & Hewitt Ltd, wall charts on the cow, and the horse, nd. [Ref: 2MRL P3/B1–2]

GLAXO WELLCOME PLC
Greenford, Greater London

History: In 1873, Joseph Edward Nathan, a Londoner who had sailed to New Zealand in 1856, set up a household supplies business, trading under the name Joseph Nathan & Co, New Zealand. A London office was opened in 1876 and in 1893 Nathan returned to England, where he incorporated the business as a limited liability company. In 1908, *Glaxo*, a dried milk product for babies, was launched. Over the next twenty years, the company became increasingly interested in health supplements and appointed a pharmaceutical chemist, Harry Jephcott, in 1919, to initiate a programme of research and development. This side of the business, which concentrated particularly on vitamins, expanded rapidly, and in 1935 was incorporated as a private limited company and wholly owned subsidiary, known as Glaxo Laboratories Ltd. Relocation to a large new plant at Greenford, Greater London, in 1936 gave Glaxo Laboratories Ltd the space and incentive to expand its pharmaceutical interests and a host of new products were developed, including vaccines, tablets and medicines. In addition, Glaxo undertook long term research in partnership with other bodies including the Lister Institute, the National Institute for Medical Research and the Therapeutic Research Corporation. By 1945 Glaxo was producing 70 per cent of the total UK supply of penicillin. After the Second World War Glaxo concentrated on pharmaceuticals, selling off its ancillary businesses to leave the parent Nathan company and one subsidiary, Glaxo Laboratories Ltd. In 1947, Joseph Nathan & Co Ltd was wound up and replaced by its subsidiary, which was incorporated as a public limited company, Glaxo Laboratories Ltd. In 1948 Glaxo marketed its first veterinary antibiotic product, penicillin cerate, to treat mastitis in cows. Other products followed and in 1952 a Veterinary Department was established to consolidate and develop the growing use of Glaxo pharmaceuticals in animal health. Dame Olga Uvarov joined the company the following year and took an active role in product development, the training of new representatives, packaging and publicity. Glaxo veterinary surgeons became involved in the clinical trials of products on farms across the country and in 1957 the company opened its own farm at Harefield, Greater London. The company's veterinary surgeons also collaborated with organisations such as the Agricultural Research Council and the National Institute for Research in Dairying, developing feedstuffs as well as animal vaccines. In 1953 nutritionists at Greenford developed *Vitablend*, Glaxo's first range of animal feedstuff additives, while 1955 saw the launch of Glaxo's first vaccine specifically for animals. Known as *Saffelin*, it was used to immunise sheep against pulpy kidney disease. *Saffelin* was followed in 1956 by *Erysilin*, a vaccine designed to combat swine erysipelas. In 1958 Glaxo entered the growing domestic animal market by developing a range of vaccines for dogs, including *Canilin* and *Lepsolin*. It was in 1958 too that Glaxo merged with Allen & Hanburys Ltd. The following year a veterinary biological project was set up in New Zealand, while Evans Medical Ltd was purchased in 1961. Glaxo and Allen & Hanburys continued to maintain separate research establishments for the next twenty years with veterinary research being carried out by Allen & Hanburys at Ware, Hertfordshire, and the medical implications of diseases being studied by Glaxo at Greenford. With a research budget of nearly £1 million, however – five times as much as that available to Allen & Hanburys – Glaxo was able to establish itself firmly within the field of veterinary research. At the end of the 1950s, an entirely new antibiotic, known as griseofulvin, was developed as the first effective treatment by mouth of skin ringworm and, following an agreement with Imperial Chemical Industries Ltd, was launched by Glaxo as *Grisovin*. Another important discovery came in the early 1960s when cortisone was found to have an effect on the metabolism of animals. This, along with its anti-inflammatory properties, opened up an enormous field of potential use. By 1963, Glaxo had developed a range of cortisone-based products including betamethasone eye and skin ointments, eye and ear drops, tablets and injections. In 1962, the company underwent a major reorganisation. Glaxo Group Ltd was constituted as the parent company and the research division of Glaxo Laboratories Ltd, based at Greenford, was incorporated as a separate company, Glaxo Research Ltd, a direct subsidiary of the Glaxo Group Ltd. Over the next decade numerous products were developed and launched. Two new vaccines appeared in 1964: *Iblin*, which protected poultry against infectious bronchitis, and *Clostrin*, used to fight a range of diseases in sheep. A contraceptive pill for dogs, launched in 1969, was followed during the 1970s by a host of new products including *Vetsovate*, a corticosteroid cream to treat animal skin conditions, *Saffan,* an anaesthetic for cats, *Oterna*, eardrops to fight otitis extrema in cats and dogs and *Betsovet*, a steroid injection aimed at alleviating sore joints in horses, dogs and cats. In 1976 cephalosporin entered veterinary medicine in the form of cerates and from this Glaxo introduced *Ceporin* and *Cepoxillin* to treat mastitis in cattle. Three years later, Glaxo's research activities at Greenford and Ware were unified under one company, Glaxo Group Research Ltd. At the same time, the veterinary business was formed into a separate company, Glaxovet Ltd, renamed Glaxo Animal Health in 1982. Glaxo Holdings plc merged with Wellcome plc in 1995 to create Glaxo Wellcome plc.

Anon, *Glaxo Wellcome: a brief history of the world's largest pharmaceutical company* (London, 1995); R Davenport-Hines and J

Slinn, *Glaxo: a history to 1962* (Cambridge, 1992); K Holland, 'Glaxo Holdings plc', *Pharmaceutical Journal*, 5 Dec 1987; H Jephcott, *The First Fifty Years: an account of the early life of Joseph Edward Nathan and the first fifty years of his merchandise business that eventually became the Glaxo group* (Ipswich, 1969); J Millen, *Glaxo from Bonnie Babies to Better Medicine* (New Zealand, 1991); C Turner, *Gold on the Green: fifty years at Greenford* (London, 1985); J Walton, *Glaxo Wellcome at Ulverston: the first fifty years* (Ulverston, 1989); N Watson, *Glaxo at Barnard Castle: a celebration* (Barnard Castle, 1994).

Records: (Historical Records), Records Centre, Glaxo Wellcome plc, 891–995 Greenford Road, Greenford UB6 0HE

Glaxo Holdings plc
Directors' meetings: minutes 1947–75, agenda and related papers 1959–67, correspondence and internal memoranda 1940s–79, nd; general meetings: minutes 1950–68, 1971–81, agenda and papers 1975–79; executive board, minutes 1951–61; transfer committee, minutes 1964–68; overseas subsidiaries committee meetings, minutes 1968–71; educational grants committee, agenda and related papers 1975–86; UK commercial committee, agenda and related papers 1978; memoranda and articles of association 1935, 1969–72; seal registers 1984–88; company secretary's papers, 1972–85; corporate papers re: co-operation with Schering Corporation Inc 1960–73, company reorganisation 1961–74, mergers 1963–64, 1971–72; preliminary announcements 1963–71; trust deed 1972; register of directors' shares 1968–75; share papers 1961–72; papers re rights issue and preference scheme 1965–74; papers re stock exchange 1959–75; shareholder correspondence 1974–79; annual reports and accounts 1963–68, 1972–80; papers re banking arrangements 1977–79; legal case studies re restrictive trade practices 1945–71; papers re industrial tribunals 1974–80; chairman's conference papers 1972; interim reports 1973–75; contracts and licences with companies 1943–73; consultancy agreements 1949–85; procedure agreements 1969–72; complaints and enquiries 1958–79; papers and correspondence re overseas subsidiaries and offices 1912–83; papers re inventions offered to company 1962–68; commercial bulletins 1973–79; files re price and income control 1967–78; correspondence with external parties 1954–80; promotional brochure 1971; register of deeds 1932–56; property papers, plans and correspondence 1939–82; pension papers 1971–74; commercial directorate bulletin 1975–76; papers re directors' retirements, nd; unlisted records 20th cent.

Glaxo Laboratories Ltd

Directors' meetings: minutes 1935–56, 1960–79, attendance books 1946–64, reports 1970–73; general meetings, minutes 1970–78; executive committee: minutes 1947–50, 1958–67, papers 1957–62; management committee (veterinary), minutes 1975–78; sealing committee, minutes 1962–77; board papers 1936–39, 1947–78; joint advisory committee, agenda, papers and minutes 1947–58, 1969–73; memoranda and articles of association 1946–55, 1962; papers re mergers 1955–60, 1974; seal registers 1938–62; debenture stock register 1966–69; papers re stocks and shares 1957–58; annual accounts 1969–78; accounts: consolidated 1969–76, legal 1969–74, general 1957–67; budgets and forecasts 1968–77; capital expenditure papers 1968–77; financial reports, incl veterinary 1975–76; papers re price increases 1973–77; papers and correspondence re sales 1959–68; papers re tax allowances 1969; customs and excise papers 1950–69; duty free bonds 1935–67; papers re rating matters 1969–79; legal papers 1950–71; licences re animal experimentation 1954–67; weights and measures legislation 1958–63; veterinary price lists and data sheets 1960–87; papers of H W Palmer re veterinary department 1952–58; papers re griseofulvin 1950s–70s; inventions offered and rejected 1962–66; product advertisements 1960, 1967; property papers: Greenford 1938, Ulverston, Cumbria 1968–78, Montrose, Angus 1966–74, general 1945–79; wages and salaries files 1969–73; personnel statistics 1968–72; job evaluations 1969–71; safety regulations for contractors 1958–61, 1969; complaints and enquiries 1973–78; sports and social club licences 1958–64; poisons register 1963; correspondence re exchange control 1942–63; misc papers and correspondence 1951–79; publications: *Guidance for Farmers Combatting Bovine Mastitis* 1951, *Glaxo in Veterinary Practice* 1952, *Glaxo Penicillin for Manufacturing Pig and Poultry Feeding Stuffs*, nd, *Penicillin for Your Pigs and Poultry* 1954, *Glaxo Veterinary Guide to Penicillin* (3rd ed) c1955; press cuttings re veterinary vaccines, dog vitamins, antibiotics, etc c1962–79; photographs 1960s–70s; unlisted records 20th cent. [Ref: GGA289; Acc98/68, 99/5, 99/400]

Glaxo Research Ltd

Minutes, agenda and papers 1963–68; agreements, share transfers and debenture correspondence 1967; annual reports and accounts 1967–68, 1975–78; accounts 1967–69; consolidated accounts 1976–77; audit papers 1967; Evans Medical and Evans Animal Division, product notices c1972–81; notices to staff 1974–79; personnel records 1975–79; correspondence with University of York 1980; statutory forms 1965–78; unlisted records 20th cent. [Ref: SP 504]

Glaxo Group Research Ltd
Veterinary development committee, minutes and agenda 1978–83; veterinary clinical trials committee, minutes 1982; mastitis working group, minutes and agenda 1983. [Ref: Acc99/27]

Glaxo International Ltd
General meetings: minutes 1966–72, agenda and related papers 1965–72; divisional meetings, minutes, agenda and related papers 1967–70; memorandum and articles of association 1965; overseas subsidiaries, minutes and papers 1966–72; misc papers and correspondence 1961–77.

Glaxo Operations UK Ltd
General meetings, minutes 1980–86; executive committee, minutes 1968; minutes, agenda and papers re other meetings 1962–82 [w]; annual accounts 1980–87; legal accounts 1962–75; consolidated accounts 1966–77, 1980–88; capital projects 1981–82; banking records 1968–78; auditor's reports 1980; customs and excise papers 1972–78; research papers 1921–67; disability pensions, board minutes 1978–87; *The Glaxo Volume* 1948–74; confidential memoranda 1963–66; biographical notes re Dr E Lester Smith 1966; misc papers and correspondence 1961–82; unlisted records 20th cent.

Glaxo Export Ltd
General meetings, minutes 1983–87; memorandum and articles of association 1983; papers re shares 1983–84; annual accounts 1983–87; capital projects, papers 1983–88; property papers 1983–85; misc papers and correspondence 1983–89.

Glaxo Allenburys Ltd
Directors' meetings, minutes 1960–72; general meetings, minutes 1968–71; memoranda and articles of association 1960–2; agenda 1960–77; attendance registers 1966–72; share certificates 1960–78; accounts 1965–74, 1978; accounting papers 1959–73; audited accounts 1962–75; reports: regional 1970–71, supplies division 1971, veterinary survey of Nigeria 1965; pension scheme, agenda and papers 1960–64; correspondence: overseas subsidiaries and agents 1950–66, internal 1965–66; statutory forms 1960–78. [Ref: GGA102, 263]

A GREAVES & SON LTD
Chesterfield, Derbyshire

History: Abraham Greaves registered as a pharmaceutical chemist in 1853 and traded in Ironville, Derbyshire, before acquiring the business of Josiah Claughton, based at 35 Low Pavement, Chesterfield, during the 1870s, naming it Greaves & Richardson. His son, Abraham Walter Greaves, registered as a chemist and druggist in 1872 and joined his father shortly afterwards. In 1902, Abraham Walter Greaves was, like his father before him, joined by his son, Sydney Chater Greaves. The business continued to trade from Low Pavement until its relocation to 3 Vicar Lane, Chesterfield, in 1980. It was incorporated as a limited liability company, A Greaves & Son Ltd, in 1983, and afterwards moved to Sycamore House, Smeckley Wood Close, Chesterfield.

'A Century-Old Chesterfield Business', *Chemist and Druggist*, vol 124, 23 May 1936.

Records: Chesterfield Public Library, New Beetwell Street, Chesterfield S40 1QN

Partnership agreement between Abraham Walter Greaves and Sydney Chater Greaves 1902; general meetings, papers 1943–44; ledgers 1905–43; Claughtons wholesale druggists, ledger 1849–52; wages, salaries and insurance books 1912–25, 1933–49; bills 1928–45; misc business papers 1920s; prescription books, some with loose press cuttings 1903–52; register of penicillin injections and account of proprietary medicines sold 1934–49; veterinary recipe books c1910–40; trade catalogues 1908, c1938; trade and professional association circulars 1933–45; correspondence c1918–46; papers re staff Christmas boxes 1918. [Ref: GRE nos. 1–110]

WALTER GREGORY & CO LTD
Crawley, West Sussex

History: Walter Gregory & Co Ltd was established in Crawley, West Sussex, during the late nineteenth century to supply animal health products to farmers in the west of England. The company was acquired by Upjohn Ltd in 1966 and dissolved in 1993.

Records: Pharmacia & Upjohn Ltd, Davy Avenue, Knowlhill, Milton Keynes MK5 8PH

Memorandum and articles of association 1965; certificate of incorporation 1965; directors' and general meeting minutes 1966–92; combined register of directors and shareholders 1966–68; registers of debtors (combined with Somerset Pharmaceuticals Ltd) 1965; correspondence re: certificate of nomination of directors 1966, shares 1966, dissolution of company 1993; share certificate 1966.

JOHNSON'S VETERINARY PRODUCTS LTD

West Bromwich and Sutton Coldfield, West Midlands

History: In 1910 Arthur Guy Johnson, a foundry clerk from West Bromwich, began to compound and supply a number of medicaments aimed at treating ailments affecting poultry, pigeons and dogs. His first three products, *Roup Cure*, *Reviving Tonic* and *Ovary Tonic* were launched in 1919 and two years later Johnson gave up his job and established himself in business as a poultry specialist, based at 13 Hope Street, West Bromwich, and trading under the name Johnson Brothers. His two sons, Arthur Howard Johnson and Raymond George Johnson, later joined him in the business. In 1926 the firm relocated to new premises at 26 Bagnall Street, West Bromwich, and by 1939 had expanded its range to twelve products. Arthur Johnson's sons acquired the business in 1945 and in 1950 incorporated it as a limited liability company, Johnson's Veterinary Products Ltd. In 1955 the company moved to a purpose built factory on the Reddicap Trading Estate, Sutton Coldfield, West Midlands. Arthur David Johnson, son of Arthur Howard Johnson, was appointed company director in 1970 and went on to become chairman and managing director in 1984.

Anon, *The History of Johnson's Veterinary Products* (unpublished typescript, 1996).

Records: Johnson's Veterinary Products Ltd, 5 Reddicap Trading Estate, Sutton Coldfield B75 7DF

Product and price list 1948; product advertisements 1922–64; customer testimonials 1934–37, 1966; circular advertising letter 1930s; letter re breakage of products during supply 1932.

LAB PAK LTD
Fillongley, Warwickshire

History: Lab Pak Ltd was incorporated as a wholly owned subsidiary of Mill House (Coventry) Ltd, a holding company owned by Jeff Thompson, in 1976. Based at Fillongley, Warwickshire, it manufactures a range of veterinary and laboratory products and distributes them to veterinary practices, colleges and research establishments across the UK. The company is also the major supplier of blood collection systems to the Ministry of Agriculture, Fisheries and Food.

Records: Lab Pak Ltd, Mill House, Mill Lane, Fillongley, Coventry CV7 8EE

Product catalogues 1975–; advertising material 1981.

OSMOND AND SONS LTD
Grimsby, North East Lincolnshire

History: Osmond and Sons Ltd was established in Grimsby in 1854. Originally the company manufactured chemicals, particularly sheep dips and animal medicines, but later diversified into a range of animal health and nutrition products. Exports were sent across the world and companies set up in Australia, New Zealand, Ireland and South Africa. The company also owned land and herds at Barnoldby, Lincolnshire. Osmond and Sons Ltd went into receivership in 1976.

Records (1): North East Lincolnshire Archives, Town Hall, Grimsby DN31 1HX

Register of members and share ledger 1909; bank pass books 1897–1911; ledger of travellers' accounts 1928–41; bought ledger c1931–40; goods received book 1938–50; export order books: New Zealand 1937–51, Dublin 1937–55, South Africa 1938–52, misc 1941–54.

Osmond and Sons (Pty) Ltd, South Africa
Day book 1943–47.

Osmond and Sons (Dublin) Ltd
Day book 1943–50.

Osmond Pharmaceuticals
Cash received book 1942–59; day book (feeding stuffs, meals, etc) 1944–75; summaries of trade 1939–41; mill books and rough notebooks re production 1935–66; company circulars to all representatives 1962–74; sales analysis file 1963–68; correspondence: Australia re stock breeding 1953–58, South Africa re veterinary and dairy supplies 1964–69, Malta 1965–70, customers 1966–67, overseas enquiries 1966–69, technical queries 1968, 1970, Dublin 1970, agricultural shows 1972; board and production meetings, minutes and papers 1970–76; photographs of commercial representatives 1920s; lists of villages and farms with totals of days worked, nd; Holland, analysis of representatives' sales 1939; travellers' agreements: Joshua William Lodge 1939, 1946–47, George Stanley McGrann 1960; address list of 20,000 top British farms 1960s; J C T Waller, representative, reports and correspondence 1974–76.

Osmond and Sons (New Zealand) Ltd
Trade labels c1924–44; dip labels c1961; misc labels c1931–70s, nd.

Osmond Estates Ltd (Barnoldby)

Ayrshire females and bulls herd book, c1931–50; correspondence re farm building improvements, etc 1940–67; Councillor L K Osmond, illuminated address 1928.

Records (2): Museum of Lincolnshire Life, Burton Road, Lincoln LN1 3LY

Books of formulae 1918–45; price list 1921; notebook 1920; booklet, *Health and Healing on the Farm*, nd.

PFIZER LTD
Sandwich, Kent

History: Pfizer Inc was established in Brooklyn, New York, in 1849 by Charles Pfizer and his cousin, Charles Erhart. At first the company focussed on the manufacture of bulk chemicals, but the emergence of antibiotics during the Second World War heralded a change of direction and transformed Pfizer Inc into an international company. Pfizer Inc became the first mass producer of penicillin and followed this success with the discovery in 1949 of the broad-spectrum antibiotic *Terramycin*. Pfizer Ltd, established as a UK subsidiary at Wear Bay Road, Folkestone, in 1952 before moving to Sandwich in 1954, expanded rapidly and by

1960 was one of the largest Pfizer operations outside the US, with over 2000 staff working across four Divisions – Pharmaceutical, Chemicals, Agriculture and Consumer, each of which had its own local board. In 1958, Kembell Bishop & Co Ltd, a British company that had enjoyed a close working relationship with Pfizer since 1936, was acquired. Kembell Bishop & Co Ltd continued to operate under its established name until its full amalgamation into Pfizer Ltd in 1968. As part of its expansion programme, Pfizer Ltd in 1955 set up an animal feed plant, primarily to exploit the growth promoting properties of *Terramycin*. This was followed in 1957 by the establishment of an Agricultural Division incorporating a small veterinary research unit that marketed animal pharmaceutical products. By the time the *Terramycin* patent expired in 1966 Pfizer Ltd was responsible for a wide range of products including several aimed at the growing animal health market. A tropical medicine research unit was set up in 1965, but scaled down again two years later. In 1971, Pfizer Central Research was formed, with sites at Groton in the US, Sandwich in the UK, Amboise in France and Nagoya in Japan, and the specific aim of discovering new products for the company's pharmaceutical, chemical and agricultural divisions. Notable successes included *Terramycin Q100* for the treatment of cattle disease, and *Paratect Bolus*, a single dose treatment for parasitic gastroenteritis in cattle, launched in 1981. In 2000, Pfizer Central Research became known as Pfizer Global Research and Development. In 1995, Pfizer Ltd acquired Smith Kline Beecham's Animal Health Division and in 2000 merged with Warner Lambert. The Animal Health Department, now known as the Veterinary Medicine Department, continues to discover, develop and market a wide range of animal medicines including vaccines, antibiotics and parasiticides for livestock, horses and pets.

Anon, *Growth Through Innovation: a brief Pfizer history* (New York, 1993); K Holland, 'Pfizer Ltd', *The Pharmaceutical Journal*, 11 Jan 1992; Jonathan Mantle, *Pfizer at Sandwich: the story of Pfizer Ltd* (London, 1994); Mines, *Pfizer, An Informal History* (New York, 1978); T Derdak (ed), 'Pfizer Inc', *International Directory of Company Histories*, vol 1 (London, 1988); Tanner, *Twenty Five Years of Innovation: the story of Pfizer Central Research* (Greenwich, 1996).

Records: Records Management Unit, Pfizer Central Research, Pfizer Ltd, Ramsgate Road, Sandwich, Kent CT13 9NJ

Pfizer Inc
Annual reports 1959–; reports to shareholders 1956–65; interim reports to shareholders 1971–73; annual meeting of shareholders, reports 1986–90;

quarterly reports 1985–96; penicillin brochure, *Chas Pfizer & Co Inc* nd; in house magazines: *Capsule* 1976–97, *Sitewize* 1980, *Pfizer World* 1996–99, *Rostrum* issues 103–107, nd, *Spectrum* issues 20–36, nd.

Pfizer Ltd
Letters patent re Sandwich site 1558; plans of Richborough site 1917–18; leases re Folkestone properties 1955–56; income tax schedule listing Pfizer properties incl site plans for Sandwich, Folkestone and Millwall 1961–64; visitor books: Pfizer Group 1961–85, Pfizer Exhibition 1986; publicity material and in house magazines: *Pfizerama* 1960–69, *Facts about Pfizer* 1965–94, *Pfizer Europe* 1968–84, *Pfizer Scene* 1969–71, 1973–97, *Insite Magazine* 1974–99, *Pfame* 1984–85, *Academic Liaison: at the chalkface* 1992–95, *Animal Health Update/Transition Update* 1995–96, *Community Newsletter* 1996–99, *Pfizer European* 1998–99; product labels c1970.

Pfizer Central Research
Annual research conference reports 1953–88.

Smith Kline Beecham Animal Health Division
Records re animal health research 1949–55.

PHARMACIA & UPJOHN LTD
Knowlhill, Milton Keynes

History: The Upjohn Pill & Granule Co was established in Kalamazoo, Michigan, US, by William and Henry Upjohn in 1885. The firm began operations in 1886 and was soon manufacturing a human medicament, the 'friable' pill, which was softer than other pills on the market, and so able to dissolve more effectively in the stomach. By the turn of the century the company was also manufacturing compressed tablets. In 1903, the business was incorporated as a private limited liability company, The Upjohn Co Inc, and increased its manufacturing and marketing activities. Between the 1920s and 1950s it conducted research and development into the prevention of human heart disease, cancer and arthritis. In 1940 a veterinary surgeon, Dr J Lavere Davidson, was employed to explore the market for veterinary pharmaceuticals. Although the Second World War slowed down development, by the late 1940s the company was manufacturing and marketing veterinary pharmaceutical products alongside its established human range. In 1952, a UK subsidiary of The Upjohn Co Inc was incorporated as a limited liability company, Upjohn of England Ltd.. Based at 4 Alford Street, London, the subsidiary manufactured and sold ethical pharmaceuticals, including corticosteroids, antibiotics, medical specialities and veterinary products. In the same year the Upjohn Co Inc produced *Teatube Neomycin*, a treatment for mastitis which revolutionised milk productivity levels in cattle. Upjohn of England Ltd relocated to a new manufacturing plant at Fleming Way, Crawley, West Sussex, in 1956 and five years later was renamed Upjohn Ltd. In 1958 the parent company was converted to a public limited liability company, The Upjohn Co Inc. Upjohn Ltd in 1966 acquired two veterinary companies supplying products to farmers in the west of England: Walter Gregory & Co Ltd and Somerset Pharmaceuticals Ltd, both of which were dissolved in 1993. In 1995 Upjohn Co Inc merged with Pharmacia AB, a Swedish company established in 1911, to form Pharmacia & Upjohn Ltd. Between 1995 and 1998 former Upjohn Ltd employees were moved from the Upjohn Ltd site at Crawley to the Pharmacia GB Ltd headquarters at Davy Avenue, Knowlhill, Milton Keynes. The company continues to be involved in the manufacture and marketing of veterinary products.

R D B Carlisle, *A Century of Caring: the Upjohn story* (US, 1987); T Derdak (ed), 'Upjohn', *International Directory of Company Histories*, vol 1 (London, 1988).

Records: Pharmacia & Upjohn Ltd, Davy Avenue, Knowlhill, Milton Keynes MK5 8PH

Upjohn Ltd
Minutes: directors' and general meetings 1952–, trustees of pension and life assurance scheme meetings 1960–66, 1969–; memoranda and articles of association 1952, 1977; correspondence re memoranda and articles of association 1972, 1977; certificates of incorporation 1981–82; change of name certificate 1961; board meeting attendance registers 1976–91; notices and proxies: directors' meetings 1974, general meetings 1974–75; registers of directors and secretaries 1954, 1967; company registration documents and correspondence 1991–94; registers: shareholders 1952–64, members and share ledger 1952–96, mortgages, nd; stock transfer forms nd; share certificate books 1952–96; correspondence re shares 1980s; annual reports 1954–95 [w]; balance sheets/profit and loss accounts 1984–95; statements of account 1991–94; balance of payments 1991; trial balances 1985, 1990, 1993; accounts 1984–95; inter-company accounts 1989–93; ledgers: sales 1990–91, 1993–94, purchases 1991; journals: costings 1991, 1993–95, sales 1988–90; expense reports: sales 1992, 1995, sales force 1993–95, external 1990–93, internal 1989–94; journals and working papers re fixed assets 1990–94; daily receipts

summaries 1992–93; cash receipts 1992, 1994; cheque requisitions 1990–91, 1994–95; banking: daily summary 1990–92, journals 1989–94, receipts and statements 1991–95, transfers 1990–94, correspondence 1992, various 1986–91; forecasts: customers 1991, exports 1993; cash postings 1990–91; catering account 1991; misc accounts 1988–95; duty and value added tax deferment statements 1990–95; taxation papers 1981–89; value added tax review 1994–95; papers re dividend taxation relief 1968, 1991; insurance policies and correspondence 1966–95; insurance papers 1984, 1988–91; insurance claims 1990–95; correspondence re: audit 1991–92, accounts 1990–95, Financial Services Act 1986; legal papers and correspondence 1983–95; affidavits re leases at Fleming Way, Crawley 1987; patent review records 1988–89; trade marks 1987–90; agreements and contracts with other companies 1960s–96; production papers and notes 1980–95; project registration files 1960, 1976–96; materials management documents 1988–95; technical support papers 1981–91; product histories and information 1986–87, 1991; correspondence with Home Office re Misuse of Drugs Act and licence to produce drugs 1990–96; advertising literature 1979–92; marketing files 1975–93, 1995; certification files 1987–91; extension works at Fleming Way, Crawley: agreement and lease 1957–64, architectural drawings 1960, 1987–91, nd, correspondence 1982–94; warehouse at Lowfield Heath, Crawley: leases 1985, 1991, architectural drawings 1988, correspondence and papers 1985–94; 12 Park Way, Crawley: land certificate and architectural drawings 1957–58, report and valuation 1958, 1965, correspondence re community charge and council tax 1991–93, photographs, nd; contracts and leases with related correspondence 1987–96; 8 Hatchfields, Cuckfield, West Sussex, tenancy agreements and inventory 1988–89; papers re: mortgages and loans 1992, construction project 1993, office expansion and renovation project 1991, 1993; inventory valuations 1991–95; pension and life assurance scheme, annual accounts 1956–95; pension trust, deeds and related correspondence 1955–; charitable trust, deeds 1960, 1979, 1987–92; papers re wages 1982–89; pension records 1977–79, 1984–94; employee survey 1981–91; office services papers 1993–95; time cards 1991–94; correspondence re: exports 1992–93, marketing 1992–93, forecasts for overseas subsidiaries 1989–94, office expansion project 1991–92; Veterinary Division: papers re technical enquiries and service 1985–91, animal health complaints 1990, animal health credit notes 1990, papers re product development 1994–97, papers re veterinary biologicals 1995, veterinary and transfer orders 1993–97.

Upjohn (Ireland) Ltd

Company registration documents and correspondence 1978–95.

PRECISION HISTOLOGY INTERNATIONAL LTD
Harleston, Norfolk

History: Precision Histology International Ltd was established by Peter Finn in 1983. Initially it concentrated on analytical work for the pharmaceutical industry, but soon expanded to include diagnostic work. Tissue samples from all over the world are processed and analysed each day. The laboratory is governed by Department of Health regulations and all processes are subject to standard operating procedures. By 1999, there were five veterinary surgeons employed on the diagnostic side while Peter Finn continued the toxicology analysis. In this capacity he is frequently called upon to act as an expert witness.

Records: Precision Histology International Ltd, Micron House, London Road, Harleston, Norfolk IP20 9BH

Annual reports 1984–; day books 1983–; laboratory books 1983–; toxicology reports 1983–; wet tissue slides 1983–; study files 1983–; papers re staff, training, etc 1983–.

L ROWLAND & CO
Wrexham

History: L Rowland & Co traded as chemists at Dolydd Road, Wrexham, during the nineteenth century.

Records: Denbighshire Record Office, 46 Clwyd Street, Ruthin LL15 1HP

Prescription books incl veterinary recipes c1828, c1859–62. [Ref: DD/DM/763/1–2]

SOMERSET PHARMACEUTICALS LTD
West of England

History: Somerset Pharmaceuticals Ltd was originally established in the west of England to exploit new aerosol technology for animals and supply veterinary products to local farmers. It was incorporated as a limited liability company during the 1950s, acquired by Upjohn Ltd in 1966 and dissolved in 1993.

Records: Pharmacia & Upjohn Ltd, Davy Avenue, Knowlhill, Milton Keynes MK5 8PH

Memorandum and articles of association 1965; certificate of incorporation 1965; directors' and general meeting minutes 1966–92; combined register of directors and shareholders 1966–68; registers of debtors (combined with Walter Gregory & Co Ltd) 1965; correspondence re: shares 1966, certificate of nomination of directors 1966, dissolution of company 1993; share certificate 1966.

STURGES
Leicester, Leicestershire

History: Henry Cooper and William Pettifor opened their chemist and druggist's store at 44 Market Place, Leicester, in c1870. Initially the business traded as Cooper & Pettifor, although it had become known as Cooper & Son by 1876. In 1878, with the arrival of William Sturges of Lutterworth, Leicestershire, the business changed its name once again, to Cooper & Sturges. Cooper moved to 15 Bartholomew Place, Leicester, some time between 1887 and 1891, leaving William Sturges at Market Place. The business remained in the Sturges family until its closure in 1961.

Records: Record Office for Leicestershire, Leicester and Rutland, Long Street, Wigston Magna, Leicester LE18 2AH

Ledger sheets 1879–84; prescription books, incl some for animals 1844–1928 [w]; veterinary prescription book 1881–90; wages book 1878–84. [Ref: 3D61]

W R SWANN & CO LTD
Sheffield, South Yorkshire

History: In 1932, Walter Swann incorporated his own razor blade manufacturing business, W R Swann & Co Ltd, as a limited liability company at Woodland Street, Sheffield, with Doris Fairweather and J A Morton as co-directors. One of the company's earliest products was named *Kleen Razor Blades*. From the outset, the company was run on socialist principles, recognising that its workers should be fairly remunerated and that their views and needs given full consideration. Consequently, the company's employees were also its shareholders, each receiving a share of the profits. In 1935, W R Swann & Co Ltd was invited to produce replaceable blades for a patented handle on behalf of a surgical house. Sales of the handle dwindled, but W R Swann & Co Ltd, not wanting to lose this business, began to manufacture its own handle, the *Swann-Morton Scalpel.* In the same year a second factory was built at Bradfield Road, Sheffield, and in 1938 building work began on a third factory at Owlerton on the edge of Sheffield. During the 1930s, the company became the first in the UK to introduce a working week of forty hours and paid annual leave for its workers. After the Second World War a further factory was opened in Scotland in an attempt to alleviate unemployment there, but closed again after only seven months. During the 1940s and 1950s, largely because of the heavy taxation on razor blades, the company shifted its manufacturing priority to surgical scalpels. It also developed an interest in blades for industrial and craft purposes and in 1951 a subsidiary company, Craft Blades Ltd, was incorporated to control this end of the market. By 1957, W R Swann & Co Ltd was producing 38 million blades and handles annually, many of which were supplied for use in the veterinary profession. The company was renamed W R Swann & Co (Holdings) Ltd in 1948, but reverted to W R Swann & Co Ltd in 1956. In 1964, the premises at Owlerton were expanded to meet the increased demand for surgical blades. Although they remained active in the management of the company until their deaths in 1980 and 1984 respectively, both Swann and Fairweather were anxious to ensure that it should never be governed by shareholders who did not work in the business. A trust was therefore set up to continue the employment ethos of its founders. Over one million surgical blades, scalpels and handles continue to be produced each day for the human and animal surgery markets.

Anon, *Swann-Morton: sixty years of achievement 1932–1992* (Sheffield, 1992).

Records: Swann-Morton Ltd, Owlerton Green, Sheffield S6 2BJ

Memoranda and articles of association 1932, 1948; change of name certificate 1948; management committee, minute book 1945–46; balance sheets and trading and profit and loss accounts 1933–34, 1944; statement of production costs and trading and financial statements 1944; ledgers 1932–33; day book 1933–34; cash books 1932–33; petty cash book 1932; supply contracts (p) 1964–65; notice re working of forty hour week, nd; notice on sterilised surgical blades, nd; press cuttings: registration of company 1932, new premises at Owlerton Green 1941, Mr Swann's award of role of honour with Sheffield Central School, nd; Mr Swann's notes and correspondence re management and production issues, politics, economics, philosophy and company history 1957–80s; wages book 1932–40; correspondence: distributors 1963–64, purchase of Bradfield engineering works 1970; photographs: Walter Swann and Doris Fairweather 1976, premises, gardens, staff and production 1932–; booklets of razor blade packaging with contents, W R Swann & Co Ltd and competitors 1930s–nd; tribute to W R Swann by staff member 1980; historical notes re Swann family 1978, nd; Swann family tree, nd.

Craft Blades Ltd
Memorandum and articles of association 1951.

TENTERDEN PHARMACY

Tenterden, Kent

History: Tenterden Pharmacy was established in 1790. S H Willsher joined the business in 1856 and went on to develop an extensive trade in extemporaneously prepared animal medicines. *Willsher's Cattle Food* was introduced in c1870 and manufactured on a large scale in adjoining premises. In 1896, Alexander Ridley acquired the pharmacy and although at first he continued to manufacture the cattle food, by 1910 it was being prepared for him by the British Drug Houses. Veterinary supplies still form part of the present pharmacy business, which is now owned by Paydens Ltd (est 1969).

H V Roberts, 'The Eighteenth Century Pharmacy at 60 High Street, Tenterden, Kent', *Pharmaceutical Historian*, October 1998.

Records: in private ownership of Mr H V Roberts, Gullivers, Main Street, Tugby LE7 9WD

Notebook re manufacture of *Willsher's Cattle Food* incl testimonials re its efficacy.

THAMES MEDICAL LTD

Lancing, West Sussex

History: Thames Medical Ltd was incorporated in February 1994 as a limited liability company by Michael Brampton at his home in Worthing, West Sussex, to supply human medical monitoring equipment to ambulance services. In June of the same year, the company began to make its own modifications to the monitors and accepted a contract to supply a monitor to the Aga Khan's veterinary surgeon, for use on his racehorses. Thereafter, the company modified and supplied monitors for use in the treatment of a variety of animals including dogs, foxes, badgers and exotic species. In 1994 the company relocated to the Winston Business Centre in Lancing. In 1996, two limited liability companies, Thames Medical Manufacturing Ltd and Thames Medical Research Ltd, were incorporated as subsidiaries of Thames Medical Ltd, and in December 1997 the former produced the company's first fully self-manufactured monitor. Thames Medical Research Ltd was a dormant company from its inception, serving as a holding company for designs and patent registrations.

Records: Thames Medical Ltd, Unit 2, Winston Business Centre, Chartwell Road, Lancing BN15 8TU

Directors' and general meetings minutes and register of shareholders 1994–; memorandum and articles of association 1994; certificate of incorporation 1994; balance sheets and profit and loss accounts 1994–; cash books 1994–; lease agreement 1994; product and service advertisements 1994–; press cuttings 1994–; photographs of products and animals receiving treatment 1994–; video recording of television news report re company 1996.

Thames Medical Manufacturing Ltd
Directors' and general meetings minutes and register of shareholders 1996–; memorandum and articles of association 1996; certificate of incorporation 1996; balance sheets/profit and loss accounts 1996–; cash books 1996–.

Thames Medical Research Ltd
Directors' and general meetings minutes and register of shareholders 1996–; memorandum and articles of association 1996; certificate of incorporation 1996; balance sheets/profit and loss accounts 1996–; cash books 1996–; patent applications, product designs and drawings 1994–.

J J THOMAS & SON
Rochdale, Greater Manchester

History: Edward Thomas was registered as a chemist and druggist at 24 Yorkshire Street, Rochdale, in 1886, and was still trading under that name in 1895. The same business later traded as J J Thomas & Son, with additional premises at 54 Drake Street and 10 St Mary's Gate, Rochdale.

Records: Rochdale Local Studies Library, Esplanade Arts and Heritage Centre, Esplanade, Rochdale OL16 1AQ

Prescription books 1902–28, 1944–63; prescription records, incl veterinary c1937–63, nd. [Ref: M/CPR/1–7]

THE WELLCOME FOUNDATION PLC
London

History: Burroughs Wellcome & Co was established in London in 1880 by the American pharmacists Silas M Burroughs and Henry S Wellcome. From 1889 a range of medicines and supplements were produced at the Wellcome Chemical Works, the company's factory in Dartford, Kent. Although Silas Burroughs died in 1895, expansion continued under the guidance of Henry Wellcome. A number of 'associated houses' were set up across the world and research laboratories established. In 1924 Henry Wellcome brought all his separate interests in manufacturing and research together into one private company, The Wellcome Foundation Ltd. This included the Wellcome Museum of Medical Science, established in 1914 and based initially at 10 Henrietta Street, London, before moving in 1932 to purpose built premises on Euston Road. Following Wellcome's death in 1936, The Wellcome Foundation Ltd was formed as a charitable foundation, with its trustees appointed the sole shareholders. Under the terms of Wellcome's will, all profits from the Wellcome Foundation Ltd were to be used by the trustees to fund medical research – particularly pharmacy and pharmacology, veterinary and tropical medicine and the history of medicine. The company's interest in veterinary medicine can be traced back to the beginning of the twentieth century. A price list produced by Burroughs Wellcome & Co in 1900 included a range of sixteen veterinary *Tabloid* brand products using morphine, digitalin, ergotinine, atropine and cocaine. Important research was carried out by the Wellcome Physiological Research Laboratories, which opened in Charlotte Street, London, in 1894 before moving to Herne Hill, Greater London, in 1898 and to Beckenham, Greater London, in 1921. The laboratories were originally established to produce large amounts of diphtheria anti-serum but in 1901 became the first private research facilities to be given official permission to carry out experimental work on live animals, a move which significantly aided their research capabilities. Further groundbreaking work was carried out in the field of tropical medicine, a subject of particular interest to Henry Wellcome. The first Wellcome Tropical Research Laboratory was opened in 1902 in Khartoum, Sudan, followed in 1907 by the introduction of a floating laboratory which carried research to hitherto inaccessible areas along the Nile. Recognising that successful research relied on co-operation from a wide range of disciplines including chemistry, protozoology, helminthology, bacteriology, biochemistry, virology and immunology, Wellcome established the Wellcome Bureau of Scientific Research (later the Wellcome Laboratories of Tropical Medicine) in 1913 to co-ordinate the work of the various institutes and laboratories within the Wellcome group. Some of the drugs to emerge from this co-ordinated research included *Pentostam*, used to fight leishmaniasis in humans and small animals, *Frantin*, which combatted nematodiriasis in lambs, *Ancaris* for hookworm in dogs and *Scoloban* for tapeworm in dogs and cats. A further impetus to veterinary research came in 1922, when Thomas Dalling MRCVS was appointed superintendent of the stable of serum-producing horses at Beckenham. Dalling had previously been one of two chief investigators at the newly established Animal Diseases Research Association, and brought with him in particular his invaluable experience of research into lamb dysentery. The research team at Beckenham did much to bring about a vaccine into this and other diseases afflicting sheep. Successful research was also carried out into 'yellows' in dogs, resulting in the development by Wellcome of the first Leptospira canicola vaccine, and into canine distemper, enabling Wellcome in 1928 to produce the appropriate prophylactics on a commercial scale, followed in 1953 by the first live distemper vaccine to be produced in Europe. In 1943, a 325 acre farm at Frant, East Sussex, was purchased and the Wellcome Veterinary Research Station set up, partly to help cope with the wartime demand for vaccines. One of its first successes was the introduction in 1946 of single dose tubes of penicillin for intramammary use against streptococcal mastitis. In the same year, a residential refresher course was set up for demobilised veterinary surgeons and proved so successful that it ran annually until 1965, attracting veterinary surgeons from across the world. In 1946, the Physiological Research Laboratories were combined with the Wellcome Chemical Research Laboratories to form the Wellcome Research Laboratories, which concentrated on medical and veterinary research. Veterinary drugs to come out of these laboratories included *Marivax*, the first officially licensed vaccine for Marek's disease, and *Thorovax*, a purified tetanus vaccine which could be injected into racehorses with minimal risk of abscesses or muscle damage. In addition, Wellcome, in collaboration with the Animal Virus Research Institute at Pirbright, Surrey, produced a vaccine for foot-and-mouth disease that is still used in over forty countries worldwide. The acquisition of Cooper McDougall & Robertson, the recognised world leader in dips and dressings, in 1959 considerably boosted Wellcome's veterinary credentials. Both companies had an anthelmintic range and shared an interest in the development of foot-and-mouth vaccines. Moreover, the acquisition of Cooper McDougall & Robertson gave Wellcome an important foothold in major overseas markets. Gradually the research interests of the two companies were merged, culminating in 1973 with the closure of the research station at Frant and the establishment at Berkhamsted, Hertfordshire, of the Wellcome Research Laboratories. In 1979, a veterinary entomology laboratory was added, which concentrated on the study of external parasites. Wellcome's position was further strengthened by the acquisition of Calmic Ltd in 1967, Hadleigh-Crowther, a specialist in dairy hygiene products, in 1969, and Macdonald Taylor, producers of surgical dressings, in 1971. During the 1970s, Wellcome's animal health business expanded rapidly and a range of new drugs were produced, including *Tribrissen* and *Trivetrin*, used to treat a range of bacterial diseases, and *Coriban*, introduced in 1971 to treat sheep for liverfluke. In 1971, the company introduced the first commercial vaccine for the control of foot-rot in sheep and followed this a few years later with *Gletvax*, aimed at preventing Escherichia. coli infections in young pigs. Wellcome also entered into licensing agreements with other companies. Oxfendazole, an anthelmintic for sheep and cattle, was jointly developed and marketed by Wellcome as *Systamex*, as were such products as *Coopex* and *Amitraz*. In 1979, Wellcome acquired Jensen-Salsbery Laboratories, a division of Richardson-Merrell Inc, US. By the 1990s The Wellcome Foundation Ltd had veterinary surgeons working in laboratories across the world – in places as far-flung as Kenya, Australia, New Zealand, South Africa, Argentina, Uruguay, Brazil and Paraguay. Money was also made available by the Wellcome Trust to fund veterinary research and education. In 1968, several specialisms were deemed priorities – parasitology, pre and post-natal studies, nutrition and metabolism. To this list were later added toxicology, dermatology and mycology. A number of veterinary scholarship and fellowship schemes were introduced and in 1979 a competitive award for research in veterinary medicine of up to £150,000 over five years for work in any field linking animal and human medicine in the UK was announced. Between 1968 and 1980, £3.5 million was spent by the Trust on veterinary research. During the 1990s the structure of the company underwent considerable alteration. In 1992, the Wellcome Trust's shareholding of the Wellcome Foundation Ltd was reduced to 40 per cent, while in 1995 Wellcome plc, parent company to the Wellcome Foundation Ltd since 1985, merged with Glaxo Holdings plc to form Glaxo Wellcome plc.

K Holland, 'The Wellcome Foundation', *Pharmaceutical Journal*, 20 Dec 1986; R R James, *Henry Wellcome* (London, 1994); G Macdonald, *In Pursuit of Excellence: one hundred years Wellcome 1880–1980* (London 1980); H Turner, *Henry Wellcome: the man, his collection and his legacy* (London, 1980).

Records (1): (Historical Records) Records Centre, Glaxo Wellcome plc, 891–995 Greenford Road, Greenford UB6 0HE

Announcement of partnership 1880; partnership disputes, correspondence and legal papers of Henry Wellcome and Silas Burroughs 1879–98; general meetings: notices/agenda 1924–40, minutes 1940s–; memorandum and articles of association 1924; statutory report 1924; agreement and papers re purchase of business in New York 1924; management committee, minutes 1941–48; secretaries' committee, minutes 1940–49; research committee, minutes 1930–45; production committee, minutes 1941–45; war production committee, minutes 1940–41; distribution committee, minutes 1945; minutes and related papers re: Wellcome Trust 1937–40, Therapeutic Research Corporation 1941–45, 1982–83, enquiry into insulin 1948; papers re overseas subsidiaries and offices: India 1885, Italy 1900–01, 1907–12, 1932–34, South Africa pre 1902, 1930–38, Egypt 1902–04, Mexico 1908, Cuba 1909, Argentina 1909–12, 1930–38, Shanghai 1912–77, US 1912–56, 1978–80, China 1924, Australia 1925–42, 1980, Montreal 1927–43, Siam 1928–30, Ireland 1939, Germany 1945–46, East Africa 1955; Wellcome Bureau of Scientific Research: general administration files c1913–23, directors' reports 1913–35, general correspondence with various members of Burroughs Wellcome & Co staff 1925–31, monthly reports of Burroughs Wellcome & Co US Experimental Research Laboratories and the Entomological Field Laboratories 1904–22, reports and minutes re research into specific drugs 1900–52, correspondence and reports 1902–75; Wellcome Historical Medical Museum: handbooks 1903–65, files re exhibitions 1927–62, correspondence with Burroughs Wellcome & Co, London and worldwide 1932–52, correspondence with Wellcome Foundation Ltd 1935–39, general correspondence 1903–64; Wellcome Chemical Research Laboratories: correspondence 1915–36, reports 1925–40, publications 1905–06, press cuttings 1925–46; Physiological Research Laboratories: reports and correspondence 1895–22, papers re registration 1900–01, publications 1903–27; Tropical Research Laboratory: legal documents 1899–1905, reports 1904–11, reports and correspondence re Khartoum laboratory 1901–40, booklet describing organisation of laboratories post 1944, publications 1921–33; share certificates 1925–43; annual reports 1940s–; balance sheet 1887; annual summaries 1889–1908;

accounts 1955; ledger, associated houses 1944–49; works journal 1935–43; cash books 1937–48 [w]; cash receipt books 1940–49; accounts of overseas subsidiaries 1950–53; overseas houses monthly estimates of sales 1950–58; bill books 1922–45; bank books 1879–90; cheque books 1879–82; notice re stamp duties 1942; correspondence re: tithes 1925–43, purchase tax 1946–48; litigation papers: general 1937–39, dangerous drugs 1942–45, prosecution under Milk Act 1917, trade marks with press cuttings of trial 1902–04; agreements re patents 1884–1900, nd; trade mark papers: licences 1936–45, oppositions and consents 1900, 1904–33, infringements 1903–45, general 1885–1943, 1946–50; papers and notes: registered designs 1898–1933, copyright 1913–41; correspondence re: patent certificates 1881–1938, compulsory licences 1938–39; monthly reports to managing director 1927–40; memoranda and circulars re management during wartime 1939–40; post-war plans 1944; laboratory notebooks 1908–33, nd [w]; chemists' diaries 1897–1909; overseas chemists' diaries 1899–1909 [w]; pharmacists' diaries 1910–40 [w]; overseas pharmacists' diaries 1910–38 [w]; medical diaries and visiting lists: 1889–1989 [w], war emergency editions 1917–19, 1941–47, service editions 1899–1940 [w], export edition 1923, overseas editions 1898–1967, 1984; nurses' diaries: 1898–1939 [w], overseas 1898–1937 [w]; formulae books and formulae 1898–1946, nd; research reports 1925–41; handbook 1945; papers, accounts and correspondence re: drugs production 1892–99, 1914–56, medicine chests 1895–1932, 1950, 1970, wood working department 1899–1904, poisons labelling 1899–1947, research laboratories 1927–43, therapeutic research 1927–28, 1982; standard production procedures, nd; developmental rejects files 1948–51; record of compressed products, nd; drugs orders and order forms 1903–08, 1922; correspondence re sale of saccharin overseas 1910, 1933; product lists: domestic 1956–69, 1981–88, export 1962–71, overseas 1960, 1977–80; patent certificates 1883–84; copyright agreements 1903–12; certificates of registration of designs 1902–33; price lists: general 1881–1959, retail 1960–68, wholesale 1960–66, retail and wholesale 1968–83, biologicals 1949–59, industrial 1969, re-agents 1958–72, hospital 1952–53, exports 1941–77, overseas 1894, 1902–69, consumer division, Crewe 1973, medical division 1974, other companies 1878, 1892; correspondence and papers re pricing and price-cutting 1888–1943; registers of advertisements 1881–91; advertising correspondence 1946; promotional poster 1943; marketing papers 1881, 1894–1909, 1933–34, 1946–54, nd; publicity: sales unit annual reports 1956–65, papers 1947–50, home sales books 1936–48; press cuttings 1891–1943, 1955–58; correspondence re marketing and public relations 1929–33, 1940–43; deeds 1889–1990; Dartford premises: conveyances 1915–42, lease and correspondence 1887–93, 1928, memorandum re acquisition 1921, plan

1928, grant of right to lay drain and cable 1916, organisation of chemical works 1898–1932, papers re print works 1937–49, valuations and inventory 1938, tenancy agreements 1948–52, rent books 1909–43, memorandum re staff safety, nd, telegram re accident 1897, correspondence and memoranda re chemical works 1946–50, correspondence re works organisation 1889, 1899, 1909, supervisor's manuals 1947, work study handbooks 1953, 1971, papers re Wellcome Club and Institute 1889–1900, press cuttings 1889–93, programmes and papers re visits to site 1890, 1905, 1932, correspondence with Dartford Urban District Council 1900–39, correspondence re land 1919–30, correspondence re water supply 1940–45, historical notes 1907–30, 1945; Gower Street, London, premises, correspondence re: sale and tenancy 1920–48, proposed new building 1944–47; Beckenham premises: directors' correspondence 1923–33, lease 1898, agreements with London County Council 1902, 1911, 1918–20, reports re construction of penicillin factory 1944–45, visitor book 1931–46, press cuttings re anti-vivisection 1919–49; Holborn Viaduct premises, correspondence re lease 1890–91; Snow Hill premises: licence to sell wines and spirits, nd, notes 1888–89, 1925, menu 1898, notice of social events and programmes 1902–08, 1920–21; 76 High Street, Marylebone, London, leases 1914–29; Euston Road premises, papers re laying of corner stone 1931; Wandsworth premises, papers and correspondence 1883–1930; inventories and valuations of estate 1938; press cuttings and promotional material re Wellcome building 1921–39; reports and general correspondence: estates department 1913–39, negotiations to lease Belmont and Carshalton serum laboratories from London County Council 1942–47; staff register 1879–1928; wages books: women 1902–37, men 1902–43; salaries book, nd; salaries and wages analysis 1950–51; letters re salaries 1885–98; staff records 1919–43; contract of employment 1897; diaries: company 1980–89, 1992–93, company appointments 1957–91, consultants' appointments 1898–1958, 1966; organisational charts of chemical works and Snow Hill head office 1914–38; notes: staff roles 1924, 1948, nurse's post 1924; card re profit sharing 1892; *pro forma* contract of employment, nd; staff accident record 1909–72; notice re female staff clothing 1904; announcement re appointment of personnel officer 1946; instructions: management 1927–37, travelling representatives 1932; correspondence re: employment 1930–40, sickness 1938–39, unemployment insurance 1912–30; *The Unicorn*, magazine 1936; *Tabloid*, monthly memoranda 1947–52; Wellcome Club: magazine 1899, programmes 1898–1905, 1920, 1949, papers re social activities 1892–95; correspondence re: drug companies 1873–1900, 1915, 1940, trade unions 1921–36, business 1880–93, 1906–41, Lederle Laboratories Inc 1935–37, internal 1927–43, foreign department 1927–40, medicine chest department 1927–40; list of business correspondence 1880–86; papers re medals, awards and prizes 1909–40; notices re deaths of presidents 1881, 1885; visitor book 1947–49; stationery samples 1931; Henry Wellcome: personal letter books 1882–1907, private letter books 1878–1907, personal and family correspondence/papers 1870–1943, general correspondence 1881–1903, business correspondence and reports 1874–1934, papers re legal matters 1903–04, will and valuation of estate incl commercial premises and assets 1880–1938; personal papers: Silas Burroughs 1878–79, 1892–98, Henry Wellcome's family 1913, 1933–58, Henry Hallett Dale 1906–32, Wellcome staff 1882–1937, 1951, 1979, nd; historical notes, articles and staff reminiscences 1905–58, 1974–80, nd; archives list pre 1945; papers, correspondence and minutes of external organisations and committees 1939–87; misc papers 1922, c1930–36; correspondence with War Office re supplies of veterinary pharmaceutical products 1914–17; Wellcome chemical works, files re packaging specifications for veterinary and human products incl vaccines 1963–69; product ratification forms re *Franocide* and other veterinary products 1934–60; Wellcome veterinary diary 1966; list of veterinary preparations 1969; dummy tablets c1970s; price lists 1941, 1943–44, 1946–55, 1957, 1960–62, 1973, 1978, 1981; printed material, incl circulars, pulls and proofs, advertisements for pharmaceutical and veterinary products, labels, press cuttings, instruction books, etc c1880–1957; photographs: Beckenham, aerial, exterior, interior, laboratories, materia medica, opening ceremonies, staff, products, 20th cent, Frant post 1943, misc incl Berkhamsted, Brockwell Hall, *Calmic*, foot-and-mouth vaccine production at Pirbright in Surrey, Kelvindale, Royal Show, animals, staff, vaccines, Tropical Research Laboratory, floating laboratory, etc 20th cent. [Ref: WA/HSW; WA/BSR; WA/HMM; WA/CRL; WA/PRL; WA/TRL; Acc99/6/7, 23, 32; Acc96/41/12; Acc96/46/5; Acc99/59; PB/129; WPH/PR3–11, 124–172]

Records (2): National Archives, Ruskin Avenue, Kew, Richmond TW9 4DU

Medical Research Council, committee papers re Burroughs Wellcome & Co and Wellcome Foundation Ltd 1913–54. [Ref: FD/1/16/919–21, 1296, 2263, 2520; FD/1/98/3702, 8614]

Records (3): Museum, Royal Pharmaceutical Society of Great Britain, 1 Lambeth High Street, London SE1 7JN

Burroughs Wellcome & Co, list of veterinary preparations 1960s. [Ref: 615.452.619]

Records (4): Museum of Lincolnshire Life, Burton Road, Lincoln LN1 3LY

Booklet on *Phenothiazwe*, a new and effective anthelmintic for sheep, horses, cattle, etc, nd.

WILLOWS FRANCIS LTD
Crawley, West Sussex

History: Burgess, Willows & Co was established in 1751 at 101 High Holborn, London, as a wholesale druggist, manufacturing chemist, distiller and oil presser. During the nineteenth century the company acquired a number of long-established London drug firms. It also at some point changed its name to Burgess, Willows & Francis, although by 1888 it was trading as Willows, Francis & Butler and describing itself as a wholesale and export druggist and manufacturer of pharmaceutical and veterinary preparations. During the late nineteenth century, Willows, Francis & Butler was appointed wholesale druggist to the Royal Veterinary College, London. In around 1904 the business was incorporated as a limited liability company, Willows, Francis, Butler & Thompson Ltd and relocated to 40 Aldersgate Street, London. By the 1930s, however, it was trading from Shacklewell Lane, Dalston, London, manufacturing and supplying human and veterinary preparations, surgical instruments and sundries. In 1949 Willows, Francis, Butler & Thompson Ltd merged with the Pharmaceutical Manufacturing Co Ltd to form a public limited liability company, Willows Francis Ltd, which went on to become a major manufacturer of ethical drugs and anaesthetics and an exporter of anaesthetics, veterinary and medical specialities, galenicals and pharmaceutical chemicals. These were produced at both the Dalston factory and at a second plant in Epsom, Surrey. By the 1970s the company had moved again, to Westhoughton, Lancashire. D W J Milligan joined the company in 1977 as its veterinary marketing director and stayed until the 1990s, eventually becoming managing director. Willows Francis Ltd was acquired by Guinness Peat in 1979 and three years later the various components of the company were separated, at which time the veterinary division was sold to the pharmaceutical company, A H Robins, although it retained the trading name of Willows Francis Ltd. In 1990, Willows Francis Ltd was sold again, this time to American Home Products Corporation Inc, and relocated to 3 Charlwood Court, County Oak Way, Crawley, where it worked closely with another subsidiary, Fort Dodge Laboratories, the second largest veterinary company in America.

The Willows Francis Ltd trading name was finally abolished in the late 1990s.

'Willows Francis: the 'original' veterinary company looks forward', *Veterinary Practice*, December 1990.

Records: in private ownership of Mr D W J Milligan, Sunnyfields, Hurston Close, Findon Valley, Worthing BN14 0AX

Product data cards 1973–74; product advertisements/data sheets c1980s; product list, nd; advertisements 1904, 1988; press cuttings: Willows Francis literary award 1979, 1981, 1989, Willows Francis veterinary student of the year award 1982, 1984, Mr Milligan 1980, acquisition by A H Robins 1983, Langhurst premises 1984; notices re Willows Francis veterinary literary award 1981, 1988; *Willowleaves*, company magazine 1978–80, 1989; A H Robins' Langhurst Report 1984; articles re company 1983–84, c1980s; historical notes and articles 1990, nd.

WILSON'S (STOWMARKET) LTD
Stowmarket, Suffolk

History: Thomas Wilson registered as a pharmaceutical chemist in 1863 and traded at Walsham le Willows, Suffolk, before entering into a partnership with William Harvey of Stowmarket in 1879. The business was incorporated as a limited liability company in 1934, after which it traded as Wilson's Ltd, although it was later renamed Wilson's (Stowmarket) Ltd and moved to Old Market Place, Sudbury, Suffolk. Wilson's (Stowmarket) Ltd ceased trading in 1980.

Records: Suffolk Record Office, Ipswich Branch, Gatacre Road, Ipswich IP1 2LQ

Sales day book 1937–52; veterinary prescription books 1924–51; poisons register 1938–54. [Ref: HC 408]

List of records of trade bodies and professional associations

BRITISH SMALL ANIMAL VETERINARY ASSOCIATION
Quedgeley, Gloucestershire

History: In September 1956 a letter appeared in *The Veterinary Record*, signed by S F J Hodgman and W B Singleton, asking anyone interested in forming a small animal veterinary association to contact them. Two months later, thirty people attended a meeting at the British Veterinary Association headquarters and a steering committee was formed. This committee met again on 2 January 1957 and the British Small Animal Veterinary Association (BSAVA) was formally established. C E Woodrow was elected chairman, while W B Singleton was appointed honorary secretary. The BSAVA's main purpose was 'to protect, foster and promote the cultural, scientific and professional interests of veterinary surgeons and practitioners engaged in small animal practice, teaching and research'. At the inaugural meeting, held at the Royal Veterinary College, London, on 7 March 1957, it was agreed that territorial regions should be established and regional chairmen elected, while the subscription for individual members was set at two guineas. By the end of that first meeting the Association had 81 members, while 150 people attended the first annual congress at the Shaftesbury Hotel, London, in March 1958. In April 1958 the BSAVA became a non-territorial division of the British Veterinary Association and two years later published the first number of its quarterly *Journal of Small Animal Practice*. The Clinical Research Trust Fund was set up by the BSAVA in 1974 to raise money for research.

Records: British Small Animal Veterinary Association, Woodrow House, 1 Telford Way, Waterwells, Quedgeley, Gloucester GL2 4AB

Minutes, correspondence, etc re establishment 1956–57; constitution (amended) c1957, 1985; lists of members 1960, 1970; membership records 1957–c1973; council, minutes, agenda, correspondence and related papers 1957–69, 1974–, resolutions 1980–85; advisory committee (executive committee until 1959), minutes, agenda, correspondence and related papers 1957–59, 1963–69, 1974–; finance committee, minutes, correspondence and related papers 1963–69, 1974–77; advisory and finance committee, minutes c1977–; scientific committee (scientific and education committee 1977–84), minutes, agenda, correspondence and related papers 1963–69, 1974–; registered animal nursing association committee, minutes, agenda, correspondence and related papers 1963–69, 1974–; publicity and public relations committee, minutes, agenda, correspondence and related papers 1963–69, 1974–; publications committee, minutes, agenda, correspondence and related papers 1963–69, 1974–; editorial committee, minute book and related papers 1969–87; education committee, minutes 1984–; other standing committees, minutes and papers 1960s–; congress: annual general meeting, minutes 1962–66, 1985–86, organising committee, minutes, agenda, accounts, programmes, related papers 1958–69, 1975–81, 1986, invoices and receipts re exhibitors and advertisers 1984, handbooks 1961–62, 1964–65, 1980–84, 1987–, scientific programmes 1958–60, 1965, 1987, copies of papers given 1988, newsletter 1990, photographs 1960s–, slides 1986, videos of proceedings 1983–84, audio cassettes of proceedings 1992; reports of meetings of officers and presidents 1963–64, 1970; symposia: Small Animal Anaesthesia, papers 1963, Canine and Feline Nutritional Requirements, programme 1964, Pet Animals and Society, papers and programme, nd, Improved Healthcare in Kennels and Catteries, proceedings, nd; regional correspondence and reports 1966–69, 1974–85; regional calendars 1979–82; regional secretaries' handbooks 1984, 1990; correspondence re: cat boxes 1972–76, specialist groups and bodies 1963–79, T M Eaton 1974–75, general 1970–78, 1985; report re small animal practice survey 1972–73; *Journal of Small Animal Practice* survey, responses 1985; profile of activities with related papers 1992–93; working party on mandatory continuing education, papers and correspondence 1976–77; euthanasia of dogs, policy statement 1982; British Veterinary Association recommended fees for part time local authority work 1982; Clinical Research Trust Fund: correspondence re survey on neutering and charity work 1985, papers re photography competition 1985, *Petsavers News* magazine 1981, misc leaflets 1982, fundraising poster 1986; establishment lists 1981–92 [w]; annual handbooks 1969, 1973, 1979, 1982, 1991–95; audio tape of transatlantic discussion with American Animal Hospital Association on orthopaedic problems 1961; *BSAVA Bulletin* 1958–60; *Journal of Small Animal Practice* 1960–; press cuttings: sheep dog trials 1963, general 1973–74.

BRITISH VETERINARY ASSOCIATION
London

History: At the first British National Veterinary Congress in July 1881, veterinary surgeons from all over the country, as well as from the army and the colonies, gathered to discuss a range of scientific and professional matters. The timing was especially appropriate, as the first Veterinary Surgeons Act was then making its way through parliament. During the meeting a veterinary surgeon called George Banham introduced his pamphlet entitled *Suggestions for the Formation of a British National Veterinary Association* and a resolution was passed stating that 'A British National Veterinary Association would be advantageous to the veterinary profession. A committee shall be formed to consider the subject and frame rules for its guidance'. The National Veterinary Association (NVA) was duly formed in 1882 with George Fleming, principal veterinary officer to the armed forces, as its first president. However, the new Association had no direct link with the various territorial associations that had been forming since 1851. Instead the NVA was a non-territorial association open to any veterinary surgeon on payment of half a guinea, and met 'in different parts of the kingdom, from time to time...under the management of a local Provisional Committee'. Within a few years, however, this system was felt to be inadequate and many began calling for a national professional association to tackle matters which did not come under the remit of the Royal College of Veterinary Surgeons. In 1909, at a meeting of the Scottish Metropolitan Veterinary Association, Professor Orlando Charnock Bradley of the Edinburgh Veterinary College called for the establishment of 'one single British Veterinary Association' into which all existing territorial societies would be incorporated as divisions. This proposal was generally supported, but the outbreak of the First World War put an end to any active planning. The idea remained, though, and at a meeting on 31 October 1919 the formation of the National Veterinary Medical Association was agreed. Charnock Bradley was elected the Association's first President. The following year the Association took responsibility for the professional publication *The Veterinary Record*, which became its official journal, reporting on meetings and discussing topical issues. At the same time the NVMA moved into its first permanent home on Buckingham Palace Road, London, although it moved to 2 Verulum Buildings, Grays Inn, in 1925 and then to 36 Gordon Square in 1937. The NVMA took an active part in the shaping of the veterinary profession, participating in the negotiations that followed the publication of the Hopkins Report in 1934 and resulted in the establishment of the Animal Health Division at the Ministry of Agriculture and Fisheries in 1938. During the Second World War, when the preservation of food supplies became vital, the NVMA Survey Scheme brought about a concentrated effort to control four major cattle conditions – mastitis, contagious abortion, Johne's disease and infertility. In 1952 the NVMA was renamed the British Veterinary Association (BVA) and two years later moved to 7 Mansfield Street, London. The

BVA today has thousands of members, 32 territorial divisions and 20 specialist divisions, all of which are represented on its Council. It regards its main functions as representing its members and campaigning for the best deployment of veterinary resources on behalf of the wider community.

Records (1): British Veterinary Association, 7 Mansfield Street, London W1M 0AT

List of past presidents and places of annual meetings/congresses 1883–1974, nd; press cuttings: centenary 1982, North of Scotland division centenary 1994, veterinary surgery 1982–91; photographs: Angus Taylor (President of the Royal College of Veterinary Surgeons) and Dr Garry Alder with plaque to William Moorcroft, unveiled at the site of his former practice in Oxford Street, London 1982; historical notes re: George Fleming, nd, William Moorcroft 1982, 7 Mansfield Street, nd, centenary celebrations 1981–82; obituary of Charles Mitchell, editor of *The Veterinary Record* between 1954 and 1971, 1990.

Records (2): in private ownership of Miss Mary Brancker, 38 Streetly Lane, Sutton Coldfield B74 4TU

Programme for centenary banquet 1982.

Records (3): in private ownership of Mr R D Locke, 4 Rathmore Road, Cambridge CB1 7AD

Photographs: annual congresses 1931–36, Lancashire division summer meeting at Harper Adams College 1932.

Records (4): Wellcome Library, Royal College of Veterinary Surgeons, Belgravia House, 62–64 Horseferry Road, London SW1P 2AF

Copies of papers given at the Veterinary Medical Association 1883–1935; misc papers 1909–14.

BRITISH VETERINARY HOSPITALS ASSOCIATION

Records: Barton Veterinary Hospital, 34 New Dover Road, Canterbury CT1 3DT

Minutes, agenda and related papers 1972–84; papers re British Veterinary Association working parties on safety at work and radiological protection 1976–80.

CENTRAL VETERINARY SOCIETY

London

History: On 11 July 1870 a meeting was held at the Royal College of Veterinary Surgeons, Red Lion Square, London, attended by twenty five veterinary surgeons, to discuss the formation of a Metropolitan Veterinary Pathological Society. The meeting followed an advertisement in *The Veterinarian* and a circular, both of which had appeared the previous March. At this initial meeting, chaired by George Fleming, it was agreed that the Central Veterinary Society, as the new Society was to be known, would hold monthly meetings 'for the purpose of promoting generally the advancement of Veterinary Science' within the London area. Annual subscriptions were fixed at one guinea. The Society was affiliated to the National Veterinary Association shortly before the First World War.

Records: Wellcome Library, Royal College of Veterinary Surgeons, Belgravia House, 62–64 Horseferry Road, London SW1P 2AF

Minutes of Council meetings 1870–48; minutes of general meetings 1955–67; rough minute book 1870–80; minutes, agenda and related correspondence 1947–55, 1958–65, 1969; reports of general meetings 1870–80, 1894–1927, 1943–47, 1949; extracts of proceedings of meetings, discussions, reports, etc 1936–43; lists of officers 1870–86, 1906–27, 1947–55, 1958–65; list of members 1965; ledger 1870–80; entrance fees and arrears 1870–80; statement of accounts 1968–69; misc accounts 1967; attendance book 1907–43; visitor book 1870–1907; lists of fellows 1870–74, 1878–79; fellows obligation book c1870; honorary secretary's outgoing letter book 1870–80; notices and directions from the British Veterinary Association 1963–68; correspondence with and re Royal Society for the Prevention of Cruelty to Animals 1965; correspondence re McCunn memorial fund 1968; reports and correspondence re British Veterinary Association representatives 1964–67; general correspondence 1964–66; contributors' papers 1962, nd; rules 1930, 1937; photograph album 1871; outline for a course of anatomical demonstrations by John Henry Steel 1878–79; address by Frank W Garnett, *A Forecast for a New Veterinary Surgeons Act* 1907; address by F Raymond, *General and Veterinary Education*, nd.

CLYDESDALE HORSE SOCIETY OF GREAT BRITAIN AND IRELAND
Glasgow

History: The Clydesdale Horse Society of Great Britain and Ireland was established in 1877 after a lengthy correspondence in the *Northern Agriculturalist.* Present at the first meeting were 'breeders, exhibitors and others interested', including Professor James McCall of the Glasgow Veterinary College. The Society aimed to maintain the purity of the breed by collecting, verifying and publishing pedigrees and investigating doubtful or suspicious pedigrees. In addition it actively encouraged the breeding of Clydesdales and to this end a stud book was produced and regularly updated. The Society also recommended veterinary inspectors for horse shows and encouraged research into conditions such as joint ill and unsoundness in mares.

Records (1): Arts Department, Mitchell Library, North Street, Glasgow G3 7DN

Council, minute books 1877–1954; general purposes committee, minute books incl agenda and financial statements 1877–1954; editing committee, minute books 1877–1945; special committees (incl scientific committee), minute books 1912–53; record book 19th cent; certificate registers 1884–1936; list of noted sires of 1886 and leading prize winners of 1885; index of mares as listed in the stud book 20th cent; subscription registers (annual members) c1940–58; register of directors 1939–70; general correspondence 1930s; report of proceedings before a committee of enquiry 1944; notes of proceedings of a deputation to the Ministry of Transport 1920; committee of enquiry into the slaughter of horses: minutes and agenda 1952–53, reports of visits to slaughterhouses by members of the committee and reports from chief constables 1949–53, misc documents used at committee 1952–53, copies of various Acts, reports, etc re horses 1911–51, first and second drafts of report 1953; catalogues for horse shows, auctions, etc 1949–70; report of proceedings in the Raeside case 1885; *The Scottish Journal of Agriculture* vol 4, no 1, 1921; *The Shire Horse for Peace or for War* 1919; Ministry of Agriculture and Fisheries report of the departmental committee on export of horses to the continent 1925; National Horse Association of Great Britain slippery roads committee, report of investigations c1920s; National Horse Association of Great Britain, first meeting of the reconstituted council 1928; Animal Breeding Research Department, Edinburgh University, report of the director 1926; Animal Diseases Research Association: research laboratory report 1924, reprint from *The*

Scotsman on opening of Moredun Institute 1927, appeal for funds 1928; Bill to regulate use of stallions for stud purposes 1918. [Ref: 891200 – SR 19, 29, 39]

Records (2): National Register of Archives (Scotland), HM General Register House, Edinburgh EH1 3YY

Private stud book 1882–1911. [Ref: NRA(S) 3698/380/6]

EASTERN COUNTIES VETERINARY ASSOCIATION
Norwich, Norfolk

History: The Norfolk and Eastern Counties Veterinary Medical Association was established in 1868. It aimed to elevate the professional and social status of veterinary surgeons in that area and provide a forum for the interchange of ideas and experiences. Meetings were held quarterly at the Norfolk Hotel, Norwich. In 1888 the Association was renamed the Eastern Counties Veterinary Medical Association in an attempt to encourage a wider membership, but later changed its name once again, to the Eastern Counties Veterinary Association.

Records: Cambridgeshire County Record Office, Shire Hall, Castle Hill, Cambridge CB3 0AP

Minutes 1868–1975; executive committee and general meetings, minutes and papers 1943–80 [w]; attendance books 1923–46, 1976–80; rules 1868, 1911, 1960, nd; balance sheets 1930–32, 1935, 1970–73; subscriptions ledger 1920–27; subscriptions receipt book stubs 1923, 1930–37; vouchers and bank statements 1931–37, 1955–58; officers' rough notes 1968–70; planning exercise re veterinary corporation scheme with general meeting minutes 1965; agreements for co-operation with Cambridge School of Veterinary Medicine re fee scales 1953, 1957; papers re local veterinary fee scales 1955–69; lecture notes on osteology 1898–99; papers re preventative medicine and the veterinary surgeon c1962; memorandum on divisional public relations officer 1962; reports and circulars: cattle diseases 1934–35, sheep diseases 1935, fur bearing animals 1935, Veterinary Advisory Scheme 1935; general correspondence and circulars 1928–79; correspondence re: rules 1952, salaries 1973–75, Royal Society for the Prevention of Cruelty to Animals' scheme for neutering cats 1972–74; history and photographs of the presidential 'jewel' and chain of office c1957, nd; designs for honorary membership certificates 1970; National Veterinary Medical Association, articles of association 1925. [Ref: R81/67]

EDINBURGH VETERINARY MEDICAL ASSOCIATION
Edinburgh

History: The Edinburgh Veterinary Medical Association has been meeting since at least 1856.

Records: Archivist, Edinburgh University Library, George Square, Edinburgh EH8 9LJ

Minute books 1873–91, 1899–1915; attendance book 1909–11; account book 1858–74; treasurer's book 1874–1910; register of members 1856–62; roll book 1893–1902; bundle of essays read before the Association 1911–14; notebook recording paper titles 1896–1915.

FEDERATION OF VETERINARIANS OF THE EUROPEAN ECONOMIC COMMUNITY

Records: Wellcome Library, Royal College of Veterinary Surgeons, Belgravia House, 62–64 Horseferry Road, London SW1P 2AF

Minutes, correspondence and papers 1974–91; liaison committee, newsletters, notes of meetings, etc 1973–75.

HIGHLAND AND AGRICULTURAL SOCIETY OF SCOTLAND
Ingliston, Edinburgh

History: The Highland Society at Edinburgh, granted a royal charter in 1787, began to play a key role in the development of veterinary education during the nineteenth century. From 1824 it awarded certificates of veterinary competence to graduates of the newly opened Edinburgh Veterinary College. In 1834 the Society was granted a new charter which allowed it to increase the scope of its activities. From that time it was known as the Highland and Agricultural Society of Scotland. The establishment of the Royal College of Veterinary Surgeons in 1844 as the newly emerging veterinary profession's sole regulatory and qualifying body was vehemently opposed by the Highland and Agricultural Society of Scotland, largely because the new College had been granted the exclusive right to award diplomas. In protest, the Highland and Agricultural Society of Scotland refused to grant any veterinary certificates from 1844. By 1848, however, the Edinburgh Veterinary College's Principal, William Dick, had fallen out with the Royal College of Veterinary Surgeons, and broken off all ties, clearing the way for certificates of veterinary competence to be awarded by the Highland and Agricultural Society of Scotland once again. In 1859 the Society announced that the students of any veterinary teacher in Scotland established under the royal sign manual would be eligible for examination for the Society's certificate, and authorised the Examining Board to take on trial any party duly qualified who applied for the Society's certificate. In 1870, the Society went a step further by allowing the students of any veterinary teacher recognised by the government to sit its examinations. However, in 1879 the Edinburgh Veterinary College ended its rift with the Royal College of Veterinary Surgeons and two years later the Highland and Agricultural Society of Scotland ceased to award certificates of veterinary competence.

A Ramsay, *History of the Highland and Agricultural Society of Scotland* (Edinburgh and London, 1879); J A Symon, *Scottish Farming Past and Present* (Edinburgh and London, 1958).

Records (1): National Register of Archives (Scotland), HM General Register House, Edinburgh EH1 3YY

Copy memoranda, proposals and drafts of revised charter 1784–1834; papers re veterinary college for Scotland incl memorial by William Dick as veterinary surgeon to the directors 1838; statement re Edinburgh Veterinary College 1845; copy of trust disposition and settlement by William Dick 1858, with codicil 1864; list of graduates 1865–67; draft agreement with Royal College of Veterinary Surgeons 1878; papers re Prevention of Infectious Diseases Among Cattle Bill 1864; papers re cattle plague 1865–66; letters and papers re Dairies (Scotland) Bill, etc 1871–1908; papers and letters re tuberculosis and tuberculin testing c1900; letters and papers re sheep scab 1905; letters and paper re enquiry into grouse disease 1906; letter from Joseph Long 'to the Flockmasters of Scotland' promoting his cures for sheep diseases, attested by Somerset farmers c1850; blank diplomas and certificates 19th–20th cent. [Ref: NRA(S) 2711]

Records (2): Staffordshire Record Office, Eastgate Street, Stafford ST16 2LZ

Letters to Duke of Sutherland re Society, incl training and employment of veterinary surgeons 1837–40. [Ref: D593/P/22/1/15]

Records (3): Moredun Research Institute, Pentlands Science Park, Bush Loan, Midlothian EH26 0PZ

Transactions of the Highland and Agricultural Society of Scotland, giving annual accounts, proceedings of meetings, etc 1865, 1867–1923, 1925–63, 1968.

Records (4): Wellcome Library, Royal College of Veterinary Surgeons, Belgravia House, 62–64 Horseferry Road, London SW1P 2AF

List of students of veterinary colleges recognised by government who have passed the examinations and obtained the certificate of the Highland and Agricultural Society of Scotland (p) 1874.

LANCASHIRE VETERINARY ASSOCIATION
Lancashire

History: The Lancashire Veterinary Association was established in 1862.

Anon, *Early Days of the LVA* (private publication, c1980).

Records (1): Lancashire Record Office, Bow Lane, Preston PR1 2RE

Minute books 1866–1963; council minute book 1905–31; attendance books 1928–60; register of members 1867–1948; cash book 1936–52; financial statements 1924–46. [Ref: DDX 1726]

Records (2): Honorary Secretary, Lancashire Veterinary Association, Barton Hall, Garstang Road, Barton, Preston PR3 5HE

Council: minutes 1931–63, 1983–, correspondence 1986–94; general meetings, minutes and related papers 1984–; papers re other meetings 1998–; correspondence: James Gourlay, president 1986–94, British Veterinary Association 1999–, Royal Society for the Prevention of Cruelty to Animals' campaign to urge owners to have their pets neutered 1991, general 1988–90; papers re Farm Animal Welfare Liaison Group 1986–88; presidential address 1953; rules 1977; papers, guides, leaflets from British Veterinary Association 1980s–90s; British Veterinary Association summary of UK legislation and other events of veterinary interest 1997–; minutes of British Veterinary Association council meetings with related papers 1998–; photograph of meeting 1932; letter from David Locke 1989, incl photographs of his family's practice 1904.

Records (3): Department of Special Collections and Archives, Sydney Jones Library, University of Liverpool, PO Box 123, Liverpool L69 3DA

Names and addresses of members (p) c1866–85. [Ref: D. 426]

LONDON VETERINARY MEDICAL SOCIETY
London

History: The London Veterinary Medical Society was established in 1813 and enjoyed close links with the Royal Veterinary College, London, until its dissolution in 1836.

Records: The Library, Royal Veterinary College, Royal College Street, London NW1 0TU

Papers and correspondence 1813–36; essays 1827–32.

NORFOLK CATTLE PLAGUE ASSOCIATION
Norfolk

History: The Norfolk Cattle Plague Association was established in 1865 during the cattle plague epidemic that was sweeping the country to compensate local farmers that had lost sheep or cattle. Following a reorganisation in 1916, any surplus annual income was divided between the Royal Agricultural Benevolent Institution and the Norfolk and Norwich Hospital for the care of agricultural workers. The Association was dissolved in 1965.

Records: Norfolk Record Office, Gildengate House, Anglia Square, Upper Green Lane, Norwich NR3 1AX

Minutes 1866–69, 1916–65; statement of facts, copy rules and valuation book 1865–66; account book 1920–65; bank statements 1932–66; passbooks 1917–32, 1953–55; notes re annual balances 1948–64; draft Charity Commission order 1966; correspondence with Charity Commissioners 1914. [Ref: SO 171/1–10; MC 974/1–3]

ROYAL AGRICULTURAL SOCIETY OF ENGLAND
London

History: At a public meeting held on 9 May 1838, the idea of forming a national society to promote and improve English agriculture was explored. Out of this emerged the English Agricultural Society under the chairmanship of Earl Spencer. Following the granting of a royal charter in 1840 the new society became known as the Royal Agricultural Society of England (RASE). The Society drew its inspiration partly from the short lived Board of Agriculture (1793–1822), although a non-political stance was firmly adopted from the outset. Its primary purpose was summed up by the Duke of Richmond, one of its principal backers and a future chairman, who regarded it as 'a matter of the greatest importance that the agriculture of the country should endeavour to profit by the discoveries of science'. A Council was formed, which met monthly, and a Committee of Management whose main purpose was to organise the annual Country Show. In addition, three members' meetings were held each year, two in London and one outside, at which reports on Council activities were read out and scientific lectures given. Two classes of membership were introduced – governors, who paid an annual five pounds subscription, and ordinary members, who each paid one pound per year. By the first general meeting membership already totalled 466, and continued to grow rapidly, reaching 6,500 by 1842. In 1841 the Society agreed to lease 12 Hanover Square, London, and three years later acquired the old Board of Agriculture's library. The highlight of the Society's calendar, however, was the Country Show. England and Wales were divided into nine divisions and the Show visited each one in turn. Prizes were awarded for livestock, new implements and crops and it is generally acknowledged that the Shows did much to improve the quality of both livestock and farming standards. From its earliest days, the RASE recognised that veterinary medicine had a vital role to play in the country's agricultural future. Indeed it was stated at the first general meeting that the society should actively seek 'to take measures for improving the Veterinary Art as applied to Cattle, Sheep and Pigs' and a sub-committee of leading veterinarians was formed under the chairmanship of William Youatt on 18 July 1838. Alarmed at the emergence of a number of contagious diseases, including foot-and-mouth (1838), pleuro-pneumonia (1841) and sheep pox (1847), and concerned at the Royal Veterinary College's emphasis on equine medicine, the RASE set about improving veterinary knowledge and education. One of its first acts was the endowment of a Chair in Veterinary Pathology at the Royal Veterinary College, London, in 1842. Although this grant was withdrawn in 1848, it was renewed in 1852 on condition that members would be able to send cattle, sheep and pigs to the Royal Veterinary College for examination and treatment and that the College would undertake to investigate certain diseases. James Beart Simonds, the first man to hold the RASE funded Professorship in Veterinary Pathology, was, in the late 1840s, also appointed Veterinary Inspector to the RASE. His duties included visiting members' farms whenever outbreaks of contagious disease occurred, and examining exhibits at the annual Country Show, to detect defects and diseases and ascertain the age of each animal. During the early years of the Show there were frequent cases of unsoundness, particularly amongst horses, but by 1869 it was no longer felt necessary to examine each horse. The RASE also supported new treatments for animal diseases. In 1851 Simonds was sent to Belgium to look at a vaccine for pleuro-pneumonia and, following his report, the Society supported trials in England. The Society also lobbied hard for legislative changes with regard to disease control. Following a serious outbreak of cattle plague in 1865, the Society's Council formed a standing committee, which put together a series of resolutions, many of which were incorporated into the Cattle Plague Prevention Act of 1866. Further lobbying brought about stricter controls on imports, including designated ports, improved quarantine provision and compulsory slaughter with compensation. However, the RASE did not forget its commitment to the improvement of veterinary education and knowledge. Grants were awarded to the Brown Animal Sanatory Institution, London, in 1875, to investigate pleuro-pneumonia, foot-and-mouth disease and anthrax, and to A P Thomas, an Oxford zoologist, in 1879 for the investigation of liver rot. RASE also offered prizes for essays on such subjects as 'Pleuro-pneumonia' (1847) and 'Abortion in Cattle' (1849). The winning essays were always published in the society's journal, which appeared thrice yearly from 1839 and twice a year from 1842. The Royal Agricultural College, which opened in Cirencester, Gloucestershire, in 1845, was supported by individual members of the RASE but received no direct support from the Society. However, from the 1860s the RASE started offering prizes to encourage the teaching of agriculture in schools. This led eventually to the introduction, under the society's auspices, of the National Diploma in the Science and Practice of Dairying in 1897 and the National Diploma in Dairying in 1900. In 1890 the Society increased its grant to the Royal Veterinary College, London, enabling a second chair, in Comparative Pathology and Bacteriology, to be established. By the beginning of the twentieth century, it was thought that the Country Show should have a permanent home. Funds were therefore raised for the purchase and equipping of land near Ealing and a private company set up to administer it. However, Park Royal Ltd held only three shows at its new ground before being dissolved in 1905. A supplemental charter awarded that same year led to a major reorganisation of the RASE. The following year, the Society's headquarters were moved from Harewood House, London, which they had occupied since 1893, to Bedford Square, London. There then followed a period of relative calm, during which the RASE gave modest amounts to research programmes in areas such as mastitis and pig breeding and promoted the idea of an animal quarantine station. In 1939 it held its Centenary Show at Windsor Great Park which attracted 4548 entries within the livestock classes. This turned out to be the last Country Show until 1947 and the outbreak of the Second World War also severely curtailed the Society's other activities. During the post-war period, the RASE found its research and advisory role reduced by the establishment in 1946 of the National Agricultural Advisory Service. In spite of this, the Society still hoped to play a role in encouraging the raising of standards amongst British livestock and the reduction of disease. With this in mind, it was announced in 1948 that only cattle from accredited herds could be shown at the Country Show. The Society also instituted an Inter-County Dairy Herd Trophy, to be awarded annually to the county that had shown the greatest progress in following the Tuberculosis (Attested Herds) Scheme for an outstanding contribution to animal health. The first winner of this award was Sir John Ritchie, Chief Veterinary Officer of the Ministry of Agriculture, for his work on the eradication of bovine tuberculosis. In 1960, the RASE leased Stoneleigh, Warwickshire, which it intended to use as an agricultural centre. The centre opened in 1962 and most of the Society's staff moved there from London in 1969. The National Agricultural Centre Advisory Board was set up in 1966 to administer Stoneleigh and included amongst its experts a representative from the British Veterinary Association. Over the next few years a number of associations moved their headquarters to Stoneleigh, including the Farm Management Association, the Meat and Livestock Commission, the National Master Farriers', Blacksmiths' & Agricultural Engineers Association, the Rare Breeds Survival Trust and the Shorthorn Cattle Society. In 1971 the government decided to base the newly formed Agricultural Development and Advisory Service at Stoneleigh, bringing an additional number of experts, including veterinary scientists, to the site. During the early 1970s, the RASE set up a number of demonstration units at Stoneleigh that allowed further research to be carried out. In the dairy unit, particular attention was given to mastitis control and metabolic profile testing, while the beef unit worked to minimise calf losses and contain diseases such as ringworm. Work carried out at the sheep unit has included the employment of ultrasonography in pregnancy testing and litter size determination, the monitoring of toxoplasma immunity in bought-in replacements and the use of progestagen sponges to induce early and synchronised breeding. From 1983 the Society has also instigated a series of International Symposia, drawing experts from all over the world to discuss a range of agricultural subjects including animal health.

W Clapperton, *Clapperton's Royal Agricultural Salisbury Handbook, Containing a Concise History of the Royal Agricultural Society of England From its Origin...* (Salisbury, 1857); N Goddard, *Harvests of Change: the Royal Agricultural Society of England 1838–1988* (London, 1988); J A Scott Watson, *The History of The Royal Agricultural Society of England 1839–1939* (London, 1939).

Records (1): Rural History Centre, University of Reading, PO Box 229, Whiteknights, Reading RG6 6AG

Charter 1840; opinion as to constitution of charter and by-laws 1875; papers re charter and supplementary charters 1904–35; opinion as to whether RASE is judicially a charity in respect of proposals to dispose of Park Royal Ltd 1905; Council: rough copy minute book 1840–87, fair copy minute book 1838–1932, agenda books 1841–1922, reports 1874–97, lists of members 1838–1900, attendances 1893–1901; finance committee: minute books 1840–47, 1850–62, agenda books 1916–62; minute books: certain general meetings 1843–44, county meetings committee incl agenda 1843–1911, general show committee 1911–32, Liverpool meetings 1841, Bristol meetings 1842, Derby meetings 1843, Cambridge meetings 1840, Southampton meetings 1844, Windsor meetings 1851, metropolitan show sites committee 1877–87, Windsor committee 1888–89, judges selection committee 1860–1947, showyard contracts committee 1865–79, showyard works committee 1878–1939, implement committee 1857–1936, farm prizes committee 1906–15, stock prizes committee 1874–1948, research committee 1922–49, chemical committee 1934–38, botanical and zoological committee 1881–1948, veterinary committee 1861–1953, special committee on potato diseases 1874–75, seeds and plants committee 1872–95, tuberculosis experiment committee 1910–14, special experiments committee 1985–89, education committee 1865–1907, national agricultural education board 1905–55, joint board for examinations in dairying 1896–97, national dairy examinations board 1928–48, journal committee 1855–1939, house committee 1844–1907, selection committee for council 1867–1938, Woburn sub-committee 1878–1921, Queen Victoria's gift fund committee 1897–1908, Jenkins memorial committee 1887–, occasional committees incl the veterinary grant committee and the horse committee 1844–60, reduction of expenditure committee 1854, French peasant farmers fund committee 1870–73, misc committees incl inspection committee for county meetings, laboratory sub-committee, cattle plague evidence committee, stock prizes committee, special stallion committee 1867–85, horse shoeing committee and abortion in cattle committee c1888–1906, Lord Vernon's committee and Sir John Thorold's committee 1872–92, hunter stallion committee 1885–90, special by-law committee 1888–89, agricultural and food products committee 1893, special committee to consider applications for increased grants from other committees 1908–13, joint chemical and finance committee and Sir Ailwyn Fellowes committee 1914, emergency committee 1916–20, dog show committee 1924–25; lists of committees 1845–68; occasional committees agenda book 1844–67; report of Sir John Thorold's committee 1888; reports and recommendations of post-war agricultural committee c1941–45; papers re: chemical committee 20th cent, journal and education committees 1938–40, publicity committee 1930s, executive *ad hoc* and special committee 1930s–40s; ordinary ledgers 1838–1965; ordinary ledger analysis book 1901–28; county meeting ledgers 1848–1930; show ledgers 1931–64; ledgers for ordinary, investment, show and farm accounts 1965–66; investment ledger 1939–70; cash books 1940–65; subscriptions 1941–51; receipts 1939–51; publications 1913–25; petty cash journal 1920–25; petty cash books 1942–66; journal combining principal and show journals 1838–57; journal 1924–64; yearly balance sheets with statements of account 1890–91, 1893–1965; monthly statements of accounts 1908–49; quarterly statements of accounts 1950–53; bank statements 1952–67; specimen farm account books 19th cent; monthly salaries books 1947–68; weekly salaries books 1947–64; expenditure registers, showyard staff 1913–60; income registers, various shows 1939–66 [w]; register of ticket sales, various shows 1953–64; statement of accounts re showyard superintendent 1898–1906; statement of accounts re showyard surveyor 1936–49; yearly statement of account, research fund 1924–53; subsidiary accounts, correspondence and papers re Woburn experimental farm c1890–1921; Harewood House: ledger 1893–1900, debenture stock records 1892–95; Hills Bequest: ledger 1896–1922, cash book 1897–1925; old superannuation fund: ledger 1915–37, cash book 1911–39, journal 1911–38; French peasant farmers ledger 1870–73; William Scott Abbott trust yearly statement of account 1964–65; registers of governors and members 1840s–; registers of subscriptions and compositions 1838–90; register of annual members and payment of subscriptions 1891–1945; legal proceedings book re arrears of subscriptions 1844; correspondence re an opinion in respect of arrears of subscriptions 1850; register of life members 1890–99; lists of members of local committees for county meetings 1895–1904; lists of subscriptions to French peasant farmers fund 1871–73; stewards' remarks 1865–1909; stewards' reprimands re stock 1888–1903; list of firms and persons excluded from shows and advertising 1887–1931; papers re National

Diploma in Agriculture examinations 1930–33, 1937–39; papers re National Diploma in Dairying 1930–39; papers re administration of examinations 1892–1944; papers re Queen Victoria gift fund 1897–; papers re long service awards 1961–64; papers re administrative reform, appointment of officers, employment 1887–1925; letter book 1838–44; letter book re articles to be published in journal 1868–69; circulars 1891–93; show and breed association papers: reports of conferences with other show and breed societies 1960–63, executive committee minutes, agenda, reports, general meeting proceedings and other papers (p) 1958–64; papers re local shows and show sites 19th–20th cent; Hills bequest agreements 1922, 1955; other agreements 1906, 1964–67; inventories and valuations of premises at Hanover Square 1870, 1888, nd; Park Royal Ltd: special show committee minute book 1902, site committee minute book 1901–04, directors' meetings minute book 1904–07, Park Royal committee minute book, incl reports of extraordinary meetings and proceedings undertaken in respect of the liquidation of the company 1904–07, report and valuation of Park Royal estate 1906, catalogues of timber sales 1905–06, notebook of sketches re buildings, etc, nd, legal agreements 1904–06, ledger 1904–07, cash book 1903–07, site cash book 1902–04, petty cash book 1903–06, journal 1904–07, expenditure register 1904–06, site wages book 1904–06, weekly site wages book 1903–05, annual report and balance sheet 1905, auctioneer's account 1905, bank pass books 1903–07; press cuttings book re Sir Walter Gilbey 1897–1910; press cuttings and photograph album re Bristol show 1913; photograph album re Windsor show 1954; photographs re Kenya show 1958; misc photographs and prints 19th cent; misc farming journals 19th cent.

Records (2): in private ownership of Dr C A Spinage, Wickwood House, Stanford Road, Faringdon SN7 8EZ

Veterinary committee circular re cattle plague, nd.

ROYAL COLLEGE OF VETERINARY SURGEONS
London

History: The Royal College of Veterinary Surgeons (RCVS) was established in 1844 by royal charter. Under the terms of the charter, veterinary medicine was formally recognised as a profession and a single co-ordinating and regulatory body created with the dual aims of enhancing the profession's status and controlling standards within veterinary education. To achieve these objectives, the RCVS intended to introduce an examination to be taken by all veterinary students on completion of their studies. Only those who passed would be admitted to the RCVS register (introduced in 1848) and entitled to call themselves 'veterinary surgeons'. Previously, certificates in veterinary medicine had been awarded by the two veterinary colleges, the Royal Veterinary College, London, (est 1791), and the Edinburgh Veterinary College (est 1823), while certificates of veterinary competence were issued to Edinburgh graduates by the Highland and Agricultural Society of Scotland. To administer the RCVS a Council was set up, with a president, six vice presidents and a secretary all elected from the membership. Six members of Council were to retire each year at the general meeting, with attendees then voting to re-elect them or select others in their place. Early meetings took place at the Freemason's Tavern before a lease was secured on 10 Red Lion Square, London, in 1853. The first examination was held in April 1844, but it soon became clear that the RCVS lacked the necessary legal powers either to compel students to take its examination, or to prevent anyone who wished to do so from practising veterinary medicine and calling himself a veterinary surgeon. Its position was further undermined by a rift with the Edinburgh Veterinary College and the Highland and Agricultural Society of Scotland. The latter, resentful at RCVS attempts to win the sole right to grant diplomas, refused to issue any certificates from 1844. But in 1848 the Edinburgh Veterinary College, offended at criticism of its examinations, disassociated itself from the RCVS entirely and persuaded the Highland and Agricultural Society of Scotland to issue veterinary certificates to its students once again. The dispute was not fully resolved until 1879, at which time the Edinburgh Veterinary College was re-affiliated to the RCVS and the Highland and Agricultural Society of Scotland agreed to cease awarding certificates from 1881 on condition that holders of its certificates would be entitled to RCVS membership. These agreements were laid down in the supplemental charter of 1879. Another supplemental charter, awarded in 1876, allowed the RCVS to create Fellows and appoint a Registrar to maintain the register of veterinary surgeons. Finally, in 1881 the first Veterinary Surgeons Act was passed which, in addition to confirming the charters, allowed the RCVS to maintain a register of unqualified 'existing practitioners', all of whom had to have been practising since at least 1876. The Act also allowed the RCVS to register the holders of colonial or foreign qualifications, to remove members' names from the register, and to bring prosecutions for breaches of the Act. Subsequent supplemental charters in 1883 and 1892 served to fix examination and registration fees and to separate the roles of members and examiners. The 1892 charter also allowed ordinary members to be appointed to the Council. Further powers were granted by a series of additional supplemental charters, awarded in 1914, 1923, 1932, 1960, 1963 and 1965, and by the passing of further legislation – the Veterinary Surgeons Act (Amendment) Acts of 1900 and 1920, and the Veterinary Surgeons (Irish Free State Agreement) Act of 1932. The Act of 1920 fixed the annual subscription fee at a guinea, thus assuring the RCVS of an income, while the 1932 Act provided both for the establishment of a Veterinary Council in Ireland and for the representation of Irish members by allowing four Irish members to sit on the RCVS Council, raising the total number of councillors to thirty six. The first woman member, Aleen Cust, was admitted to the Royal College of Veterinary Surgeons in 1922. The introduction of a new Veterinary Surgeons Act in 1948 brought about significant changes. Under its terms the RCVS no longer had the power to examine veterinary students. Instead, the four existing veterinary colleges at London, Edinburgh, Glasgow and Liverpool, along with two newly created ones at Bristol and Cambridge, were integrated into universities and their degrees recognised as the qualification which allowed veterinary surgeons to practise as Members of the Royal College of Veterinary Surgeons (MRCVS). The RCVS's role from this time forward was to be a supervisory one. The Act also finally banned all unqualified and unregistered persons from practising veterinary surgery, although a supplementary register was created allowing those who had been practising for seven out of the previous ten years to continue carrying out certain minor treatments. To reflect the changes brought about by the Act, it became necessary to alter the composition of the RCVS Council. After that time, the Council was made up of twenty elected members, with another four members appointed by the Privy Council, twelve university appointed members and four representatives of the profession in Ireland. At the same time, the Council's disciplinary powers were transferred to a statutory committee. The Veterinary Surgeons Act of 1966 replaced all previous legislation, although some of the provisions of the 1948 Act were re-enacted, and granted the RCVS additional powers governing temporary registration and disciplinary proceedings, including the introduction of a Preliminary Investigation Committee. This was followed in 1967 by a new supplemental charter that swept away all previous charters with the exception of the original charter of 1844. The new charter was concerned largely with administration, with rules on the appointment of Fellows and admission of new members. It also allowed the Council to award diplomas or certificates to those training as veterinary nurses or veterinary specialists, signalling the increased role that the RCVS would go on to play in the provision of continuing professional development. The RCVS Trust Fund, set up in 1958, raises funds for the College library and does much to enable the RCVS to actively support veterinary education and research. Both the Act of 1966 and the charter that followed it were revised in 1980 to allow holders of approved European Economic Community veterinary qualifications to become members of the RCVS. In 1999, the Council voted to allow lay people to sit on its Preliminary Investigation Committee.

E Boden and J MacArthur Clark, *Challenges for Change: RCVS Charter 150 Symposium* (London, 1994).

Records (1): Wellcome Library, Royal College of Veterinary Surgeons, Belgravia House, 62–64 Horseferry Road, London SW1P 2AF

Royal charter 1844; grant of arms 1844; supplemental charters 19th–20th cent; correspondence and papers re charter and supplemental charters 1841–1931; drafts (3) of the petition c1840; letters from those wishing to add their names to the memorial presented to the government in support of the formation of the RCVS 1840; copy of the charter as professed to be altered by the governors of the Royal Veterinary College 1846; memorial addressed to Sir G Grey re Royal Veterinary College's opposition to charter 1850; petitions 19th–20th cent; proposals of amendments to by-laws c1849; copies of by-laws 1890–95; correspondence re by-law 62 applications 1955–56; index to by-laws and resolutions, nd; annual general meeting: minutes, reports, names of those attending 1845–50, 1852–78, lists of members present 1883–1963; report of the proceedings at a special general meeting 1893; *Registers of Members* 1852, 1860s–; card index of members c1844–1960; Council: minute books 1840–, agenda for quarterly meetings 1880–1917, draft minutes of meetings 1898, nd, minutes and agenda for various Council and committee meetings 1949, report of special meeting 1896, reports of quarterly meetings 1896, 1898, 1900; annual reports 1845–; report re preparation of *Register of Members* c1850; nominations, correspondence and papers re elections 1942–54; attendance book 1924–53; attendance book for Council and committees 1908–49; amendments to by-laws 1931–67; opinions 19th–20th cent; correspondence and papers re setting up and running of Council Club 1951–66; files re election of committees, ceremonial costume, witness fees, artificial insemination officers, London Veterinary Medical Society special fund, International Labour Office c1940s; examination committee: minutes 1887–1938, correspondence re Polish applications 1945–47, papers 1932–34; registration committee: minutes 1886–1938, standing orders re procedure, nd, sub-committee papers and letters re boarding kennels run by veterinary surgeons 1935–36, sub-committee minutes, memoranda, etc re People's Dispensary for Sick Animals 1939; parliamentary committee: minutes 1915–38, reports, agenda, etc 1964–67, general correspondence and papers 1976–78; college fund committee, minutes 1873–84; finance committee, minutes

1886–1915; finance and general purposes committee, minutes 1915–38; honours and prizes committee, minutes 1915–37; examination fees sub-committee, papers 1946–48; preliminary investigation and advisory committee, minutes 1954–63; disciplinary committee, minutes 1955–58; Indian Veterinary Service special committee, minutes 1923–26; India and Egypt sub-committee, papers 1945–47; sub-committee on publication of the Loveday report, papers 1938, 1945–46; commercial veterinary services committee, minutes, agenda, etc 1970–72; RCVS/British Veterinary Association joint European Economic Community committee, papers, etc 1967–72; minutes of special committees 1918–38; 10th International Veterinary Congress organising committee, minutes, agenda, accounts 1911–14, 1916, 1920, 1922–28; 11th International Veterinary Congress, minute books 1928–31; 14th International Veterinary Congress, minute book 1947–49; organising committee's attendance book for 10th, 11th and 14th International Veterinary Congresses 1911–49 [w]; Dr Bullock's rough minute books 1929–43, 1946–47; rough minute books 1888–1914, 1942–47; copies of minutes from various committees 1935–42; attendance books for various committees 1949–78; Trust Fund: minutes of general and executive council meetings 1964–91, agenda, annual reports, balance sheets 1988–91; account summary 1844–1928; treasurers' accounts 1841–1928; accounts 1891–96, 1951–56, 1958; journals 1862–1943; ledgers 1897–1963; ledger for hire of rooms to Central Veterinary Society and other veterinary associations 1895–1933; cash books 1897–1958, 1978–82; petty cash books 1932–51; petty cash sheets 1984–89; bank statements re Robert Daubney fund 1983–89; bank statements re appeal 1989–91; correspondence re Bill Hiddleston award fund account 1987–92; register of student fees 1940–44; examination fees account books 1945–53; estimated receipts and expenditure re examinations 1954–57; accounts for students' and examiners' fees 1904–10; account book for examiners' fees and expenses 1934–58; record of examiners' fees 1934–54; statements of accounts for corporation duty 1916–55 [w]; invoice book 1909–15; ledger with details of entertainment fund for 10th International Veterinary Congress 1912–14 and later congresses 1925–31; accounts, correspondence, estimates, etc re funding of 10th International Veterinary Congress 1909–24; members' subscriptions to the 10th Congress 1914; petty expenses book for Veterinary Tribunal 1918–19, International Veterinary Congress 1922–35 and International Veterinary Congress entertainment fund 1921–29; petty cash receipts 1958–60; schedule of accounts 1954–60; misc papers re accounts 1957, nd; library: cash account 1955, cash book 1955–64, ledger 1955–64, budgets and estimates 1952–55, expenditure book 1986–92, memorial library fund statements of receipts and payments 1956–60; misc papers re: Fitzwygram prize

1928–40, Walley memorial prize and Williams memorial prize 1940–50; correspondence re payment of fees arrears 1922–39; building extension fund contributions, nd; record of appeal donations 1978–86; valuation of investments 1956; papers re investments 1915–25; quotations for new diplomas for degree graduates 1955; war damage claims 1941–48; papers and correspondence re investments, taxes, etc 1920–41; statement of accounts re trust funds with related papers 1910–20; registrars' outgoing letter books 1954–; secretarys' outgoing letter books re: general 1862-1943, Veterinary Tribunal 1918–19; registrar/secretarys' correspondence and papers re: appeals to Privy Council by those rejected as members after the Veterinary Surgeons Act (1881) 1883–84, tuberculosis experiments 1891, Worshipful Company of Farriers' registration scheme 1893, 1919, 1944–46, Veterinary Surgeons Amendment Bill 1907–08, 1919–20, regulations, examinations and syllabus re diploma in veterinary science medicine c1909–20, production and distribution of milk 1913–c1933, appeals for Army Veterinary Corps recruits and petrol rationing during First World War 1914–18, curriculum c1915–29, reciprocity with South Africa 1915–43, entrance of de-mobbed soldiers (with list of entrants) 1918, Indian Civil Veterinary Department 1920–29, meat inspection 1921–27, Irish Free State 1924–30, 1932, standardising of colour and marking descriptions of horses c1925–30, appointment of examiners 1925, 1933, 1936, 1938–40, 1942, 1944–47, Colonial Veterinary Service 1927–30, recruitment, pay and services of veterinary surgeons to Malaya and Kenya 1927–30, finance 1928–44, third interim report of the local government and public health consolidation committee and Draft Food and Drugs Bill and Pharmacy and Poisons Act 1930–38, veterinary investigation officers 1930–43, patent veterinary medicine 1933–34, People's Dispensary for Sick Animals 1933–37, non-payment of fees 1934–57, conduct of final examinations under the five year curriculum 1936–37, veterinary education and Ministry of Agriculture and Fisheries 1937–39, allowances to those giving evidence in indictable cases 1939, Royal Society for the Prevention of Cruelty to Animals Bill 1939–40, veterinary colleges 1940, Privy Council 1940–42, forms of certificate to be given to members in insurance claims 1942–43, examination syllabuses 1944–47, Middle and Far East sub-committee on Indian officers training at British veterinary colleges 1945–48, MRCVS applications from India and Burma 1946–49, matriculation to Irish universities 1947, entrance requirements to veterinary courses 1947, Veterinary Surgeons Act 1948, MRCVS application of Ahmed Farid of Egypt 1948–49, civil service commission 1948–50, 14th International Veterinary Congress 1949–52, Veterinary Surgeons Act 1965–66, statutory registration bodies 1967–78, British Small Animal Veterinary Association 1968–77, appearance of veterinary surgeons in advertising photographs 1969–70, specialisation sub-committee 1969–71, care of laboratory animals 1969–73, representation 1969–75, working party looking at soundness of horses 1971–77, European Liaison Group for Agriculture 1972–75, parliamentary bills 1973–75, ova transplants 1975–76, Council of Professional Bodies 1976–80, general c1891–1921, 1924–35, c1950–86; correspondence and papers re: Highland and Agricultural Society of Scotland 1882–1909, British Institute for Preventative Medicine 1894–1904, notification of contagious disease 1895, meat inspection 1897–1935, preliminary educational examinations 1898–1932, reciprocity with Australia, South Africa, India, Egypt 1899, c1918–37, South African War memorial tablet 1902, Melbourne University veterinary degree 1909–17, veterinary provision overseas (mainly colonial) c1912–48, examinations in secondary schools 1913–18, military service 1914–18, Department of Agriculture and Technical Instruction for Ireland staff salaries c1915–21, veterinary research 1921–23, investigations into unregistered veterinary surgeons 1927–41, Agricultural Research Association 1930–36, Australian and South African qualifications 1931–35, proposed Royal Society for the Prevention of Cruelty to Animals hospital and effects of People's Dispensary for Sick Animals proposed scheme for free veterinary treatment in Liverpool 1932–33, report of cattle diseases committee of economic advisory council 1933–34, establishment of Cambridge Veterinary School 1934–44, use of signboard by members 1936–37, British Broadcasting Corporation 1937–39, British Standards Institution 1937–49, revision of examination syllabus 1941, Colonial Advisory Council of Agriculture and Animal Health 1941, Veterinary Educational Trust 1943–47, Victoria Veterinary Benevolent Fund covenants 1946–54, agreement with the Irish Republic 1964–79, Young Farmers' Clubs stockmanship examinations 1965–69, staff 1965–79, college newsletter 1968–87, European Economic Community re veterinary medicines, pesticide residues and animal feedstuffs 1972–79, European Community secondary legislation 1976–78, European Association of UK Professions 1980–82, affiliated schools 20th cent; incoming letter books 1868–69, 1877–78; misc correspondence and papers 1897–c1950; Professor Wooldridge's papers re Red Cross Agriculture Fund 1940; Veterinary Surgeons Act 1881: letters 1881, list of appeals to Privy Council 1883, register of those who applied to be reinstated 1890–1904, registers of those rejected 1880s–90s, restorations to register 1901–49; papers re Veterinary Surgeons Act (Amendment) Bill (1920) 1918–22; Veterinary Surgeons Act 1948: papers incl copies of draft 1941–42, copy of president's letter to members of the parliamentary committee considering the Bill and their replies 1948, correspondence with Ministry of Agriculture and Fisheries 1946–48; government reports re Veterinary Surgeons Bill (1966) 1966; copies of Corporation Bills with related correspondence and papers re amendments to clauses on slaughterhouses and meat inspection 1926, 1936–38, 1949–52; Slaughter of Animals Bill and related correspondence 1927–32; correspondence re Agriculture Act 1937 and Northern Ireland Veterinary Surgeons Bill 1934–38; private Bills with limited correspondence 1930s; correspondence re Bill to exempt veterinary surgeons from serving on juries c1935; misc correspondence re parliamentary bills 1928–29, c1971–77; copies of People's Dispensary for Sick Animals Bill 1933–34; misc papers re Medicines Act 1968; misc parliamentary papers c1915–19; papers, etc re: Sir Frederick Smith and Miss Aleen Cust fellowships 1956–76, Williams memorial prize 1902–07, 1951–52, Walley prize 1900–50, Bursary prize 1903–04, 1908, Steel medal 1896–1944, Jubilee memorial fund 1903–39; Fitzwygram prize, lists of eligible students with marks obtained 1905–20; record of examinations 1844–90; report of examinations 1869–1917; report of first examinations 1873–1917; record of first examinations 1873–1920; record of final examinations 1890–1920; examination record sheets 1920–52; examination papers 1925–59; index to report of first examinations, nd; index to report of final examinations, nd; reports of the practical examinations of students from the Royal Veterinary College, London 1871–85; records of fellowship examinations 1893–1930; students exemption register book 1939–49; list of Royal Veterinary College students who provided birth certificates 1899–1906; registers of school certificates enabling students to enter university: British students 1948–50, overseas students 1948–61; record of education certificates 1935–48; educational certificate indexes, nd; record of students c1894–1940s; examination book, giving the name of each student and indicating whether they passed or failed 1888–1909; notebook indicating pass/fail of students in examinations 1888–1909; misc statistics on student numbers, numbers passing, etc 1904–10; applications for exemption from the preliminary examination by ex-servicemen 1919; instructions for the conduct of examinations, nd; correspondence and papers, incl deeds, of Messrs Hedges & Davis, solicitors, re administration of the Acton, Brixton and Hampton estates 1894–1931 [w]; correspondence re properties offered to RCVS and rejected 1954–57; plans for various unspecified buildings, nd; correspondence re building works, furniture supply, etc 1946–51; correspondence re 18 Victoria Avenue, Harrogate 1940–44; papers re renting out of basement and top flat in Red Lion Square 1957; papers, letters and estimates re maintenance and repair works at 10 Red Lion Square 1925; 11th International Veterinary Congress, programmes, tickets, menus, etc 1930; 12th International Veterinary Congress, preliminary programme 1934; 14th International Veterinary Congress, correspondence, papers, programmes, notebook re programme, list of delegates, photographs, etc 1949–51; list of veterinary nurse applications 1986; Animal Nursing Auxiliary Trainee applications 1962–69; charts and diagrams re final report of the Royal Commission on Tuberculosis 1915; postage books 1946–76; list of people appointed to veterinary schools worldwide c1880–1958; notes on disease, anatomy, treatment, etc by J F Kendall, Chief of Technical Staff c1920s; responses to RCVS survey to establish division of veterinary surgeons' time between small animal, equine and livestock work with related papers 1971; circulars and other papers re proposed new appendix in *Register of Members* and *Directory of Practices* listing holders of post-graduate qualifications c1974; completed forms re census on unqualified practice 1939–44; obituary book 1868–84; index to letter book commencing 1966; list of veterinary surgeons using motor cars, nd; memorandum on reorganisation and finances of Royal Veterinary College, London, 1936; registers of complaints, mostly against unqualified practitioners 1889–1929; list of those ineligible to practise as veterinary surgeons under Veterinary Surgeons Act (1881) 1882; letters re registration 1912; register showing when members gained their diplomas 1794–1843; library accessions register 1950–81; biographical information on various prominent veterinary surgeons for presentations, etc 1930s; notes to chairmen 1964–70; submission forms re visitation to Western College of Veterinary Medicine 1977; veterinary surgeons' death certificates 19th–20th cent; returns from regiments giving farriers' names, qualifications, scales of fees, etc 1912–13; application by Harvard University for recognition of diploma 1890; petition re pension for children of the late William Hunting 1914; guest list, menu, etc for jubilee dinner 1894; law and animal experimentation working papers 1975–76; petition re People's Dispensary for Sick Animals' mobile vans and Medicine Act Regulations 1975–76; Irish Free State, correspondence, statements of accounts, lists of members who had paid fees c1932–46; historical collection accessions book 1953–57; report by W S Petrie, Honorary Secretary of the Association of Veterinary Inspectors re veterinary staff of Ministry of Agriculture and Fisheries 1924; Society for the Study of Animal Breeding sub-committee report on embryo transfer with particular reference to cattle late 1970s; testimonials for Mashuk Ali Salutin and Ayoub Khan Salutrie of Meerut c1915; album with synopsis of career of Colonel Ernest Albert Le Souef of Western Australia, backing up his fellowship application incl letters, photographs, etc 1934; photographs of staff, veterinary surgeons, animals, annual dinners, events, etc 19th–20th cent; prints, certificates, etc 19th–20th cent; press cuttings 1924–32, nd; notes for an article on Delabere Pritchett Blaine 1927–29; letters to Professor James McQueen from Frederick Smith 1894 and John Gamgee 1893; brief history of McQueen's career 1896; Ministry of Labour leaflets on career choices, incl veterinary surgery 1931, 1938, 1945; papers re research on Dr John Adam McBride MRCVS, author of *Anatomical Outlines of the Horse* 20th cent; Society of Veterinary Officers, minutes 1933–38; Ontario Veterinary College: calendar 1945–46, curriculum 1946; Association of Agriculture, memorandum and articles of association 1947; misc booklets from American universities 1939–47; American Veterinary Medical Association, membership directory and constitution 1936; Punjab Veterinary College, Lahore, prospectus 1930; Bihar and Orissa Veterinary College, Patna, India, syllabus 1936.

Records (2): Archives and Manuscripts, Wellcome Library for the History and Understanding of Medicine, 183 Euston Road, London NW1 2BE

Council's annual reports 1963–64.

Records (3): The Library, Royal Veterinary College, Royal College Street, London NW1 0TU

Charter of incorporation, petitions and correspondence c1844.

Records (4): in private ownership of Miss Mary Brancker, 38 Streetly Lane, Sutton Coldfield B74 4TU

Memorandum re draft Veterinary Surgeons Act (Amendment) Bill 1943; presidential statement on progress of Veterinary Surgeons Bill 1948; presidential circular re abolition of unqualified veterinary practice 1951.

Records (5): in private ownership of Mr R D Locke, 4 Rathmore Road, Cambridge CB1 7AD

Photographs: 11th International Veterinary Congress banquet, London 1930, 12th International Veterinary Congress banquet, New York 1934, RCVS Presidents' luncheon, London 1935.

ROYAL PHARMACEUTICAL SOCIETY OF GREAT BRITAIN
London

History: The Pharmaceutical Society of Great Britain was established in 1841 by Jacob Bell at 17 Bloomsbury Square, London, to regulate the pharmaceutical profession and to set up a system of registration for pharmacists. It received a royal charter in 1843, but was not granted the use of the word 'Royal' in its title until 1988. The Society was primarily concerned with the examination and registration of pharmacists and the enforcement of legislation relating to human pharmaceuticals and the sale of medicines and poisons. In addition it had a lesser involvement in the field of animal health. From the 1940s, the Society's Council considered various aspects of animal health and veterinary medicine and a number of committees with an interest in veterinary medicine, including a veterinary committee, were formed. In 1988 a specialist Animal Medicines Division was established in response to a European Economic Community directive on the sale and manufacture of medicated feedstuffs and animal medicines. The Division today is responsible for ensuring that the manufacture and sale of medicated animal feedstuffs through agricultural merchants, saddlers and feed distributors meets legal requirements. It does this through a national team of six inspectors.

Records (1): Museum, Royal Pharmaceutical Society of Great Britain, 1 Lambeth High Street, London SE1 7JN

Council: correspondence and committee minutes re drafting of statement on veterinary advertising 1973–74, reports and correspondence with Royal Society for the Prevention of Cruelty to Animals and others re policy of euthanasia of small animals 1957–60; committee on veterinary practice by unregistered persons, minutes and reports 1947–48; branch representatives of pharmacists engaged in supply of veterinary and agricultural preparations, minutes 1953, 1960–62; veterinary committee, minutes 1954–64; joint veterinary pharmaceutical committee: minutes 1954–64, correspondence with Association of the British Pharmaceutical Industry, British Veterinary Association, Ministry of Agriculture, Fisheries and Food, Royal College of Veterinary Surgeons 1953–77; joint committee on use of antibiotics in animal husbandry and veterinary medicine (Swann Committee), working party minutes 1970–73; minutes and papers re meeting with Association of the British Pharmaceutical Industry on distribution of veterinary pharmaceutical products 1970–71; notes and correspondence re distribution of penicillin products for veterinary use 1953; papers and correspondence re: companies, veterinary associations and Ministry of Agriculture, Fisheries and Food re distribution of veterinary medicines 1939–57, views on Penicillin Bill and Act 1947, Therapeutic Substances (Prevention and Misuse) Bill and regulations on use of procaine penicillin in animal feedstuffs 1953, 1947–55, secretary and registrar's department re *British Veterinary Codex* 1949–69, illegal sale of antibiotics to farmers and in animal feedstuffs 1967–77, Swann Committee 1968–73, correspondence with Association of the British Pharmaceutical Industry re distribution of veterinary medicines 1968–74, objection to agreement between Ministry of Health and manufacturers to confine supplies of injectable methylamphetamide to hospitals without consulting Society and to British Veterinary Association's proposal to supply the drug direct to veterinary surgeons 1968–70, future of *British Pharmaceutical Codex* and *Veterinary Codex* 1968–78, Department of Health and Social Security incl re animal test certificates 1970–71, agricultural and veterinary legislation 1971–77, distribution of animal medicines under Medicines Act 1968 incl maps and statistics showing number of pharmacies engaged in agricultural and veterinary general practice 1971–76, Society's role in enforcement of Act and regulations re prevention of misuse and illegal sales of veterinary antibiotics 1971–82, enforcement, investigations and prosecutions re illegal supply, sale and use of veterinary antibiotics 1976–77; correspondence, extracts of committee minutes, bills and publications re Society's views on attempts to change law on animal experimentation 1973–76; correspondence and inspectors' reports re sale of animal medicines containing poisons at horse shows 1977; correspondence re control of production of veterinary biological products 1945–53; booklet re diploma in agricultural and veterinary pharmacy 1982; Allstock Products Ltd, catalogue of veterinary and medical cod-liver oil 1935; British Distributors of Animal Medicines Association Ltd, classified products list 1979; Benjamin Morris Edmonds, Lowestoft, Suffolk, *A Lecture on the Composition Properties and Effects of the Atmosphere Upon the Animal and Vegetable Kingdom* 1838; Fannin & Co Ltd, catalogue of veterinary instruments, books and drugs 1953; Miles Leagh, Ramsey, Isle of Man, annotated copy of Francis Slater's *Every man His Own Farrier* containing recipes 1824; L F Newman, *A Country Horse Doctor's Notebook* 1959. [Ref: 121/41/12/3.1–4, 10, 14, 16D; 170/45/46; 204/24/77, 84, 86; 351/2–3, 5, 5/1.4–7, 5/5, 9, 9/1, 10, 13, 13/1, 14; 975.2; 2874; G21/26; IRA.1996.178, 342, 451; M1/9/13, 18.1, 18.2; 665.214.1; 615.452:619:914.2; IRA.1997.059, 615.46/7:619(085.6); IRA.1997.093.2, 619.1]

Records (2): Animal Medicines Division, Royal Pharmaceutical Society of Great Britain, 1 Lambeth High Street, London SE1 7JN

Animal medicines division annual reports, incl statistical details of agricultural merchants, saddlers and manufacturers of medicated animal feedstuffs 1988–.

SCOTTISH METROPOLITAN VETERINARY ASSOCIATION
Edinburgh

History: The Scottish Metropolitan Veterinary Association was formed in Edinburgh during the mid to late nineteenth century with the purpose of bringing together local veterinary surgeons to discuss the issues affecting their profession. It was at a meeting of the Scottish Metropolitan Veterinary Association in 1909 that Orlando Charnock Bradley of the Edinburgh Veterinary College called for the establishment of 'one single British Veterinary Association' into which all existing territorial societies would be incorporated as divisions.

Records: Archivist, Edinburgh University Library, George Square, Edinburgh EH8 9LJ

Minute books 1888–1962; veterinary assistant's group, minute book and related correspondence 1962–69.

SOCIETY OF WOMEN VETERINARY SURGEONS

History: The Society of Women Veterinary Surgeons was established in 1941 as a non-territorial division of the British Veterinary Association to consider the role of women within the veterinary profession. It focussed particularly on the special problems faced by those who had to combine family commitments with career development and aimed to make it easier for women who had temporarily left the profession to retrain. The Society also wished to promote scientific development within the veterinary profession and to encourage continuous education for all women veterinary surgeons. Meetings were held two or three times a year and a newsletter published twice a year. In 1969 the Society of Women Veterinary Surgeons Charitable Trust was set up. Inspired by the Society's first president, Miss Joan O' Joshua, it aimed to provide financial help for women veterinary surgeons and students. Although trustees were appointed by the Society's Council, the trust itself remained a separate body. The Society of Women Veterinary Surgeons was dissolved in 1990.

Records: Wolfgar Veterinary Surgery, Wolfgar, Cheriton Bishop, Exeter EX6 6HH

General meetings: minutes 1989, attendance book 1975–90; rules and regulations, nd; correspondence and papers re dissolution 1990;

membership application forms (blank), nd; general correspondence 1989–90; newsletters 1986–87.

VETERINARY DEER SOCIETY
London

History: The Veterinary Deer Society was established in 1981 to provide a forum for the discussion and exchange of ideas on all matters relating to deer.

Records: c/o British Veterinary Association, 7 Mansfield Street, London W1M 0AT

Minutes 1981–; balance sheets/profit and loss accounts 1981–; correspondence 1981–; photographs 1981–; press cuttings 1981–.

VETERINARY DEFENCE SOCIETY LTD
Knutsford, Cheshire

History: At a meeting of the Liverpool Veterinary Medical Association in 1865, Ephraim Alfred Friend led a discussion on the legal responsibilities of veterinary surgeons which resulted in a recommendation that a society be formed which could offer legal defence and insurance to veterinary surgeons. On 6 September 1865, therefore, the Veterinary Mutual Defence Society was established, with Robert Lucas of Liverpool as its first president. Although the Society was concerned primarily with legal defence, it also served a benevolent function, offering financial aid to the widows and orphans of veterinary surgeons and to those unlucky enough to sustain injuries which left them unable to work. In recognition of this side of its work the society was renamed the National Veterinary Benevolent & Mutual Defence Society (NVBMDS) in 1867. Although ostensibly a national organisation, the benevolent activities of the NVBMDS were limited to those living in the north of England, a restriction which led in 1897 to the establishment of a rival society, the Victoria Veterinary Benevolent Fund (VVBF), in London. During the twentieth century differences of opinion between the two societies subsided and they frequently worked alongside each other. In 1973, NVBMDS was renamed the Veterinary Defence & Benevolent Society, although most of its resources were being concentrated on defence work. Five years later the VVBF took over all the Veterinary Defence & Benevolent Society's benevolent functions and was renamed the

Veterinary Benevolent Fund. The Veterinary Defence & Benevolent Society was renamed the Veterinary Defence Society Ltd in 1979 and is now based at 4 Haig Court, Parkgate Estate, Knutsford.

R D Locke, 'The Origins of Benevolence in the Veterinary Profession', *The Veterinary Record*, 27 Sept 1997.

Records: in private ownership of Mr R D Locke, 4 Rathmore Road, Cambridge CB1 7AD

Programme of toasts at first annual dinner 1866; centenary brochure 1965.

VETERINARY HISTORY SOCIETY

London

History: The Veterinary History Society was established in 1962 to encourage an interest in, and the study of, the history of veterinary medicine. In the first few years there was a membership of around thirty but by the 1990s this number had increased to sixty. At least two meetings are held each year and since 1973 the Society has aimed to produce a bi-annual bulletin.

Records: Wellcome Library, Royal College of Veterinary Surgeons, Belgravia House, 62–64 Horseferry Road, London SW1P 2AF

Committee minutes and agenda 1996–; programmes for meetings with related correspondence 1962–66, 1969–87; correspondence re: establishment 1962, bulletin 1996–98, subscriptions 1997–98; list of officers and committee members 1974–75.

VETERINARY MEAT HYGIENE GROUP

History: Following a correspondence in *The Veterinary Record* a meeting of veterinary surgeons involved in meat inspection was held on 27 October 1974. Out of this meeting emerged the Veterinary Meat Hygiene Group which aimed to forge links between veterinary surgeons and others involved in the production of food from animal origin, to work for the establishment of a centrally operated and integrated Meat Hygiene Service under veterinary supervision and to increase the overall standard of meat hygiene in the UK. In 1977 the Group merged with the Veterinary Public Health Association.

Records: Mr Jason Aldiss, Eville & Jones, Century House, 1275 Century Way, Thorpe Park, Leeds LS15 8ZB

Minutes of executive and general meetings with related papers 1974–76; attendance book 1975–77; correspondence and papers, incl some re amalgamation with the Veterinary Public Health Association 1974–79.

VETERINARY MEDICAL ASSOCIATION

London

History: The Veterinary Medical Association was established in 1836 as a discussion group for veterinary surgeons and students of the Royal Veterinary College, London. It had no connection to the London Veterinary Medical Society which was dissolved that same year. Nor was the Veterinary Medical Association formally connected to the Royal Veterinary College, London, although most of its meetings were held on college premises and its membership was derived largely from former or current staff and students.

Records: The Library, Royal Veterinary College, Royal College Street, London NW1 0TU

Council minute book 1866–84; general meetings minute book c1866–84; rules 1836, 1844; membership list c1836–64; correspondence and papers re formation 1836–41; donations book 19th cent; essays 1836–41, c1866–88.

VETERINARY PUBLIC HEALTH ASSOCIATION

History: At the British Veterinary Association Annual Congress in Glasgow on 19 August 1960, a meeting to discuss veterinary food hygiene was announced. The meeting, chaired by Professor A Robertson and attended by twelve people, led to the establishment of the Association of Veterinary Food Hygienists. Horace Thornton of Newcastle upon Tyne was elected the Association's first chairman while G S Ferguson of Edinburgh was appointed its secretary. The Association intended from the outset to be a technical body, facilitating and encouraging the exchange of information and ideas between all members of the veterinary profession engaged in food hygiene, with particular reference to meat and milk hygiene and technology. It also hoped to improve the level of training for those working in public health. In September 1963 the Association changed its name to the Veterinary Public Health Association (VPHA), incorporating the Veterinary Public Health Division of the British Veterinary Association. In 1977 the VPHA, which had been suffering considerable financial difficulties, merged with the Veterinary Meat Hygiene Group. The VPHA remains a division of the British Veterinary Association and has a wide remit including meat hygiene, quarantine, slaughterhouses and epidemiology. Meetings of Council are held four times a year while scientific meetings (formerly referred to as general meetings) are held twice a year.

Records: Mr Jason Aldiss, Eville & Jones, Century House, 1275 Century Way, Thorpe Park, Leeds LS15 8ZB

Council, minutes, agenda and related papers 1962–; general meetings, minutes, agenda and related papers 1960–83; scientific meetings, reports 1984, 1987–89; papers re attendance at Council and general meetings 1974–77; attendance book, 1977–94; papers re questionnaire on poor attendance at meetings, nd; correspondence and papers re membership 1970–74, 1982–83, 1990–97; papers re proposed visits to Heinz and Walls 1971; Royal Society of Health Congress, VPHA sessions/symposia, papers re: Anthrax 1964, Fish 1970, Disposal of Animal Residues 1971, Pets, Friend or Foe? 1972, Are Hormones a Hazard? 1973, Ante-Mortem Stress and Animal Welfare 1974; correspondence and papers re VPHA sessions at British Veterinary Association Congress 1968, 1970–71; British Veterinary Association, committee minutes and related papers 1971–77, 1989, 1993–94; secretary's papers and correspondence re: role of the veterinary officer in local government 1965, meat regulations 1965–67, meat inspection and slaughterhouses 1966–92, salaries and fees for meat inspectors and local government veterinary officers 1969–71, Swann Committee 1970–71, Association of Public Health Inspectors working party on food hygiene 1971, Harry Steele-Bodger scholarship 1972–73, local government reorganisation 1972–74, World Veterinary Association 1972–75, drug residues in food analysis 1973–77; European Union of Veterinary Food Hygienists, reports, proposed constitution, reports on attendance, etc 1973–80, 1984; Ammerdown Group, report on the transport and slaughter of livestock 1980–81; correspondence with Ministry of Agriculture, Fisheries and Food re: welfare of farmed deer 1987, *World Health Organisation Guide to the Diagnosis, Treatment and Prevention of Anthrax* 1987, Transport Group 1990, animal by-products regulation

1993, bovine spongiform encephalopathy 1990–96, toxoplasmosis 1991, ante-mortem inspection 1990–92, tuberculosis and badgers 1993–98, control of importation of animals 1992–94, Royal Institute of Public Health and Hygiene 1990–91, Society of Food Hygiene Technology 1991, animal welfare 1984–97, Humane Slaughter Association 1991–93, students and training 1991–97, Official Veterinary Surgeons Group 1987–91, identification of sheep and goats 1996–97, Health and Safety Executive 1990, Meat and Livestock Commission 1990–97; correspondence with: Parliamentary Food and Health Forum 1990–95, Food Standards Agency 1998, British Veterinary Association 1990–97, Royal College of Veterinary Surgeons 1990–97; consultative documents 1990–97; papers re Association of Veterinary Food Hygienists incl report of round table conference on meat hygiene and inspection 1970s; revised constitution 1994; papers re revision of constitution 1992–93; association rules 1978, 1985; blueprints of association's objectives, nd; cash book 1975–93; press cuttings 1994; newsletter 1993; American Veterinary Medical Association report on veterinary services in disasters and emergencies 1987; misc leaflets, offprints, etc c1970s–80s; misc papers re Pig Veterinary Society 1978; misc papers re Central Veterinary Society, incl rules, minutes, etc 1972–77.

VETERINARY RESEARCH CLUB
London

History: On 29 January 1924 a meeting was held in Piccadilly, London, to discuss the formation of a Veterinary Research Club 'consisting of Members of the Veterinary Profession who are engaged wholly in research in connection with animal diseases'. Attending the meeting were its convener Major George W Dunkin, Professor J B Buxton, Captain T J Bosworth, Thomas Dalling, H Roscoe Allen, R Glover and R L Cownell. It was agreed that a Council should be formed, composed of the men named above, and that monthly meetings should allow papers on various aspects of animal disease research to be presented. Like the Medical Research Club, all papers were to be unpublished at the time of presentation. Dunkin was elected the first president, while Roscoe Allen was appointed honorary secretary. Membership at first was restricted to veterinary surgeons actively involved in research, the first non-veterinary members not being admitted until 1931. The 1932 rules stated that there were to be no more than forty ordinary members and a maximum of ten associate members (non-veterinary surgeons engaged in research), although the number of ordinary members was increased to sixty in 1945. In 1968 all restrictions were ended and membership was opened up to veterinary and non-veterinary alike, up to a total of 150. Subscriptions were set at 5/- for ordinary members and 2/6d for associate members until 1948 when all members were charged 10/-. Meetings were held on the second Friday of alternate months, although this pattern was somewhat disrupted during the Second World War. The Club in the beginning was non-political in nature, although it was listed as a non-territorial division of the National Veterinary Medical Association in 1927. But by the late 1930s it was becoming more difficult to avoid involvement in the politics of veterinary research, particularly with the publication of the first Loveday Report in 1938. In 1945, therefore, a proposal was put forward for the establishment of an Association of Veterinary Teachers and Research Workers, sponsored by the Veterinary Research Club and open to all veterinary laboratory workers and teachers. The Association's first meeting was held in 1946 and by 1948 it too had affiliated to the National Veterinary Medical Association, a move which allowed the Veterinary Research Club to withdraw once again from any political involvement.

I H Pattison, 'A History of the Veterinary Research Club 1924–1974', *The Veterinary Record*, vol 94, no 6, 9 Feb 1974.

Records: Archives and Manuscripts, Wellcome Library for the History and Understanding of Medicine, 183 Euston Road, London NW1 2BE

Minutes of meeting called by Major George W Dunkin to discuss the formation of a Veterinary Research Club 1924; minutes of general and council meetings 1924–74. [Ref: GC/50]

WEST OF SCOTLAND VETERINARY MEDICAL ASSOCIATION
Glasgow

History: The West of Scotland Veterinary Medical Association was established in Glasgow during the nineteenth century and gave local veterinary surgeons the opportunity to meet on a regular basis and discuss both local and national issues affecting their profession.

Records: James Herriot Library, University of Glasgow, Faculty of Veterinary Medicine, Bearsden Road, Glasgow G61 1QH

Minute books 1912–29, 1932–46; list of minimum fees and related correspondence 1919–20; notes of meetings 1919–20.

WORSHIPFUL COMPANY OF FARRIERS
London

History: The origins of the Worshipful Company of Farriers can be traced back to 1356. In that year, the Mayor of the City of London, voicing a general concern at the harm being done to horses by unskilled persons, called upon all farriers within a seven mile radius of the City of London to form a Fellowship to govern their trade. Although little is known of the Company's history over the next three centuries, virtually all the early records having been destroyed in the Great Fire of 1666, it undoubtedly continued to develop. In 1674 the Company received its charter from Charles II and in 1692 was raised to the status of Livery Company of the City of London. The Company was run along similar lines to other livery companies with a Court, made up of a Master, three Wardens and between ten and twenty Assistants, which met quarterly. Court meetings were held at the hall of the Inn-Holders in College Street, although it is thought that the Company may have had its own hall, Trinity Hall, off Aldersgate Street, at one time. The Master and Wardens were elected annually by the Court while records were passed from Clerk to Clerk. Wishing to establish complete control over London's farriers and to stamp out quackery, the Company decreed that every farrier and shoesmith within the seven mile boundary was expected to serve a seven year apprenticeship, then register with the Company. This proved virtually impossible to enforce, although from the 1750s the Court became more active – initiating numerous prosecutions and extending its control over the large numbers of continental farriers coming to London at that time. Links were also made with related organisations. In 1848, the Company met a delegation from the Royal College of Veterinary Surgeons to establish what steps could be taken for their mutual advantage, and in 1876 offered prizes for essays on the treatment of horses to students at the Royal Veterinary College, London, and to those studying for their Membership of the Royal College of Veterinary Surgeons qualification. As the nineteenth century came to a close, however, the numbers of apprentices began to fall and concerns were raised that horses were being damaged by inadequately trained men. In 1890, therefore, the Company launched its Scheme for the Examination and Registration of Shoeing Smiths, supported by both the Royal Agricultural Society of England and the Royal College of Veterinary Surgeons. Although some 10,000 farriers were examined and registered over the next eighty five years, the fact that the scheme was voluntary meant that the Company's powers to fight low standards remained limited. Compulsory registration was not introduced until the Farriers (Registration) Act (amended in 1977) was passed in 1975. This led to the establishment of the Farriers Registration Council, which maintained a register of all those entitled to practise as farriers and had the power to act against the unqualified or incompetent. Entrants to the trade were compelled to complete an apprenticeship and to pass either the Company's Diploma Examination or the Army Farriery Trade Test Class II. The Company also started its own apprenticeship scheme in the 1950s and trained some 300 farriers before it was superceded in the 1980s by the Farriery Apprenticeship Scheme funded by the Services Commission. The Company continues to support education by providing prizes and grants and funding a Youth Exchange Scheme. Relations with the veterinary profession have always been friendly and representatives from the Royal College of Veterinary Surgeons sit on the Farriers Registration Council.

L C F Robson, *The Farriers of London. being an account of the Worshipful Company of Farriers as described in the records of the Company* (Leeds, 1949); L B Prince, *The Farrier and his Craft. the history of the Worshipful Company of Farriers* (London, 1980); A G W Scott, *The Company, The Craft and The City* (London, 1990).

Records: Manuscripts Department, Guildhall Library, Aldermanbury, London EC2P 2EJ

Copy of the charter granted to the company by Charles II 1674; copies of the ordinances 1356, 1675; copies of documents re re-establishment of the livery 1692–1724 and various legal points arising from the charter and ordinances 1758–1867; oath of a Freeman, nd; copies made c1600 of two orders of the court of aldermen re the company 1356, 1599; copy of act of common council re employment of foreigners 1557; copy of the will of John Sowle 1572; general memoranda c1400–1619; court minute books 1718–1962; book of fines for non-attendance of the Master, Wardens and Assistants at court meetings 1825–76; Masters', Wardens' and Assistants' declaration books 1884–1974; register of Assistants, recording dates of offices of Master and Warden served, trades and places of abode 1749–1868; register of members of the livery who served the office of steward, recording trades and places of abode 1739–1864; liverymens' declaration book 1933–58; registers of Freemen, giving dates of admission to freedom, places of abode, trades and offices served 1709–1869; register of Assistants 1733–68; registers of livery 1733–76; registers of freedom admissions (stamp duty books) 1755–1949; Freemens' declaration book 1921–51; registers of apprentice bindings 1619–1811; register of apprentice bindings with account of orphan's duty 1694–1862; quarterage books 1794–1802; audited Masters' account books 1725–1973, incl inventories of stock, ground rents, books and moveable goods 1876–1932 and annual accounts and balance sheets 1940–47; ledgers 1932–72; petty cash book 1942–48; account book containing alphabetical lists of members making payments for quarterage, functions, fines and court luncheons 1951–58; Clerk's out-letter book 1846–77; papers re company's return to the Municipal Corporation commissioners 1833–37; papers re Bill for the Better Regulation of the Corporation of the City of London 1858; copy list of books and other items delivered by Moulden to the company, endorsed with rough notes re date of company's foundation as given in the case submitted to T Chambers 1850; Christ's Hospital, Robert Mellish's gift: deeds, leases and associated papers re 10 messuages with appurtenances in the parish of St Botolph without Aldersgate 1551–1823. [Ref: Ms. 5534, 2890, 5523, 5532, 8035, 5529, 5530, 21106, 5528, 5525, 5524, 21105, 5526, 5527, 5531, 5522, 21380, 21381, 21382, 5533, 21383, 21384, 21385, 13473]

YORKSHIRE VETERINARY SOCIETY

Yorkshire

History: In September 1863 Edward Coleman Dray, a veterinary surgeon based in Leeds, held a meeting at his home to discuss the setting up of a local veterinary society. After a further meeting the following month, open to all practitioners within a fifty mile radius of Leeds, the Yorkshire Veterinary Medical Society was formed. Dray was elected president and William Williams, later Principal of the Edinburgh Veterinary College, was appointed secretary. At first, the quarterly meetings were held in Leeds, which boasted good rail connections and large hotels, but from 1888 it was decided to hold meetings at various locations across the county, although the annual general meeting continued to be held in Leeds. Meetings gave practitioners the opportunity to discuss issues of both local and national interest, while distinguished veterinary surgeons were invited to give papers on relevant subjects, such as cattle plague, milk fever, education and relations with the Royal Society for the Prevention of Cruelty to Animals. In 1919, the Society was affiliated to the newly established National Veterinary Medical Association. The word 'Medical' was dropped from the Society's title in 1952. The East Yorkshire Clinical Club, set up in 1970 under the auspices of the Society, was well supported at first, but its numbers gradually fell away and the Club was dissolved some years later. The Yorkshire Veterinary Society continued to flourish, however, its initial membership of fifteen increasing to 212 by 1980.

A Wilson, *A History of the Yorkshire Veterinary Society 1863–1980* (private publication, 1980).

Records: West Yorkshire Archive Service, Chapeltown Road, Sheepscar, Leeds LS7 3AP

Minute books 1863–1979; council minutes 1903–08, 1915–68; attendance books 1888–1952, 1970–77; rule books 1863–1966; list of officers 1948–57; honorary associate certificates, nd; report of joint meeting with Yorkshire branch of Society of Medical Officers of Health 1932; papers re co-operation with Royal Society for the Prevention of Cruelty to Animals 1929–32; guides to fees 1956–66; general correspondence 1863–65, 1901–10, 1954–57; annual dinner cards 1896–1914 [w]; funeral cards 1934–37; rules for: Lancashire Veterinary Association 1863, North of England Veterinary Medical Association c1870, West of Scotland Veterinary Medical Association c1870; National Veterinary Association, proceedings of 10th general meeting 1892; letters, memorandum and articles of association re formation of National Veterinary Medical Association 1907–32; George Banham's leaflet re scheme for National Veterinary Medical Association 1881. [Ref: Acc 2385]

List of records of national government

BOARD OF AGRICULTURE

London

History: The Board of Agriculture was established by royal charter in 1793. Funded by the Exchequer, it aimed to improve the farmer's knowledge of livestock health by gathering and publishing information on a number of diseases including swine fever. The Board ceased to exist after 1822.

Records: Museum of English Rural Life, University of Reading, Whiteknights, Reading RG6 2AG

Copy of charter 1793; minute books: rough copy 1797–1822, fair copy 1798–1819, North of Trent 1798–nd, various committees 1794–99; register of members 1793–1819; register of letters received 1793–1822; letter books 1793–95, 1810–22; treasurer: ledger 1794–1820, cash account, Smith, Payne & Smith 1793–1820; Agricultural Society, treasurer's cash book 1793–1820; misc agricultural surveys, reports, etc 19th cent.

BOARD OF TRADE

London

History: The original Board of Trade, largely concerned with plantations, was dissolved in 1782, but the continuing need to regulate Britain's trade with her colonies as well as with North America and France led in 1784 to the establishment of a new Board of Trade within the Privy Council. The Board's responsibilities altered considerably during the course of the nineteenth and twentieth centuries as it became increasingly involved in matters of commerce, industry and overseas trade. In 1844 it assumed responsibility for the newly established Railway Board and from 1867 was involved in the awarding of charters. Under the terms of the Bankruptcy Act of 1883 and the Companies (Winding Up) Act of 1890 the Board of Trade was also given responsibility for the administration of insolvencies in England and Wales. From 1916 it administered the registration of business names, and in 1925 assumed responsibility for both the registration and custody of deeds of arrangement, as well as for the accounts of trustees appointed by the deeds and the supervision of official receivers. Other responsibilities granted to the Board included the awarding of patents, trade marks and copyright, the administration of weights, measures and merchandise marks and control over monopolies, mergers and restrictive practices. In 1970 the Board of Trade merged with the Ministry of Technology to create the Department of Trade and Industry.

Records: National Archives, Ruskin Avenue, Kew, Richmond TW9 4DU

Papers and correspondence re Royal Veterinary College of Scotland charter 1868; files re dissolved companies: Albert Veterinary College Ltd 1865, Herron's Veterinary Shoeing Forges Ltd 1895, Phoenix Veterinary Company Ltd 1897, Veterinary Radiant Heat Syndicate Ltd 1901, Veterinary Medicine Company Ltd 1905, British Veterinary & Legal Aid Association Ltd 1905, Phoenix Veterinary Supplies Ltd 1908, Churchill's Veterinary Sanitorium Ltd 1909, Scientific Veterinary Supply Association Ltd 1910, Vetrex Veterinary Food Ltd 1911, National Veterinary Medical Association of Great Britain and Ireland Ltd 1921, Veterinary Medicines Company Ltd 1922, Pugh's Veterinary Medicines Ltd 1945; National Veterinary Medicine Association of Great Britain and Ireland Ltd, application for exemption under Section 2(2) Companies Act 1921; registration of MRCVS under Business Names Act (1916) 1922; report on supply of veterinary services in relation to restrictions on advertising 1976; files re bankruptcies: C E L Harwood, veterinary surgeon 1931–32, P J Cauntley, veterinary surgeon 1961–70; files re Restrictive Trade Practices Act 1968 section 4, Pesticides Safety Precautions Scheme and Veterinary Products Safety Precautions Scheme 1969. [Ref: BT22/2/3; BT31; BT58/70/COS/2994; BT58/70/COS/2994; BT169/98; BT226/4646; BT357/32]

BRITISH RAILWAYS HORSE SECTION: CAMDEN (SOUTHERN AREA) VETERINARY DEPARTMENT

London

History: Although horses were used to pull the first trains in the late eighteenth and early nineteenth centuries, by the 1830s and 1840s steam-powered locomotive engines had taken their place. However, the arrival of steam power actually increased the number of horses employed by the railway companies as goods and people had to be transported to and from stations and equipment shunted within the yards. Among the numerous railway companies that emerged during this time were the Midland Railway (est 1844), the London & North Western Railway (est 1846) and the Lancashire & Yorkshire Railway (est 1847). In 1923 some 123 separate railway companies were amalgamated into just four company groups – the London Midland & Scottish Railway (which included the Midland Railway, the London & North Western Railway and the Lancashire & Yorkshire Railway) the London & North Eastern Railway, the Great Western Railway and the Southern Railway. Following nationalisation in 1948, responsibility for these four groups and all minor railways passed to the Railway Executive, which operated under the British Transport Commission, and the railways were divided into six regions for operational purposes. The following year, the horse stud was substantially reorganised. A chief veterinary surgeon and horse superintendent were appointed, with overall responsibility for some 8700 horses, and additional officers employed in London, Birmingham, Manchester and Glasgow. The purchase and sale of horses was centralised, as was the veterinary hospital and the shoeing and harness facilities. By 1964, when the last horses were withdrawn from the railways, the depot at Camden, London, had assumed responsibility for horses in all regions as far north as Manchester.

Records: National Archives, Ruskin Avenue, Kew, Richmond TW9 4DU

Books of instructions, Birmingham depot, former Midland Railway 1885–1918; disposal books for horse depot, Curzon Street, Birmingham, London & North Western Railway, later London Midland & Scottish Railway 1919–59; shoeing and veterinary accounts, Birmingham area 1949–64; register of horses in central area, Birmingham book 1948–53; register of disposal of horses, Birmingham book 1954–59; register of new horses received at Liverpool depot, London & North Western Railway 1880–1924; stock price book, harness and other horse depot materials from London & North Western Railway depot, Park Lane Station, Liverpool c1888; register of horses purchased, Manchester depot, Lancashire & Yorkshire Railway 1918–20; register of sick horses, Derby depot, London Midland & Scottish Railway 1938–50; register of sawdust and straw supplied to horses at Camden depot 1948–64; accounts book, Camden depot and Southern Area 1949–64; accounts record book, all regions 1951–64; register of horses, Camden depot 1951–64; daily working book, Camden depot 1955–64; horse stock record book, all regions 1949–63; British Transport Commission area book, all regions 1953–59; registers of horse sales, all regions 1949–64; register of four weekly returns of horses sold, all regions 1949–62. [Ref: AN35]

BURMA OFFICE

London

History: The Burma Office was established in 1937 after the separation of Burma from India. It was abolished in 1948 when Burma was granted full independence.

Records: Oriental and India Office Collections, British Library, 96 Euston Road, London NW1 2DB

Papers re replacement of Indian Agricultural Service and Indian Veterinary Service in Burma 1938–39 [Ref: M/3/442]; grant of additional pay to A J Kelly during privilege leave on vacating post of Deputy Assistant Director of Veterinary Services, Burma 1938–39 [Ref: M/3/597]; papers re extension of tenure of appointment of Director, Army Veterinary Services, Army in Burma 1939 [Ref: M/3/708]; papers re reconstruction of the veterinary department 1943 [Ref: M/3/1530]; veterinary estimates 1943–45 [Ref: M/ 3/1419]; economic department: papers re establishment of veterinary consultative body for Far East 1945–47 [Ref: M/4/364], veterinary equipment for south east Asia 1946 [Ref: M/4/617]; papers re veterinary services 1946–47 [Ref: M/4/2846]; papers re recruitment of agricultural and veterinary engineers 1946, 1948. [Ref: M/4/1420, 2260]

COLONIAL OFFICE

London

History: The Colonial Office was established in 1854 with its own Secretary of State and a number of geographically defined departments. In 1907 the Office was divided into two Divisions – the Crown Colonies Division, concerned with British dependencies, and the Dominions Division which took responsibility for dominion affairs and imperial conferences. The latter went on to become the Dominions Office in 1925, although until the late 1930s the post of Secretary of State for each of the two departments was usually held by the same person. While the Colonial Office grew steadily during the 1930s the granting of independence to numerous colonies in the period following the Second World War led to a corresponding decline in power as responsibility for relations with former colonies passed to the Commonwealth Relations Office. Additionally, responsibility for overseas aid and development passed to the Department of Technical Co-operation in 1961 while in 1962 responsibility for relations with Northern Rhodesia and Nyasaland passed to the Central

African Office. In 1966 the Colonial Office and the Commonwealth Relations Office were merged to form the Commonwealth Office.

Records: National Archives, Ruskin Terrace, Kew, Richmond TW9 4DU

Bahamas Humane Society, vacancy for veterinary surgeon 1938; appointment of veterinary surgeon in Barbados 1927–28; P T Saunders, Director, Indian Veterinary Service, pension rights 1935; proposed Ceylon Institute of Veterinary Research 1947; Cyprus, papers re creation of office of director of veterinary and stock services, organisation of service, etc 1927–40; Falkland Islands, closure of experimental farm and stock department, appointment of veterinary officer, etc 1928–33; eligibility of Australia and New Zealand graduates for appointment in Colonial Veterinary Service 1927–28; Fiji, vacancies for veterinary officers 1938–40; Gambia: veterinary report 1939, difficulties over export of eggs and poultry because of veterinary regulations 1950–51; Gibraltar, appointment of veterinary officer 1937; Gold Coast: private practice for veterinary officers 1928–31, veterinary department staff 1934, 1937; form and submission of annual departmental reports 1935–37; annual departmental reports 1941; colonial veterinary scholarship scheme 1935–42; Royal (Dick) Veterinary College, Edinburgh, Diploma in Veterinary Tropical Medicine 1935–39; recognition of veterinary qualifications obtained in the dominions 1935–36; International Veterinary Bureau 1936, 1938; future position of Royal Veterinary College, London 1936; practice of veterinary surgery by foreigners incl Jewish referees in the dominions 1937–41; reciprocity with South Africa on qualifications of veterinary surgeons 1937; Royal Veterinary College, London, Diploma in Tropical Veterinary Medicine 1938–40; International Veterinary Congress 1938; allocation of work on animal husbandry in Malaya between agricultural and veterinary departments 1938; Imperial Veterinary Conference, minutes 1938; grant from colonial development fund re Diploma in Tropical Veterinary Medicine 1939–40; Tanganyika: files re veterinary department staff 1927, 1932–36, claim for allowances by Oscar Hopgood 1927, veterinary stock farm, Njombe 1933–34, annual report 1927, 1934; Federated Malay States: petitions re veterinary services 1927–28, papers re appointments to veterinary service 1929–30, 1933–34, veterinary services 1930–31, recognition of Indian veterinary colleges diplomas 1931, 1936–37, annual reports 1934–35, appointment of Malays to higher posts 1936, proposed scheme for veterinary laboratory 1950–51; veterinary convention between Iraq and Turkey 1929; Palestine: appointment of Captain Idenden to post of Veterinary Officer, Frontier Force 1926, dismissal of a veterinary officer for neglect of duty 1928, legislation re veterinary surgeons 1928–29, vacancy for a senior veterinary officer 1937, department of veterinary services 1946; Empire Marketing Board: grant to D A Gill for study in UK 1927–30, grant to Colonial Office and Veterinary Research Laboratory for immunisation of cattle against gall sickness before export 1932–33; Northern Rhodesia, revision of veterinary department salaries 1929; Kenya: veterinary services for nature reserves 1930–31, veterinary surgeons ordinance 1930, Mazabuka agricultural and veterinary research station 1933, 1938–40, veterinary department annual reports 1938–43, 1949, report of Financial and Economic Commission 1938, application for grant 1945–48, Central African Council agricultural veterinary and forestry committee 1947–48, colonial development and welfare schemes for veterinary services and research 1947–51, Rockefeller Foundation declines financial aid for veterinary research 1931–32, proposed retention of O Dixon as veterinary officer 1933, proposed separation of agricultural and veterinary departments 1937, veterinary department staff 1929, 1937–43, delegation of power to Director of Veterinary Services to waive or reduce charges in respect of laboratory products 1940; West Africa: exchanges between French and British West African colonies re publications 1930–31, representations of the National Veterinary Medical Association 1936, staff position within agricultural and veterinary departments 1943, liaison with the French authorities 1949–51, vacancies in veterinary division of Nigeria 1958–59; Nigeria: employment of staff 1927–31, veterinary department report 1926–29, files re veterinary department 1944–47; Zanzibar, report on visit to examine cattle industry 1942; East Africa: central veterinary research 1927–29, co-ordination of veterinary research 1934–48, 1954, Makerere College veterinary department 1944–49, establishment of a post-graduate school at Kabete for the Colonial Veterinary Service 1947–49, comment on the veterinary department annual report for Kenya 1950, report of delegation to East Africa enquiring into training of Africans for Veterinary Service 1960–62, visit of veterinary expert to East Africa 1951; files re personnel and scholarships 1932–33, 1937–42; file re unification of Colonial Veterinary Service 1934–35; conditions of service in Colonial Veterinary Service 1937–38; estimates for veterinary supplies for Far East 1944–45; file re West Indian Veterinary Conference 1948; qualifications for practising in Colonial Territories 1950–52; papers re training for locally born officers 1946–51; papers re veterinary education 1960–61; file re Transvaal Veterinary School 1921; file re scholarships 1934–52; research department: insecticide research on veterinary problems in East Africa 1948, establishment of East African Veterinary Research Organisation 1946–49, transfer of production of sera and vaccines from Kabete to Kenya Veterinary Department 1949, committee of enquiry to investigate failure of certain vaccines produced by East African Veterinary Research

Organisation 1949, East African Veterinary Research Organisation annual report 1948, research schemes involving grants 1948, East African Veterinary Research Organisation erection and equipping of an Animal Diseases Section and Biological Production Section at Muguga, North Kenya 1949–52, request for grant for Naivasha Veterinary Research Station 1949–50, proposed West African Veterinary Research Organisations 1950–52, East African Veterinary Research Organisation financial provisions 1954–57, West African Institute for Trypanosomiasis Research co-operation with the Veterinary Department Northern Nigeria 1956, misc papers re East African Veterinary Research Organisation 1960–61; West Indian Royal Commission, official memoranda re veterinary, forestry and fishery questionnaire 1938–39; Central Africa, file re agricultural and veterinary research 1950–51; commission to enquire into service, salary scales, etc of colonial government staff, submissions and memoranda from veterinary department 1945–48; Central Africa and Aden, general staff position in Nyasaland Veterinary Department 1951; general policy re veterinary training courses and recruitment 1952–53, 1960–61; scheme for expansion of North Borneo Veterinary Department 1954–55; West Indies: report of veterinary committee of advisory council 1952–53, veterinary committee of British Caribbean Advisory Council 1954–56; file re East African Conference on Veterinary Education 1961; representations against provisions of Ramage report 1962–63. [Ref: CO23/622, 28/307/5, 28/314/16, 54/1003/7, 67/223/7, 67/232/5, 67/234/6, 67/255/10, 67/290/11, 78/178/5, 78/180/15, 78/191/11, 78/194/2, 83/179/12, 83/186/4, 83/225/9, 87/249/13, 87/269/6–7, 91/504/7, 96/682/19, 96/716/2, 96/734/10, 323, 533, 554, 583, 618, 691, 717, 730, 733, 758, 795, 822, 850, 852, 859, 865, 877, 885/50, 892/1/3, 927, 950, 952/9/3, 963/36, 963/88, 963/134, 963/166, 1015/21, 1017/2, 1017/637, 1017/671, 1030/186, 1031/792, 1031/1884, 1045/811, 1048/6]

DEPARTMENT FOR THE ENVIRONMENT, FOOD AND RURAL AFFAIRS

London

History: Following the demise of the first Board of Agriculture in 1822, the monitoring of livestock in Britain became somewhat lax despite the increased risks posed by the introduction of free trade in 1846. Regulation was largely restricted to local by-laws which, where they existed, were concerned with the seizure and destruction of unsound meat and did not apply to live animals, Smithfield Market being the notable exception. The authorities, therefore, were ill-prepared to cope effectively with the outbreak of cattle plague that swept the country in 1865. In an effort to control the disease, a temporary Veterinary Department was set up within the Privy Council in October 1865 to co-ordinate the work of inspectors and carry out a programme of eradication. The following April, responsibility passed to the newly created Cattle Plague Department, again within the Privy Council, and again intended to be only a temporary body. Its work was aided by the passing of the Cattle Plague Prevention Act of 1866, which allowed local authorities to appoint inspectors with the power to enter any premises thought to be infected with plague and to arrange for the slaughter and disposal of infected animals. This was followed by a series of Contagious Diseases (Animals) Acts and Orders that widened the Department's scope considerably. The 1869 Contagious Diseases (Animals) Act, for example, included measures aimed at dealing not only with cattle plague, but with a host of other diseases including pleuro-pneumonia, sheep pox, foot-and-mouth disease, sheep scab and glanders, while the Transit Orders of 1870 and 1871 limited the number of ports through which animals could pass and ensured a higher standard of travelling and quarantine facilities. From a hastily assembled temporary body, therefore, the Department rapidly developed into a permanent fixture, which by 1871 was employing two senior veterinary officers and eighteen full time veterinary port inspectors. Local authorities employed another 1450 inspectors, of which 372 were veterinary surgeons. From 1874, the Department also employed travelling inspectors and produced an annual *Return of Proceedings* containing details of disease outbreaks, imports and exports and compensation costs. Weekly returns of disease outbreaks were published in the *London Gazette* from 1875. By the early 1880s, however, there was a feeling that more could and should be done. With the country in the grip of depression, and the population still increasing, the pressure to produce food was never greater, whilst the development of refrigeration was making the importation of meat from across the world a reality. In 1883, therefore, the Veterinary Department was renamed the Agricultural Department of the Privy Council and took over responsibility for the publishing of agricultural returns from the Board of Trade, although the Inland Revenue Department continued to collect the returns. The first detailed statistics were published in 1884. In 1888 a departmental committee looking at pleuro-pneumonia and tuberculosis in livestock recommended that the administration of the Contagious Diseases (Animals) Acts be concentrated in a single department. This led to the Board of Agriculture Act of 1889 and the establishment of the Board of Agriculture (Board of Agriculture and Fisheries from 1903), which incorporated the Agricultural Department of the Privy Council as a Veterinary Department. In 1894 a separate Animals Division was established, and two years later the veterinary staff was constituted separately as a Veterinary Department. These measures, together with the Contagious Diseases (Animals) Act of 1894, gave the Board of Agriculture wide-ranging powers with regard to the handling of animal diseases, the benefits of which were quickly felt. An outbreak of foot-and-mouth disease in 1892 was quickly stamped out, and Britain was declared free of pleuro-pneumonia in 1898. Although a separate Board of Agriculture was set up in Scotland in 1911 and a similar Department established in Northern Ireland in 1921, the control of contagious diseases throughout the UK continued to be the responsibility of the Board of Agriculture in London. Following the appointment of Stewart Stockman as Chief Veterinary Officer in 1905, the Department greatly increased its veterinary laboratory services and research work. A key development was the opening of the Central Veterinary Laboratory (CVL) at Weybridge, Surrey, in 1917. During the 1920s, the CVL was chiefly concerned with the diagnosis of scheduled diseases, research on foot-and-mouth disease and poultry work. After the Second World War, however, it expanded from five departments to thirteen, including a centre at Lasswade near Edinburgh and a Cattle Breeding Centre in Reading. Additionally, an experimental station, later known as the Animal Virus Research Institute, was established at Pirbright, Surrey, in 1925. In 1919, the Board of Agriculture was reconstituted as the Ministry of Agriculture and Fisheries while the Veterinary Department was renamed the Diseases of Animals Branch. In 1935 the Ministry was given responsibility for administering the newly introduced Tuberculosis (Attested Herds) Scheme, involving the routine inspection of herds and dairies by veterinary inspectors. Following the Agriculture Act of 1937, the Diseases of Animals Branch at the Ministry was replaced by an Animal Health Division which brought together the various veterinary services into a nationally co-ordinated service of veterinary inspectors. Under the new system, the country was divided into 22 areas, each under the charge of a superintending inspector, and 78 divisions (mainly along county lines) under the charge of a divisional inspector. Further reorganisation came in 1946 with the transfer of the Veterinary Investigation Service, whose thirteen officers, mainly based at agricultural colleges, carried out diagnostic work on cattle, sheep and pig diseases as well as research work on poultry diseases, to the Ministry. In 1950 the Contagious Diseases (Animals) Act of 1894 and its amendments of 1896, 1903, 1910, 1927 and 1935 were replaced by a new Diseases of Animals Act. By 1955, therefore, when the Ministry of Agriculture and Fisheries became the Ministry of Agriculture, Fisheries and Food, the Animal Health Division was made up of two organisations: the Inspectorate, responsible for the prevention, control and eradication of animal diseases, and the Veterinary Investigation Service, which provided a routine diagnostic service for veterinary surgeons and employed 1500 full time staff and a further 1700 on an *ad hoc* basis. In 1958 the Animal Health Division was reorganised, partly due to the rapid expansion of its work, while in 1963 the Inspectorate was re-designated Veterinary Field Services. Under the new system, the senior Deputy Chief Veterinary Officer was appointed Director of Veterinary Field Services under the Chief Veterinary Officer, with two Deputy Directors based in London and a third at the Scottish Office in Edinburgh. In 1971 the whole veterinary service was incorporated within the newly created Agricultural Development and Advisory Service, which also brought together the National Agricultural Advisory Service, the Agricultural Land Service, the State Veterinary Service and the Drainage and Water Supply Service. Subsequent developments have included the introduction of a computerised Veterinary Investigation Diagnosis Analysis as well as a Zoonoses Order Data System and the establishment in 1972 of an Epidemiology Unit. Further extensive reorganisation of the Animal Health Division was carried out during the 1980s and 1990s, reflecting growing concerns about food safety, scientific advances and the introduction of new legislation. By 1992 there were six Divisions within the Ministry of Agriculture, Fisheries and Food: a Meat Hygiene Division (formed 1982), an Animal Health (Disease Control) Division which dealt with all notifiable diseases except salmonella and bovine spongiform encephalopathy, an Animal Health (International Trade) Division concerned with the import and export of live animals and genetic material including that relating to artificial insemination and embryo transfer, an Animal Welfare Division with responsibility for animal health on farms, markets and in transit, an Animal Health (Zoonoses) Division for the control of salmonella in poultry and an Animal Health Resource Management Division giving administrative support to the other Divisions. In addition there was a new Animal Health and Welfare Veterinary Section with responsibility for animal health schemes, particularly bovine spongiform encephalopathy, tuberculosis and brucellosis, and the importation of domestic animals. Following a serious outbreak of foot-and-mouth disease in 2001, which resulted in the slaughter of over four million animals, the Ministry of Agriculture, Fisheries and Food was replaced by the Department for the Environment, Food and Rural Affairs.

Anon, *Sixty Years Veterinary Investigation Service 1922–1982* (London, 1982); J W R Pearce, L P Pugh, J Ritchie, (eds), *Animal Health: A Centenary 1865–1965* (London, 1965); S Foreman, *Loaves and Fishes: an illustrated history of the Ministry of Agriculture, Fisheries and Food*

1889–1989 (London, 1989); J Winnifrith, *Ministry of Agriculture, Fisheries and Food* (London, 1962).

Records (1): National Archives, Ruskin Avenue, Kew, Richmond TW9 4DU

Correspondence and papers re agricultural education and research, created largely by National Agricultural Advisory Service and predecessors 1888–1963; correspondence and papers re animal health, incl legislation and measures to control importation and movement of animals, containment and elimination of disease, creation of Central Veterinary Laboratory 1876–1972; working files of Central Veterinary Laboratory re investigations into animal diseases, reports and papers of the Agricultural Improvement Committee, Agricultural Research Council, Agricultural Research Institutes (Scotland), Animal Health Trust and Veterinary Investigation Centre, papers on international veterinary health 1924–67; correspondence and papers re State Veterinary Service Chemistry Department 20th cent; files re import and export of breeding livestock and semen, particularly controls to ensure health of livestock strains in UK, and compliance with other states' regulations concerning veterinary control of imported livestock 1945–71; publications: journals produced for and by staff of Animal Health Division, incl *The State Veterinary News* and *The State Veterinary Journal* 1945–84, *Medium*, the technical journal of the veterinary laboratories 1968–84; working instructions circulated to full time veterinary officers re diseases of animals, welfare of livestock, export and import of animals, etc 1934–89; files re statutory and voluntary methods of improving the safety of agricultural workers and others who might be endangered by dangerous farming practices, especially pesticides 1926–79; files from various Animal Health Divisions re general animal health and welfare issues, incl disease prevention and elimination, regulation of imports, certification of exports, cruelty, preparation and implementation of legislation, regulations and schemes, organisation of State Veterinary Service and research 1942–75; files re agricultural, food, and veterinary attachés based in British embassies, the permanent delegate to the United Nations Food and Agriculture Organisation in Rome, agricultural missions to other countries 1947–71; records re operations of Central Veterinary Laboratory incl individual research and project working papers and policy, production of vaccines, post-mortems and diagnoses, testing of therapeutic substances and research into causes and control of diseases of farm livestock 1948–81; files re administration of the Central Veterinary Laboratory and the Veterinary Investigation Service incl papers re committee and management meetings, conferences, staffing, procedures and annual reports of Veterinary Investigation Centres 1954–75; Animal Health Division responsibilities for control of veterinary medicines under the Medicines Act 1968 1968–87 [Ref: MAF33, 35, 188, 189, 192, 248, 249, 259, 284, 287, 290, 364, 386, 416]; amounts paid to inspecting veterinary surgeons 1869 [Ref: MAF7/3]; veterinary committee reports 1928–30 [Ref: MAF34/322]; Economic Advisory Council standing committee on scientific research, memorandum on regulations governing sale of proprietary insecticides, fungicides and veterinary preparations sent by the Ministry 1932–40 [Ref: MAF36/309]; veterinary laboratory, main files 1934–39 [Ref: MAF39/45,46]; Agriculture Act 1937, files re: superannuation position of transferred local authority veterinary officers 1936–45, establishment of State Veterinary Service 1937–42 [Ref: MAF39/47, 48]; Treasury approval of additional veterinary inspectors to be employed in connection with outbreaks of foot-and-mouth disease 1922–35 [Ref: MAF39/151]; Central Veterinary Laboratory, Weybridge, Surrey, papers re staffing 1940–48 [Ref: MAF39/420]; veterinary advisory aids committee, minutes of meetings 1949–52 [Ref: MAF45/47]; veterinary surgeons, requirements of agriculture and HM Forces 1943–45 [Ref: MAF47/128]; files re licensing of stallions, fees payable to veterinary surgeons 1911–37 [Ref: MAF52/57]; veterinary inspections, co-ordination of arrangements by importing countries 1949–50 [Ref: MAF83/2466]; inter-departmental committee on slaughterhouses, consultations with British Veterinary Association 1953–55 [Ref: MAF88/555]; agricultural and veterinary supplies for relief 1943–46 [Ref: MAF97/1266, 1267]; veterinary certificate for Faroes re whalemeat 1948–53 [Ref: MAF101/124]; reports of veterinary surgeons on hygiene in whaling industry 1949–54 [Ref: MAF101/214]; Eastern Region Veterinary Service, staff inspections 1962–72 [Ref: MAF105/530]; British Veterinary Association/National Agricultural Advisory Service liaison committee, papers re animal feedstuffs industry 1964–74 [Ref: MAF106/38, 69–71]; working party on regional laboratories and veterinary investigation centres and pilot exercise 1973–74 [Ref: MAF106/149, 150]; East Midlands Regional Office, veterinary development policy 1971–73 [Ref: MAF106/156]; Veterinary Investigation Centre, Longbenton, Tyne & Wear, file re accommodation 1974–79 [Ref: MAF107/240]; South East Veterinary Investigation Service, file re reorganisation and complement 1964–71 [Ref: MAF108/104]; Divisional Veterinary Officers: annual reports 1961–64 [Ref: MAF108/125], minutes 1966–75 [Ref: MAF108/126]; Veterinary Field Service, staff inspection 1965–66 [Ref: MAF109/247]; Veterinary Investigation Centre, Truro, Cornwall, staff inspection 1965–70 [Ref: MAF109/249]; papers re veterinary study groups 1965–72 [Ref: MAF109/286]; Agricultural Development and Advisory Service, veterinary service staff inspections 1973–76 [Ref: MAF109/333, 334]; review of veterinary service staffing complement 1970–71 [Ref: MAF109/357]; Regional Veterinary Study Group, minutes and papers 1965–72 [Ref: MAF110/423, 424]; Agricultural Development Advisory Service, staff inspections 1971–74 [Ref: MAF110/442, 448, 449]; Chester, staff inspections 1972–73 [Ref: MAF110/452]; file re Leeds and Liverpool Veterinary Investigation Centres 1964–68 [Ref: MAF111/95]; British Veterinary Association/Agricultural Development and Advisory Service committee on regional liaison, papers re animal feedstuffs industry 1961–77 [Ref: MAF111/110, 111]; papers re veterinary education in Wales 1946–50, 1959–63 [Ref: MAF112/790, 791]; Local Veterinary Inspectors, general correspondence 1962–73 [Ref: MAF112/1176]; Bangor Veterinary Investigation Centre, reports of inspection 1960–71 [Ref: MAF112/1177]; Cardiff Veterinary Investigation Centre, reports of inspection 1960–71 [Ref: MAF112/1178]; file re veterinary inspection of markets approved for sale of imported animals 1963–76 [Ref: MAF112/1187]; files re joint committee on use of antibiotics in animal husbandry and veterinary medicine 1961–69 [Ref: MAF113/565, 566]; joint meetings of veterinary officers and advisory nutrition chemists, minutes 1960–65 [Ref: MAF114/614]; papers re co-operation between National Agricultural Advisory Service and the veterinary service 1965–71 [Ref: MAF114/819]; proposal to establish research institute at West Grinstead as part of Royal Veterinary College, London, field station 1946–49 [Ref: MAF117/87]; instructions and procedure for guidance of veterinary surgeons 1948–50 [Ref: MAF121/1]; Stallion Licensing Panel, appointment of veterinary surgeons 1953–70 [Ref: MAF121/22]; licensing of bulls, referees and Local Veterinary Officers' fees and expenses 1934–61 [Ref: MAF121/25]; stallion licensing scheme, instructions and procedure for guidance of veterinary surgeons 1957–71 [Ref: MAF121/32]; British Veterinary Association, papers re supervision of artificial insemination centres 1942–60 [Ref: MAF124/33, 34]; Central Veterinary Laboratory files re: proposed purchase of land 1953–58 [Ref: MAF142/264, 285], effect of proposed M25 motorway 1949–65 [Ref: MAF144/107, 108], catalogue of brucella strains 1981 [Ref: MAF217/74], professional staff 1948–55 [Ref: MAF224/73, 74], director and deputy director posts 1948–63 [Ref: MAF224/140], review of organisation 1954–58 [Ref: MAF224/186], organisation and complement 1955–66 [Ref: MAF224/234–236], Whitley committee 1956–67 [Ref: MAF227/75], lease of Manor Farm 1960–61 [Ref: MAF255/1067], capital grants re poultry diseases research 1922–29, capital expenditure 1923–28 [Ref: MAF54/72, 74, 75]; papers re protection of animals in markets 1963–66 [Ref: MAF142/469]; Cod Liver Oil and Veterinary Oil (Control) Order 1943–47 [Ref: MAF154/352];

Divisional Veterinary Officer's annual reports 1963–76 [Ref: MAF175/15, 16]; veterinary officers stationed in South America, diplomatic status 1951–64 [Ref: MAF184/30]; Civil Service Pay Research Unit, survey of veterinary service 1959–61 [Ref: MAF184/139]; papers re age distribution, veterinary service 1960–70 [Ref: MAF184/160]: loan of veterinary staff at Agricultural Research Council for trials of foot-and-mouth vaccine 1961–63 [Ref: MAF184/195]; departmental committee of enquiry into recruitment of veterinary profession 1962–69 [Ref: MAF184/226]; proposed refresher courses for veterinary surgeons returning from HM Forces 1945–46 [Ref: MAF198/9]; Royal College of Veterinary Surgeons' veterinary courses 1948–52 [Ref: MAF198/12]; bibliographical references to brucella in veterinary scientific publications 1982 [Ref: MAF217/75]; veterinary books, a subject guide 1983 [Ref: MAF217/78]; Animal Health Division, files re: veterinary staff 1948–64 [Ref: MAF224/47, 48, 160–163], veterinary reorganisation 1957–59 [Ref: MAF224/242], staff inspections 1962–70 [Ref: MAF224/375]; Lasswade Veterinary Laboratory, papers re professional staff 1948–55 [Ref: MAF224/73, 74]; Veterinary Investigation Centres, papers re organisation and complement 1955–1962 [Ref: MAFF224/233]; proposed new Veterinary Investigation Centres 1955–60 [Ref: MAF224/237]; technical advisors on meat inspection, proposed merger with veterinary service 1957–59 [Ref: MAF224/257]; veterinary laboratories and investigation service, proposed new posts 1958–60 [Ref: MAF224/268]; Medicines Act 1968, inclusion of veterinary medicines 1965–70 [Ref: MAF224/325]; Royal College of Veterinary Surgeons, British Veterinary Association, staff inspections 1964–70 [Ref: MAF224/424]; Royal College of Veterinary Surgeons, general papers 1960–66 [Ref: MAF225/159]; papers re veterinary services 1956–58 [Ref: MAF227/91]; *Veterinary Hygiene* by P T and D W B Sainsbury, working papers 1964–66 [Ref: MAF227/251]; submission on reorganisation of the veterinary service 1957 [Ref: MAF227/344]; veterinary advisory aids committee, meetings 1948–67 [Ref: MAF240/19–22]; agricultural defence planning, Animal Health Division incl wartime veterinary organisation 1951–59 [Ref: MAF250/162]; role of veterinary surgeons in war 1958–59 [Ref: MAF250/222]; restriction of supplies by veterinary surgeons 1963–64 [Ref: MAF251/426]; warning by veterinary surgeons re withholding of milk by farmers 1963–64 [Ref: MAF251/427]; Local Veterinary Inspectors, export certification irregularities 1958–66 [Ref: MAF254/13]; Veterinary Surgeons Act 1948, report of committee on licences 1953 [Ref: MAF255/52]; report re animal health services in Great Britain 1955–58; file re animal health future veterinary programme 1959–60 [Ref: MAF255/894]; Antarctic whaling expeditions, reports of food veterinary surgeons 1947–50 [Ref: MAF256/105]; papers re imports of meat and meat products from France incl public health and veterinary regulations 1969–76 [Ref: MAF276/379, 389]; arrangements for work at slaughterhouses by veterinary service 1958–64 [Ref: MAF282/47]; papers re meetings with European Economic Community officials re veterinary directives 1964–68 [Ref: MAF282/85, 86]; imported food regulations, reports on overseas visits by veterinary staff 1964–74 [Ref: MAF282/130–133]; British Veterinary Association, veterinary certificates and grading for cattle 1957–67 [Ref: MAF294/140, 221]; Animal Health Division, wartime veterinary organisation 1964–65 [Ref: MAF355/10]; veterinary products safety precautions scheme, notification of *Dosopak No 3*, Day, Son & Hewitt Ltd 1964–65 [Ref: MAF364/8]; Export of Horses (Veterinary Examination) Order 1966, excepted cases, etc 1965–67. [Ref: MAF369/34–36]

Records (2): Archives and Manuscripts, Wellcome Library for the History and Understanding of Medicine, 183 Euston Road, London NW1 2BE

Board of Agriculture Veterinary Department, annual reports 1890–93; Contagious Diseases (Animals) Acts, the Markets and Fairs (Weighing of Cattle) Acts, annual reports 1906–08, 1912–15, 1917–18, 1920–21; report on animal health services in Great Britain 1966; report by joint committee on antibiotics in animal feedstuffs 1962; Hannah Dairy Research Institute, annual reports 1971, 1973.

Records (3): in private ownership of Miss Mary Brancker, 38 Streetly Lane, Sutton Coldfield B74 4TU

Second report of the Loveday Committee on veterinary education in Great Britain 1944.

Records (4): in private ownership of Mr R D Locke, 4 Rathmore Road, Cambridge CB1 7AD

Photographs: Divisional Veterinary Officers Conference, Cirencester 1970, Eastern Region Conference, Cambridge 1982.

DEVELOPMENT COMMISSION
London

History: The Development Commission was established under the Development and Roads Improvement Funds Acts of 1909 and 1910 specifically 'to promote the economic development of the UK'. Eight commissioners were appointed by royal warrant with the power to recommend the granting of funds from the Development Fund to government departments, local authorities, universities and other institutions. Agriculture was an important part of the Commission's remit and in 1911 a comprehensive scheme for the reinforcement of agriculture in the United Kingdom was produced. Together with the Board (later Department then Ministry) of Agriculture, the Commission rapidly became the major source of funding for agricultural research. A standing Agricultural Committee on agricultural science was set up and run by the Commission until 1931 when its functions were transferred to the newly created Agricultural Research Council. In 1946 the Commission's remaining functions relating to agricultural research, advisory and education services were transferred to the Ministry of Agriculture and Fisheries.

Records: National Archives, Ruskin Avenue, Kew, Richmond TW9 4DU

Papers re establishment of Agricultural Research Council 1920; A D Hall, memorandum on veterinary research and education 1913; Ministry of Agriculture and Fisheries correspondence and papers re: veterinary investigation work 1941–43, position of veterinary investigation officers at provincial advisory centres as affected by establishment of State Veterinary Service 1938–45; South Eastern Agricultural College, Wye, Kent, papers re equipment for new veterinary laboratory 1938; Veterinary College, New Haw, Surrey, papers re: purchase of Coombelands Farm 1934, extension of buildings 1935–38; Royal (Dick) Veterinary College, Edinburgh, papers re: extension of premises 1935–41, accommodation for women students 1942–43, renewal of heating system nd; University of Liverpool, papers re: veterinary education and research 1944–45, veterinary investigation work 1941–46; Royal Veterinary College, Institute of Animal Pathology, papers re: maintenance 1941–46, purchase of property at Streatley 1944; Central Veterinary Laboratory, Weybridge, papers re: purchase of part of Coombelands estate 1941–43, research schemes 1941, establishment of an artificial insemination centre 1943; Department of Agriculture for Scotland, papers re: appointment of veterinary investigation officers 1941–46, adoption of buildings on the Craibstone estate of North of Scotland Agricultural College to provide working accommodation for veterinary investigation officer 1946, establishment of a field station by Glasgow Veterinary College 1945–46, additional laboratory accommodation and equipment for Glasgow Veterinary College 1946. [Ref: D4/4, 91, 476, 478–481, 484, 486, 490, 491, 494, 498, 500, 502–505, 923–925]

DOMINIONS OFFICE
London

History: The Dominions Office was established in 1907 as the Dominions Division of the Colonial Office with responsibility for relations with Canada, Australia, New Zealand, the Irish Free State, Southern Rhodesia and South Africa, as well as the territories of the Bechuanaland Protectorate, Basutoland and Swaziland and a number of territories in the Western Pacific. In 1925 the Dominions Division became the Dominions Office with its own Secretary of State, although the post until 1939 was generally held jointly with the Colonial Secretary. Its responsibilities included financial matters, the development of infrastructure and the provision of British experts to train local personnel, including veterinary surgeons, generally in the lead up to a country's independence. The Dominions Office was renamed the Commonwealth Relations Office in 1947 and merged with the India Office shortly afterwards.

Records: National Archives, Ruskin Avenue, Kew, Richmond TW9 4DU

Bechuanaland Protectorate: papers re veterinary staff 1930–36, agricultural and veterinary department correspondence 1937–42, representations from British Veterinary Association re salaries for veterinary officers 1954–55; Swaziland: papers re veterinary staff 1930–31, 1936, agricultural and veterinary department correspondence 1937–42, proposals for a levy on trek sheep 1951, appointment of Principal Veterinary Officer 1956; Basutoland papers re: agricultural and veterinary staff 1930–36, agricultural and veterinary department 1937–43, agricultural and veterinary matters 1940, creation of a veterinary division 1950–51; Basutoland, Bechuanaland Protectorate and Swaziland papers re: general principles 1943–46, organisation and staffing 1943–46, appointment of Director of Agriculture 1943–46, separation of posts of Advisor and Director 1943–46, Mr Leckie's increased emoluments 1943–46, approval for adoption of title 'Director of Agriculture and Livestock Services of the Three Territories' 1943–46, appointment of A C M Vingerhoets as Stock Inspector 1943–46, B B Murcott, employment as

Agricultural and Livestock Officer 1943–46, Fort Cox Agricultural School, report by Leckie 1943–46, colonial agricultural policy 1943–46; Republic of Ireland: veterinary agreements 1949, 1954, papers re registration and control of veterinary surgeons 20th cent; recognition of South Africa's veterinary degree 1933–36; South African Veterinary Service correspondence 1937; Ministry of Labour pamphlets on choice of career series, veterinary surgery 1938; veterinary officer's correspondence 1938; file re veterinary services in New Zealand 1943–46. [Ref: DO35/344, 372, 379, 448, 480, 602, 716, 907, 908, 918, 1109, 1159, 1173, 1174, 1178, 4033, 4035, 4440, 4441; DO118/68, 105]

FOREIGN OFFICE
London

History: Prior to 1782 responsibility for foreign affairs was divided between two Secretaries of State. In 1782, however, a separate Foreign Office was formed with its own Secretary of State. At first there were only two departments, North and South, but the number of departments grew as the office's responsibilities increased to cover such matters as commerce, news and cultural relations. In 1946, the Information Department of the Foreign Office took over the functions of the Ministry of Information, becoming actively involved in the organisation of sponsored visits, exhibitions and international conferences.

Records: National Archives, Ruskin Avenue, Kew, Richmond TW9 4DU

Papers re international veterinary convention 1929; ratification of veterinary convention by Turkey 1938: report and comments 1941, ratification by Turkey and Iraq 1941, 1943; file re International Veterinary Congresses 1947–48; veterinary convention, Geneva 1938; vacancy for veterinary officer in China 1939; Latvian-Polish veterinary convention 1937; veterinary consultative body for the Far East 1946; papers re Food and Agricultural Organisation project to set up a demonstration area in the Middle East to cover land use, hygiene, preventative medicine and veterinary work 1950; Russian veterinary experts in Afghanistan re outbreak of rinderpest in Herat region 1950; Portuguese veterinary certificates not recognised by British authorities 1950; arrangements to accommodate Ministry of Food Chief Veterinary Advisor during his official visit to Rome 1950; report of UK veterinary experts visit to Hungary 1955; Department of Agriculture report on Veterinary Section 1926; report on Conference of Federated Malay States and Straits Settlement re veterinary surgeons, Kuala Lumpur 1927;

Veterinary Services, director's monthly report 1947; sanitary and veterinary supplies to Germany and Austria 1945–46; Ministry of Agriculture and Fisheries, veterinary department, informal reports 1946; Iraq, veterinary agreement with Lebanon 1948; establishment of Cyrenaican veterinary department 1950–51; establishment of Tripolitanian veterinary department 1950–51. [Ref: FO286/1082; FO370/647, 826, 1574, 1382; FO371/23517, 23610, 26669, 58161, 81944, 83096, 89473, 89670, 116396; FO628/42, 43; FO643/406; FO1015/406, 713; FO1015/425, 733; FO1020/335]

HM TREASURY
London

History: The Treasury manages the public revenue and controls its expenditure by government departments. Civil Service pay and conditions form part of the Treasury's responsibilities, although this function did pass to the Civil Service Department between 1968 and 1981. Additionally, the Treasury was responsible for the University Grants Committee until 1963, and for approving advances from the Development Fund until 1971.

Records: National Archives, Ruskin Avenue, Kew, Richmond TW9 4DU

Board of Agriculture and Fisheries, files re: J W T Moore, veterinary inspector, superannuation, temporary re-employment, remuneration 1913, increase of annual grant to Royal Veterinary College, London 1914, remuneration of local veterinary surgeons for services during outbreaks of swine fever 1916, revision of scale of fees for Local Veterinary Inspectors 1919, schemes for training ex-servicemen in veterinary science, etc 1919, expansion of scheme for fostering light horse breeding, arrangements for the demobilisation of army horses, boarding out, veterinary attendance, reorganisation of staff, livestock branch 1920; Board of Agriculture and Technical Instruction for Ireland, files re: salary of veterinary inspectors at ports, definition of 'approved service' 1910, S Adamson, temporary veterinary surgeon, compensation for injury 1914, G J Bell, temporary veterinary surgeon, payment of medical expenses for illness contracted while on duty 1914, T S Ashbee, senior veterinary inspector, pension 1916, F C Ryan, veterinary inspector deceased, gratuity to representatives 1919, G W Tyson, veterinary inspector, gratuity to dependants 1919, recommendations by Royal College of Veterinary Surgeons for improvement of veterinary staff pension arrangements 1919; Colonial Office files re: Major C C Boileau, stock inspector, Veterinary

Department East Africa, gratuity to widow 1911, improvement of pay and prospects of veterinary officers, Uganda 1914; War Office files re: terms of employment for civilian veterinary surgeons 1883, warrants and promotions 1883, rates of pay and travelling allowance for civil veterinary surgeons temporarily employed in the event of mobilisation 1912, increase of peacetime establishment of Army Veterinary Corps 1912, annual cost of appointment of staff to Territorial Force Veterinary Service 1913, H T Locke, horse keeper, Army Veterinary Hospital, Romsey, Hampshire, compensation for injury 1917, Major J J Phillips, Remount Depot, Romford, Essex, compensation for injury 1919, T Wright, veterinary surgeon, pension to widow 1919, pay and retired pay of officers of the Royal Army Veterinary Corps 1920–21, new rates of pay and conditions of service 1924–46, rates of pay for veterinary specialists in the services 1941–53; W H Brooke, compensation claim against Birmingham Corporation for loss of office as veterinary surgeon 1913; Local Government Board, Ireland, abatement of motor car duty for veterinary surgeons using their vehicles for professional purposes 1914; Development Commission files re: grants to Board of Agriculture and Fisheries for improvement of light horse breeding 1911, 1916, appointment of an advisory committee on research in animal breeding 1912, grant from Development Fund for establishment of scholarships in agricultural and veterinary sciences, establishment of milk recording societies, improvement of livestock, veterinary examination at ports for imported animals, staff arrangements 1914, establishment of a Research Institute in Animal Nutrition, Leeds 1914, grant to Board of Agriculture and Fisheries for improvement of livestock, annual report 1919, implementation of Selborne committee's recommendations 1920, grant to University of Aberdeen/North of Scotland Agricultural College for research on animal nutrition 1920, maintenance of Veterinary College Research Institute in Animal Pathology 1922–24, grant to Liverpool University for instruction and research in veterinary science 1924–35, grants for rebuilding of Royal Veterinary College, London 1926–35, grant to Central Veterinary Laboratory, Weybridge, for special research schemes 1941; Chief Secretary's Office Ireland, waiver of Home Office fees on transfer of control of Royal Veterinary College, Ireland, to the care of the Department of Agriculture and Technical Instruction for Ireland 1915; Ireland: Veterinary Department, establishment matters 1879, estimates for inspection at ports 1879–80, cost of inspection to be charged to cattle diseases fund 1879, temporary appointment of constables as ship inspectors, continued employment of assistants for disinfecting duties and to establish a station 1883; Privy Council files re: inspection of animals brought to London 1879, scheme for re-arrangement of system 1879, increase of personal allowances for inspectors 1879, personal allowance of Mr Holmans 1879, establishment of Agriculture Department 1883, reorganisation and reduction of staff 1883; claim by Penilee Live Stock Co Ltd against Stewart Stockman, Chief Veterinary Officer, Ministry of Agriculture, Fisheries and Food 1924; Board of Agriculture (Scotland) files re: loans to Royal (Dick) Veterinary College, Edinburgh 1925, maintenance grants for veterinary colleges 1925–27; Iraq, uniform allowance for veterinary assistants in the levies 1923; reports of technical co-ordinating committee on medical veterinary stores 1924–39; maintenance grants for veterinary colleges, Scotland 1930–32, 1934–35, 1937–41; Royal Veterinary College, London, grants in respect of purchase of property 1931–44; appointment of special committee to consider grants to veterinary colleges 1935–37; file re Colonial Agricultural and Veterinary Scholarship Schemes 1925–42; Ministry of Agriculture and Fisheries files re: employment of veterinary and hay inspectors and staff in connection with foot-and-mouth disease 1919–26, Chief Veterinary Officer and Director of Veterinary Research, telephone facilities at private residence 1919–27, Central Veterinary Laboratory, revision of staff on expansion 1921–42, fees in veterinary laboratories re post-mortem and other examinations of poultry 1934–40, position of Local Veterinary Inspectors transferred from local authorities 1937–38, remuneration of veterinary inspectors employed re exportation of horses 1937–41, requirements for experimental officers, assistants and laboratory attendants at veterinary laboratories 1946–53, application of Civil Service Arbitration Tribunal award no 381 to veterinary officers 1960–61, veterinary grades pay research survey 1960–62, special merit promotion for scientific and research classes in veterinary laboratories 1961–62; F S Clay, veterinary inspector, compensation for foot-and-mouth contracted while attending outbreaks 1922; veterinary officers, Northern Ireland, half of pre-establishment staff to reckon for pension 1925; Dr W H Andrews, Director of Veterinary Laboratory, pension position on appointment as Director of Imperial Bureau of Animal Health 1928; file re remuneration of consulting veterinary surgeons 1924–48; file re history of veterinary officer class 1953–58. [Ref: T1/11180, 11195, 11311, 11348, 11379, 11386, 11413, 11500, 11525, 11538, 11580, 11610, 11615, 11629, 11630, 11645, 11649, 11667, 11687, 11754, 11894, 11924, 11993, 12087, 12275, 12304, 12330, 12358, 12360, 12406, 12430, 12456, 12492, 12562, 16665, 16810, 17148, 15073, 15628, 15323, 16646, 13405, 14720; T161/5, 51, 194, 215, 230, 245, 515, 643, 645, 651, 771, 880, 888, 967, 980, 1014, 1045, 1065, 1153, 1427; T162/1, 585, 616, 754, 844; T164/56/17; T164/80/13; T164/168/4; T213/148; T214/8, 284, 1167, 1224, 1270, 1343; T217/167]

HOME OFFICE
London

History: Until 1782 responsibility for internal and foreign affairs was shared by the two principal Secretaries of State. But in 1782 the work was divided between them, one taking charge of home affairs while the other concentrated on foreign matters. Over time, the Home Office accumulated numerous responsibilities in the areas of public health, including warrants, poisons, markets and fairs, vivisection, prevention of cruelty to and protection of animals, firearms licensing, law and order, naturalisation, the employment of foreign nationals and the status of citizens of the Irish Republic.

Records (1): National Archives, Ruskin Avenue, Kew, Richmond TW4 9DU

New Edinburgh Veterinary College, papers re affiliation to Royal College of Veterinary Surgeons 1858–59; Albert Veterinary College: papers re affiliation to Royal College of Veterinary Surgeons 1865, use of title royal refused 1865; New Veterinary College, Edinburgh, application for royal warrant to affiliate to Royal College of Veterinary Surgeons granted 1873; Royal Veterinary College, London, papers re: assuming of infirmary title and royal arms 1882, examination of police horses 1892–1914, objection to vivisection licence remaining in force for their premises after licensee has left 1910, papers re opening of new buildings by George VI 1936–47, new charter of incorporation 1936, supplemental charter 1936–47; papers re: power under Highways Acts to remove cattle found on roads to common ground 1864, smallpox in sheep, Southease, East Sussex 1865, allowances to expert witnesses 1866, government refusal to prosecute or pay expenses of prosecution re poisoning of animals at Ely 1867, dealing with owners of dogs known to have been bitten by a rabid dog but allowed to be at large 1868, precautionary measures in Great Britain re smallpox in sheep on the continent 1868–69, burial of carcasses of cattle washed ashore 1868–69, reward offered re poisoning of cattle of James Diamond of Tavistock, Devon 1869, employment of and fees for veterinary surgeons called in cruelty cases 1889–1905, fees for veterinary surgeons re disposal of animals injured or ill in the streets 1889–1906, Patrick J Howard's claims against War Office for services as a veterinary surgeon, refused 1903–07, Royal College of Veterinary Surgeons' charter 1914, establishment of veterinary staff, Ireland 1923, establishment of a veterinary laboratory in Northern Ireland 1924, criticism of penalties imposed for cruelty to animals, removal from police list of names of veterinary surgeons censured for false evidence in prosecution cases with memorandum on reported torture of mouse 1924–28, naturalisation and nationality of foreign veterinary surgeons 1943, liaison between police forces, veterinary surgeons and local inspectors of Royal Society for the Prevention of Cruelty to Animals and extension of police training to include veterinary practice and use of humane killers 1948; letter from Wakefield proposing legislation to control movement and muzzling of dogs, etc 1870; William Williams, complaint re professors of veterinary medicine not being authorised to sign certificates 1900; Nottingham & Nottinghamshire Veterinary Association, royal title refused 1908; People's Dispensary for Sick Animals: papers re veterinary qualifications of officials and liability for payment for veterinary services in street accidents 1920–43; application by J Moore, ex veterinary inspector, for increase in pension 1923–24; Ireland: papers re Council of Ireland Services (Veterinary and Fishery) Fund 1923–24, registration and control of veterinary surgeons and the Veterinary Surgeons (Irish Free State) Bill (1931) 1928–31; subsistence allowances paid to veterinary inspectors, exchequer and audit department queries 1923–25; veterinary officers' subsistence claims, Northern Ireland 1924–25; Isle of Man, papers re government veterinary inspector's appointment, salary and pension 1927–46; Royal Canine and Veterinary Infirmary, royal title refused 1928; Jersey, Channel Islands, law re practice of veterinary medicine and surgery 1939–40; general policy re eligibility of veterinary surgeons to act as signatories to licences and certificates, protection of laboratories 1950–52; advisory committee on the administration of the 1876 Cruelty to Animals Act, appointment of veterinary surgeon 1952; policy re frequencies allocation to veterinary surgeons 1955–60; application from veterinary surgeon at Woburn Wild Animal Kingdom for possession of hypodarts, granted 1970–80; charters of incorporation, veterinary colleges 20th cent; petition from William Smith to Prince Regent for appointment as veterinary surgeon to the Shrewsbury regiment of Yeomanry Cavalry, nd. [Ref: HO44/49; HO45/2446, 2446, 7574, 7712, 8041, 8099, 8144, 8168, 8299, 8394, 6672, 7397, 7756, 9351, 10004/A49913, 10006/A50090, 10285/107935, 10453/B13085, 10429/A53895, 21436, 19976, 18581, 11715, 14241, 20422, 22229; HO144/101/A19552, 329/B10869, 327/B10250, 1025/166707, 965/B20568, 22331, 9949; HO213/343; HO255/93; HO267/132, 147, 200, 438; HO285/24, 77; HO288/129; HO348/13]

Records (2): Archives and Manuscripts, Wellcome Library for the History and Understanding of Medicine, 183 Euston Road, London NW1 2BE

Returns to House of Commons from veterinary inspectors showing numbers of experiments performed on living animals 1878, 1884–85, 1887–88, 1891, 1893–95, 1897–1904, 1906–11, 1925, 1927–38.

INDIA OFFICE

London

History: By the mid eighteenth century the East India Company, established by royal charter in 1600, was a powerful body that controlled much of the trade throughout southern and eastern Asia from its base in Calcutta, India. The Company also began forming its own native armies in Bengal, Madras and Bombay from the 1750s, and by 1824 had created 27 cavalry and 174 infantry regiments, as well as a European corps of artillery and infantry. This steady increase in power alarmed the British government who created the Board of Commissioners for the Affairs of India (the Board of Control) in 1784 specifically to supervise the Company's activities. In 1801 the East India Company set up a stud committee to improve the breeding of horses for use in its cavalry regiments. William Moorcroft, an English veterinary surgeon trained at Lyon, France, was appointed Superintendent of the Stud in 1808. Veterinary surgeons were regularly appointed to the various cavalry and artillery regiments from 1826 and entered under the patronage system; being 'recommended' by members of the Company's Court of Directors or the Board of Control. Following the Mutiny of 1857, both the East India Company and the Board of Control were abolished and responsibility for the administration of India passed to the newly created India Office, based at Whitehall. At the same time, the European corps was dissolved, although the native armies continued until the new Indian Army replaced them in 1895. The first Indian veterinary college opened in Bombay in 1883 and was quickly followed by others at Lahore, Calcutta, Madras and Patna. The India Office remained responsible for the administration of India until India and Pakistan were granted independence in 1947, after which the India Office was dissolved and its remaining functions transferred to the Commonwealth Relations Office.

A Farrington, *Guide to the Records of the India Office Military Department* (London, 1982); M Moir, *A General Guide to the India Official Records* (London, 1988).

Records: Oriental and India Office Collections, British Library, 96 Euston Road, London NW1 2DB

East India Company

Stud committee: minutes 1801–09, 1818–32 [Ref: L/MIL/5/459–461], correspondence 1801–09 [Ref: L/MIL/5/462], account book 1807–12 [Ref: L/MIL/5/463], veterinary surgeons' descriptions of horses embarked for India 1818–57 [Ref: L/MIL/5/464], copy correspondence and proceedings re breeding of cattle and horses in India 1794–1806 [Ref: L/MIL/5/465], half yearly reports from India re imported English stallions 1842–45 [Ref: L/MIL/5/466], report of the stud commission in India 1851. [Ref: L/MIL/5/467]

Records of the Board of Commissioners for the Affairs of India

Papers re decision to allow Monsieur de L'Etang to enter the service of the Nawab of Oudh as Superintendent of the Nawab's stud and veterinary surgeon 1766–1809 [Ref: F/4/312/7127]; papers re training establishment for veterinary students at Baliganj, Calcutta, incl returns of students 1796–1824, nd. [Ref: F/4/738/20145, F/4/889/23120]; papers re appointment of J T Hodgson as veterinary surgeon to the Governor General's Bodyguard, and decision to allow him to select and train eight assistant apothecaries as veterinary surgeons for the Light Cavalry Regiments 1821 [Ref: IOR/F/4/661/18358]; papers re failure of experiment to introduce Merino sheep to India and decision to distribute the flock at Sabathu among the Hill Chiefs and transfer flock at Dehra Dun to care of J T Hodgson, veterinary surgeon at Hapur 1829–32 [Ref: F/4/1340/53334]; papers re management of Hapur Stud Farm incl investigation into accusations brought by officers of the stud and the consequent dismissal or transfer of staff incl J T Hodgson, veterinary surgeon 1833–34. [Ref: F/4/1517/59944]

Accountant General's Records

Joseph Stevenson, veterinary surgeon, mentioned on roll of subscribers to Madras Military Fund 1825. [Ref: L/AG/23/10/1]

Economic Department

Papers re International Veterinary Bureau convention 1921–31 [Ref: L/E/9/1371]; papers re India's part in creation of an International Veterinary Office to deal with contagious diseases of animals 1927, 1932–38. [Ref: L/E/9/1372]

India Civil Veterinary Administration

Public proceedings incl re veterinary matters 1838–1870 [Ref: P/186–187]; proceedings re studs, cattle breeding and cattle disease 1871–89 [Ref: P/675, 677, 941, 1332, 1684, 2059, 2279, 2524, 2730, 2981, 3219, 3449]; proceedings re horse breeding and agricultural stock 1890–94

[Ref: P/3680, 3910, 4133, 4361, 4571]; proceedings re civil veterinary administration 1895–1923 [Ref: P/4767, 4983, 5213, 5444, 5669, 5901, 6137, 6366, 6598, 6832, 7074, 7343, 7619, 7902, 8179, 8461, 8719, 8965, 9216, 9466, 9727, 9959, 10181, 10379, 10603, 10847, 11051, 1986, 11341]; Bombay Revenue proceedings re civil veterinary service 1928, 1931. [Ref: P/11678, 11916]

Military Department

Bengal Army: draft and copy memoranda and correspondence by James Salmond, military secretary incl re Bengal Stud Department 1816 [Ref: L/MIL/5/431/420], original and copy correspondence re appointment of veterinary surgeon John Hodgson, and on proposed changes to veterinary establishment 1816–24 [Ref: L/MIL/5/395/160a], copy correspondence and proceedings on provision of horses in England for Bengal and Bombay Stud Departments 1817–24 [Ref: L/MIL/5/388/112a], copy proceedings and correspondence of William Moorcroft, Bengal Stud Superintendent, re trip to Central Asia to purchase horses 1819 [Ref: L/MIL/5/378/32], copy correspondence and proceedings on Indian Veterinary Establishments, especially Madras, with copy Madras veterinary medicine indents 1819–27 [Ref: L/MIL/5/388/112], copy reports and accounts of Bengal Stud Committee 1821–23 [Ref: L/MIL/5/389/120], veterinary surgeons' papers, consisting of petitions, certificates of age, testimonials and related correspondence 1826–59 [Ref: L/MIL/9/433], extracts from military letters to Bengal and committee of correspondence minutes on appointment of veterinary surgeons 1825–39, lists of vacancies and appointments of veterinary surgeons 1843–58, printed copy of Royal College of Veterinary Surgeons' charter of 1844 with covering letter 1848, list of veterinary surgeons in Company's service 1850, lists of rank of veterinary surgeons c1852 [Ref: L/MIL/9/434], register of appointment certificates incl for veterinary surgeons 1856–61 [Ref: IOR/L/MIL/9/286], statements of service and/or leave out of India re John Whitmore Garrad, veterinary department, nd [Ref: L/MIL/10/85 ff.294–295, L/MIL/10/78 f.129], Archibald Turnbull, veterinary department, nd [Ref: L/MIL/10/86 f.218, L/MIL/10/78 f.47, L/MIL/10/82 f.21], Mathew Joseph Marshall, veterinary department, nd [Ref: L/MIL/10/89 ff.204–206, L/MIL/10/82 f. 175], Edwin John Batt, veterinary department, nd [Ref: L/MIL/10/94 f.185, L/MIL/10/82 f.241], William P McDermott, veterinary department, nd [Ref: L/MIL/10/75 ff.105–106], George Kettlewell, veterinary department, nd [Ref: L/MIL/10/75 ff.282–283], John Field, veterinary department, nd [Ref: L/MIL/10/77 f.33], Robert Walter Murray, veterinary department, nd [Ref: L/MIL/10/77 ff.128], William Johnson, veterinary department, nd [Ref: L/MIL/10/77 ff. 203–204], Henry Charles Hulse, veterinary department, nd [Ref: L/MIL/10/77 ff.294–295], Isaac Bicknell, veterinary department, nd [Ref: L/MIL/10/79 f.56], Archibald Campbell Williams, veterinary department, nd [Ref: L/MIL/10/79 f.119], Henry Dawson, veterinary department, nd [Ref: L/MIL/10/80 ff. 96–97], James Quallett, veterinary department, nd [Ref: L/MIL/10/84 ff.77–78]; British Army: British Veterinary Department, Indian Establishment, register giving rank and date of appointment, index 1871–1913 [Ref: L/MIL/15/21]; Indian Army, files re horse breeding operations and Army Remount Department 1851–1927 [Ref: L/MIL/7/9626–9716]; Remount Department, reports etc 1874–1939 [Ref: L/MIL/17/5/2169–2184]; regulations re Veterinary Department 1887, 1900, 1909, 1916, 1925, 1935 [Ref: L/MIL/17/5/591]; field service departmental code, veterinary 1894 [Ref: L/MIL/17/5/766]; supplement to field service departmental code, veterinary 1894 [Ref: L/MIL/17/5/767]; field service manuals, mobile veterinary section 1927, 1935 [Ref: L/MIL/17/5/768, 769]; field service manual, veterinary evacuating station 1928 [Ref: L/MIL/17/5/770]; Veterinary Services Department: notes re working of mobile veterinary sections 1920 [Ref: L/MIL/17/5/2363], statistical and general reports 1921–45 [w] [Ref: L/MIL/17/5/2361], rules for admission of Indians to commissioned rank in Indian Army Veterinary Corps 1934 [Ref: L/MIL/17/5/2362], notes on camel management 1926 [Ref: L/MIL/17/5/2364], veterinary manual (war) India 1934 [Ref: L/MIL/17/5/2365], handbook of contagious and infectious diseases in animals 1936 [Ref: L/MIL/17/5/2366], defence of animals against gas 1942 [Ref: L/MIL/17/5/2367]; supplementary instructions, remount and veterinary 1919 [Ref: L/MIL/17/5/2407]; statistical returns re horses 1884–1908 [Ref: L/MIL/7/13235–13242]; files re veterinary department in India 1859–1927 [Ref: L/MIL/7/830–921]; Madras Army: statements of service and/or leave out of India re George Western, veterinary department, nd [Ref: L/MIL/11/79 f.161, L/MIL/11/89 f.85, L/MIL/11/92 f.24], James Thacker, veterinary department, nd [Ref: L/MIL/11/82 f.207], Frederick George Shaw, veterinary service, nd. [Ref: L/MIL/11/85 f.261, l/MIL/11/89 f.95, L/MIL/11/92 f.24]

Services and General Department

Indian Veterinary Service: regulations 1920–28 [Ref: L/SG/7/655], papers re modification of cadre 1924–47 [Ref: L/S&G/7/377], papers re change in designation of certain posts 1925–36 [Ref: L/S&G/7/378], papers re special pay attached to certain posts 1925–40. [Ref: L/S&G/7/379]

LASSWADE VETERINARY LABORATORY

Penicuik, Midlothian

History: Lasswade Veterinary Laboratory was established by the Ministry of Agriculture and Fisheries in 1938 to carry out agglutination testing and post-mortem examinations of poultry under the Accredited and Poultry Improvement Schemes of the Department of Agriculture. Previously these services had been provided by the Royal (Dick) Veterinary College, Edinburgh, but the introduction of the Agriculture Act 1937 had prompted fears of administrative difficulties. After lengthy consultations with various officials, Eskgrove House, near Lasswade, Midlothian, was purchased in 1938 for £3900. The old house was converted into a laboratory, additional buildings were built in the grounds and the whole site was officially opened in 1939 with J E Wilson, formerly responsible for poultry work at the Royal (Dick) Veterinary College, as Officer in Charge. Although originally intended only to service schemes within Scotland, the difficulties of movement in wartime led to Eskgrove being given responsibility for poultry work from the six northern counties of England from 1941. The laboratory also from this time offered a fee-paying service to farmers who were not part of the accredited scheme. In 1947 the production and issue of fowl pox vaccine was transferred from the Central Veterinary Laboratory, Weybridge, Surrey, to Lasswade and remained there until it was moved to Wye, Kent, in 1950. Lasswade's first full time research worker in poultry diseases was appointed in 1952, after which the research and development work expanded. In addition to poultry, the laboratory undertook investigations into the causes of mortality in wild birds. In 1959, at the request of the British Trust for Ornithology, it was agreed that members throughout Britain might submit carcasses of wild birds for examination. Lasswade also assumed responsibility for post-mortems during the enquiry into the decline of the red grouse and for birds dying at the Royal Scottish Zoological Society. From early 1961 Eskgrove became responsible for haemagglutination testing for Newcastle disease antibodies in Scotland and the North of England. The laboratory's scope was first extended beyond birds in 1945 with the setting up of a large animal unit which carried out investigations into bovine tuberculosis until 1964 and sent weekly supplies of S19 Brucella abortus vaccine to the Central Veterinary Laboratory at Weybridge, Surrey, for bottling and issue between 1945 and 1949. To accommodate this growth, additional land was purchased during the late 1940s and 1950s and new buildings erected to provide isolation facilities, brooder houses, loose boxes, post-mortem rooms, incubator rooms and a lecture theatre. Specialists and post-graduate students came from across the world while poultry disease diagnostics were taught to final year students at the Royal (Dick) Veterinary College. By 1980 the laboratory had also acquired two out-stations, a smallholding twelve miles from Eskgrove with sheep and poultry production units and a poultry disease experimental unit four miles from the main site. In 1971 the laboratory was divided into six units – avian and mammalian pathology, bacteriology, brucella, clinical pathology and microbiology. The brucella section was responsible for testing all samples within the Brucellosis Eradication Scheme in Scotland and the north of England. A support service to the Scottish Veterinary Investigation Centres operated from 1973, chiefly in histopathology but also offering clinical pathology and microbiology. In 1985 it was decided to close Lasswade Laboratory and Eskgrove was sold. However, pressure from the Scottish Office, the Scottish Veterinary Investigation Service and other interested parties brought about a change of heart and a much-reduced laboratory was opened at the Bush Estate, Penicuik, in 1986. In 1988 additional staff were recruited to carry out the work generated by new legislation relating to salmonella infection in poultry. The laboratory also assumed responsibility for the diagnosis of bovine spongiform encephalopathy in Scotland and continues to carry out a centrally-funded research and development programme into spongiform encephalopathies. In 1990 Lasswade Veterinary Laboratory became part of the new executive agency, Veterinary Laboratories Agency. In 1998 the laboratory was moved to the Pentlands Science Park, Penicuik. By 1999, twenty-five staff were employed at the laboratory, offering research and diagnostic services relating to diseases of farmed livestock and wildlife.

Anon, 'The Veterinary Laboratory Lasswade', *State Veterinary Service*, vol 22, 1967; G Mackenzie, *History of the Lasswade Veterinary Laboratory* (private publication, 1999); J E Wilson, 'An Account of Development at Eskgrove 1938–1961', *State Veterinary Service*, vol 17, 1962.

Records: Lasswade Veterinary Laboratory, Pentlands Science Park, Bush Estate, Penicuik EH26 0PZ

Annual reports 1974–84; register of files c1952–82; copy of particulars for the sale of Eskgrove 1985; photographs: staff at work and on outings, staff clubs, W Gordon in the post-mortem room, Eskgrove incl old canteen and games room, building of new laboratories, grounds c1940–.

MEAT RESEARCH INSTITUTE

Bristol and Norwich, Norfolk

History: The Meat Research Institute was formed in 1968 at Langford near Bristol under the control of the Agricultural Research Council, later known as the Agricultural and Food Research Council. In 1986 the Meat Research Institute merged with the Food Research Institute and the National Institute for Research in Dairying to form the Institute of Food Research. The laboratory at Langford was closed in 1990 and by 1999 the entire Institute of Food Research was based in Norwich under the auspices of the Biotechnology and Biological Sciences Research Council.

Records (1): National Archives, Ruskin Avenue, Kew, Richmond TW9 4DU

Files re: establishment 1955–63, finance 1961, Meat Industry (Scientific Research Levy) Order (1963) 1962–67. [Ref: CAB124/1552–1555; ED188/223; MAF88/666; MAF246/115; MAF256/265, 269–271; MAF275/59–60]

Records (2): in private ownership of Miss Mary Brancker, 38 Streetly Lane, Sutton Coldfield B74 4TU

Programme to celebrate opening of Institute by Elizabeth II 1968.

MEDICAL RESEARCH COUNCIL

London

History: The Medical Research Council owed its creation largely to the Royal Commission on Tuberculosis (1901–11), which in 1908 recommended the formation of a permanent body dedicated to medical research. To fund the new body it was suggested that a Sanatorium Benefit, at the rate of one penny per person, be included in the National Insurance Act of 1911, which could then be used to fund research not just into tuberculosis but a whole range of diseases. The Medical Research Committee that emerged in 1913, made up largely of scientific experts, was charged with devising various research plans and estimating their expenditure. Until 1919 all such plans were passed to the National Health Insurance joint committee for its opinion but thereafter they were referred to the Ministry of Health. In 1920 a royal charter reconstituted the Medical Research Committee as the Medical Research Council, with responsibility for instigating and funding biomedical research. Various amendments were made to the charter over the decades that followed, and a new charter was granted in 1966. Most of the Medical Research Council's research was carried out at the National Institute for Medical Research, established in 1914, and at the Clinical Research Centre, which operated from 1967 until 1994. A network of over forty units was also built up, each concentrating on a particular area of research. Between 1939 and 1961 the Medical Research Council also administered the Public Health Laboratory for England and Wales.

Records: National Archives, Ruskin Avenue, Kew, Richmond TW9 4DU

Veterinary Therapeutic Substances Act, Diseases of Animals Act 1935: report on international biological standards, correspondence with League of Nations Health Section 1930–35, correspondence re standardisation of therapeutic substances for veterinary use 1938–50, correspondence with Ministry of Agriculture and Fisheries re control and standardisation of veterinary therapeutic substances 1941; correspondence with Empire Marketing Board re veterinary research in South Africa 1928–30; reports re review of veterinary and medical mycology 1951–54; correspondence with Royal College of Veterinary Surgeons 1921–54; scientific sub-committee, reports on antibiotics and on animal feedstuffs with and without veterinary prescription 1960–61; informal conference for medical and veterinary workers in mycology, minutes 1954–55, 1957–63; Swann Committee: terms of reference 1967–69, reports 1968, report on control of antibiotics 1969–70, timetable and publication of report 1968–71, meeting with Smith, Kline and French about nitroforans 1970–72, papers and notes re informal group to submit advice to Council 1968, agenda for meetings held 1969; Page committee: report, notes and correspondence 1989–90; working party on clinical and veterinary sciences, minutes, agenda and papers 1985; papers re legal action by J Bleby, veterinary surgeon, against magazine *Titbits* 1968–70; veterinary products committee, papers, notes and correspondence re intake of synthetic oestrogens in the diet 1970–73; consultative document re protection of persons against ionising radiations arising from veterinary use 1983; correspondence and papers re Royal Commission into Relations of Human and Animal Tuberculosis 1901–11. [Ref: FD1/1008–1010, 4330, 4331, 4765, 5048, 8227, 8245, 8248, 8250, 8254, 8258, 8260, 9262, 8265, 8267, 8269; FD7/899–903, 1621, 1622, 2506, 2905; FD9/938, 1392; FD22; FD23/1599, 4643]

MILK MARKETING BOARD

London

History: During the 1920s a number of Milk Recording Societies were established to measure and record the yield and quality of milk on a county by county basis. The information gathered was intended to help both farmers and breeders make better decisions regarding the selection and breeding of their herds. Most Societies were dissolved after 1943, when the National Milk Records Organisation, sponsored by the Ministry of Agriculture and Fisheries and run by the Milk Marketing Board, was launched. This new organisation provided information on milk yields, butterfat and protein content on a national scale, allowing a more comprehensive strategy for improving the quality of the nation's milking herds to be developed. An additional measure aimed at improving the quality of the nation's cattle was the establishment of two artificial insemination centres in 1942. Over the next few years a number of these centres were opened across England and Wales and responsibility for them eventually passed to the Breeding and Production Division of the Milk Marketing Board. A Bureau of Records was also formed to maintain the records relating to cattle breeding and to make the information available to breed societies and individual cattle breeders on payment of a fee. In 1962 the Low Cost Production Service was introduced. Farmers who enrolled received twelve visits over the course of a year during which their milk production costs were monitored and compared with those of neighbouring farms. At the end of the year each farmer received an annual report detailing the costs and returns for his herd. From 1965 it was possible to have a costing done to cover an entire farm. To reflect this expansion, the Low Cost Production Service was renamed Farm Business Services in 1967. In 1990 the Breeding and Production Division moved from its base at Thames Ditton, Surrey, to new offices at Crewe, Cheshire. Later the same year its name was changed to Genus. Genus became a separate public limited company in 1994 when the Milk Marketing Board ceased to operate. The National Milk Records became a limited company in 1997.

Records (1): National Archives, Ruskin Avenue, Kew, Richmond TW9 4DU

Milk recording year book 1924; registers of dairy cattle with authenticated milk records 1924–26, 1928; Staffordshire Milk Recording Society, first official handbook 1926; papers re consideration and establishment of national service 1937–47; files re policy development and administration, incl re National Milk Records advisory committee

1943–81; annual reports 1947–91 [w]; correspondence re annual reports 1944–76; accounts 1943–74; technical sub-committee reports and minutes 1943–69; central advisory committee on artificial insemination, files re: improved breeding of cattle 1933–81, identification of cattle 1934–76, establishment and operation of artificial insemination centres 1936–62, talks 1940–63, proposed artificial insemination centre sites 1943–51, purchase and hire of bulls 1945–75, fees 1945–81, accounts 1946–67, conception rates 1946–75, veterinary research 1948–81, bull layoff accommodation 1951–78, deep freeze semen 1952–57, research into oestrus (heat) synchronisation in cattle 1952–79, storage of semen by private breeders 1954–79, Scott-Brown case re claim that Milk Marketing Board herd was infected with vibrio foetus 1955–60, breeding statistics 1958–67, ova transplants, embryo transfers 1959–90, statistics re business trends 1962–77, bull licensing 1963–65, operational structure for liquid nitrogen frozen semen programme 1963–70, sales promotion 1966–68, strategy 1967–69, semen stock control 1969–70, consultations re regulations, livestock quality controls on bulls 1976–77, R Newcomb's dissertation on investigation of factors affecting superovulation, egg recovery and transfer in cattle 1979; artificial insemination centre advisory committees, papers 1944–81; specimen forms for artificial insemination centres 1945–47; Whiligh Cattle Breeding Centre: advisory committee minutes 1946–71, papers 1944–74; Beccles Cattle Breeding Centre, minutes of meetings 1946–74; meetings of chairmen of cattle breeding centres: minutes 1947–69, reports 1964–79; Cattle Breeding and Production Division: annual reports 1951, 1956–89, reports by breeding and production research unit and others 1950–64, 1968–72, 1975–81, general files 1943–69; National Dairy Herd Census, reports 1955, 1970; forms used for milk recording 1942–73; lactation certificates 1943–74; recording register 1954–73; standard instructions for recorders 1957–70; National Milk Records Guide 1987; mastitis: files re research and control 1937–79, misc reports, conferences, etc 1971–90; Bureau of Records files re: establishment and operations 1943–74, investigation work 1946–66, services to breed societies 1946–76, co-operation with Scottish Milk Marketing Board on dairy bull progeny tests 1948–76; relative breeding values, contemporary comparisons and improved contemporary comparisons: methods of rating bulls 1950–79, lists of bulls showing ratings 1955–64, 1969; breeding research papers 1959–68; foot-and-mouth disease: papers re committee of enquiry re epidemic 1968–69, milk code of practice 1970–80, general files 1928–67; Worcester Veterinary Laboratory, papers re technical services 1970–82; files re: training for recorders 1926–57, meat marketing 1934–65, cattle sales and prices, incl Milk Marketing Board shows and sales 1934–81, milk machine testing 1935–77, recording for goats 1936–72, feeding stuffs incl prices, rationing 1937–40, 1946–60, milk recording in Scotland 1941–74, milk production campaign 1942–47, Victory Churn Contest, Inter-County Dairy Herd Trophy 1942–70, milk weighing methods and equipment 1942–81, identification of cattle 1943–75, recorders' visits 1943–77, branch committees 1943–77, testing methods and equipment 1943–77, butterfat testing 1943–79, annual conference 1943–80, experimental form of recording 1944–54, progeny testing of artificially inseminated bulls 1944–67, veterinary research into cattle diseases 1944–81, solids-not-fat and protein testing 1945–74, Low Cost Production Service (later Farm Management Services) 1945, 1962–82, grass drying 1946–58, branch annual general meetings 1946–73, grassland management 1946–81, importation of bulls incl Charolais 1946–82, policy re semen exports and imports 1946–82, regional organisation 1948–76, misc dairy husbandry projects 1948–63, farm investigations 1948–80, British Field Products Ltd, independent investigation 1952–54, Felin Fach pilot scheme 1952–57, beef progeny testing incl Beef Improvement Programme, Warren Farm 1952–77, Private Milk Records Scheme 1953–79, export of live cattle, especially calves 1953–81, private breeders' bull proving scheme 1955–76, butterfat testers' bulletin 1956–63, British Semen Exports Ltd 1959–75, Farm Management Recording Scheme 1962–79, Controlled Milk Records scheme 1963–75, liberalisation of artificial insemination regulations, do-it-yourself artificial insemination, quality control 1963–81, monthly recording by statement 1964–75, Dairy Progeny Testing Scheme, incl Jersey Improvement Project, Ayrshire breeding schemes, etc 1965–82, beef situation, etc 1967–76, brucellosis eradication 1970–77, pregnancy diagnosis from milk samples 1971–79. [Ref: JV10]

Records (2): Archives and Manuscripts, Wellcome Library for the History and Understanding of Medicine, 183 Euston Road, London NW1 2BE

Breeding and Production Organisation, annual reports 1979–80, 1983–84.

MINISTRY OF AGRICULTURE, NORTHERN IRELAND
Belfast, County Down

History: Although ultimate responsibility for the control of contagious disease remained with the Ministry of Agriculture and Fisheries in London, responsibility for the administration of all Contagious Diseases (Animals) Acts dating from 1894 passed to the newly created Ministry of Agriculture for Northern Ireland in 1921. Any outbreaks of diseases such as fowl pest, sheep scab, bovine tuberculosis and foot-and-mouth were to be reported to the Ministry, which would then take the appropriate measures including the slaughter and restriction of movement of animals. In 1949, the Tuberculosis (Attested Herds) Scheme, underway in England since 1935, was introduced to Northern Ireland and the Ministry arranged for the routine testing of animals by veterinary inspectors, the slaughter of those animals that failed the tests and the payment of compensation to owners. This was followed in 1953 by the transfer to the Ministry from local health authorities of the sheep dipping scheme, which required that all sheep be dipped annually in a Ministry-approved sheep dip. The Ministry also controlled the importation and exportation of animals and birds via an official quarantine station. The Gosford Advisory Committee, set up in 1961, advised Ministry officials on various poultry testing schemes at the poultry progeny testing station at Gosford, Co Armagh, while the Cattle Improvement Committee, established in 1970, recommended measures to improve the efficiency of cattle production.

Records: Public Record Office of Northern Ireland, 66 Balmoral Avenue, Belfast BT9 6NY

Proposed legislation re control of poultry disease 1930–37 [Ref: AG/16/9/2/1268]; Anthrax Order (Northern Ireland) 1932, papers 1930–60 [Ref: AG/33/55/1]; Chief Veterinary Officer's report re outbreak of foot-and-mouth disease 1931–32 [Ref: AG/16/10/1/1625]; papers re sheep dipping 1934–59 [Ref: AG/53/1–4]; proposed legislation to prevent docking and nicking of horses 1938–66 [Ref: AG/33/12/1/38]; East Twin Island quarantine station, policy 1944–66 [Ref: AG/33/2/3/16]; Control of Dogs Order (Northern Ireland) 1958, 1959, 1961, policy 1952–65 [Ref: AG/33/8/20/4]; correspondence with Ulster Society for the Prevention of Cruelty to Animals re proposals for new legislation 1957–65 [Ref: AG/33/14/10/59]; cabinet memoranda re proposed legislation to restrict exports of live animals 1960–65 [Ref: AG/33/15/2/60]; Gosford Advisory Committee, minutes and related papers 1961–82 [Ref: AG/62/1/1–4]; cattle improvement committee, minute book 1970–79. [Ref: AG/63/1/1]

MINISTRY OF HEALTH

London

History: The Ministry of Health was established under the Ministry of Health Act in 1919 and allocated various powers and responsibilities previously held by the Local Government Board, the National Health Insurance Commissions for England and Wales and the Privy Council. Although the new Ministry's duties initially included the regulation and inspection of all food, milk and pharmaceutical products, most of these functions were gradually transferred to other bodies including the Ministry of Agriculture and Fisheries. Consequently, by 1951 the Ministry of Health's area of responsibility was restricted to the provision of human health services. In 1968 the Ministry of Health became part of the newly created Department of Health and Social Security.

Records: National Archives, Ruskin Avenue, Kew, Richmond TW9 4DU

Diseases of Animals (Tuberculosis) Order 1925, inspection of cows by veterinary surgeon 1925–26; arrangements made by Dr Llewellyn Williams (Welsh Board of Health) and Mr Hatfield (Ministry of Agriculture and Fisheries) re introduction of an improved technique for carrying out tuberculosis tests in cattle by veterinary officers 1929–61; Diseases of Animals Act 1935, papers re tuberculin and other substances used for veterinary purposes 1930–35; economic advisory council cattle diseases committee, veterinary inspection of dairy cattle by urban district councils 1933; papers re National Veterinary Medical Association's scheme for utilising services of the veterinary profession re milk 1934–36; Public Health Inspector, veterinary surgeon qualifications 1934–35; Dr Morgan's report on visit to Argentina, Uruguay and Brazil to investigate methods of veterinary inspection of animals and their products for export to Great Britain 1935; papers re proposed state service for veterinary inspection of cattle 1936–37; files re veterinary inspection of cattle, supervision of food, drugs and milk supplies 1936–42; Milk (Special Designation) Regulations 1943, veterinary examination of accredited herds 1943; Veterinary Surgeons Bill, proposals and consideration of amendments re provision of animal organs and tissue for transplantation to human patients 1965–66; papers re inspections by veterinary officers for export 1965–69; Poultry Meat (Hygiene) Regulations 1976, reports re appointment of a joint working group to review future relationships between Association of Meat Inspectors, British Veterinary Association and Environmental Health Officers 1976–77; papers re veterinary products committee, investigation into acceptable safety levels of antibiotic residues found in milk incl submission to ministers, briefs, correspondence, minutes of meetings 1976–82; papers re proposals to establish a European Economic Community scientific veterinary committee incl membership nominations, correspondence and minutes of meetings 1976–88; Central Military Service Tribunal and Middlesex Military Service Tribunal, Veterinary Tribunal, minutes and papers, nd. [Ref: MH47/4; MH52/142, 372, 480; MH56/72, 86, 150, 373; MH58/124; MH79/351; MH96/275; MH148/270, 828, 894, 934; MH150/393]

PRIVY COUNCIL OFFICE
London

History: The Privy Council originated in those groups of men who advised medieval kings on the administration of the state. By the fifteenth century, when the Council first acquired its name, the monarch was relying heavily on the Privy Council to carry out the day to day execution of both foreign and domestic policy. In the early part of the seventeenth century the Privy Council Office emerged to carry out the Council's administrative work, generally via a system of committees and commissions. Although some of these had only a short lifespan, others evolved into permanent departments or ministries. A series of Acts from 1848 gave the Privy Council the power to impose Orders relating to the importation, movement and slaughter of diseased animals. From 1868 the Privy Council also regulated the sale of poisons, although this function passed to the Home Office in 1933. The most significant developments, however, followed a severe outbreak of cattle plague that swept the country in 1865. To deal with the crisis, a temporary Veterinary Department was set up within the Privy Council to co-ordinate the work of inspectors and carry out a programme of eradication. The following April, responsibility passed to the newly created Cattle Plague Department, again within the Privy Council, and again intended to be a temporary body. The Department's work was aided by the passing of the Cattle Plague Prevention Act of 1866, which allowed local authorities to appoint inspectors with the power to enter any premises thought to be infected with plague and to arrange for the slaughter and disposal of infected animals. By 1870, the Veterinary Department had developed into a permanent fixture, employing travelling inspectors and producing an annual *Return of Proceedings*, with details of disease outbreaks, imports and exports and compensation costs, and annual reports recording its work. Further powers were accrued over the next twenty years as numerous Contagious Diseases (Animals) Acts and Orders were introduced and the Veterinary Department continued to expand. In 1883 it was renamed the Agricultural Department of the Privy Council. Five years later, a departmental committee looking at pleuro-pneumonia and tuberculosis in livestock recommended that the administration of the Contagious Diseases (Animals) Acts be concentrated in a single department. This led to the Board of Agriculture Act of 1889 and the establishment of a Board of Agriculture, which incorporated the Agricultural Department of the Privy Council as a Veterinary Department. The Privy Council, however, continued to play a role in the development of the veterinary profession. Under the terms of the Veterinary Surgeons Act of 1881 it was given the power to hear appeals from those veterinary surgeons that had had their names removed from the professional register by the Royal College of Veterinary Surgeons. Its role in agriculture was revived in 1931 when the newly established Agricultural Research Council was placed under the supervision of a Privy Council committee, remaining there until its transfer to the Department of Education and Science in 1965.

A V Dicey, *The Privy Council* (London, 1880); A Fitzroy, *The History of the Privy Council* (London, 1928).

Records (1): National Archives, Ruskin Avenue, Kew, Richmond TW9 4DU

Papers re cattle plague 1865–66; papers re establishment and running of Veterinary Department 1866–76; appeals against removal from professional register: misc 1883, J Howard 1896–97, J B Gresswell 1907, H J Cooke 1907; appeal of Alexander Wynd against refusal to register him as a colonial practitioner 1899; Ordinance no 4 re degrees in veterinary medicine and surgery with amendments 1905; papers re holding of examinations at Liverpool Veterinary College by Royal College of Veterinary Surgeons 1905; papers re Veterinary Surgeons Bill incl correspondence on Royal College of Veterinary Surgeons' supplemental charter, Veterinary Surgeons Act 1881 and Veterinary Surgeons Act (Amendment) Act 1920 1907–21; appeal of H R Seddon, Melbourne University, against refusal by Royal College of Veterinary Surgeons to register him 1916–17; complaint by unregistered practitioners of interference by veterinary surgeons 1922–23; Royal College of Veterinary Surgeons: papers re relaxation of provisions of charters and by-laws under the Chartered and Other Bodies (Temporary Provisions) Act 1940, appointment of J Henderson Stewart as member of council 1950; Royal Veterinary College, London, files re: directions under Chartered and Other Bodies (Temporary Provisions) Acts, supplemental charter 1941–46, appointment to council 1946, appointment of Dr J Edwards to council 1951–52; Veterinary Surgeons (Irish Free State Agreement) Act 1932, restrictions on entry to UK of Irish trained veterinary surgeons 1942; appeal of Dr S Mylej against refusal to register him as a foreign practitioner 1949; Veterinary Surgeons Act 1948: appointment of Privy Council nominees to council of Royal College of Veterinary Surgeons 1945–49, direction under section 1 for recognition of Bachelor of Veterinary Medicine and Science degree at University of Edinburgh 1948, Order approving form of application for registration in supplementary register 1948–49, direction to University of Glasgow under section 3 1949, direction under section 1 for recognition of

Bachelor of Veterinary Science degree at University of Liverpool 1950, application of section 4 to students of veterinary medicine and surgery at University of Edinburgh 1950–51, direction under section 1 for recognition of Bachelor of Veterinary Medicine degree at University of London 1952. [Ref: PC1/2889; PC8; PC9; PC12]

Records (2): Archives and Manuscripts, Wellcome Library for the History and Understanding of Medicine, 183 Euston Road, London NW1 2BE

Privy Council Veterinary Department, annual reports 1872–75, 1878–79.

ROYAL ARMY VETERINARY CORPS

Aldershot, Hampshire

History: Prior to the establishment of the Army Veterinary Service in 1796, the overall management and care of army horses rested with the Quartermaster, who ordered the shoeing and, along with the farriers, carried out back inspections while on the march. By the end of the eighteenth century, however, there was growing concern at the large numbers of horses being lost through disease, ignorance or neglect, a situation not helped by the paucity of military stables, which led to horses being scattered all over the country. In 1795, therefore, as an experiment, William Stockley was appointed as veterinary surgeon to the 1st Fencible Cavalry for six months. His success, together with a serious outbreak of glanders in Kent early in 1796 which resulted in the slaughter of many horses, precipitated the appointment of Edward Coleman, Principal of the Veterinary College, London, as Principal Veterinary Surgeon to the Cavalry and Veterinary Surgeon to the Board of Ordnance (Artillery). On Coleman's advice, part of the stables at Woolwich, Greater London, was set aside as a hospital and a resident assistant, John Percivall, appointed. It was further agreed that a veterinary surgeon should be attached to each cavalry regiment and that the army should defray the costs of up to six men per year at the Veterinary College, London. After three years training these men would then join the army as veterinary surgeons. When some within the army baulked at the thought of waiting three years for veterinary assistance, especially as both men and horses were urgently needed for the Napoleonic Wars (1793–1815), Coleman advertised for medically qualified men whom he offered to train in three months, a move that outraged those who were endeavouring to raise the standard of veterinary care and establish a veterinary profession. The first veterinary surgeon to be appointed to the army was John Shipp, who joined the 11th

Light Dragoons in 1796. A further sixteen veterinary surgeons were appointed the following year and by 1801 the total had reached forty-four. These men did much to improve the health of the horses in their care, largely by implementing changes in diet and stable hygiene. In around 1804, the Royal Horse Infirmary was opened at Woolwich and acted as a hospital, veterinary store and research station. In 1805 a warrant detailing pay and conditions for veterinary surgeons within the Ordnance Service was introduced. This was followed in 1807 by a similar warrant for veterinary surgeons serving in cavalry regiments. Frederick C Cherry, who succeeded Coleman as Principal Veterinary Surgeon in 1839, worked hard to improve the pay and allowances of veterinary surgeons. He also introduced a record of treatment, to be kept alongside the registers of sick and lame horses maintained by the Artillery since 1802 and the Cavalry since 1818. The *Regulations for the Performance of Veterinary Duties* of 1853, the earliest Regulations to have survived, further established the role of the veterinary surgeon. Many of the clauses remained unchanged well into the twentieth century. But despite these developments the Service's wartime record remained poor, as the Crimean War (1854–56) clearly demonstrated. By 1856 there were sixty four veterinary surgeons in the Army Veterinary Service, of which forty three were in the Crimea. But a lack of co-ordinated organisation still resulted in much unnecessary suffering and loss amongst horses on active service. The first attempt to formulate an organisation for the Army Veterinary Service in wartime was not made until the *Regulations for the Supply of Military Stores to an Army in the Field* were published in 1866. These dealt primarily with shoeing but also stipulated that a veterinary surgeon must be provided for every 400 transport horses and that a reserve of veterinary surgeons should be available to replace casualties. The introduction of sick depots in Abyssinia the following year saw a concerted effort to deal with animal casualties for the first time. The appointment of James Collins as Principal Veterinary Surgeon in 1876 led to further changes. First, Collins had his office recognised as part of the War Office, and relocated to Pall Mall, London. Then, realising that poor pay and the prospect of long service in India made recruitment difficult, he proposed placing all veterinary officers in one department and stationing them for fixed periods in the various military districts, including the Foreign Service. This scheme was turned down but in 1878 a new warrant was issued which effectively abolished the regimental system of veterinary care in all but the Cavalry. Additionally, all new entrants had their service limited to an initial ten years, with no more than four officers being selected for retention annually thereafter. Pay and allowances were increased, with new recruits receiving £250 per annum. The efficiency of the Service in wartime was addressed by new Regulations which stipulated that an executive officer was to have charge of 250 animals, while there was to be an administrative officer for every 3000 animals. In addition, one Farrier Quartermaster Sergeant was to be appointed for every 500 animals and one Farrier Sergeant and one shoeing smith for every 50 horses or mules. Arrangements were also made for the provision of field veterinary hospitals, known as remount depots. Further Regulations, published in 1881, provided for a veterinary depot with stores for up to six months under the charge of a Purveyor. Although these new systems did much to improve efficiency, real progress was hampered by the necessity to use up existing supplies of outdated equipment and by the continued shortage of recruits. It was partly with this latter problem in mind that the Army Veterinary School was opened at Aldershot, Hampshire, in 1880. As well as providing training for probationary veterinary surgeons and opportunities for research, the School instructed officers in the selection of remounts and the treatment of simple cases when no veterinary surgeon was available. In 1888 the Army Vaccine Institute was set up at the School and over the next twenty two years produced enough lymph vaccine to supply two million people. The regimental veterinary system within the Cavalry was finally abolished in 1881, following the recommendations of a War Office Committee led by Frederick Fitzwygram. From this time the Army Veterinary Service became known as the Army Veterinary Department. In 1892 a Civil Veterinary Department for India was created, made up partly of seventeen officers transferred from the Army Veterinary Department. The Boer War (1899–1902) highlighted both the advances made by the Army Veterinary Department and its weaknesses. A new Veterinary Field Equipment Chest, introduced in 1897, proved to be a great success while conditions for horses being transported by sea were markedly improved. But both sick and healthy horses continued to be held at hospitals that also acted as remount depots. Inevitably disease spread and calls for independence from the Remount Department became more urgent. The Warrant of 1903 created an Army Veterinary Corps, made up initially of non-commissioned officers and men already employed on veterinary service but including from 1906 the officers of the Army Veterinary Department. With the Corp's creation came reorganisation. New Standing Orders and Regulations were compiled, and hospitals opened at Aldershot in Hampshire, Bulford in Wiltshire, and the Curragh in Ireland. Around this time too, the veterinary service added to its responsibilities by taking over the inspection of both stock for slaughter at military abattoirs and dairies and dairy stock supplying milk to the veterinary hospitals. In 1911, a reserve of stores was established, which greatly alleviated the fears over lack of equipment which had dogged the service during previous campaigns and did much to ensure that it was better prepared to cope with the conflict of 1914–18. But while the volume of work greatly increased, the staff remained the same – a Director-General (formerly the Principal Veterinary Surgeon) and a Deputy Assistant Director-General. Their position was strengthened, however, by the granting of independence from the Remount Department in 1913. From that time, the Directorate was able to function more freely, being responsible only to the Army Quartermaster General. In 1912 a record office was opened at Woolwich. The following year a Veterinary Field Unit was instituted to serve as a connecting link between troops in the field and veterinary hospitals while agreement was reached over the staffing of the Army Veterinary Corps (Territorial Army), set up in 1907. All these changes meant that the Service was well prepared for war when hostilities broke out in 1914. A total of 1668 officers and 41,755 men served in the Army Veterinary Corps during the First World War and, with the help of supplemental aid from the Royal Society for the Prevention of Cruelty to Animals, they were able to work in hospitals equipped to the most modern standards. In 1918, in recognition of the role the Corps had played in the war, it was granted the title Royal Army Veterinary Corps. The war, however, did highlight the Corps' chronic shortage of farriers, their numbers having decreased steadily since the introduction of machine-made horseshoes in 1885 and a general decline in the number of horses. To counteract this, four Schools of Farriery were established in 1915. During the 1920s and 1930s, there were cutbacks across the Service as the army became increasingly mechanised and more local personnel were enlisted overseas and the Royal Army Veterinary Corps' main role became one of support to the army in the policing of trouble spots such as Ireland, Turkey, China, Palestine and the Indian frontiers. Additionally, it provided reinforcements for duty in the Sudan, Egypt and India. At home, the Service was consolidated by the forming of associations such as the Old Comrades Association (1920), the Royal Army Veterinary Corps Officer's Club (1920), the Corps Golf Club (1924) and the Point-to-Point Association (1925), and by the establishment of the *RAVC Journal* (1929). During the 1930s, however, with the prospect of war becoming ever more likely, attention turned once again to Europe. Preparations were made for possible mobilisation, while in 1936 research was initiated into the protection of animals caught up in chemical warfare. The overall need for animals during the Second World War was relatively small, although a considerable number of pack animals were required to overcome the difficult terrain in Burma and Italy. A combined veterinary and remount organisation acted to purchase and deliver pack animals and oversee their veterinary care and replacement. Dogs, however, were used in far greater numbers than hitherto. A trial establishment of four dogs was opened at Aldershot in 1940, quickly followed by further training schools at Ruislip,

London, and Potters Bar, Hertfordshire. Overall, some 6000 dogs were donated by members of the public during the Second World War, while others were taken from canine shelters. The army's commitment to the dog increased in 1947 with the establishment of a War Dog Training School at Melton Mowbray, Leicestershire, followed by further training units in Malaya, Kenya and Cyprus. Together these schools provided training in the main types of dog use – guard, messenger, casualty detection, tracker, infantry patrol and mine and arms detection. In 1958 the Army Guard Dog Units in Cyprus, Singapore and Hong Kong were transferred to the Royal Military Police. Although the Royal Army Veterinary School had closed in 1938, its research interests were taken over by the newly established Royal Army Veterinary Corps Laboratory which tested new treatments, produced vaccines and supplied the Royal Army Medical Corps with blood and serum. Research work was restricted after 1945, but the Laboratory continued to develop its research into the effects of nuclear, bacteriological and chemical warfare on animals, while the Ministry of Defence sponsored post-graduate study for veterinary officers. The army's increasing reliance on dogs also stimulated further research into canine diseases such as haemolytic streptococci, distemper, leptospirosis and filariasis. In 1960 a Royal Army Veterinary Corps officer was attached to the Medical Research Council Radiobiological Unit at Harwell, Oxfordshire. Additionally, in 1951 a division of the British Veterinary Association was formed within the Royal Army Veterinary Corps, which allowed both retired and serving officers to take part in British Veterinary Association Councils and keep abreast of the new developments within veterinary science. Although the Royal Army Veterinary Corps' overall future looked increasingly uncertain in the decades following the Second World War, the Corps continued to develop. Its Regimental Headquarters was established at Melton Mowbray in 1989, while in 1991 the Defence Animal Centre was formed by the amalgamation of the Royal Air Force Police Dog School with the Royal Army Veterinary Corps Centre. A Royal Army Veterinary Corps (Territorial Army) Veterinary Officer Pool was formed in 1986, based at Melton Mowbray, and its officers were used extensively in support of the regular cadre, a use of the Territorial Army that became generally accepted throughout the army following the 1997 Strategic Defence Review. In 1997, the pool was able to provide two suitably qualified veterinary officers for the Army Civil Affairs Group – a newly raised body made up of representatives from a range of professions able to offer expert advice and assistance in both civil and military emergencies. In 1995, with the demise of the Department of the Vice-Adjutant General, the Royal Army Veterinary Corps became a Corps within the Army

Medical Services and the Directorate of Army Veterinary and Remount Services became part of the Army Medical Directorate.

L J Blenkinsop and J W Rainey, *History of the Great War Based on Official Documents: veterinary services* (London, 1925); J Clabby, *The History of the Royal Army Veterinary Corps 1919–61* (London, 1963); F Smith, *A History of the Royal Army Veterinary Corps: 1796–1919* (London, 1927); F Smith, *A Veterinary History of the War in South Africa 1899–1902* (London, 1919).

Records (1): Army Veterinary & Remount Services, Army Medical Directorate, Gallwey Road, Aldershot GU11 2DG

Army Veterinary Department, annual and statistical reports 1879–1906; Aldershot Army Veterinary Association, minutes 1895–1938; notebooks: disease, histology, pathology 1898, nd; veterinary officer's black list c1900–18; minutes of evidence taken before the court of enquiry on the administration of the Army Remount Department 1902; record of officers and their horses 1904–10; register of horses 1905–nd; Army Veterinary Corps Orders 1905; Army Veterinary Service statistical reports: Northern Command 1906–07, Burma Division 1906–07, Eastern Command 1906–07, 9th Secunderabad Division 1906–07; notebook re horses and mobilisation 1910; Royal Army Veterinary School: photographs 1910–61, nd, lecture notes on care of laboratory animals, nd, list of chemicals used in the pharmacy, nd; Army Veterinary and Remount Services: records of members 1914–18, Regulations and Instructions 1960, papers re role in Second World War 1961, papers re development and diversification 1981; Remount Purchase Commission, memoranda re embarkation orders First World War 1914–18; British Remount Commission, Canada branch, memoranda re postings 1914–18; information on the recruitment of grooms for the Expeditionary Forces Overseas field veterinary hospital during First World War 1914–18; report on the purchase of horses and mules by the British Remount Commission in Canada and US 1914–19; record of officers 1914–19, 1914–45; list of soldiers killed in First World War (p), nd; notebook with lists of drugs 1916; British East Africa, technical reports 1916; benevolent fund ledgers 1919–38; Army Veterinary Corps, India, Standing Orders 1920; Old Comrades Association: minutes 1920–47, cash book 1947–nd, list of members, nd; misc accounts 1930–38; registers of officers 1930s; remount book 1930s; record of dogs offered during Second World War 1939–45; record of dogs donated during Second World War 1939–45; Army Remount Department account books 1939–48; F E Gibson, notes on remounts in Lebanon during Second World War 1940–45; finance ledger 1943–47;

correspondence with Major R F Wall, sent to US to buy mules for the British Army 1940s; typed reports re epizootic lymphangitis 1940s; Department of Army Veterinary and Remount Services Conference, minutes 1977, 1979; quarterly report by Major J F P Clemanger 1983; correspondence and memoranda re Corps matters 1984–89; report on future of joint service dog school 1985; analysis of dog food, nd; x-ray registers, nd; form F718, animal account and forage running account (blank), nd; Lieutenant Colonel Green, notes on organisation of the Army Veterinary Service at home and abroad on the outbreak of war, nd; War Office reports: manoeuvres held in the neighbourhood of Salisbury 1898, foreign manoeuvres 1911, unit animal and animal ration accounting 1953; pamphlets: *Detail of the Sets of Harness Required for the Various Natures of Service Pattern Vehicles* 1915, *Guide to Assist Officers on the Preparation and Despatch of Specimens for Examination by Royal Army Veterinary Corps Laboratories* 1954, *Instructions for Handling Infective Materials* 1957, *Instructions on the Duties of the Royal Army Veterinary Corps*, nd; notes on a lecture by Lieutenant Colonel J Bleby in 1989 to commemorate a lecture of the same title given in 1889 by E E Bennett, incl copies of both lectures; Lieutenant Colonel Willder, notes and typescript of lecture given to Cambridge Military Hospital Clinical Meeting 1977; plans and reports re development of Melton Mowbray site 1978; photographs of staff, buildings, animals, etc 1980s–90s; press cuttings: demobilisation of horses 1918–19, horses 1925–39; career leaflet 1972; recruitment pamphlet 1977; prospectus 1979–80; Sydney H Slocock, surgery, medicine notebooks from Royal Veterinary College, London 1912; Animal Diseases Research Association report on grass sickness 1929; papers submitted to Veterinary Public Health Association scientific meetings 1980s–90s; misc papers collected by G R Durrant, nd; memoranda, etc re jubilee 1953; notes and documents re history of Corps, nd; *RAVC Journal* 1929–72.

Records (2): The Army Medical Services Museum, Keogh Barracks, Ash Vale, Aldershot GU12 5RQ

Roll of veterinary officers in Boer War 1899–1902; Army Veterinary Store: price lists 1914, 1917, 1943, letters re mobilisation 1948–53; casualty list of Army Veterinary Corps officers (copy) 1914–19; misc papers re veterinary hospital 1914–19; Henry E Hunt, notebook on acarid experiments 1914–19, 1952; veterinary field case books (unused) 1915–16; misc letters 1916–19, 1935, 1963, 1986; field message book 1917; horse complaints and treatments 1917–55; notebook on mallein testing of animals, Portuguese Corps 1917; war diary of veterinary services in Zhob Force, India, with additional papers re instructions for the veterinary officer and veterinary section of the operation 1919; copy of letter issued by Imperial Institute of Veterinary Research, Mukhtesar re bursatti 1925; correspondence and reports re anti-gas leggings for horses 1925–42; veterinary reports on horses and mules 1926–43; letters and papers re instructions for the protection of animals against gas warfare 1927–44; case history sheets, elephants 1929; animal inoculation register 1929–81; notes with photographs re collection of blood from camels 1935; letters and reports re: horse respirators 1936–44, anti-gas ointments 1937–44, anti-gas equipment for horses and dogs 1938–42, chemical warfare 1939–46, pigeon diseases 1942–46, dog respirators 1943–45, insecticides 1944–47, animal management 1945–46, veterinary matters at Chemical Defence Experimental Establishment, Porton Down, Wiltshire 1945–51, effects of smog on animals 1952; papers and photographs re European bison 1938–46; veterinary reports on combat conditions 1939–43; veterinary officer's wallet and field message book 1939–45; war estimates of veterinary units in the army 1940–45; papers re equitation training 1940–45; letters and papers re use of blood transfusions for horses 1942–43; papers, reports, etc re Indian Army Veterinary Centre, Ambala 1942–46; letters and reports re treatment of phosphorus burns on mules 1944; correspondence and papers re Kippen cattle poisoning 1946; letters, reports and papers re 7th and 9th Tripartite Conferences on Toxicological Warfare 1952–54; Lieutenant Colonel D F G Smith: register of experiments 1952–57, reports on horses and dogs c1952–53; horse purchase books 1953–63; veterinary reports on easinophil counts 1955; instructions for use of autocautery no 2807 1955; register of remounts purchased 1961–67; record book, civilian farriers and veterinary bills passed for payment 1962–69; registers of sick mules, Hong Kong 1963–65; equipment lists 1964; register of animals 1965–67; papers re complete horse feed trial 1970–71; animal history sheets (samples) 1975–85; papers re Army Dog Training Unit 1976–83; correspondence re early days of no 1 Army Dog Training Unit 1982, incl photograph 1946; correspondence re medals awarded to veterinary surgeons 1986; correspondence re veterinary surgeons in the Indian Mutiny 1986; reports: uniform horse equipment for the army 1855, technical reports 1882, 1898, 1916–17, horse breeding in Turkistan and Trans-Caspia 1908, camel diseases 1909, 1911, War Office reorganisation of the Army Veterinary Department 1910, veterinary arrangements at the cavalry concentration at Gurgaon 1910, treatment of surra in camels 1920, Captain J Bell on railway accident at Adavoyle 1921, committee on light breeding scheme 1923, committee on remount duties 1936, annual administrative report of Army Veterinary Service in India 1936–38, committee on organisation of army veterinary services 1937, Indian Army Veterinary Corps Centre 1942–46, equine and canine nerve gas casualties c1950, observations on sweating in the horse 1955, study into future of service dog training 1989; John Shipp: veterinary college certificate (copy) 1796, commission (copy) 1797; Samuel Newman, commission 1799; Michael F Healey, commissions 1873, 1879; Henry Lewis, attestation paper for enlistment 1915; Captain C W B Sikes, mentioned in dispatches certificates 1917–18; Major Herbert Laurie, warrant of appointment as MBE 1918; Sergeant Major Briggs, School of Farriery pass, nd; John Storey, typed account of service 1969; Edward Stanley, veterinary surgeon to the 5th Lancers, papers (copies) re life and work 1980; Lieutenant Colonel Badcock, typed account of service life and hunting experiences c1890–1950; Veterinary Officer William Dunlop Smith, correspondence and article 1986; obituaries: Major K I Barlow 1988, Dr E A Gray 1989, Colonel George Barnett 1989, Brigadier J J Plunket 1990, Albert Victor Franklin (draft), nd; Staff Sergeant George Hayes: references 1911–21, plan for operating table for horses c1911–20; Private R A Huxham, transcript of diary c1918; misc personal papers: Major Harold Irwin 1912–19, Sergeant Alfred Cherry 1914–19, Staff Sergeant G Parker 1914–19, Private William George Monger 1914–19, Major Frank Chambers 1915–19, Major E J Burndred 1915–25, Private W Jones 1919, Private J R Smith 1919, Sergeant P G Briggs c1928–44, Ex Staff Sergeant J Swarbrick 1939–45, Captain B Morris 1940–45, 1950, Lieutenant Colonel L H B Poer 1942–43, 1987, Lieutenant Colonel V G Hinds 1943–45, Captain A R Thomas 1943–48, W S Gale 1946–61; *RAVC Journal* committee: minute books 1929–72, papers and correspondence 1962–66, list of subscribers c1966; Old Comrades Association (Doncaster), minute books, account books, etc 1947–81; papers re hockey team 1942–44, golfing society 1958–61; maps of Belgium and France used during First World War 1914–19; plans: Aldershot camp 1966, proposed veterinary hospitals at Aldershot 1911 and Catterick Camp 1924, proposed museum at Melton Mowbray 1979, decontamination bath 1940, kennels 1956–67, Porton Down Camp c1945; specification for 'Budd's Farriery Training Apparatus' 1915–17; photographs: animal complaints, tests, etc incl mustard gas lesions c1916–18, training centre 1963, misc re staff, animals, equipment, farriery, overseas, veterinary procedures, etc 19th–20th cent; x-ray plate, navicular disease c1970; pamphlets, etc: *The Structure of the Horse's Foot and the Principles of Shoeing* 1892, *Horses for the Army – A Suggestion* 1902, *Veterinary Corps Orders* 1905–16, *Standing Orders* 1906, 1930, 1960, *Field Service Manual Veterinary India* 1908, *Cavalry Training* 1912, *Types of Horses Suitable for Army Remounts* 1912, 1920, 1924, *The King's Regulations and Orders for the Army* 1914, *An Appeal to All Horse Lovers* c1915, *Feeding Stuffs as Applied to the Management of Army Horses* 1918, *Knight's Painless Horseshoe Nail* 1919, *The Empressment of Horses etc in Time of National Emergency* 1924,

Veterinary Regulations India 1925, 1935, 1937, military manuals re apprentice tradesmens' entrance exams 1931, *Handbook of Saddle and Harness Makers* 1932, *Veterinary Manual (War) India* 1934, *Regulations re Admission to Commissioned Rank* 1936, *Remount Regulations* 1937, *Remount Manual (War)* 1937, war office circulars re veterinary matters 1939–46, *Regulations for the Army Veterinary Services* 1943, training notes for infantry patrol dogs c1945, account (copy) of the training of horses for the Coronation 1953, *Guide to Assist Veterinary Officers on the Preparation and Dispatch of Specimens to RAVC Laboratory* 1954, training pamphlets 1959–61, *Vocabulary of Army Veterinary Stores* 1963, *Instructions for the Use of Army Horses* 1966, *The History and Development of Stredabed* incl a letter and copies of reports on stredabed and its use 1979, notes on machine made horseshoes, nd; veterinary instrument catalogues: Baird and Tatlock 1954, Arnold & Sons 1954, Medical Supply Association 1955; articles: *From the Past – The Dick Vets OTC* 1979, Colonel George Barnett, *History of Indian Army Veterinary Corps Centre 1942–46*, nd, article based on a lecture given by E E Bennett in 1889 on *Employment of Dogs for Military Purposes*, nd; *Dunkirk Veterans Association* magazine 1966; press cuttings of Royal Army Veterinary Corps in Palestine 1939–45; scrap books and photographs re Army Dog Training Unit Hong Kong 1970s–80s; tape of radio broadcast re John Shipp ceremony 1988; lecture and press cuttings re *Remounts for the British Army* 1902; misc press cuttings and scrapbooks 20th cent; annual reports, rules, etc re Foxhounds Association of India 1930–47; photographs and press cuttings re Narbudda Vale, Peshawar Vale Hunts 1927–30; misc programmes, orders of service, Christmas cards, etc 20th cent; notes on history of veterinary corps 1899. [Ref. Boxes V1–41]

Records: (3): National Archives, Ruskin Avenue, Kew, Richmond TW9 4DU

War Office files re: plans, sections and elevations of proposed ordnance and veterinary establishment for Royal Artillery 1813, Veterinary Surgeon General, appointment to be held by an army veterinary surgeon 1839, report of Herbert committee on appendix to report on supply of stores to army in the field 1863–65, royal warrant reconstructing Army Veterinary Department 1876–78, medals and awards 1878–1918, papers re embarkation and disembarkation 1879–80, 1885–86, 1889–98, proposal to establish a reserve of veterinary surgeons for use in emergencies 1880–81, report of Sir F Fitzwygram's committee on organisation of Veterinary Department, incl minutes, correspondence, opinions and recommendations 1880–85, warrants and promotions 1883, proposed formation of three field veterinary hospitals 1901–02, final recommendations 1901–02, instruction of officers in tropical veterinary medicine 1903, Army Veterinary Department colonels to be designated Army Veterinary Staff and other officers amalgamated with Army Veterinary Corps 1905–06, scheme for organisation of Army Veterinary Reserve 1906, formation and organisation of Veterinary Department (Territorial Army) 1907–10, appointment and promotion of officers 1908–09, provision of sick horse attendants in peace and for a reserve on mobilisation 1911–14, increase of peacetime establishment 1912, history and development 1914–19, pay and retired pay of officers 1920–21, new rates of pay and conditions of service 1924–46, committee on organisation of Army Veterinary Services, report 1936, formation of committee to investigate Army Veterinary Services in view of mechanisation 1936–38, military handbook vol 5 1936–45, Army Veterinary School, training and military education 1939, army veterinary and remount services, amalgamation 1940–42, army veterinary services during operations against Japan 1943–45, extracts from orders of battle 1946, dress items 1948–72, alliance with Pakistan Remounts Veterinary and Farms Corps 1954, committee on future of Royal Army Veterinary Corps, report 1957–58, army veterinary and remount services during Second World War 1961, Army Veterinary and Remount Services, director's report 1964; F Raymond, experiments on horses for influenza 1891; Cavalry Brigade Mobile Veterinary Sections, war diaries 1918–19, 1944–45; Ministry of Agriculture and Fisheries, papers re demobilisation of army horses 1920; regular officers' retired pay 1920–29. [Ref: HO144/329/B10869; PIN15/2139; T1/11413; T1/12087; T1/12304; T1/12562; T1/14720; T161/5; T162/844; WO25/3510, 3512–3519; WO32/4505, 4506, 6545, 6027–6029, 6031, 6032, 6668–6672, 7021, 9882, 15566, 16563, 17047, 17909; WO33/35, 1460; WO43/722; WO78/2521/1; WO95/4512, 4517, 5391; WO100/53, 60, 81, 84, 96, 100, 108, 230, 355; WO106/388A, 482; WO108/157; WO146/1/102; WO170/3776–3779, 7379–7384; WO203/1229, 1435, 1744; WO212/504; WO279/550; WO305/2855; WO329/2104–07, 2292, 2303, 2503, 2919, 2920, 2942, 2955, 3238, 3239, 3270, 3272]

Records (4): National Army Museum, Royal Hospital Road, Chelsea, London SW3 4HT

Frederick Cherry, letter to Lieutenant General Sir Henry Clinton forwarding copy of his *Observations on Army Forges* 1817; General Sir William John Codrington, Commander in Chief in the Crimea: papers re duties of staff veterinary surgeons 1854 and pay of staff veterinary surgeon Cherry 1855 [Ref: 6807/377–1–Bundle 1; 6807/377–2–2nd folder], returns of medical and veterinary stores shipped to the Crimea 1854 [Ref: 6807/377–3–Bundle 1], letters from London re allowances for veterinary surgeons and permission for probationary veterinary surgeons to wear regimental uniform 1856 [Ref: 6807/378–1–Bundle 2; 6807/378–3], charge for farrier to be accounted for 1855 [Ref: 6807/377–2–2nd folder], letters from London re claims for farrier's tools and pay of farriers and farrier majors in the Crimea 1855–56 [Ref: 6807/378–1–Bundle 1; 6807/378–1–Bundle 2]; James Rowe, veterinary surgeon, Dorset Yeomanry: Lord Lieutenant's commission 1871, certificate of freedom of Borough of Weymouth 1902; W E Adams, Army Veterinary School, Aldershot: treatise on the horse and its diseases 1891, notes of lectures on horse management incl anatomy and illness of horses, treatment of wounds and injuries and list of drugs employed 1895; Field Marshall William Riddell, Lord Birdwood, manuscript extract from Bombay Command Order announcing that he has passed a course of instruction at the Army Veterinary School, Poona 1896 [Ref: 67–7/19–113]; Brigadier J J Plunket, Colonel Commandant 1914–18, memoirs, nd; *RAVC Journal* 1929–55, 1961–64; recruiting pamphlets and leaflets 1972–82. [Ref: 7507–2; Acc 8207–28; ARC 9102–134, 7207–24–1/2; Acc 8311–81]

Records (5): Imperial War Museum, Lambeth Road, London SE1 6HZ

Captain W Fyrth, veterinary surgeon, diary giving details of service 1914; Major H Kirk, account of his service during First World War; Lieutenant Colonel F C O'Rorke, diary of service 1914–18; E G Barrett, diary written whilst stationed at various French ports, giving details of duties incl receiving and checking deliveries of horses from US for use by Allied armies 1915–16; W G Smith, discharge certificate and papers 1916; A W Bradbury, memoir re service as trooper with Hertfordshire Yeomanry, incl spell at Egyptian veterinary hospital 1916–18; diary of unnamed officer 1916–19; field message book containing messages to Veterinary Officer commanding 51st Mobile Veterinary Section, 256th Brigade, re treatment of sick and wounded horses 1917; 2nd Lieutenant E M P Fisher, transcript of letters written home during service with 36th Divisional Ammunition Column, incl details of period spent on veterinary course 1917–18; J Storey, veterinary surgeon, typescript reminiscences re enlistment, training at Woolwich and service in Egypt and Gibraltar 1919–32, 1969. [Ref: 74/99/1; 76/160/1; 97/4/1; 74/8/1; 80/30/1; PP/MRC/54; Misc. 1453, 846, 521]

Records (6): Liddell Hart Centre for Military Archives, King's College London, Strand, London WC2R 2LS

Lieutenant Colonel Kenneth H Cousland, Royal Field Artillery 1914–18, detailed account of his military career, incl reproductions of photographs and extracts from his letters home and diary 1974 [Ref: GB0099 KCLMA Cousland]; official papers, orders and regulations, South African Field Force and Natal army incl re welfare of horses and appointment of veterinary surgeons 1895–1900. [Ref: Hamilton 2/4/1–13]

Records (7): Liddle Collection, Brotherton Library, Leeds University, Leeds LS2 9JT

W K Stuart, Veterinary Officer, 19th Mobile Veterinary Section, 2nd Royal Naval Brigade, diary 1915; H V Hughes: *Report of the Purple Cross Service for Wounded and Sick Army Horses* 1916, typescript recollections of career to 1961; Thomas Dalling, Army Veterinary Corps, no 2 field veterinary hospital: commissions 1916, 1921, 1927, photograph albums showing officers, troops, farriers, horses, veterinary hospitals, etc 1914–18, dispatches certificate 1917, memorial from entertainment corps c1918; L Moore: war diary incl veterinary work (p) 1917–18, misc papers re Imperial Camel Corps 20th cent; 7th Veterinary Hospital, Forges les Eaux, France, horse and mule statistical returns 1917–18; photograph of unidentified member of Royal Army Veterinary Corps 1918.

Records (8): Bedfordshire and Luton Archives and Record Service, County Hall, Cauldwell Street, Bedford MK42 9AP

Call up papers of Robert Brookbanks, Biggleswade, Bedfordshire, to Army Veterinary Corps 1916 [Ref: Z 1039/1/1]; postcard photograph of two [Army Veterinary Corps] privates with a small boy c1916. [Ref: Z 1039/2/1]

Records (9): Ministry of Defence, Defence Records 2, Bourne Avenue, Hayes UB3 1RF

This archive is not open to the public. On payment of a fee, however, statements of service can be provided to researchers who give the following information: name and number of the person in question, year of discharge, consent of the data subject or, if deceased, proof of their death and consent of their next of kin.

Personnel records 20th cent.

SCOTTISH EXECUTIVE RURAL AFFAIRS DEPARTMENT
Edinburgh

History: The Board of Agriculture (Scotland) was established under the Smallholder(s) Scotland Act 1911, primarily to encourage the setting up of smallholdings. At first its main functions were the compilation of agricultural statistics, the aiding of agricultural education and research, organisation and co-operation within agriculture and the promotion of agriculture as well as forestry and other rural industries. The Board became a Department in 1928, under the Secretary of State for Scotland, and its role expanded greatly from 1939 as the need for home produced food intensified. Following the publication of the Report of the Royal Commission on Scottish Affairs in 1954, responsibility for animal health in Scotland was divided between the Department of Agriculture and Fisheries for Scotland (DAFS) and the Ministry of Agriculture, Fisheries and Food. The former took responsibility for numerous aspects of animal health work in Scotland from 1955 including the administration of the Tuberculosis (Attested Herds) Scheme, while the latter retained control over epidemic diseases, veterinary staff appointments and the Lasswade Veterinary Laboratory. DAFS also assumed responsibility for the importation of animals via Scottish ports and the Glasgow quarantine station, but it was agreed that policy decisions surrounding such issues should be managed jointly. The Department assumed an active role in livestock improvement work, formulating and administering grant and service schemes, for example maintaining stud farms near Inverness, which lent bulls and rams to crofting communities, controlling artificial insemination, licensing bulls, boars and stallions and considering applications for permission to export and import livestock. Between 1968 and 1970, the Department formed a joint committee (the Swann Committee) to examine the use of antibiotics in animal husbandry and veterinary medicine. In 1991 the Department of Agriculture and Fisheries for Scotland was renamed the Scottish Office Agriculture and Fisheries Department and changed its name again in 1999 to the Scottish Executive Rural Affairs Department.

Anon, *The Scottish Office: a guide to the structure and functions of the Departments of the Secretary of State for Scotland* (Scottish Information Office Factsheet); Anon, *A Handbook on Scottish Administration* (Edinburgh, 1956).

Records: National Archives of Scotland, HM General Register House, Edinburgh EH1 3YY

Animal health files re control of diseases incl bovine tuberculosis, foot-and-mouth, anthrax, rabies, fowl pest, sheep scab, scrapie, warble fly, swine fever, etc, import, export and quarantine of animals, administration of calf vaccination, pig and poultry schemes 1886–1991; education, research and intelligence files re all aspects of agricultural education and research incl advisory services, agricultural surveys and activities of agricultural colleges, veterinary colleges and research institutes 1899–1991; provisional Order re Royal (Dick) Veterinary College, Edinburgh 1952; files re: Veterinary Products and Treatments Bill 1958–64, protection of veterinary workers from exposure to ionising radiation 1958–89, registration of Young's veterinary products for sale abroad 1959–65; Veterinary Services, files re: bovine tuberculosis eradication plan 1959–62, committee of enquiry into veterinary recruitment 1962–66, future organisation of services 1966–73; study group re application of results of veterinary research, notes of meetings and draft report 1964–65; Swann Committee: minutes and correspondence 1968–69, constitution, general papers and correspondence 1968–69, papers re appointment of members 1968, evidence submitted 1968–69, confidential evidence and papers 1968–69, drafts of report incl notes and summary of evidence 1968–69, final report 1968, report and action following 1969–70, inter-departmental working party minutes re consideration of report and implementation of recommendations 1969–71, papers re publication of report 1969, comments by agricultural organisations and feedstuffs manufacturers 1969–70; committee of enquiry into the veterinary profession, papers re establishment, members and evidence submitted 1969–74; file re veterinary investigations 1970–71; Scottish Senior Veterinary Officers, minutes and papers 1975–86. [Ref: AF070; AF072; HH080/00882]

VETERINARY LABORATORIES AGENCY

Weybridge, Surrey

History: The Veterinary Laboratories Agency's origins can be traced back to 1894 and the establishment of a veterinary diagnostic service in a single basement room at the back of 4 Whitehall Place, London. The Veterinary Department of the Privy Council, set up in 1865 after an outbreak of cattle plague swept the country, had initially used facilities at the Royal Veterinary College, London, for diagnostic backup. However, an outbreak of swine fever in 1893 finally convinced the Board of Agriculture that it needed its own diagnostic laboratory service. Following the Swine Fever Order of 1893, which instructed inspectors to send samples from suspected swine fever cases to London for analysis, a room at the Board's headquarters was converted to accommodate swine fever pathology. The Laboratory's remit quickly expanded to cover a range of animal diseases, however, rendering this facility inadequate. In 1906, therefore, it moved to Sudbury, Greater London, and moved again in 1908 to Alperton Lodge, Wembley, London. By that time the Laboratory was carrying out research into various conditions including contagious abortion, scrapie, Johne's disease and bracken poisoning as well as continuing to provide confirmatory diagnoses of scheduled diseases. Its role expanded still further after the outbreak of war in 1914 forced Britain to produce her own supplies of vaccine to replace those previously imported from the continent. Once again the lack of space became an issue and so the government in 1914 made available £28,650 to buy and develop a forty acre site at the Moat Farm Estate, Addlestone, near Weybridge, Surrey. The Central Veterinary Laboratory (CVL), with five laboratories, loose boxes, further animal housing and a special building for the production of swine fever anti-serum finally opened in 1917. Six veterinary officers were seconded from the Board of Agriculture and worked under Sir Stewart Stockman, who combined the dual roles of Chief Veterinary Officer and Director of Research. In 1918, the diagnostic service was called upon to deal with an outbreak of rabies, re-awakening an interest in rabies research. After Stockman's death in 1926, his duties were divided between J J R Jackson, who became Chief Veterinary Officer, and W H Andrews, who was appointed Director of Research. During the 1930s, the laboratory's facilities were expanded to include three new blocks: one for the production of tuberculin used in the diagnosis of tuberculosis in cattle, one for diagnosis and research into poultry diseases and a third for the production of a vaccine against brucellosis. Two neighbouring farms were also bought to house the CVL's livestock. Following the Agriculture Act of 1937, all veterinary investigation functions previously carried out by local authorities were transferred to the Animal Health Division of the Ministry of Agriculture and Fisheries, resulting in an increase in the CVL's research staff from fifteen to twenty six between 1936 and 1942. At the same time, five distinct research departments were established: Bacteriology, Biochemistry, Parasitology, Pathology and Poultry Science. A satellite laboratory was also set up at Lasswade, near Edinburgh, to monitor the health of Scottish poultry. The outbreak of war in 1939 brought additional changes. The threat of biological warfare meant that the new brucellosis research block was used instead to build up and renew reserves of anthrax vaccine. Female technical staff were employed for the first time. Further building work carried out after the war provided the CVL with accommodation for the new Biological Products and Standards Department, opened in 1956, and new buildings for the Parasitology and

Biochemistry Departments, completed in 1964. By 1956, the original five research departments had been increased to eight. The Virology Department formally separated from the Bacteriology Department in 1952 and went on to play a crucial role in the eradication of swine fever. In 1961 the CVL achieved recognition by the World Health Organisation as the Third International Laboratory for Laboratory Standards and has remained a reference centre for the storage of standard preparations of a range of vaccines and sera of veterinary importance. The Laboratory also played an important role during major outbreaks of foot-and-mouth disease in 1967 and 2001 and in the bovine spongiform encephalopathy crisis from 1986. In 1990 it became an Executive Agency of the Ministry of Agriculture, Fisheries and Food, a move which allowed it to manage its own affairs with greater freedom than hitherto and to make its surveillance, research and laboratory services available to the private sector for the first time. In 1995, the CVL and the Veterinary Investigation Centres were merged to form the Veterinary Laboratories Agency. Under the new system, the central research and diagnostic functions of the Weybridge laboratories were able to complement the work of the regional laboratories working with farmers and practitioners at a local level.

Anon, 'The Weybridge Veterinary Laboratory During the Second World War', *Veterinary History*, vol 8, nos 3 & 4, 1995; Anon, *Sixty Years Veterinary Investigation Service, 1922–1982* (London, 1982); Anon, 'Central Veterinary Laboratory Weybridge Golden Jubilee 1917–1967', *State Veterinary Journal*, May 1967; Anon, 'The Central Veterinary Laboratory Weybridge 1917–1967', *The Veterinary Record*, 1967; S Foreman, *Loaves and Fishes: an illustrated history of the Ministry of Agriculture, Fisheries and Food 1889–1989* (London, 1989); J W R Pearce, L P Pugh, J Ritchie, (eds), *Animal Health: A Centenary 1865–1965* (London, 1965).

Records (1): Veterinary Laboratories Agency, New Haw, Addlestone, Weybridge KT15 3NB

Annual report of the veterinary department (animal health services from 1948) 1881–89, 1897–; 2nd interim report of the Royal Commission appointed to enquire into the relations of human and animal tuberculosis 1907; report of departmental committee to enquire into the requirements of the public services with regard to officers possessing veterinary qualifications 1913; correspondence and papers re building and furnishing of the veterinary laboratory 1914–18; staff signing in book 1924–26; inoculation book kept by Captain Doyle 1927–39; visitor books 1929–76;

papers re pathological and bacteriological laboratory assistant association 1937–39; case book, tuberculosis order 1938 (unused); order book 1939; laboratory equipment issue book 1943–44; veterinary laboratory staff lists 1945–46, 1964, 1967–72, 1976–77; Veterinary Investigation Service, conference reports 1947, 1949–71 [w]; glanders file 1950–64; indoor technical staff records of examinations 1952; chemical stock check 1952; laboratory book re cattle 1950s–60s; correspondence re setting up of 3rd International Laboratory for Biological Standards 1961–63; staff lists for Weybridge, Lasswade and Reading 1965–70; book recording signatures of those taking part in golden jubilee 1967; draft report of Rayner Review 1981; correspondence and papers from Dr A G Pierce re his article on Weybridge during Second World War 1993; Reading Artificial Insemination Scheme, advisory committee minutes, nd; Dr Stapleforth: photographs taken on trip to Soviet Union 1955, papers re working party on animal husbandry in Istanbul 1957, papers re World Health Organisation expert committee on zoonoses 1958, papers re Cento Seminar on brucellosis, Turkey 1960, drawings to commemorate his retirement 1963, obituary notice, etc 1968, slides, portrait, nd; catalogue for Beck's microscopes 1939; Veterinary Laboratory Research Club: executive committee, minutes 1945–65, general meetings, minutes 1945–71, 1973–78, notices of meetings, lists of officers, staff, etc 1949–64, secretary's reports, programme outlines, etc 1971–74; Technical Staff (later Scientific Officers) Conference, minutes and agenda 1949–75; Veterinary Laboratory Sports and Social Association: programmes, lists of competitors, results and related correspondence 1951–52; photographs: staff, buildings, laboratories, equipment, animals, etc 20th cent; photographs and commentary cards on illness and treatment of Ching-Ching the panda 1980; 8mm films: border disease of lambs 1971, test for aflatoxin in groundnuts, cobalt cure for pining sheep, nd; gaslight lantern plates: horses c1937, graphs and tables of average infection of guinea pigs with brucella abortus c1945, mastitis and brucellosis in Hanover, mastitis, various microscopic organisms, nd; slides of CVL site and work stations, nd; group study slides and notes on various veterinary subjects incl fasciolasis, pig mortality, bovine mastitis, etc, nd; slides re: salmonella in pigs 1961, salmonella 1967, various veterinary subjects, nd, interior of laboratories and library 1987–88; printing block giving charts and tables re experiments in bovine contagious abortion vaccines, nd; misc drawings 20th cent; press cuttings: retirement of Professor G Brown as Chief Veterinary Officer 1893–94, visit to laboratory of representatives of Allied Nations 1943, 'What Weybridge is doing for the Farmer' 1953; invitation, menu and correspondence re Albert Norman centenary dinner 1982; poster of Bob Bevan at work, nd; centenary brochure 1994; golden jubilee celebration leaflets 1967.

Records (2): National Archives, Ruskin Avenue, Kew, Richmond TW9 4DU

Files re: correlation between fluorescence and biological activity 1961–67, collaborative research on mycotoxicoses 1963, vaccine production building scheme and modification to Block A 1974–82. [Ref: AY4/2816, 2879; CM37/10]

Records (3): Archives and Manuscripts, Wellcome Library for the History and Understanding of Medicine, 183 Euston Road, London NW1 2BE

Chief Veterinary Officer's annual report 1913.

List of records of local government

History: Prior to 1866 there was little obligation on local authorities to make adequate provision for the prevention and containment of animal disease. They could pass by-laws or regulations but these applied only to meat and fish and did not include live animals. Only after a serious outbreak of cattle plague in 1865 were local authorities compelled to do more. Under the terms of the Cattle Plague Prevention Act 1866, every local authority had to appoint inspectors with the power to enter any premises thought to be infected. If cattle plague was found, the local authority was to arrange for the slaughter of all infected animals, compensate the owners and ensure that the premises were adequately disinfected. In order to administer the Act effectively, most local authorities set up cattle plague committees. The 1866 Act, though, was followed by a whole series of Acts and Orders that increased the local authorities' responsibilities still further, notably the Contagious Diseases (Animals) Act 1878 which made the employment of veterinary inspectors compulsory. At first, responsibility for administering these Acts and Orders lay with the Quarter Sessions, but following the Local Government Act of 1888 responsibility passed to the newly created County and Borough Councils who appointed Local Veterinary Inspectors to inspect dairies, cow sheds and markets on their behalf. Additionally, the Local Veterinary Inspectors enquired into reported cases of cattle plague, pleuro-pneumonia, sheep pox, foot-and-mouth disease, sheep scab, swine fever, glanders and rabies, all under constant supervision from travelling inspectors sent out by the Board of Agriculture. After the Contagious Diseases (Animals) Act of 1894 became law the Board of Agriculture became the central authority in the handling of animal disease. Local authorities, though, were bound to enforce any Orders the Board made and to appoint veterinary inspectors with full powers to seize all animals, carcasses or organs considered diseased or unfit for human consumption. The Tuberculosis (Attested Herds) Scheme, introduced into England and Wales in 1935, involved Local Veterinary Inspectors in routine inspections of herds and dairies. Following the passing of the Agriculture Act 1937, ultimate responsibility for all local government veterinary services passed to the Ministry of Agriculture and Fisheries. Local authorities, however, still employed Chief Veterinary Officers and inspectors who maintained licensing and hygiene standards in dog boarding and breeding kennels, riding stables and pet shops. They also inspected slaughterhouses, meat plants, ports, markets and railway stations and carried out ante and post-mortem examinations on animals intended for human consumption.

ARGYLL COUNTY COUNCIL
Inveraray, Argyll & Bute

Records: Argyll and Bute Council Archives, Area Office, Manse Brae, Lochgilphead PA31 8QU

Executive committee (under contagious diseases board), minute books 1866–1921 [Ref: CA/3/17]; booklet of instructions to constabulary re cattle plague 1866. [Ref: CSC/1866/2]

BARROW IN FURNESS COUNTY BOROUGH COUNCIL
Barrow in Furness, Cumbria

Records: Cumbria Record Office, 140 Duke Street, Barrow in Furness LA14 1XW

Memoranda books incl slaughterhouse licenses 1888–1902; lease for slaughterhouse 1913; veterinary inspector's letterbook 1915–38; registers of samples re animal inoculation tests 1931–44, 1949–59, 1968–74; register of condemned carcasses 1939–50; veterinary correspondence: proposed cattle market 1886–87, slaughterhouses 1902–25, nd, cattle market committee 1930s, abattoirs and cattle market 1954–64; veterinary aid to Russia fund: minutes, statement of account and correspondence 1942. [Ref: Ba/C 5/1/5, 16–17, 21, 26, 37–38, 41; Ba/C 7/4; Ba/H; Ba/T; BD TB Box 216; BDB 17/8/1–2, 15; BDX 278/20]

BEDFORDSHIRE COUNTY COUNCIL
Bedford, Bedfordshire

Records: Bedfordshire and Luton Archives and Record Service, County Hall, Cauldwell Street, Bedford MK42 9AP

Quarter Sessions' papers re appointment of inspector, killing, burial and other duties re cattle plague 1749 [Ref: QSR1749/76]; bill for advertisement re horned cattle and Woburn Fair 1751–73 [Ref: QSR 1751/73]; diseases of animals sub-committee, papers 1866–1947 [Ref: AG/Sub2]; notification of diseased animal returns 1880–94 [Ref:

AO/A1/1/1–47]; Board of Agriculture and Fisheries, annual reports of proceedings under Contagious Diseases (Animals) Acts, Markets and Fairs (Weighing of Cattle) Acts 1885–1920 [Ref: AO/A1/2/1–22]; procedures under Contagious Diseases (Animals) Act 1890 [Ref: QAV4/2]; Board of Agriculture: special report of veterinary department on pleuro-pneumonia in Britain 1890–91 [Ref: AO/A1/3/2], Director of Veterinary Department's annual report 1891 [Ref: AO/A1/3/1]; returns re outbreaks of swine fever 1899–1923 [Ref: AO/A1/4/1–7]; return re swine fever control 1908 [Ref: BML10/74/8 (iii)]; references to work of veterinary inspectors used by agricultural committee 1920–43 [Ref: AO/C3/1–12]; correspondence and papers re appointment of County Veterinary Inspector and Assistant Veterinary Officer 1935–36 [Ref: GPV24, 27]; Agricultural Officer's correspondence incl references to veterinary officers' fees and appointments 1938–39. [Ref: AO/C4/4]

BERKSHIRE COUNTY COUNCIL
Reading

Records: Berkshire Record Office, Shire Hall, Shinfield Park, Reading RG2 9XD

Police chief constables' reports to the executive committee under the Contagious Diseases (Animals) Acts 1878–1927. [Ref: Q/APR/1/1–3]

BIRKENHEAD COUNTY BOROUGH COUNCIL
Birkenhead, Merseyside

Records: Wirral Archives Service, Town Hall, Hamilton Street, Birkenhead CH41 5BR

Town Clerk's department, health committee, papers re appointment of veterinary officer incl list of duties 1930. [Ref: B/163/65/6, 7]

BIRMINGHAM CITY COUNCIL VETERINARY DEPARTMENT
Birmingham, West Midlands

Results: Birmingham City Archives, Central Library, Chamberlain Square, Birmingham B3 2HQ

Birmingham City Council Veterinary Department, minutes, reports, correspondence and inspections c1914–30s. [Ref: unlisted loc.X27]

BUCKINGHAMSHIRE COUNTY COUNCIL
Aylesbury, Buckinghamshire

Records: Buckinghamshire Records and Local Studies Service, County Hall, Aylesbury HP20 1UU

Correspondence re payment of police costs in an appeal against conviction by Stony Stratford magistrates under the cattle plague legislation 1866–67 [Ref: Q/AP/109/9–49]; Sir T F Fremantle, bundle of reports re cattle plague 1866–69 [Ref: D–FR/108/8]; printed proceedings of the committee on contagious diseases of animals 1877. [Ref: D13/27]

BURY BOROUGH COUNCIL
Bury, Greater Manchester

Records: Bury Archive Service, First Floor, Derby Hall Annexe, Edwin Street, Bury BL9 0AS

Horse and cartage committee, minutes and related correspondence 1876–1902 [Ref: ABU/T689, 1300]; cattle plague committee, minutes 1877–1934. [Ref: ABU/T127]

BUTE COUNTY COUNCIL
Rothesay, Argyll & Bute

Records: Argyll and Bute Council Archives, Area Office, Manse Brae, Lochgilphead PA31 8QU

Buteshire cattle diseases board, minute book 1866–89 [Ref: CB/1/4]; notice re prevention of cattle plague 1866.

CHELTENHAM BOROUGH COUNCIL
Cheltenham, Gloucestershire

Records: Gloucestershire Record Office, Clarence Row, Alvin Street, Gloucester GL1 3DU

Annual report of the director of the veterinary department to the Board of Agriculture with statistics of the various animal diseases 1893. [Ref: CBR/C3/2/1/4/3]

CHESHIRE COUNTY COUNCIL
Chester, Cheshire

Records: Cheshire Record Office, Duke Street, Chester CH1 1RL

Professor Delepine, memorandum on anthrax presented to diseases of animals acts committee 1905 [Ref: CHeX3]; County Veterinary Service, annual reports 1934–36 [Ref: CHeX14]; report on construction of cow sheds and dairies 1938 [Ref: CHeX16]; memorandum of evidence to the committee of enquiry on foot-and-mouth disease 1968. [Ref: CHeX23]

CORPORATION OF LONDON CATTLE MARKETS
Deptford and Islington, London

History: In 1855 the Corporation of the City of London opened a Metropolitan Cattle Market in Islington for the sale and slaughter of livestock. This replaced the cattle market at Smithfield, which re-opened as a dead meat market in 1868. As well as supplying animals to local butchers, however, the Islington market also acted as a distribution centre for livestock. Dealers came from cities such as Birmingham as well as from towns along the south coast to purchase sheep and cattle, which they would then take back for sale in their local markets. By 1865 about 20 per cent of the estimated 5500 cattle passing through the market each week went to other parts of the country for slaughter. Imported livestock was also being brought in to Islington from Europe, although the fact that they were allowed to mix freely with the domestic beasts gave rise to considerable concern. The cattle plague epidemic of 1865–67 led to stricter controls over the importation of livestock. Under the Contagious Diseases (Animals) Act 1869, countries which had suffered recent outbreaks of infectious disease were listed as 'scheduled' and allowed to land their animals only at specified ports. In London, the Foreign Cattle Market was established at Deptford in 1871 specifically for the reception, sale and slaughter of imported animals. It was a relatively small concern during the early 1870s as it received animals from only a limited number of countries, except during the years when the numbers of 'scheduled' countries were high, for example in 1872 and 1877 when there were outbreaks of cattle plague in Europe. After the passing of the Contagious

Diseases (Animals) Act 1878, however, business at Deptford increased, since the Act stated that all imported livestock was to be landed only at designated wharves for immediate slaughter unless the government was sure there could be no danger of disease. After 1890, the numbers of domestic animals being sent to Islington began to fall, largely due to high rail charges, the growth of small markets and the development of the chilled and frozen meat trade. The Foreign Cattle Market, Deptford, also went into decline as imports of European cattle and sheep ceased by 1900 and those from North America, which were in any case landed mostly at Liverpool, ended in 1914. The market at Deptford closed in 1910, although the Islington market continued until 1964.

P E Jones, *The Corporation of London. its origins, constitution, powers and duties* (Oxford, 1950); R Perren, *The Meat Trade in Britain 1840–1914* (London, 1978).

Records: Corporation of London Record Office, PO Box 270, Guildhall, London EC2P 2EJ

Metropolitan Cattle Market, Islington: cattle markets committee, minute books 1872–74, 1893–1964, cattle markets sub-committee, minute books 1875–92, cattle markets committees and sub-committee, papers 1872–1937, 1941–64, cattle markets committee, annual reports of clerks, superintendents and veterinary inspectors 1885–1964 [w], reports re positions of clerk, superintendent and veterinary inspector, nd, inspectors' report books 1864–1901 [w], record of condemned carcasses 1899–1910, return of Corporation appointments incl reference to James King, veterinary surgeon 1908, list of duties and appointment of W G Barnes as veterinary inspector 1910, recommended salary increase for J R Hayhurst, veterinary inspector 1922, annual reports of chief veterinary inspector 1921–62 [w], joint report of clerk, superintendent and veterinary inspector upon sundry matters connected with the market 1900, officer's and clerk's committee reports on petitions re salary of A C Lloyd, assistant veterinary inspector 1929, 1935, and J R Hayhurst, veterinary inspector 1928, delegation of functions to veterinary officer, Geoffrey Stuart Wiggins 1976, 1981, poster re cattle plague 1866, poster re selling and marking of cattle 1866, poster re tolls, dues and payments, nd; Foreign Cattle Market, Deptford: papers, minutes and correspondence 1868–75, notebook with brief committee meeting minutes 1872–74, report on veterinary department 1873, plans 1872, nd, by-laws 1872–73, *London Gazette* articles re opening 1871, report by market committee 1870, papers re sale of building and material 1872, posters re opening 1871 and proposed abolition and conversion into docks 1875. [Ref: Printed Reports

A/3B, 6S, 7A, 15E, 23D, 25X, 27L, 30B, 30K, 32H, 35E, 36R, 44L, 52H, 93E; B/46J; C/17B, L; Market Files Box 1; Delegations Box 1.12, 2.2; Misc.MSS.315.1, 315.3, 316.3–4]

DERBYSHIRE COUNTY COUNCIL
Matlock, Derbyshire

Records: Derbyshire Record Office, County Hall, Matlock DE4 3AG

Derbyshire Quarter Sessions, certificates of fitness to keep slaughterhouses not for butchers' meat 1787–1823 [Ref: QS]; misc papers re cattle plague in Derbyshire 1866; Bakewell Petty Sessions diseases of animals sub-committee, minutes 1857–76 [Ref: D232]; contagious diseases act committee, Derby, records 1869–79 [Ref: D4538]; Bolsover urban district council horse committee, records 1924. [Ref: D1486]

DEVONSHIRE COUNTY COUNCIL
Exeter, Devon

Records: Devon Record Office, Castle Street, Exeter EX4 3PU

Diseases of animals (formerly cattle plague) committee, minute book 1866–86. [Ref: QS/86/3]

DUMFRIESSHIRE COUNTY COUNCIL
Dumfries, Dumfries & Galloway

Records: Dumfries & Galloway Archive Centre, 33 Burns Street, Dumfries DG1 2PS

Contagious Diseases (Animals) Act, administrative minutes, Sanquhar 1870–91 [Ref: SANQB 2/3]; Board of Agriculture, order and returns re swine fever in Dumfriesshire 1895–96 [Ref: BH2/1/8]; press cuttings re foot-and-mouth disease 1952 [Ref: GGD 203/1]; pamphlets re animal husbandry, incl statutes re animal health 1955–83. [Ref: GGD 203/2]

EAST RIDING COUNTY COUNCIL
Beverley, East Riding

Records: East Riding Record Office, County Hall, Beverley HU17 9BA

Cattle plague central committee, minute book 1866–78 [Ref: QAD/1]; cattle plague account book 1866–89. [Ref: QAD/2]

EAST SUSSEX COUNTY COUNCIL
Lewes, East Sussex

Records: East Sussex Record Office, The Maltings, Castle Precincts, Lewes BN7 1YT

Papers re cattle plague, being mainly letters from Privy Council giving orders, granting licences for markets and dealing with compensation claims 1866–69 [Ref: QAV/611]; cattle plague executive committee, minutes 1884–88 [Ref: QAV/6/2]; county veterinary officers' reports included in: Brighton County Borough, baths and washhouses and animal diseases committee, minutes 1885–99 [Ref: DB/B 17/11–14], diseases of animals acts committee and diseases of animals acts sub-committee of county agricultural committee, minutes 1889–1953 [Ref: C/C 11/6/1; C/C 11/59/9–10], Newhaven urban district council sanitary committee, minutes 1935–38. [Ref: DL/D 19/20]

EDINBURGH CITY COUNCIL, VETERINARY SECTION
Edinburgh

History: In 1913 Councillor Bruce Lindsay, prompted by a letter from the Association of Veterinary Officers of Health in Glasgow, proposed in a motion of Council that the City of Edinburgh should establish an independent veterinary department. However, the Town Clerk recommended that any veterinary staff should form a section within the Public Health Department rather than an independent department, reasoning that their duties were 'closely identified with the public health of the City'. The section was duly established in 1913 as a staff of four veterinary surgeons working under a Chief Veterinary Inspector who reported to the Medical Officer of Health. In 1975 control of the Veterinary Section passed to the Environmental Health Committee.

Records: Edinburgh City Archives, City Chambers, High Street, Edinburgh EH1 1YJ

Cattle plague: first report by Commissioners appointed to enquire into the origin of cattle plague 1865 [Ref: inventory box 00 01 01 283A], misc prints 1865–79 [Ref: inventory box 00 01 01 283A], returns in accordance with Contagious Diseases (Animals) Acts 1887 [Ref: inventory box 00 00 87 283C]; Sanitary Department, reports re inspection of meat and abattoirs 1898–1973 [Ref: SL140/1/1–33]; town council treasurer's committee, files re Veterinary Department 1929–59; establishment committee, file re Veterinary Department 1962–75; public health committee: remits incl letter re outbreak of fever in a dairy herd at Rosehall 1875, report on sanitary inspection of dairy at Mid Hermiston 1880, letter re sale of milk from infected dairy herds 1881, report on West Dalry piggeries 1885, copy of Dairies, Cow Sheds and Milkshops Order 1885, report of departmental committee appointed to enquire into pleuro-pneumonia and tuberculosis in the UK 1888, Bailie Russell's notes on tuberculosis 1888, monthly reports on unsound meat seized at slaughterhouse 1888–89, letter announcing deputation of cattlemen concerned with disposal of cattle infected with tuberculosis 1888, reports on seizure of condemned carcasses at slaughterhouses and communication of infectious disease by contaminated milk 1888, motion by Councillor Anderson on reporting on seizure of unsound meat 1888, returns showing number of outbreaks of pleuro-pneumonia conlagiosa traceable to animals from Cumbria 1888–89, duties of inspector and assistant inspector of markets 1889, draft job description for assistant inspector of markets 1889, report on slaughterhouses 1889, report on seizures of unsound meat 1890–91, letter notifying visit of a deputation from Glasgow to investigate procedures for inspection of carcasses 1890, motion by Bailie Russell as to market inspectors re inspection of meat 1891, regulations for dairies, cow sheds and milkshops 1893, report of intention to appoint an Inspector of Dairies 1893, annual report by Inspector of Dairies 1894, letter indicating intention of committee to appoint a veterinary inspector 1895, representation on mange in dairies 1896, letter from Principal Dewar of the Royal (Dick) Veterinary College, Edinburgh, opposing amendments proposed by Glasgow to Public Health Bill 1896, report on condition of byres in Portobello 1896, applications and testimonials of twelve candidates for post of Inspector of Markets 1897, report on seizure of diseased live animals 1897, representation and letter re tuberculous cow at Leith slaughterhouse 1900, letter from horse slaughterer requesting renewal of licence 1902, letters from Board of Agriculture, Edinburgh and Leith Dairymen's Association and Local Government Board and reports by Veterinary Inspector and Medical Officer of Health re importation of frozen boneless meats and offal 1905–06, minutes 1907–75, resolution passed by Association of Veterinary Officers of Health on tuberculosis in milk supply 1911, tuberculosis order from Board of Agriculture and Fisheries re disease in animals and letters re its enforcement 1913, printed list of applications for post of Chief Veterinary Inspector 1914, report on proposed Veterinary Department 1914, Veterinary Department report 1915, letter from Chief Veterinary Inspector requesting release for military service 1915, letters from Veterinary Department re need to increase milk supply 1915, report on first years of Veterinary Department 1916, memorandum re duties of market, veterinary and other inspectors 1898, motion by Councillor Lindsay re Veterinary Department, memorandum for sub-committee of markets committee 1914; reports: Town Clerk on motion by Councillor Bruce Lindsay re proposed Veterinary Department 1914, progress reports 1930–63, Minister of Health and veterinary surgeon re pasteurisation of milk 1931, Minister of Health and Chief Veterinary and Sanitary Inspectors re Glasgow's enquiry as to Edinburgh's co-operation in obtaining powers re certified and/or tuberculin tested milk 1931, Minister of Health and Veterinary and Sanitary Inspectors to public health committee re plant-pasteurisation of milk 1931, duties of Veterinary Inspector 1944. [Ref: DRT 12; ES/A37; SL26; SL123; C4:7, 9; C7:14, 31–33; K1:7]

ESSEX COUNTY COUNCIL
Chelmsford, Essex

Records: Essex Record Office, Wharf Road, Chelmsford CM2 6YT

Quarter Sessions' contagious diseases (animals) committee, minutes 1869–89; contagious diseases (animals) executive committee, minutes 1889–1920; agriculture committee: diseases of animals sub-committee, minutes 1920–47, Beacontree division sub-committee, minutes 1888–98, 1900–01, 1910–12; agricultural committee, minutes 1927–46; diseases of animals committee, minutes 1947–64; joint advisory sub-committee of diseases of animals sub-committee and public health and housing committee, minutes 1934–39; Petty Sessions: Dunmow division, contagious diseases (animals) act sub-committee, minutes 1879–1915, Ongar division, contagious diseases (animals) sub-committee, minutes 1905–14, South Hinckford division, Braintree branch, cattle plague papers 1865–66; Orders in Council re foreign animals not subject to slaughter or quarantine 1884–85; County Treasurer's accounts re expenditure under Cattle Plague Prevention Act 1867–68, 1878; registers of cattle premises 1879–86; returns, correspondence and press notices re cattle plague 1866–67, 1869–79; compensation vouchers to owners of slaughtered animals 1866, 1874–80. [Ref: C/MD/1–3, 1/1–10, 4–5, 7/1–6, 8/1–4, 8/1/1; Q/ACm/33–35; Q/Amd; Q/FAc 9; P/DM/1; P/HZ/4; P/NM/3]

FLINTSHIRE COUNTY COUNCIL
Hawarden, Flintshire

Records: Flintshire County Record Office, The Old Rectory, Hawarden CH5 3NR

Papers re cattle plague 1865–66 [Ref: D/E/2747]; Quarter Sessions, Orders re cattle plague 1866 [Ref: D/E/1303]; Flintshire County Council, Clerk's papers: animal diseases incl veterinary inspection of cattle markets 1919–43 [Ref: FC/C/6/264–95], appointment of veterinary surgeons 1921–24 [Ref: FC/C/6/24], veterinary services 1937 [Ref: FC/C/6/26]; regulations re sheep dipping 1932. [Ref: D/DM/1033/3]

GLASGOW CORPORATION
Glasgow

Records: Glasgow City Archives, Mitchell Library, North Street, Glasgow G3 7DN

Committee on diseases of animals acts: minutes 1878–99 [Ref: C2/25], papers 1864–1916 [Ref: D–TC 8/11], accounts 19th–20th cent [Ref: D–CC 3/23], general papers 19th–20th cent [Ref: D–TC 6/62]; committee of Scotch local authorities, Contagious Diseases (Animals) Act 1878, minutes 1883–91 [Ref: C2/91]; circular to Scotch local authorities re proposed appointment of a representative board 1868 [Ref: MP 19/581, 585]; report by Professor McCall on 1869 Contagious Diseases (Animals) Act 1873 [Ref: MP 3/241 and D–TC 14/2/36/103]; report by sub-committee as to working of 1869 Contagious Diseases (Animals) Act 1876 [Ref: MP 1/132 and D–TC 6/285]; report by Superintendent of Public Parks in Glasgow 1878 [Ref: MP 4/643]; abstract statements of receipts and disbursements 1879–87 [Ref: MP 16/1]; by-laws for foreign animals wharves at: Pointhouse 1879 [Ref: MP 5/92, 97,100 and D–TC 14/2/36/119, 127,137], Plantation 1880 [Ref: MP 6/102], Shieldhall 1886 [Ref: MP 32/347]; memorandum by Town Clerk re rules and regulations suggested by Sanitary Authorities re dairies, milkshops, etc 1880 [Ref: MP 7/66]; memorandum as to working of Contagious Diseases (Animals)

Act 1878 and carrying out relative orders of Privy Council 1882 [Ref: MP 9/704]; circular requesting local authorities of Scotland to appoint representatives to a conference in Glasgow 1883 [Ref: MP 9/708]; minute of conference of representatives and resolutions 1883 [Ref: MP 9/716]; resolutions of local authorities on 1878 Contagious Diseases (Animals) Act 1883–84 [Ref: MP 9/740–744, 748, 752, 756, 758, 766, 762]; draft form of petition to House of Commons for amalgamation of local authorities 1884 [Ref: MP 9/68]; declaration forms for animal owners (blank) 1884 [Ref: MP 9/774–780]; declaration forms for inspector (blank) 1884 [Ref: MP 12/143–156]; remarks by Professor McCall on diseases which render the meat of cattle, etc unfit for human consumption and prejudicial to public health 1884 [Ref: MP 10/621]; notice to owners of horses, etc as to provisions of Contagious Diseases (Animals) Act 1878 re glanders and farcy 1886 [Ref: MP 14/291]; paper by Professor McCall on contagious pleuro-pneumonia in cattle 1887 [Ref: MP 18/50]; epitome of evidence taken by committee of Highland and Agricultural Society of Scotland on pleuro-pneumonia 1887 [Ref: MP 18/62]; minute of conference between sub-committee of health of Glasgow and local authority of Paisley, Renfrewshire, on tuberculosis in cattle with report by Professor McCall and minute of executive committee of Glasgow local authority thereat 1887–88 [Ref: MP 17/301]; report by Professor McCall and Dr Russell on tuberculosis in cattle 1888 [Ref: MP 17/314A]; report by Dr Littlejohn to Board of Supervision on bovine tuberculosis 1888 [Ref: MP 18/58]; report by departmental committee appointed to enquire into pleuro-pneumonia and tuberculosis in the UK 1888 [Ref: MP 19/589]; local authority of Paisley, Renfrewshire: circular with related documents re proposed meeting with Privy Council on tuberculosis 1888 [Ref: MP 17/305], memorandum to Secretary for Scotland and opinions of authorities re tuberculosis 1888 [Ref: MP 17/307]; report by Dr Russell on prevention of disease 1895 [Ref: MP 28/960]; minutes of executive committee of the local authority and sub-committee on glanders 1897–98 [Ref: MP 30/12]; memorandum by Sir Herbert Maxwell, Mr Harcourt Clare and Mr Cook-Trench 1898 [Ref: MP 30/106]; report of royal commission appointed to enquire into administrative procedures for controlling danger to man through the use as food of the meat and milk of tuberculous animals 1898 [Ref: MP 30/78]; reports by Professor McCall 1898–1900 [Ref: MP 30/63]; reports by Professor McCall on glanders 1898, 1900 [Ref: MP 31/565]; report by Professor McCall on rabies and glanders 1899 [Ref: MP 30/996]; report of departmental committee appointed by Board of Agriculture to enquire into and report upon the working of Contagious Diseases (Animals) Acts in as far as they relate to glanders 1899 [Ref: MP 30/52]; report of conference of local authorities in Glasgow on prevention of tuberculosis in relation to meat and milk supply 1900 [Ref: MP 30/109]; necessity for tuberculosis test by Principal Dewar, Edinburgh 1900 [Ref: MP 32/912]; deletion and disposal of cows with tuberculosis 1900 [Ref: MP 32/964]; interim report by Professor McCall to executive committee of the local authority 1900 [Ref: MP 30/36]; memorandum and reports by General Manager of Tramways Department on an outbreak of glanders in Corporation Tramways Department stud and mallein tests in connection therewith 1900 [Ref: MP 30/40,44]; report by veterinary surgeon to the Corporation tramways on glanders outbreak 1900 [Ref: MP 30/46]; report by Corporation bacteriologist re glanders 1900 [Ref: MP 30/50]; report of conference of local authorities in Scotland in relation to meat and milk supply held in Glasgow 1900 [Ref: MP 32/851]; veterinary surgeons' reports re prevention of cruelty to animals 1904–14 [Ref: T–PAR 1]; veterinary surgeon's reports to the Corporation 1906–14 [Ref: C2/1]; proceedings, correspondence, etc re enquiry by Board of Agriculture into charges for Irish cattle at Merklands cattle wharf 1913 [Ref: D–TC 6/61]; duties of and regulations for veterinary inspectors under Milk and Dairies (Scotland) Act 1914 [Ref: C 7/2]; Corporation veterinary surgeon's report re handling and distribution of milk in Canada and US 1926 [Ref: D–TC 14/2/18]; report on bovine tuberculosis 1931 [Ref: D–TC 14/2/21/1347]; report on International Dairy Congress, Copenhagen 1931 [Ref: D–TC 14/2/21/1372]; veterinary inspector's reports re 1925 tuberculosis order 1933 [Ref: D–TC 14/2/22]; memorandum re bovine tuberculosis 1934 [Ref: D–TC 14/2/22/1447]; Highland and Agricultural Society of Scotland: printed conditions for Society in Glasgow 1882 [Ref: D–TC 6/270], minutes of Town Council and other papers re Society's Show in Glasgow 1888 [Ref: MP 19/739], papers re centenary 1922. [Ref: PAV 1/III/18]

GLASGOW MARKETS AND SLAUGHTERHOUSES TRUST
Glasgow

History: The Markets and Fair's Clauses Act 1847 and the Glasgow Markets and Slaughterhouses Act 1865 together enabled the Market Commissioners in Glasgow to appoint an Inspector of Provisions to inspect and seize unsound meat in their markets. Responsibility for inspection, given first to the police, was passed to the Sanitary Inspector in 1867 before being returned to the police again in 1890. But while these measures ensured that Corporation markets were inspected, there was no regulation governing the inspection of private markets. Consequently, there was persistent agitation for a better system of meat and milk inspection during the 1870s and 1880s, especially as the spectre of tuberculosis still loomed large. The Glasgow Markets and Slaughterhouses Trust was set up in an attempt to regularise the inspection of private markets.

Records: Glasgow City Archives, Mitchell Library, 201 North Street, Glasgow G3 7DN

Minutes 1871, 1876–83, 1891–93; abstracts of account 1846–90; invoice book 1884–86; correspondence and papers re inspection of meat 1877, 1885–93; correspondence and papers re by-laws 1864–93; papers, plans, notices, etc re expansion of markets and slaughterhouses, tenders, licensing of jobbers and porters, proposed change of market day, etc 1850–94; general trust correspondence and papers 1874–83, 1891–93; report by sub-committee on diseased meat 1882; report of sub-committee appointed to make enquiries and report with regard to the inspection of dead meat 1891; returned questionnaires re proposed change of market day 1886; book of reference for alteration plans 1864; list of cattle salesmen c1870s; notebook detailing slaughtering dues at market for Milton Street and Moore Street 1864; inventory of machinery, furniture, etc 1913. [Ref: F4]

GLOUCESTERSHIRE COUNTY COUNCIL

Gloucester, Gloucestershire

Records: Gloucestershire Record Office, Clarence Row, Alvin Street, Gloucester GL1 3DW

Diseases of animals sub-committee, minutes 1889–1964. [Ref: CAD/M]

GODMANCHESTER BOROUGH COUNCIL

Godmanchester, Cambridgeshire

Records: Cambridgeshire County Record Office, Shire Hall, Castle Hill, Cambridge CB3 0AP

Privy Council veterinary department, circular re infectious diseases of animals 1881 [Ref: G/14/14]; letters from Whitehall re diseases of animals 1882. [Ref: G/14/13]

GRIMSBY BOROUGH COUNCIL
Grimsby, Lincolnshire

Records: North East Lincolnshire Archives, Town Hall, Town Hall Square, Grimsby DN31 1HY

Diseases of animals committee, minutes 1904–10. [Ref: 1]

HAMPSHIRE COUNTY COUNCIL
Winchester, Hampshire

Records: Hampshire Record Office, Sussex Street, Winchester SO23 8TH

Quarter Sessions: order book incl a conviction for cruelty to animals 1850 [Ref: Q1/42], account books incl re cattle disease 1866–90 [Ref: Q10/1/5, Q10/3/5–6]; Winchester city cattle diseases prevention committee, minutes 1866–70 [Ref: W/B5/10/3]; notice warning about cattle plague in Basingstoke 1866 [Ref: 8M62/99]; Winchester local board cattle diseases committee, minutes 1879 [Ref: W/B4/7]; resolutions of executive committee re Contagious Diseases (Animals) Act 1889 [Ref: 38M49/CC6/1–2]; committee reports re contagious diseases of animals 1889 [Ref: 38M49/CC5/4–5]; minutes of special committee for appointment of County Veterinary Officer 1935 [Ref: H/CX1/48/2]; results of tuberculosis and brucellosis tests and licences for movement of pigs 1950s–74 [Ref: 22M92/205, 211]; file re proposed veterinary inspection and animal health centre, Itchen Abbas 1964–71. [Ref: 39M73/DDC488]

HASTINGS COUNTY BOROUGH COUNCIL
Hastings, East Sussex

Records: East Sussex Record Office, The Maltings, Castle Precincts, Lewes BN7 1YT

Diseases of animals (executive) committee (formerly cattle plague committee 1865–68 and cattle diseases committee 1881–94), minutes 1865–68, 1881–92, 1919–66. [Ref: DH/B 19/8–10; DB/B 33/1–6; DH/B 29/1–2]

HEREFORDSHIRE COUNTY COUNCIL
Hereford, Herefordshire

Records: Herefordshire Record Office, Old Barracks, Harold Street, Hereford HR1 2QX

Return of the inspectors for Fownhope listing owners of horned cattle in the parish 1755 [Ref: Q/AD/1]; agriculture and diseases of animals standing joint committee, reports 1904. [Ref: A63/IV/51/2]

HERTFORDSHIRE COUNTY COUNCIL
Hertford, Hertfordshire

Records: Hertfordshire Archives and Local Studies, County Hall, Hertford SG13 8EJ

Accounts and vouchers re contagious diseases of animals returns 1866, 1873–75; correspondence and reports re removal of animals 1868–69 [Ref: QS/Misc/B/42]; agriculture and contagious diseases of animal returns 1872–74 [Ref: QS/Misc/B/32–33, 40–41]; letter books containing copies of letters from the Clerk of the Peace re contagious diseases of animals 1880–94 [Ref: QS/Misc/B/43]; Dacorum division, *Handbook of the Acts and Orders Relating to the Diseases of Animals* 1894–1945. [Ref: PS/6/10/16]

HOVE BOROUGH COUNCIL
Hove, East Sussex

Records: East Sussex Record Office, The Maltings, Castle Precincts, Lewes BN7 1YT

Contagious Diseases (Animals) Act notices book 1896–1908. [Ref: DO/A 36/3]

HUNTINGDONSHIRE COUNTY COUNCIL
Huntingdon, Cambridgeshire

Records: Cambridgeshire County Record Office, Shire Hall, Castle Hill, Cambridge CB3 0AP

Contagious diseases (animals) acts committee, minute books 1902–20 [Ref: HCC/M/19/1–2]; contagious diseases (animals) acts sub-committee, minute books 1920–39. [Ref: HCC/M/20/1–2]

ISLE OF WIGHT COUNTY COUNCIL
Newport, Isle of Wight

Records: Isle of Wight County Record Office, 26 Hillside, Newport PO30 2EB

County Assistant Inspector, notebook entitled 'Foot-and-Mouth Disease' 1870–1885. [Ref: AC 98/48]

KENT COUNTY COUNCIL
Maidstone, Kent

Records: Centre for Kentish Studies, County Hall, Maidstone ME14 1XQ

County executive sub-committee on diseases of animals (later committee on diseases of animals), minutes 1875–1900 [Ref: Q/GCol/1–2]; veterinary services joint sub-committee of agricultural committee, minutes 1934–38. [Ref: CC/MC/34/5]

KINGSTON TOWN COUNCIL
Kingston upon Thames, Greater London

Records: Kingston Museum and Heritage Service, North Kingston Centre, Richmond Road, Kingston upon Thames KT2 5DE

Regulations made under the Sheep Scab Order of 1928 by the markets and baths committee of the town council acting as the executive committee under the Contagious Diseases (Animals) Act (1894) 1932. [Ref: KT/9/4]

LANCASHIRE COUNTY COUNCIL
Preston, Lancashire

Records (1): Lancashire Record Office, Bow Lane, Preston PR1 2RE

Returns of places infected with cattle plague 1866; licences to hold markets, exhibitions and sales 1867–68; returns made by Manchester under Contagious Diseases (Animals) Act c1870; letter from Veterinary Department to deputy Clerks of the Peace, Preston, re foot-and-mouth disease incl cutting from September edition of *The Veterinarian* 1875; John Bromley and Son of Lancaster, veterinary surgeons, accounts for work done for cattle plague committee 1878; executive cattle plague committee, minutes 1889–1910; Amounderness, Blackburn and Leyland sub-committee, minutes 1889–93; Lonsdale sub-committee, minutes 1889–93; Salford sub-committee, minutes 1889–93; West Derby sub-committee, minutes 1889–93; diseases of animals advisory committee, minutes 1904–1919; diseases of animals acts committee acting sub-committee, minutes 1905–08; agriculture committee diseases of animals sub-committee, minutes 1920–47; county livestock and horse breeding sub-committee, minutes 1921–32; diseases of animals and small-holding committee, minutes 1951–72; county horse breeding committee, minutes 1911–20; rabies standard operating procedure, nd. [Ref: QAC; QAP/3848/34; QSP/3973/54; QSP/4031/5–6; CC/CNM; CC/CNS; CC/DAM; CC/DAS; CC/CDM; CC/CKM; CC/HRM; LCC 18/1]

Records (2): Rawtenstall Library, Haslingdon Road, Rawtenstall, Rossendale BB4 6QU

Memoranda, circulars and correspondence re Contagious Diseases (Animals) Acts 1920s–40s; Diseases of Animals Acts Tuberculosis Orders, correspondence and quarterly statements 1925–38; rodent control workable area committee, minutes and correspondence 1940s–50s. [Ref: Rc 352.4/Rc 352.4 RAW]

LEICESTERSHIRE COUNTY COUNCIL

Leicester, Leicestershire

Records: Record Office for Leicestershire, Leicester and Rutland, Long Street, Wigston Magna, Leicester LE18 2AH

File on proceedings re distemper amongst horned cattle 1748–52 [Ref: QS35/2/1]; handbook of laws and regulations re contagious and infectious diseases among animals 1875 [Ref: QS35/2/2]; cattle plague executive committee, minutes 1878–89. [Ref: QS35/1/2]

LINCOLNSHIRE COUNTY COUNCIL
Lincoln, Lincolnshire

Records: Lincolnshire Archives, St Rumbold Street, Lincoln LN2 5AB

Abstract of information and correspondence re distemper among horned cattle 1748–50. [Ref: KQS/B/3]

LONDON COUNTY COUNCIL
London

History: London County Council was created along with sixty other local authorities by the Local Government Act 1888. The Council replaced the Metropolitan Board of Works (est 1855) and administered an area that was made up of what had previously been parts of Middlesex, Surrey and Kent. Among the responsibilities that passed to the new authority was enforcement of the Contagious Diseases (Animals) Acts. As the Metropolitan Board of Works had been constantly troubled by outbreaks of diseases such as glanders, cattle plague, pleuro-pneumonia and foot-and-mouth, the new Council appointed ten veterinary inspectors to its Public Control Department in 1889. Each was responsible for a district and each was paid £1, 1/ per day plus travelling expenses. As London and its suburbs became more built-up, however, and the policy of slaughtering diseased and contact animals took effect, the outbreaks of disease became fewer. While 2300 cases of glanders were reported in 1899, for example, by 1912 this had fallen to 172. Further duties were conferred by the Public Health (London) Act 1891, including the inspection of anything intended as food with the power to destroy unsound material and the control of dairies and cow sheds. Cow sheds and dairies had been subjected to annual registration under the Metropolis Management (Amendment) Act 1862 and the Council continued this policy. In 1888 there were some 720 cow-houses in London, but the numbers fell steadily, reaching 225 by 1908 and 36 by 1938. In 1904 the Council was granted the power to order the slaughter of any cow suspected of suffering from tuberculosis and to pay compensation to its owner. In 1933 responsibility for the licensing of cow sheds passed to the metropolitan borough councils. Following the Agriculture Act 1937, all local authority veterinary work, including the inspection of cattle, was transferred to the Ministry of Agriculture and Fisheries. The Council, though, continued to employ two lay inspectors to carry out checks on the large numbers of animals coming into London by road and rail. They also visited travelling circuses to check on the condition and welfare of their animals.

Additionally, the Council arranged for veterinary surgeons to make annual visits to London's riding stables and report on the health of their horses.

Records: London Metropolitan Archives, 40 Northampton Road, London EC1R 0HB

Public Control Department: public control committee (sanitary and special purposes committee before 1892), minutes 1889–1965, agenda 1889–1963, presented papers 1889–1965; veterinary surgeons for Public Control Department, subject and policy files 1930–40; departmental committee report 1922; foot-and-mouth disease: general papers 1922–27, press cuttings 1937–61; papers re report of committee on the slaughtering of livestock 1932–33; papers re departmental committee of enquiry into cruelty to British wildlife 1949; anthrax: papers re incident of 1959, general papers 1893–1960; glanders: infringements and incidents 1892–1964, general papers 1892–1912, 1914–52; parasitic mange, general papers 1911–38; rabies and hydrophobia, infringements and incidents 1895–1963, general papers 1896–1938; fowl pest, general papers 1948–60; Control of Dogs Orders and Dogs Act 1906, general papers 1897–1963; Importation of Dogs and Cats Orders: infringements and incidents 1937–63, general papers 1923–62; sheep scab: infringements and incidents 1895–1941, general papers 1920–54; Sheep Pox Order, general papers 1938–52; Johne's disease, general papers 1930–37; destruction of carcasses, general papers 1892–1955; slaughterhouses, general papers 1899–1963; slaughter of horses, general papers 1951–56; slaughter of pigs, general papers 1953–58; transit of animals orders, general papers 1924–60; transit of calves orders, general papers 1955–63; animals (sea-transport) orders, general papers 1930–32; exported cattle protection order 1957, general papers 1957–64; overcrowding of animals in railway trucks, general papers 1955–64; transit of unfit animals by rail, general papers 1957–59; transit of bulls by rail, incidents 1956–60; British Railways guide to staff, general papers 1934–53; transit of small livestock by passenger train, general papers 1952–57; removal of bulls and unfit animals from railway premises to cattle markets, general papers 1928–59; transit of animals by road, general papers 1955–64; records of stock carried by road 1957; importation of animals, general papers 1922–63; horses from Ireland order 1954, general papers 1954; Protection of Animals Act 1911, general papers 1911–59; Pet Animals Act 1951, general papers 1926–61; Animals Boarding Establishments Act 1963, general papers 1957–63; Cruelty to Animals Act 1876, general papers 1925–53; Protection of Birds Act 1954, general papers 1953–57; Markets (Protection of Birds) Order 1964, general papers 1964; Animal Cruel

Poisons Act 1962, general papers 1955–63; notices for public display re regulations 1905–14; misc reports 1893–1933; veterinary attendance on animals at hospitals and establishments of council public health and mental hospitals departments, general papers 1932–37; handbook of orders re diseases of animals to 1965. [Ref: LCC/CL/PH/1/15; PC/ANI/1; LCC/MIN/7236, 9566–9987]

LONDON PORT HEALTH AUTHORITY
London

History: The Sanitary Authority of the Port of London was established by the Corporation of London under the terms of the Public Health Act of 1872 and given responsibility for carrying out checks on imported animals to ensure that they were disease free and for administering quarantine procedures. Although the Public Health (London) Act 1891 created sanitary authorities for London under the supervision of the London County Council, the powers of the Corporation of London as a port sanitary authority were preserved. In 1908 the Sanitary Authority of the Port of London was renamed the London Port Health Authority. Through the Port Health Authority, the Corporation is also responsible for the Animal Quarantine Station at Heathrow Airport, and as such deals with the wide variety of animals and birds imported into the United Kingdom each year.

Records: Corporation of London Record Office, PO Box 270, Guildhall, London EC2P 2EJ

Medical officers of health for the Port & City of London, annual reports 1848–1978; medical officer of health for the Port of London, monthly reports 1880–84; public health committee, minute books, report books and papers 1866–1956; Port of London sanitary committee (later Port of London health committee and Port & City of London health and social services committee), minute books, report books and papers 1872–; royal docks bacteriological meat examination book 1966–73; royal docks detention books 1965–70; Animal Quarantine Station, Heathrow airport: by-laws 1976–, notes on prevention and control of rabies, nd.

MANCHESTER CITY COUNCIL
Manchester, Greater Manchester

Records: Manchester Central Library, Local Studies Unit, St Peter's Square, Manchester M2 5PD

Contagious diseases animals committee, Newton Heath: minutes 1887–88 [Ref: M10/19/6/21], regulations 1886 [Ref: M173/1/4/1]; Manchester Transport Department, correspondence re veterinary service and carriage of animals on buses 1901–46. [Ref: M29 325A, 347A]

MIDDLESEX COUNTY COUNCIL
London

Records: London Metropolitan Archives, 40 Northampton Road, London EC1R 0HB

Clerk's Department: veterinary inspectors' fees and conditions of service 1909–65 [Ref: MCC/CL/DA/001–002], veterinary inspectors' monthly accounts 1961–65. [Ref: MCC/CL/DA/003–004]

MONMOUTHSHIRE COUNTY COUNCIL
Monmouth, Monmouthshire

Records: Gwent Record Office, County Hall, Cwmbran NP44 2XH

Resignation of G W Lewis as county veterinary surgeon 1875 [Ref: QS/P&R 0085–8]; diseases of animals committee, minute books 1937–74. [Ref: unreferenced]

NORTH YORKSHIRE COUNTY COUNCIL
Northallerton, North Yorkshire

Records: North Yorkshire County Record Office, Malpas Road, Northallerton DL7 8TB

Orders in Council, Acts and papers re distemper in horned cattle 1747–54 [Ref: MIC 2038]; accounts, correspondence and papers re cattle plague, foot-and-mouth disease and other diseases 1865–89 [Ref: MIC 2038,

2040, 2043]; minute books of the committee appointed under the Contagious Diseases (Animals) Acts 1869–89. [Ref: MIC]

NOTTINGHAMSHIRE COUNTY COUNCIL
Nottingham, Nottinghamshire

Records: Nottinghamshire Archives, County House, Castle Meadow Road, Nottingham NG2 1AG

Letters re outbreak of distemper 1783 [Ref: C/QAD/7–9]; rules of Cattle Plague Association for Rushcliffe, Thurgarton and Broxtowe incl insurance proposal by James Swinton 1865 [Ref: C/QAD/4–6]; sessions order establishing committees for the prevention of cattle plague 1866 [Ref: C/QAD/10]; papers re cattle plague 1866–1900 [Ref: C/QAD/11–15]; Worksop petty sessions, minutes of local committee for administering Contagious Diseases (Animals) Acts 1880–83 and area sub-committee re same 1889–96. [Ref: C/PS/WD/1/1]

OXFORDSHIRE COUNTY COUNCIL
Oxford, Oxfordshire

Records: Oxfordshire Record Office, St Lukes Church, Temple Road, Cowley, Oxford OX4 2EX

Order of Quarter Session's executive committee appointing chief inspector, inspectors and veterinary inspector under the Contagious Diseases (Animals) Act 1878 [Ref: QSA/2]; Order of Quarter Session's executive committee making new resolutions 1879. [Ref: QSA/3]

RETFORD CATTLE PLAGUE COMMITTEE
Retford, Nottinghamshire

Records: Nottinghamshire Archives, County House, Castle Meadow Road, Nottingham NG2 1AG

Ledger of farmers' claims and compensation 1866–67. [Ref: DD.ME 3/53]

RUTHIN BOROUGH COUNCIL
Ruthin, Denbighshire

Records: Denbighshire County Record Office, 46 Clwyd Street, Ruthin LL15 1HP

Papers re livestock, control of cattle plague and other infectious animal diseases 1865–66, 1875, 1883–85 [Ref: Ruthin QSD/AD/1–18; QSD/FS/6/1–2]; receipts and disbursements, cattle plague rates 1867 [Ref: Ruthin QSD/FR/3/1]; contagious diseases (animals) executive committee, papers 1883–88. [Ref: Ruthin QSD/AC/2/1–3]

SHROPSHIRE COUNTY COUNCIL
Shrewsbury, Shropshire

Records: Shropshire Records and Research Centre, Castle Gates, Shrewsbury SY1 2AQ

Appointment of inspector of hides and skins, Bridgnorth 1800 [Ref: 4478/3/1]; public notices incl local by-laws re slaughterhouses 1853, 1855, confinement of all dogs due to suspicion of 'canine madness' 1853 [Ref: DA2/990/4/4/20–21, 43–44]; slaughterhouse returns and correspondence, blank notices re deceased or unsound cattle 1854 [Ref: DA2/819/2/50–65]; cattle plague: report of special committee 1865 [Ref: 53/53], circular re spread of cattle plague 1865 [Ref: DA2/9990/4/7], rate book 1866 [Ref: P7/B/1/3/1], notice of levying of rate 1866 [Ref: P7/B/1/3/2], relief for those suffering effects of cattle plague 1866 [Ref: P315/L/4/15], special cattle plague rate book 1866 [Ref: P318/Fiche 438–443], cattle plague accounts 1866–67 [Ref: QF/7], assessment book, incl cattle plague rate account 1866–67 [Ref: QF/10/1/5], cattle rate assessment book 1867 [Ref: P75/V/1/1], police committee order for additional constables for cattle plague duty 1884 [Ref: QA/6/4/6/27]; bundle of returns and correspondence under the Contagious Diseases (Animals) Act 1869–71 [Ref: DA2/804/2]; papers re contagious diseases in animals 1869–73 [Ref: DA2/866/2]; correspondence and papers re cattle diseases 1869–76 [Ref: DA2/866/1]; agreement surrendering powers to Salop County Council re contagious diseases in animals 1887 [Ref: DA1/151/75]; foot-and-mouth disease: message from Minister of Agriculture, Fisheries and Food to farmers whose stock have been slaughtered c1968 [Ref: 6175/D/6/4/6], Ministry of Agriculture, Fisheries and Food leaflet to farmers who have lost stock c1968 [Ref: 6175/D/6/4/7], Ministry of Agriculture, Fisheries and Food, list of precautions to be taken 1967 [Ref: 6175/D/6/4/25], Diseases of Animals Act 1950, Foot-and-Mouth Disease of 1928 (Article 19), Order, withdrawal notice, Oxon Hall 1968 [Ref: 6175/D/6/4/26, 6175/D/6/4/36], treasurer's report to Shelton House committee 1968 [Ref: 6175/D/6/4/27], B J Whittingham, County Chairman of National Farmers' Union, letter to W R Howell 1968 [Ref: 6175/D/6/4/28], *Shropshire County News Bulletin* 1968 [Ref: 6175/D/6/4/32]; veterinary study groups, Welsh and West Midland regions: 'Avoid Disease when Restocking' 1968, 'Brucellosis and Restocking' 1968 [Ref: 6175/D/6/4/33–34]; extract from annual report of Veterinary Department of Privy Council Office re importation of animals, nd. [Ref: 327/5/12/6/36]

SOMERSET COUNTY COUNCIL
Taunton, Somerset

Records: Somerset Archive and Record Service, Obridge Road, Taunton TA2 7PU

Cattle plague accounts 1866–89 [Ref: Q\AD/6, 7]; diseases of animals executive sub-committee, minutes 1867–1946 [Ref: C\SH\DA/1–9]; draft orders under Contagious Diseases (Animals) Act 1869 [Ref: Q\AD/8]; diseases of animals reports 1881–1924 [Ref: C\SH\DA/10, C\SH\G\A/16d]; general orders from Board of Agriculture 1894–1914 [Ref: C\SH\DA/12]; local and temporary orders from Ministry of Agriculture and Fisheries 1895–1920 [Ref: C\SH\DA/11]; diseases of animals committee, minutes 1963–69 [Ref: C\SH\G\B/35]; Ilminster petty sessions, Orders in Council and by Quarter Sessions incl reports and correspondence 1865–86 [Ref: D\PS\ilm/10/1–2]; Wincanton petty sessions, contagious diseases (animals) sub-committee, minutes 1878–81, 1886–93 [Ref: D\PS\winc/6/1, 2]; Wilton petty sessions, contagious diseases (animals) sub-committee, minutes 1878–1923 [Ref: D\PS\wil/4/3]; Dunster petty sessions, contagious diseases (animals) sub-committee, minutes 1882–1952; [Ref: D\PS\du/4/3]; Wiveliscombe petty sessions, diseases of animals sub-committee, minutes 1904–52 [Ref: D\PS\wiv/4/1]; Taunton petty sessions, contagious diseases (animals) sub-committee, minutes 1906–42. [Ref: D\PS\tau/4]

STROOD RURAL DISTRICT COUNCIL
Strood, Medway

Records: Medway Archives & Local Studies Centre, Civic Centre, Strood ME2 4AU

Leaflets re humane design of slaughterhouses c1939 [Ref: SRDC/226]; applications for renewal of slaughterhouse licences 1939–45 [Ref: SRDC/226]; Clerk's correspondence re public health matters incl animal slaughter, disposal of animal waste, myxomatosis, meat inspections and contagious diseases 1945–47, 1952–58 [Ref: SRDC/221, 234]; photographs of public health inspectors examining and disinfecting slaughterhouses, a granary and a mobile food shop, nd. [Ref: SRDC/91/14–17]

SURREY COUNTY COUNCIL
Guildford, Surrey

Records: Surrey History Centre, 130 Goldsworth Road, Woking GU21 1ND

Quarter Sessions: comparative statement of number and market value of diseased animals slaughtered by direction of inspectors in Kingston upon Thames district between August and November 1865 as appears in compensation returns and inspectors' reports 1865 [Ref: QS5/1/3A]; general cattle plague committee, minutes 1866–69 [Ref: QS5/14/1]; executive committee for the purposes of the Contagious Diseases (Animals) Acts of 1869 and 1878, minutes 1869–78; minutes and returns of expenditure under 1878 Act to the Agricultural Department, Privy Council Office 1886–88 [Ref: QS5/14/2–6]; County Council: executive committee under Contagious Diseases (Animals) Acts of 1878 and 1894, minutes 1889–1923 [Ref: CC767/32/1–3, CC767/33/1–5]; diseases of animals sub-committee of agricultural committee, minutes 1924–38 [Ref: CC767/36/2/1–3]; notice books under Contagious Diseases (Animals) Acts 1937–89 [Ref: CC580/1–10]; Chief Veterinary Officer's annual report 1930. [Ref: CC228/1/142]

WARWICKSHIRE COUNTY COUNCIL

Warwick, Warwickshire

Records: Warwickshire County Record Office, Priory Park, Cape Road, Warwick CV34 4JS

Contagious diseases (animals) executive committee, reports 1870–89 [Ref: QS/2/2/15]; report of executive committee on remuneration of Clerk of the Peace for work in connection with Contagious Diseases (Animals) Act 1871 [Ref: QS/2/2/23/5]; papers re Contagious Diseases (Animals) Acts 1873–93. [Ref: QS/86/1–20]

WEST SUSSEX COUNTY COUNCIL

Chichester, West Sussex

Records: West Sussex Record Office, County Hall, Chichester PO19 1RN

Quarter Sessions' committee, papers re cattle disease 1877–89; contagious diseases (animals) executive committee, minutes 1889–1920, Lower Arundel division local sub-committee minutes 1898–1916, Steyning division local sub-committee, minutes 1902–08; Arundel division local sub-committee, minutes 1911–14; county agricultural committee, minutes 1920–38, 1947; county agricultural committee and sub-committee, minutes 1939–46; county agricultural committee: county livestock committee, minutes 1913–16, county livestock and light horse breeding sub-committee, minutes 1920–21, diseases of animals sub-committee, minutes 1920–47, county veterinary joint sub-committee, minutes 1934–38; diseases of animals committee, minutes 1950–60; agricultural and small holdings committee, agenda papers 1970–73; Director of Agriculture's Department, Chief Officer's reports 1920–26, 1929–30; Chief Veterinary Officer's first annual report 1936; West Sussex war agricultural executive committee, circulars, reports and returns 1938–43; tuberculosis records 1913–14, 1925–38; Tuberculosis Order 1925. [Ref: QAV/6/W2; WOC/CM11/1–4; WOC/CM83/1–2, 7, 10; WDC/AG1/1/1; WDC/AG4/1/1; SCC959–65, 971, 1018–20, 1078, 1081]

WILTSHIRE COUNTY COUNCIL
Trowbridge, Wiltshire

Records: Wiltshire & Swindon Record Office, County Hall, Trowbridge BA14 8JG

Printed Orders, Acts, correspondence and returns by the Clerk of the Peace 1848–80 [Ref: A1/621/3]; correspondence, printed circulars and notices, reports by the Chief Constable and the executive committee to the Quarter Sessions, records of cattle slaughtered and other papers 1865–86 [Ref: A1/621/5]; minutes of the cattle plague committee and subsequent contagious diseases of animals committee with printed dues for inspectors 1866–81 [Ref: A1/621/2]; printed handbooks of regulations re Contagious Diseases (Animals) Acts, pamphlets re prevention and cure of cattle plague and annual reports of the Agricultural Department 1869–86 [Ref: A1/621/4]; printed notices declaring areas either infected or free of disease 1875–88 [Ref: A1/621/1]; Trowbridge urban district council, veterinary surgeon's report re Surveyor's horses 1877 [Ref: G15/1/48]; printed notices declaring individual farms either infected or free of disease 1879–88 [Ref: A1/620]; accounts 1879–88. [Ref: A1/715]

WORCESTERSHIRE COUNTY COUNCIL
Worcester, Worcestershire

Records: Worcestershire Record Office, County Hall, Spetchley Road, Worcester WR5 2NP

Quarter Sessions' papers re cattle diseases 1865–66 [Ref: 128]; Contagious Diseases (Animals) Act 1878 and the New Orders in Council 1878 [Ref: 498 BA 8681/241 item 40]; by-laws re cattle market auction sales 1891, 1907 [Ref: X496.5 BA 10576, items 9 and 23]; cattle plague folder containing orders of Board of Agriculture re Contagious Diseases (Animals) Acts, incl re swine fever, anthrax, muzzling of dogs, etc and notices about movement of animals, closure of markets, etc late 19th–early 20th cent [Ref: X496.5 BA 11769/11 (ii)]; conditions for sale of cattle at markets 1960s [Ref: 705:507 BA 11, 439/2 (i)]; cattle market, Bromsgrove, reports, plans, correspondence, etc 1960s [Ref: 705:507 BA 11439/2 (ii)]; Ayrshire cattle, inventory details of buyers, correspondence, etc re sale 1964. [Ref: 705:507 BA 11439/2 (iii)]

List of records of education and research establishments

ANIMAL HEALTH TRUST

Newmarket, Suffolk

History: The Animal Health Trust (AHT) was established in 1942 by Walter Reginald Wooldridge. Wooldridge qualified as a veterinary surgeon in 1924 but quickly came to realise that although animals were sometimes suffering unnecessarily because their illnesses were not being diagnosed, the situation was unlikely to improve unless the amount of funded research was substantially increased. His concerns were echoed by the Loveday Committee, which in 1938 recommended that more resources be made available for research. The outbreak of war in 1939 placed an even greater strain on the nation's veterinary surgeons, as food supplies became more important than ever and each new outbreak of disease was guaranteed to stretch the economy's already limited resources still further. Although the Ministry of Agriculture and Fisheries was unable to act, Wooldridge used his position as President of the National Veterinary Medical Association to announce in 1942 the formation of the Veterinary Educational Trust. The Trust, set up with donations from the Royal College of Veterinary Surgeons and the National Veterinary Medical Association, appointed thirteen trustees and a Council of Management – including five out of the six Loveday Committee members. The Duke of Norfolk agreed to act as Chairman. Further financial contributions were made by the horseracing fraternity, which recognised that improved veterinary services would reduce infertility, abortion, early death and career ending injuries, so saving them enormous sums of money. In 1943 Messrs Tattersalls launched the Bloodstock Industry Fund to raise money specifically for the Veterinary Educational Trust. There were two further boosts in 1946 with the offer from Lady Yule of the use of her Newmarket stable, Balaton Lodge, and the purchase of Lanwades Park on favourable terms from Major Durham Matthews. One of the first steps taken by the Equine Research Station, which opened at Balaton Lodge in 1947, was the introduction of a course in stud management. In 1948, the Veterinary Educational Trust became the Animal Health Trust (AHT), and, although it continued to serve its original purpose of reducing mortality rates among animals by increasing knowledge and fighting disease, it also began to explore the possibilities of disease prevention. Extensive research programmes, designed to improve methods of rearing animals with a greater resistance to disease, were introduced, and three new centres were established. The Canine Health Centre (later the Small Animal Centre), set up in 1948 with support from the National Greyhound Racing Society and the Kennel Club, had a number of significant successes, including the discovery of how progressive retinal atrophy, or night blindness, was genetically transmitted in red setters. The Poultry Research Station, established at Houghton Grange in 1948, also scored a significant early success with the introduction of artificial insemination. The Farm Livestock Research Centre, set up in 1957, was also based at Houghton Grange before moving to Lilystone Hall, Essex, where it closed in 1971. Money, however, was always tight, and in 1955 the Agricultural Research Council bought Houghton Grange and all its equipment on condition that the AHT contribute a third of the Station's future running costs. The Equine Research Station continued to flourish, however, and in 1961 the Gladys Yule Surgical Wing was opened, boasting the most advanced equine veterinary complex in the world at that time, including operating and pre-operating examination theatres as well as various laboratories. Also in 1961, the Equine Forensic Laboratories were opened, prompted largely by the Norfolk Report into a series of doping scandals in the late 1950s. One of its first contributions was a survey on behalf of the Porchester Committee into an outbreak of Kebsiella in 1963, the findings of which provided much of the information for the report that followed in 1966. The AHT received its royal charter in 1962 but by 1964 was again in financial trouble and had to rely heavily on the support of individuals and the Home of Rest for Horses in order to survive. Its programme of research and grants continued, however, with pioneering work being carried out in the fields of eye treatment, virology, neuro-surgery and oncology. With the increased movement of horses following the removal of trade restrictions within the Common Market in 1992, the AHT became actively involved in devising tests to prevent the introduction into Britain of previously unknown diseases. It also worked closely with Cambridge University, looking especially at oncology among cats and dogs. By 2000 the Trust was operating a multi-disciplinary centre at Lanwades Park in Newmarket under the corporate title Animal Health Trust. It was acknowledged to be a world leader in animal genetics, and played a leading role within the international consortium that published the genome linkage map of both the dog and the horse. It is currently working on the genome map of the cat. These developments have led to the introduction of a number of DNA tests for inherited diseases, such as progressive retinal atrophy in setters, and severe combined immunodeficiency disease in Arabian horses. In conjunction with the

Humane Genome Sanger Centre in Cambridge, the Trust is now working to identify the genetic basis for lymphoma cancer in both dogs and humans.

R Onslow, *A History of the Animal Health Trust* (private publication, 1992).

Records (1): Library, Animal Health Trust, Lanwades Park, Kentford, Newmarket CB8 7UU

Annual reports 1947–; annual scientific reports 1988–; minutes and related papers re Council of Management and various committees 1970s–; correspondence 1960s–; promotional film on work of AHT 1982–85.

Records (2): in private ownership of Miss Mary Brancker, 38 Streetly Lane, Sutton Coldfield B74 4TU

Report re formation of the Veterinary Educational Trust 1942.

Records (3): Archives and Manuscripts, Wellcome Library for the History and Understanding of Medicine, 183 Euston Road, London NW1 2BE

Annual reports 1949–50, 1953, 1986.

HERIOT-WATT UNIVERSITY
Edinburgh

History: Amongst the courses at the School of Arts established in Edinburgh in 1821 was a series of farriery lectures given by William Dick, who went on to open the Edinburgh Veterinary College in 1823. In 1852 the School of Arts was renamed the Watt Institution, after James Watt the inventor, but changed its name again in 1885 to Heriot-Watt College after receiving an endowment from a trust bequeathed to the city of Edinburgh by George Heriot, formerly goldsmith to James VI. In 1902 the College became a Central Institution, part-funded by the Scottish Education Department, specialising in science and engineering. After receiving university status in 1966, it was renamed Heriot-Watt University. Between 1973 and 1992, the university gradually moved from central Edinburgh to a purpose built campus at Riccarton, on the edge of the city.

Records: Heriot-Watt University Archive, Records Management & Museum Service, Riccarton, Edinburgh EH14 4AS

First report of the School of Arts 1821; second directors' report, incl reference to lectures on farriery given by William Dick 1823; detailed syllabus of lectures on farriery given by William Dick 1822–23. [Ref: SA1/1/1–2]

LISTER INSTITUTE
London

History: In 1889 a committee was set up to investigate the possibility of establishing a British Pasteur Institute, leading two years later to the incorporation of the British Institute for Preventative Medicine (BIPM). A site was acquired at Chelsea in 1893 and the first phase of building completed in 1898. Although a merger with the Sanitary Institute was suggested in 1893, it was with the College of State Medicine (est 1886) that the BIPM ultimately joined forces with later that same year. In 1894 the Institute produced its first batch of therapeutic diphtheria anti-toxin and established a Serum Department at Sudbury, Greater London. To raise much needed funds for research the Jenner Memorial Fund was set up in 1896, while in 1898 the 1st Earl of Iveagh donated £250,000. Lord Lister became chairman of the governing body in 1898 and president in 1904. The following year the BIPM changed its name to the Jenner Institute of Preventative Medicine, although after only four years this was changed to the Lister Institute of Preventative Medicine. A further site was purchased at Elstree, Hertfordshire, in 1902, to which the Serum Department moved in 1903. Although the Lister Institute was admitted as a school of the University of London in 1905, its future was never certain. Proposals were put forward in 1913 which, had they had been carried, would have seen the Institute form part of a new National Institute for Medical Research. The following year the Institute also rejected a merger with the Medical Research Council. In spite of this uncertainty, however, the Institute continued to expand. A Vaccine Lymph Department, established in Cornwall in 1915, continued until 1935, while in 1919 a national collection of type cultures was established. One of the Institute's most notable successes occurred in 1929, when Professor A Harden was awarded the Nobel prize in Chemistry for his work on alcoholic fermentation. During the Second World War the Medical Research Council Blood Research Unit was set up at the Institute. In the later twentieth century there was considerable reorganisation. The laboratories at Chelsea were closed in 1975, followed by the vaccine and sera laboratories at Elstree in 1978. In 1981 a Scientific Advisory Committee was set up to consider applications for the support of research in biomedical sciences, signalling the Institute's new purpose as a grant-making body. As a result, the Council was dissolved in 1982 and the memorandum and articles of association amended.

H Chick, M Hume, M Macfarlane, *War on Disease: a history of the Lister Institute* (London, 1971); L Hall and N Morgan, 'Illustrations from the Wellcome Institute Library: the archive of the Lister Institute of Preventative Medicine', *Medical History*, no 30, April 1986.

Records: Archives and Manuscripts, Wellcome Library for the History and Understanding of Medicine, 183 Euston Road, London NW1 2BE

Annual reports and accounts 1895–1986; minute books: Council of the College of State Medicine 1886–93, acting committee/executive committee of proposed Institute 1890–91, general meetings 1891–1959, British Institute for Preventative Medicine Council 1891–1900, Jenner (later Lister) Institute of Preventative Medicine Council 1901–82, Jenner Institute of Preventative Medicine Governors 1899–1982, building committee 1894–96, finance committee 1895–1936, house committee 1900–03, academic studies committee 1900–02, 1949–73; correspondence and papers re establishment 1889–99; correspondence and papers re College of State Medicine 1886–94; papers re Sanitary Institute 1892–93; papers re animal experiment protests 1889–99; correspondence of Lord Lister 1893–1912; Lord Lister's letters to Dr George Dean 1893–1908; correspondence and papers re organisation and administration 1896–1982; papers re diphtheria anti-toxin 1894; notes on the Serum Department, Sudbury and Elstree 1899, 1904; report on anti-plague serum 1900; correspondence and papers re supply of anti-plague serum 1901–05; testing records: meningo testing books 1916–42, meningococci testing books 1931–33, pneumonia testing books 1931–46, tetanus testing books 1937–53, misc testing books 1907–16, 1922–38, general notes on testing 1904–19, calendar of tests 1920–28; post-mortem books 1924–31; papers re production and distribution of serum and lymph vaccine 1894–1950; correspondence and papers re various research projects 1891–c1940; relations with outside bodies and individuals 1891–1975; papers re property 1820–1971, nd; correspondence, papers, etc re Institute's history 1898–1996, nd; correspondence and misc papers re individuals 19th–20th cent; pamphlets 19th–20th cent; photographs: staff, property, animals, disease, etc 20th cent. [Ref: SA/LIS/A–S]

MOREDUN RESEARCH INSTITUTE
Bush Loan, Midlothian

History: The Animal Diseases Research Association (ADRA) was born out of a public meeting held in Edinburgh on 17 March 1920. Its objective, as stated at the first meeting held the following month, was 'to promote, or assist in promoting, experimental and other research concerning the diseases of farm livestock and of other animals whose health affects that of farm livestock'. District committees were formed to promote the new Association amongst farmers and landowners and a joint committee of investigation set up to determine research priorities. Additionally, two Chief Investigators were appointed, Professor S Gaiger and Thomas Dalling, both of Glasgow Veterinary College, who between them visited every landed proprietor with livestock in Scotland in an effort to enlist support. Members paid an entrance fee of one shilling per score of sheep or sixpence per head of horses and cattle, to a maximum of £10. Annual subscriptions ranged from £1 for large farmers to 2/6- for shepherds and stockmen. The Association's early research base was at Glasgow Veterinary College, which made available a research laboratory and two accessory rooms, a histology laboratory, stabling, a small animal house, sheep quarters and an office. This soon proved inadequate, however, so in 1923 thirty six acres of land were purchased at Moredun, Edinburgh. After extensive building works paid for by an £18,000 grant from the Development Commission and a donation of £10,000 by Falconer Wallace, the Moredun Institute was opened in 1926 with Professor Gaiger as its first Scientific Director. Early the following year a mobile field laboratory was added to the Institute's resources. Meanwhile, in 1923, an agreement on funding had finally been reached with the Board of Agriculture by which the Board would contribute twice the amount raised annually by the ADRA. Diseases to which priority were given in the Institute's early days included braxy, trembling, scrapie, lamb dysentery and grass sickness, while investigations were recommended into sheep and cattle mastitis, tuberculosis and bovine abortion. But while the Institute made some significant advances – notably the development of vaccines for braxy and lamb dysentery during the 1920s and for louping-ill in 1936 – all efforts to understand and cure grass sickness remained elusive, although a tour of the Blairgowrie district of Perth & Kinross by the mobile laboratory in 1928 did yield valuable data. Gradually, new buildings were added, additional staff engaged and the research boundaries expanded to include such diseases as grass staggers and pine, the latter in collaboration with the Rowett Research Institute and the Macauley Institute for Soil Research. In addition, a Mastitis Research Unit was established at Fenton Barns, East Lothian, in 1944, although it closed after just four years. In 1947, Tower Field near Roslin, Midlothian, was acquired. However, the Second World War curtailed the Institute's research, and in some areas work ceased altogether. In spite of this, by 1949 the Institute's Scientific Director, Dr J Russell Greig, was able to point out that of the sixteen major problems affecting sheep and causing heavy losses to farmers, nine could now be controlled and two more partly controlled, while four of the eight main cattle diseases could be prevented or quickly cured and three largely prevented. Over the next thirty years, the Institute continued to expand. A Department of Parasitology was opened in 1955, followed by a new Microbiology building in 1962, a Metabolism and Radioisotope unit in 1964 and a new Pathology block in 1973, quickly followed by a Gnotobiotic unit and a new Biochemistry building. The period between 1970 and 1985 was also a golden one in terms of research, with notable successes in sheep pneumonia and scour in lambs and calves. Work continued into a range of conditions, including louping-ill, Johne's disease, jaagsiekte, malignant catarrhal fever, foot-rot, copper and other trace element imbalances and ovine abortion. By the 1970s, however, work on scrapie had passed largely to the Animal Breeding Research Organisation and in 1983 all scrapie work was transferred to the new Neuropathogensis Unit in Edinburgh. Research into grass sickness recommenced in 1971, funded in part by the Horserace Betting Levy Board, while in 1987 the Equine Research and Grass Sickness Fund was established. In 1973, following discussions with the Council of the Scottish Agricultural College, the Moredun Institute agreed to provide specialist diagnostic services in sheep neuropathology, metabolic profiles for sheep and cattle and virological diagnosis for the Scottish Veterinary Investigation Service. These services were further developed over the years, as was the Institute's reputation as the deer disease centre for Europe. Decreased funding during the 1980s, however, meant that the ADRA had to look increasingly toward the commercial sector. Consequently, in 1987 the ADRA became the Moredun Foundation, and the Moredun Research Institute was established as a wholly owned subsidiary. Additionally, a Trust Fund was set up which in turn created Moredun Animal Health Ltd, focussing on creating products that could be marketed via commercial companies. In 1988, the Moredun Research Institute moved to Pentlands Science Park, Bush Loan.

K Angus, *A History of the Animal Diseases Research Association 1920–1990* (private publication, 1990).

Records (1): Moredun Research Institute, Pentlands Science Park, Bush Loan, Midlothian EH26 0PZ

Animal Diseases Research Association: minutes of first meeting 1920, visitor book 1926–99, annual report and accounts 1928–73; scientific reports 1985–; livestock books 1926–50; laboratory day books 1926–30, 1959–64, 1969–76; files re grass sickness survey incl returned forms noting occurrences and individual case histories, associated reports and paperwork 1967–71; correspondence re: investigations into ovine scrapie 1917–44, Dr Greig's investigations into ovine abortion 1921–40, pine experiment 1930–45, general 1928–44; correspondence and papers re scrapie experiment at Twiglees Farm 1938–43; *Veterinary Journal* 1887–91, 1896–1948; photographs: laboratory at Gilmerton Road 1926, service room at Gilmerton Road c1926, official opening of the Moredun Institute 1927, delegates at the Imperial Agricultural Research Conference 1927, mobile field laboratory 1928, nd, post-mortem yard and post-mortem room c1930, the first library at Gilmerton Road c1930, Dr D R Wilson's laboratory c1930, building work [at Gilmerton Road?] 1953, hill sheep farming committee c1955, constant temperature room for the culture of insect and helminth larvae 1959, the Duke of Edinburgh at the Institute 1962, Scientific Directors: Mr W A Pool (1926–29), Dr J Russell Greig (1929–53), Dr J T Stamp (1953–77), Dr W B Martin (1977–84), Dr Ian Aitken (1985–97), external views of ADRA, nd, external and aerial views of the Moredun Institute, Gilmerton Road, before and after extension, nd, animal accommodation at Gilmerton Road, nd, laboratories, nd, library, nd, Professor W L Williams of Cornell, nd, Theiler, nd, Eichorn, Manninger, Marek, John Mohler and J R G, nd; maps showing individual farms in Roxburghshire (annotated) c1930; maps showing grass sickness incidence in: Scotland c1935, Berwickshire 1935, Fife and Angus c1935, Atholl, Perth & Kinross and Badenoch, Highland c1935, Perthshire c1935, Deeside (Aberdeenshire) c1935, England and Wales 1940; misc annotated maps presumably used in fieldwork, nd.

Records (2): Archives and Manuscripts, Wellcome Library for the History and Understanding of Medicine, 183 Euston Road, London NW1 2BE

Annual reports 1960–61.

ODIHAM AGRICULTURAL SOCIETY
Odiham, Hampshire

History: On 16 May 1783 six men met at The George Inn, Odiham, hoping to establish a society which would encourage the development of agriculture and industry in the town and its surrounding area. Out of this meeting emerged the Odiham Agricultural Society, with forty seven members each paying a subscription of 2/6- per annum. One of the Society's first acts was to organise a ploughing match for subscribers' servants. Always on the look out for ways to improve agriculture, the Society encouraged the cultivation of turnips in Hampshire by acquiring Norfolk turnip seed from the Bath Agricultural Society and selling it on to its subscribers, and actively campaigned for the enclosure of wasteland. Perhaps the Society's most lasting contribution, however, was its involvement in the establishment of the Royal Veterinary College, London. At a Society meeting in August 1785 it was agreed, 'that Farriery is a most useful science and intimately connected with the Interests of Agriculture; that it is in a very imperfect neglected state and highly deserving the attention of all friends of Agricultural economy'. With this in mind, the Society had by 1788 raised enough money to send two boys to the veterinary college at Alfort near Paris. But in 1789, before any further steps could be taken, Granville Penn, a member of the Odiham Society, met Charles Benôit Vial de St Bel, a French veterinarian keen to establish a veterinary college in England, and a whole new plan was formed. With the backing of the Odiham Society, Penn set about raising the necessary funds for a college in England. A London Committee was formed, which first met in November 1790. By February 1791 the Committee had agreed to call itself 'The Veterinary College, London'. At this point the Odiham Society withdrew from the scene. Long term interest in the Society was not sustained and it ceased to meet after 1796.

Anon, *Queries relating to Agriculture, submitted by the Society at Odiham in Hampshire, for the encouragement of that art, to the High Sheriffs of the under-written Counties, etc* (Reading, c1800); M Gotelee (ed), *A Record of the Past History of the Town, Park, Manor, Hundred and Castle of Odiham* (Odiham, 1932).

Records: Southampton Archives Office, Civic Centre, Southampton SO14 7LY

Orders agreed at general meetings 1785; lists of subscribers 1783–95; copies of letters received 1783–91. [Ref: D/LY 25/1–3]

ROSLIN INSTITUTE
Roslin, Midlothian

History: The National Animal Breeding and Genetics Research Organisation (Animal Breeding and Genetics Research Organisation from

1947) was established in 1945 on the recommendation of the Agricultural Research Council and the Agricultural Councils of the UK joint committee, set up to examine the future direction of research in animal genetics and breeding. The new Institute was located alongside the Institute of Animal Genetics on the University of Edinburgh campus under the directorship of Professor R G White. Over the next few years several farms were acquired for field research and large scale breeding experiments in East Lothian, the Scottish Borders, Staffordshire and the Dee Valley in Wales. Following Professor White's retirement in 1950, Dr H P Donald and Professor Waddington were appointed co-directors, Donald taking responsibility for the Animal Breeding Section while Waddington concentrated on the Animal Genetics Section. The two sections were formally separated in 1951, with Donald being appointed director of the renamed Animal Breeding Research Organisation (ABRO) and Waddington director of what became known in 1957 as the Agricultural Research Council Unit of Animal Genetics within Edinburgh University's Institute of Animal Genetics. This latter unit was disbanded in 1980. In 1964 the ABRO moved into a new building next to the Institute of Genetics, which it shared with the Commonwealth Bureau of Animal Breeding and Genetics. During the 1970s and early 1980s, its research parameters were expanded to include genetics and molecular biology. At the same time the network of farms was reduced, with the Welsh farm being sold in 1981, followed by one of the Borders farms in 1990 and the Staffordshire farm at the end of the 1990s. Meanwhile, the Agricultural Research Council Poultry Research Centre had been established in 1947 under the Directorship of Dr Alan Greenwood, formerly Acting Director of the Institute of Animal Genetics, and based in new buildings next to the Institute of Animal Genetics. Several of Centre's staff were recruited from the Poultry Section of the University of Edinburgh's Institute of Animal Genetics and an outstation was set up at Bush, Midlothian. Originally concerned with genetics and breeding the Centre soon expanded its remit to include welfare, anatomy, biochemistry and physiology. The Poultry Research Centre moved to the village of Roslin, Midlothian, in 1980. In 1986 the Animal Breeding Research Organisation, the Institute of Animal Physiology, Cambridge, and part of the Poultry Research Centre were merged to form the Institute of Animal Physiology and Genetics Research, but, following the publication in 1992 of a report drawn up by a committee chaired by Professor W V Shaw, the Edinburgh and Cambridge Research Stations were separated once again, with that in Edinburgh re-emerging in 1993 as the Roslin Institute, under the directorship of Professor Grahame Bulfield, previously head of the Edinburgh Research Station. In 1995, the Roslin Institute was incorporated as a non-profitmaking organisation with its own governing body. Funding was provided by the Ministry of Agriculture, Fisheries and Food, the European Union, the Meat and Livestock Commission, the Milk Development Council and the Biotechnology and Biological Sciences Research Council with additional funds coming from other public and private organisations. Much of the research now carried out at the Roslin Institute focuses on molecular and quantitative genetics of farm animals and poultry science. During the late 1990s, the Institute successfully produced 'Dolly', the first clone to be successfully produced from the cells of an adult mammal. It is now a recognised centre for the study of genomics with a number of livestock genome mapping databases. In addition, the Institute is undertaking a number of major programmes relating to the biology of reproduction, developmental biology and growth, and animal welfare and behaviour.

G W Cooke (ed), *Agricultural Research 1931–1981: a history of the Agricultural Research Council and a review of developments in agricultural science during the last fifty years* (London, 1981); F A E Crew, 'The Genealogy of the Poultry Research Centre, Edinburgh', *British Poultry Science*, 12, 1971; M McKeen, *A Brief History of Roslin Institute* (www.roslin.ac.uk 1999); R G White, *The Origin and Early History of ABGRO* (unpublished manuscript, 1965).

Records (1): Roslin Institute, Roslin BioCentre, Midlothian EH25 9PS

Animal Breeding Research Organisation annual reports 1963–86; Poultry Research Centre, annual reports 1965–86; Roslin Institute, annual reports 1994–.

Records (2): National Archives, Ruskin Avenue, Kew, Richmond TW9 4DU

Files re accommodation for sheep at Roslin incl: payments, note of visit 1983, feasibility study 1982, feasibility report 1984, estimated final accounts, costs payments, correspondence 1977–87. [Ref: FD11/75–77]

ROWETT RESEARCH INSTITUTE
Aberdeen

History: The Rowett Research Institute was established as the Institute for Research in Animal Nutrition in 1913 by the Development Commission and the Scottish Education Department and administered by a joint committee appointed by the North of Scotland Agricultural

College and the University of Aberdeen. First located in a basement of Marischal College, Aberdeen, the generosity of three principal benefactors allowed the Institute to expand during the 1920s. John Quiller Rowett, a London businessman, gifted the crofts of Bridgefoot and Redpool and donated £10,000 towards the building of laboratories. Walter A Reid, the Institute's principal benefactor, gifted the library and the director's house, while J Duthie Webster's gift enabled the Institute to set up the Duthie Experimental Stock Farm. Although initially involved in the study of animal nutrition, under its first director, John Boyd Orr, the Institute broadened its remit to include human nutrition in Britain and beyond. In 1945, Boyd Orr was succeeded by Sir David Cuthbertson. Under Cuthbertson and Sir Kenneth Blaxter, who took over in 1965, the work of the Institute was greatly expanded. The Institute is presently administered by a governing body made up of representatives appointed by the Secretary of State for Scotland, the University of Aberdeen, the Royal Agricultural Society, the Confederation of British Industry and various learned societies. It aims to increase understanding of the biochemical and physiological aspects of animal nutrition and growth and interaction with reproduction, and to investigate aspects of human nutrition.

D P Cuthbertson (ed), *Progress in Nutrition and Allied Sciences Marking Fifty Years of the Rowett Research Institute* (Edinburgh, 1963); W R H Duncan and J A Crichton, *Windows & Worthies: artistic and cultural works in Strathcona House and the Reid Library* (Rowett Research Institute, 1997); D F Smith, 'The use of team work in the practical management of research in the inter-war period: the case of John Boyd Orr at the Rowett Research Institute near Aberdeen', *Minerva*, vol 37, 1999; D F Smith, 'The Agricultural Research Association, the Development Fund, and the Origins of the Rowett Research Institute', *Agricultural History Review*, vol 46, 1998; D F Smith, 'The Early Institutional and Scientific Development of the Rowett Research Institute', in A Adam, D F Smith and F Watson (eds), *To the Greit Support and Advancement of Helth* (Aberdeen History of Medicine Publications, 1996).

Records: Rowett Research Institute, Greenburn Road, Aberdeen AB21 9SB

Minutes 1962–81; annual reports re studies in animal nutrition and allied sciences 1945–53, 1960–; University of Aberdeen and North of Scotland Agricultural College joint committee on research in animal nutrition, minute books 1913–62; farm management minute book 1925–38; staff meetings and meetings of heads of departments, minute book 1922–34; draft scheme for Craibstone Animal Nutrition Research Institute, minute book 1919; alcohol record book 1920–54; papers and technical communications published by the Commonwealth Bureau of Animal Nutrition 1933–70 [w]; joint committee interim report on Institute for Research in Animal Nutrition 1919; papers and correspondence re John Boyd Orr 1937–71; papers and correspondence re staff, research, etc c1930s–; wages and salaries books for Rowett Research Institute, Strathcona House and Duthie Farm 1921–63; copies of theses c1922–40; collected papers and theses from Enzymology Department 1937–68; maps and plans of grounds and buildings 1923–70; photographs and slides incl staff, buildings, events, experimental work, etc 1913; press cuttings and press reports 1922–80s; papers and articles re historical development 20th cent. [Ref: RRI; DML; DPC; DSC; JBO]

ROYAL (DICK) VETERINARY COLLEGE, EDINBURGH
Edinburgh

History: The establishment of this, the first veterinary college in Britain outside London, was due very much to the vision and determination of one man, William Dick. Dick (1793–1866) initially worked alongside his father as a smith and farrier, but also found time to attend John Barclay's lectures on anatomy at Edinburgh University as well as lectures on medicine and chemistry. In 1817 he enrolled at the Veterinary College, London, and after obtaining his diploma the following year returned to his native Edinburgh. At that time there were estimated to be no more than a dozen qualified veterinary surgeons in Scotland, since few could afford the fare to London, the cost of living there for a protracted period or the expensive class fees. During the early 1820s, Dick began lecturing in veterinary science at the newly established School of Arts. By this time, the idea of a veterinary college had already been raised, notably by the Lord Provost of Edinburgh, William Arbuthnot, who in around 1821 had asked the University of Edinburgh to establish a Chair in Comparative Anatomy. Although the University turned down Arbuthnot's idea, it did suggest that a veterinary college be set up with the support of the Highland Society at Edinburgh (later the Highland and Agricultural Society of Scotland). A committee was formed, with John Barclay as its Convener, which in due course recommended that a veterinary course be set up with William Dick as lecturer. Dick's first lecture was given on 24 November 1823 at the Calton Convening Rooms. During the first session forty six lectures, covering the diseases of horses, sheep and cattle, were given to twenty five students, each paying up to two guineas, backed up by clinical sessions at the Dick forge in Clyde Street. During the 1825–26 session, the course was extended to three lectures a week and students were also admitted to classes at the university medical school. Examinations were held at the end of each session and certificates issued by the Highland and Agricultural Society of Scotland to those that passed which declared them 'qualified to practise the veterinary art'. From 1829, all lectures were held at Clyde Street. To accommodate the expanding curriculum and student numbers the premises were extended in 1833, largely at Dick's expense, to include a lecture room, museum, dissecting room, infirmary and forge. Clinical material was provided by Dick's private practice and his 'pauper patients'. The course's growing reputation was enhanced by the government's decision in 1838 to allow Edinburgh graduates to apply for appointments as veterinary surgeons in both the army and the East India Company. From 1844 the college was affiliated to the newly established Royal College of Veterinary Surgeons, but in 1848 it severed all links with the College, choosing once more to offer its own certificate of veterinary competence through the Highland and Agricultural Society of Scotland. Relations with the Royal College of Veterinary Surgeons remained strained for many years, the Highland and Agricultural Society of Scotland in 1876 going so far as to apply to the Privy Council for a charter which would allow them to grant a regularised veterinary diploma. In 1879, however, a settlement was reached by which holders of the Society's certificate were admitted to membership of the Royal College of Veterinary Surgeons. In return, the Society agreed not to hold veterinary examinations after 1881. The middle years of the nineteenth century also proved difficult in other ways. John Gamgee, who had been appointed Dick's assistant in 1856, left within a year following a violent dispute and set up the New Edinburgh Veterinary College in Drummond Street as a direct rival to his former employer's college. The New Edinburgh Veterinary College eventually moved to London in 1865 where it reopened as the Albert Veterinary College. Following Dick's death in 1866 a trust was set up to fund the college with the Lord Provost, Magistrates and Council of the City of Edinburgh all being nominated trustees. William Williams was appointed Principal in 1867 but left in 1873 after a series of disputes. Like Gamgee before him, Williams set up a rival college, the New Veterinary College, Edinburgh, based at Gayfield House. Unlike Gamgee, however, Williams succeeded in taking with him all but nine of the students, as well as the entire staff and the college library, thus leaving the future of Dick's college in considerable doubt. Happier times returned, however, following the appointment of Thomas Walley as Principal in 1875 and the Royal (Dick) Veterinary College as it was known from 1874 was able to gradually increase its student numbers and develop its curriculum. In 1905, management of the college passed from the trustees to a Board of Management. At the same time endowments by Alexander Inglis MacCallum and the trustees of Mary Dick's (sister of William) estate provided for two new Chairs in Pathology and Bacteriology & Physiology. The following year the college was incorporated as The Royal (Dick) Veterinary College, Edinburgh, and the University of Edinburgh was asked to take steps to obtain the power to grant degrees in veterinary science. The Royal (Dick) Veterinary College eventually became an integral part of the University of Edinburgh in 1951, with full faculty status from 1964. The Board, meanwhile, had turned its attention to the growing accommodation problem. After some discussion, land was purchased at Summerhall in 1908 and classes transferred there from Clyde Street in 1916. From 1962, the college operated from two sites. Although the main base continued to be at Summerhall, the Easter Bush Veterinary Centre was opened at Roslin, Midlothian, allowing students to work with farm animals and horses within a rural setting. The faculty was reorganised in 1986 into four departments: Preclinical Veterinary Sciences, Veterinary Pathology, Veterinary Clinical Studies and Tropical Animal Health, while in 1992 the Faculty of Veterinary Medicine was incorporated within the faculty group of Medicine and Veterinary Medicine.

L Auchterlonie, *Sixty Years Back: some light-hearted reminiscences of a Royal 'Dick' Veterinary College graduate* (unpublished typescript, 1868); O C Bradley, *History of the Edinburgh Veterinary College* (Edinburgh, 1923); M Sewell, 'The Royal (Dick) School of Veterinary Studies', *The Veterinary Record*, vol 141, no 9, 30 August 1997.

Records (1): Archivist, Edinburgh University Library, George Square, Edinburgh EH8 9LJ

Researchers should note that access to recent records, ie those covering the last seventy five years, is subject to the prior agreement of appropriate university staff, in accordance with University policies and legislation.

Board of management, minute books 1905–51; Council, minute books 1908–51; board of studies in veterinary medicine: minutes and papers 1974–91, general correspondence 1987–93; property, law and finance committee, minutes 1921–27; education committee, minutes 1924–49; finance committee, minutes 1928–50; veterinary college committee, minutes and papers incl proposals for field station 1953–57; veterinary hospital users committee, minutes 1962–64; Summerhall refectory users committee, minutes, papers, etc 1962–89; buildings committee field station sub-committee (field station buildings committee from 1968), minutes, agenda, papers 1963–93; faculty committee, minutes, papers, etc 1964–; special lectures committee, correspondence, papers, etc 1965–83; postgraduate studies committee, minutes, etc 1965–92; Wellcome research accommodation committee, minutes, reports, papers 1966–84; faculty buildings committee, Summerhall sub-committee (Summerhall buildings committee from 1968), minutes, plans and papers 1966–86; staff appointments committee, minutes, papers 1967–76; faculty standing committee on extra-mural clinical instruction, minutes, agenda, papers 1967–97; board of studies committee on faculty diplomas, minutes, papers, etc 1968–71; higher degree committee, minutes and papers 1968–81; faculty development committee: minutes 1969–71, papers 1964–69, 1984–85; faculty special committee on the survey of examinations, reports, etc 1969–73; faculty recurrent expenditure committee, minutes, agenda, papers 1970–90; staff/student liaison committee, minutes, agenda, papers 1971–85; educational policy committee, minutes, papers 1973–74, 1989–96; library committee, minutes, reports, etc 1974–91; equipment committee, minutes, correspondence, requests for equipment, etc 1974–94; teaching, learning and assessment committee, correspondence and papers 1975–86; vacation grants committee, papers 1975–89; undergraduate selection committee: acceptance/rejection sheets 1976–86, general 1986–87; curriculum standing committee, minutes, agenda, etc 1977–90; faculty further education committee, agenda and papers 1978–84; field station refectory committee, minutes, memoranda, etc 1978–89; audio-visual aids committee: minutes, reports, etc 1979–90, report of working party with questionnaires, statistics 1984–88, deputations and recommendations re facilities 1969–84; honorary degrees committee, minutes, reports, etc 1980–91; special committee on membership of faculty, reports, etc 1981–82; concessions committee, papers 1983–93; development committee working party, minutes, agenda, papers 1985–90; faculty computing committee, minutes and papers 1985–93; readerships committee, minutes, correspondence, etc 1985–93; university development committee (later estates and buildings committee), minutes, agenda, papers 1986–91; academic policy committee: minutes 1987–90, agenda 1987–89, papers and correspondence 1983–90; entrance arrangements committee, minutes, agenda and related papers 1987–91; senatus postgraduate studies committee, minutes, agenda, papers 1987–94; recruitment policy committee, minutes, agenda, papers 1988–91; procedure of chair committees incl personal chair's committee and honorary professorships 1988–93; buildings committee, papers and correspondence 1988–95; curriculum review committee, minutes, papers 1990–91; academic planning and resources committee, minutes and associated papers 1990–96; central management group, minutes, agenda, papers 1991–94;

academic staff promotions committee, correspondence and papers 1991–96; entrance arrangements and requirements and undergraduate selection committee, papers 1992–93; University Grants Committee, correspondence and papers re visits 1961–86; abstracts of accounts 1906–51; ledger 1943–48; cash books 1913–34; treasurer's cash book 1934–51; Bradley presentation fund cash book 1937; cashed cheques 1938–40; income tax and war stock records c1945; weekly wage books for laboratory assistants, grooms, clerical staff, cleaners 1914–37; class fees books 1938–44; wage record cards 1943–55; trial balance book 1948; account book (due) 1904–07; petty cash book 1948–51; physiology department, invoices/receipts 1960–64; extension appeal subscription book 1936, 1939; papers re external examiners' fees, etc 1984–92; lists of staff, vacancies, etc 1964–81; applications and papers re appointments and promotions 1970–72, 1978–98; late working book 1986–87; general correspondence 1969–74, 1984–93, correspondence re non-academic staff and laboratory technicians 1976–82; correspondence re appointment of director of Centre for Laboratory Animals 1980–81; papers and correspondence re staff houses 1974–89; correspondence, etc re retirement presentation to Professor Iggo 1990; correspondence re honorary fellowships, professorships 1964–93; correspondence and papers re election of Dean and Associate Dean 1966–93; papers re Principal and Dean's Group 1989–90; Association of Lecturers, general correspondence 1957–65; personnel files c1930–79; papers re Dean's meetings with Principal 1985–91; Dean's correspondence 1972–93; papers re meetings of heads of departments 1965–82; reports to university Secretary by senior administrative officer 1969–78; annual reports of departments to faculty 1970–88; departmental correspondence and papers: Veterinary Medicine 1948–86, Animal Health 1951–86, Physiology 1952–86, Veterinary Anatomy 1952–86, Veterinary Pharmacology 1953–85, Veterinary Pathology 1953–86, Biochemistry 1964–86, Tropical Animal Health 1964–92, Veterinary Surgery 1971–86, Veterinary Clinical Studies 1988–92; Pathology Laboratory Animal Unit, correspondence and papers 1965–75; correspondence of Anatomy Department professors 1972–79; correspondence re directors of studies 1986–93; correspondence, etc re election of Rector 1957–97; Dr O Charnock Bradley , papers, incl testimonials c1906–43; Professor Henry Dryerre: experimental physiology notebook 1916, correspondence and notes 1922, 1926–36, 1942, nd, notes, etc re aetiology of milk fever 1924–35; F J Elliott, teaching notes c1955; Professor A Iggo: Master of Agricultural Science thesis with notes 1947, experiments notebooks 1957–59, reprint requests, etc 1956–60, undergraduate notebooks, nd; Professor Alan Ramsey Muir, correspondence, etc 1960s–74; Professor J S Spreull, correspondence 1972–77; Universities Central Council on

Admissions, circulars and related papers 1978–94; report and correspondence re faculty animal house and workshop 1981–82; correspondence, etc re: charges for alcohol and methylated spirits 1938–84, regent scheme 1958–83, Edinburgh for Rural Economy 1964–91, Faculty of Veterinary Medicine Research Fund 1964–93, visits to college 1966–91, European Economic Community grants 1968–88, 150th anniversary 1972–73, safety and accidents 1977–93, Centre for Laboratory Animals 1978–87, Centre of Tropical Veterinary Medicine 1978–89, care of animals re Animals (Scientific Procedures) Act 1987, 1984–92, 40th anniversary reunion of the 1950 graduating class 1989–90; correspondence with: research councils 1959–83, Royal Society of Health 1964–76, Horserace Betting Levy Board veterinary advisory committee 1971–92, British Veterinary Association 1978–86; Royal College of Veterinary Surgeons: Council minutes 1985–93, related papers 1976–93, veterinary practice teaching unit committee, reports, etc 1969–79, heads of schools meetings, agenda, reports, etc 1978–93, visitations 1952–90, proposed course on veterinary radiology 1963–66, prizes 1978–84, general correspondence 1977–97; quinquennial estimates 1962, 1966–76; correspondence and papers re: Swann report 1970–77, relationship with University of Pennsylvania 1975–91, Riley report 1988–89; Secretary's working files c1908–48; general faculty correspondence 1977–91; general departmental correspondence 1981–83; student registers 1866–91, 1901–15; student declaration/matriculation books 1866–71, 1890–1915, 1928–42; student fee registers 1886–1904, 1918–36; list of graduates 1911–78 [w]; graduate records 1954–; analysis of applications and acceptances 1961–69; student numbers and statistics except matriculation 1960–82; entry of students into each year, progress and statistics 1986–88; papers, correspondence re admissions 1985–86; seeing practice records 1996–98; Tropical Veterinary Medicine graduate files c1956–69; PhD graduate files 1967–72; Master of Science student files c1956–69; student questionnaire returns 1988; papers re unsatisfactory students 1958–86; estimates for students' books, instruments and special clothing 1964–69; correspondence re student wastage 1967–81; student record cards c1943–55; roll book 1962–74; registers: Physiology I and II 1974–83, Veterinary Physiology 1953–63, 1982–84, 1st year class register 1983–87, 2nd year class register 1983–87; Veterinary Students Council, papers and correspondence 1974–89; student notebooks 19th–20th cent; class lists: pathology 1883–1913, physiology 1884–1912; graduation album 1951–54; Diploma in Veterinary Medicine & Science degree: examination record 1953–61, professional examination results 1953–86, 1st–3rd professional pass lists 1953–87, examination papers 1955–75, correspondence and papers 1964–90; correspondence and papers re teaching of: Veterinary Jurisprudence 1964–77, Poultry Diseases 1971–75;

statistics for teaching time 1981–87; Diploma in Veterinary Science: proposals, etc 1971–72, correspondence re examinations 1989–95, examination results 1952–82, class examination papers 1940–89; Bachelor of Science: Biology examination papers 1928–53 [w], Anatomy examination papers 1922–73 [w], sectional classes, timetables and reports 1976–84, Animal Management, examination arrangements and results 1971–85; Diploma in Tropical Animal Production and Health, examination results 1975–84; Diploma in Tropical Medicine, examination results 1956–73; Doctor of Science degree: example file 1963–77, final professional pass lists 1962–86; Master of Science in Diagnostic Veterinary Pathology, arrangements and results for examinations 1973–78; Master of Science in Veterinary Public Health, correspondence 1973–79; boards of examiners, papers 1978–84; card index of physiology lectures 1937–38; suggested curricula c1941–48; correspondence and papers re curricula 1957–74; correspondence and papers re: centenary postgraduate fellowship 1950–93, Faculty of Veterinary Medicine scholarship fund 1953–89, Carnegie Trust 1958–85, Peter Wilson bequest lecture 1959–92, Association of Fish Meal Manufacturers research award in animal nutrition 1961–79, Commonwealth Bureau of Animal Health prize 1962–86, Sir William Y Darling prize and bequest 1965–85, vacation research scholarships 1966–93, McCaughey prize 1968–84, postgraduate scholarships 1972–83, Birrell Gray travelling scholarships 1972–89, Stewart McDougal prize 1974, William Mawlum Ogilvy gold medal and prize 1974–75, Charnock Bradley memorial lecture 1976–89, William Dick memorial lecture 1976–93, Wellcome Trust awards 1987–91, undergraduate vacation scholarships 1988–89, misc fellowships, scholarships, bursaries and prizes 1986–93, legacies and bequests 1962–87; unnamed architect's plans 1914; Alan Reiach, Eric Hall and Partners, architects: plans for Block B at Easter Bush 1968, report to be put before Summerhall development project sub-committee 1968, brochure outlining plans carried out, with photographs, showing alterations to Summerhall, Edinburgh, and Leahurst Veterinary Field Station, Liverpool c1970s, notes of meetings, plans, etc 1960s–70s; plans, files, etc re development and equipping of Block D 1960s–70s; university works department, plans incl veterinary field station, Centre for Tropical Veterinary Medicine, Summerhall c1958–86; long term planning proposals for Summerhall and Easter Bush 1971; correspondence and plans re Hope Park Church renovations 1979–87; plans re building of sheep unit at Dryden 1984–85; drawings re Summerhall by Lorimer & Matthew, architects c1960s; correspondence, plans and papers re development of Summerhall and veterinary field station 1958–87; correspondence re works in Anatomy and Embryology departments 1951–72; works department, general correspondence 1950–84; Estates and Buildings department plan re proposed layout of upgrading at Summerhall 1990; prospectus for a new small animal hospital c1994; college practice: day books 1874–1942, ledgers 1873–1909, cash books 1907–43, records of charges 1914–28, receipts cash books 1930–48 [w], payments cash books 1907–28, invoice books 1907–42; pathology practice: cash book 1947–48, receipts cash books 1914–41; Leith Forge ledger 1913–16; photographs and prints of staff, students, sports teams, buildings, open days, exhibitions, etc 19th–20th cent; slides of Shields' paintings of cattle, nd; lantern slides of rooms c1916; glass negatives of laboratory, etc, nd; three cases of glass negatives re sheep, cattle, dentition, horses, nd; films: ear cleaning endiscope, spaniel, labrador, cat and alsatian, nd, ear operations on a poodle and Yorkshire terrier, nd; audio tape of William Dick memorial lecture 1969; original artwork for *Anatomy of a Dog*, nd; figures illustrating the paper 'On the Abdominal Viscera of Cercocebus Fuliginosus and Lagothrix Humboldti' by O C Bradley, nd; drawings, photographs and proofs for *Regional and Applied Anatomy of the Domestic Animals* vol 1 by John Alexander Taylor 1951–54; drawing of the arteries, veins and nerves of the horse by Richard Carter, veterinary surgeon, nd; caricature of Professor Richard Owen and men of the new system by R H Laurie 1827; diagram of the proportions of an Arabian quite on a new system by R H Laurie 1827; folder of pathology drawings 1880s–90s; radiographs, nd; pyelograph of the dog's kidneys, nd; Hope Park Free Church roll of honour for 1914–18 war; certificates: Alexander Robertson 1844, George Beattie 1850, James Slater 1852–53, Highland and Agricultural Society of Scotland 1857, nd, William Morris 1864, John Cordell c1874, Andrew Reid c1880, John Beattie 1882–83, W G Gurndred 1899–1900, Harry Leitch Torrence 1911, 1914, misc 19th–20th cent; prospectuses 1877, 1885–1904; college calendars 1911–37 [w]; university calendars 1965–72 [w]; handbook commemorating transfer to new building 1916; college constitution, nd; proofs with handwritten corrections for *The Remarkable Gamgees* by R D'Arcy Thompson c1974; legal papers and correspondence re Dick Trust 1876–1904; copies of letters by William Dick 1841–79; copy of *North British Agriculturalist* incl an account of a meeting of the Town Council of Edinburgh to appoint professors to the Chairs of Anatomy and Cattle Pathology 1871; copy of address by Thomas Walley to Lord Provost, Magistrates and Town Council of Edinburgh re student disturbances of 1887; letters by Thomas Walley re examinations in veterinary subjects 1891–92; charter of incorporation 1906; extract of matriculation of arms 1978; press cuttings: Lulu the terrier injected with germs 1961, field station architecture 1964–71, arson attacks at field station 1991–92, misc 1923–29, c1960–62; William Stokoe, veterinary columnist and broadcaster: press cuttings 1950s–60s, film scripts c1960s, glass negatives, nd, notebook possibly for after dinner speeches, nd; poster, 'Vetting Your Pets', nd; menus and magazines for final year dinner 1956–65, 1968–80; clinical club: papers presented 1949–51, annual dinner menu 1936; staff social club, account book and papers c1962–65; athletic club, records c1960s–70s; riding club, minutes 1938–69; soccer club, minutes 1965–75; correspondence, etc re Student Alumnus Association 1958–91; staff luncheon club, visitor book 1958–67; biological club, members and visitor book 1908–11; menu and guest list for reunion dinner 1990; British Veterinary Association Congress, booklet of events and menu for banquet 1965; letter from John Gordon to Sir Charles Jordan re a calculus 'found in the gall-bladder of an aged cow' 1838; notebooks of recipes c1848, nd; research notes on fat metabolism in sheep 1934–44.

Records (2): The Library, Royal (Dick) School of Veterinary Studies, Summerhall, Roslin EH9 1QH

Notes on lectures on the anatomy, physiology and pathology of the horse delivered by E Coleman at the London Veterinary College, taken down by William Dick [1817–18]; W Gavin, lecture notes and notes from reading on veterinary subjects, Edinburgh Veterinary College 1844–48; J Henderson, notes of lectures on veterinary subjects delivered by T Walley and Professor J McFadyean and on botany at the Royal (Dick) Veterinary College 1888–91; notes of lectures on toxicology and therapeutics, materia medica, etc c1890. [Ref: Vet Lib MS3, 4, 6–22]

Records (3): Edinburgh City Archives, City Chambers, High Street, Edinburgh EH1 1YJ

Report on Professorship of Comparative Anatomy and Veterinary Physic and Surgery 1816; Dick trust: sederunt books 1866–77, misc papers and letters 1866–90, letters from Malcolm MacGregor 1868, rules and regulations 1898, agreement re college 1905, transfer of property 1908; accounts, etc 1866–83; draft charters 1867; letters from John Graham and presentation of veterinary surgeon's memorial re charter 1867–68; veterinary college council, minute book 1870–73; packet of receipts for disbursements 1874; John McKendrick, Professor of Physiology, letter of resignation 1876; Dick trust sub-committee minute books 1883–1905; memorial of opinion of counsel, statements, etc re disturbance by veterinary students at examination 1887; report by Dick College sub-committee on report by Council of Royal College of Veterinary Surgeons 1887; note of accounts to reconstruct college 1888; prospectus 1888; memorandum by trustees re proposed incorporation of an Edinburgh College of Agricultural Science 1891; conditions of management 1895;

documents re college constitution 1906; memorandum re duties of secretary and treasurer 1906; complaints re diseases of animals 1913–32; town council treasurer's committee files re Royal (Dick) Veterinary College 1930–57; city chamberlain's file on sheep dog trials at Braidburn Valley arranged with the college for the Lord Provost's Benevolent Fund 1939. [Ref: 62 Upper; 86 Upper; Bundle 16, 100U; Bundle 25A; Murrayburn 261B, 265B, 283B, 284B, D30:2; C1:8; C2:13–14; C3:1–2; J1:7; J70:9]

Records (4): Edinburgh Room, Edinburgh Central Library, George IV Bridge, Edinburgh EH1 1EG

William Dick: occasional papers on veterinary subjects 1869, trust disposition, settlement and codicil 1858, 1864; New Edinburgh Veterinary College, syllabus 1863–64; prospectus 1888; calendars 1923–50 [w]; programme for centenary celebration bazaar, Music Hall, George Street 1923; *The Centaur*, magazine of the Royal (Dick) Veterinary College 1933–66 [w]; bill to confirm provisional order under Private Legislation Procedure (Scotland) Act 1936 re University of Edinburgh (Royal (Dick) Veterinary College) 1951; Order Confirmation Act 1951.

Records (5): Wellcome Library, Royal College of Veterinary Surgeons, Belgravia House, 62–64 Horseferry Road, London SW1P 2AF

Calendar 1942; examination papers 1955–57, 1961–62.

ROYAL VETERINARY COLLEGE, LONDON
Camden, London

History: This, the oldest of the six British veterinary colleges, was established at Camden Town, London, in 1791. Much of the early pressure to form a college came from the Odiham Agricultural Society, which as early as 1785 was calling for a more scientific treatment of animals and had begun raising money with the intention of sending boys to the veterinary college at Alfort near Paris. However, a chance meeting between Granville Penn, one of the Society's members, and Charles Benôit Vial de St Bel, a graduate of the Lyon Veterinary College, led to a much more ambitious plan being put forward, namely the establishment of a veterinary college in Britain. A London Committee of the Odiham Agricultural Society was formed in 1790 and immediately set about raising the necessary funds. In February the following year the Committee adopted the name 'The Veterinary College, London' and appointed St Bel as its Principal. At a further meeting, held in April, the Duke of Northumberland accepted the presidency while eight vice presidents, eighteen directors and fifteen honorary members were elected. The first students entered the College in 1792 and the first certificate was awarded in 1794, allowing its recipient, Edmund Bond, to 'practise the veterinary art'. Just as the College was finding its feet, however, St Bel, very much the driving force behind the venture, died, reputedly from glanders. The difficulty was deciding how best to replace him, since the only qualified British veterinary surgeon at that time, William Moorcroft, who had trained for a year at Lyon, had little desire to leave his successful practice in London's Oxford Street. Eventually Moorcroft agreed to a joint professorship with a physician called Edward Coleman. Within a short time, however, Moorcroft had returned to his practice, leaving the running of the veterinary college entirely in the hands of Coleman. During Coleman's long reign – he remained until 1839 – he made no attempt to implement St Bel's vision of a three year course providing training and education on the anatomy, physiology and diseases of all domesticated animals. Instead Coleman was content to let standards slip by shortening the length of the course, lowering the entry requirements, concentrating almost exclusively on equine medicine and refusing to allow veterinary surgeons to sit on the examinations board. By the late 1820s critical articles were appearing in the newly established veterinary publications, *The Farrier and Naturalist* and *The Veterinarian*, while in Edinburgh William Dick was attracting widespread support for his rival college. Little in the way of change was achieved during Coleman's lifetime, and any hope of reform following his death in 1839 was quickly dashed by the appointment of William Sewell, Coleman's assistant since 1799. Other appointments, however, proved more rewarding – particularly that of James Beart Simonds as the first Professor of Cattle Pathology in 1842, a post funded by the Royal Agricultural Society of England. The establishment of the Royal College of Veterinary Surgeons in 1844 was an additional boost for those seeking reform, since it set out to raise educational standards and control entry to the profession. Simonds, Principal between 1872 and 1881, was in charge when the Veterinary College was awarded its first royal charter of incorporation in 1875, although the patronage of George IV had ensured its future as The Royal Veterinary College since as far back as 1826. Simonds also oversaw the foundation of the Cheap Practice Clinic in 1879. Known in later years as the Poor People's Out-Patients Clinic, it was aimed particularly at people who could not afford either the Royal Veterinary College's annual subscription or the fees charged by private practices. During the centenary year of 1891 a student union was formed along with a student journal *The Students' Record*. In the same year John McFadyean joined the staff as

Professor of Pathology and Bacteriology. McFadyean went on to become Principal in 1894 and during his long reign was actively involved in a number of major developments, including the acquisition of the College's first x-ray machine in 1895 and the construction of a Research Institute in Animal Pathology (later the Department of Pathology and Infectious Diseases) in 1924. The latter's production of tuberculin and mallein on a commercial scale provided a much-needed boost to the College's finances. Lack of finance was a constant problem, however, and the situation became desperate in 1927 when the College buildings were officially declared unsafe. Frederick Hobday, who had just succeeded McFadyean as Principal, immediately launched the Giant Nosebag Appeal, which raised a total of £135,000. This, combined with a £150,000 government grant, allowed the Royal Veterinary College to buy the freehold of its Camden site and initiate a large-scale construction programme from 1935. The new buildings were formally opened in 1937 by George VI. To complement them, the Beaumont Animals' Hospital, paid for with a legacy, was opened in 1932 to continue the work of the Poor People's Out-Patients Clinic. During the Second World War the College, with the exception of the Beaumont Animals' Hospital, was evacuated to Streatley, West Berkshire. In 1949, the Royal Veterinary College became a University of London school, although the retention of its federal structure allowed it a greater than usual degree of independence. It continued to have its own Council and a full time Principal who was appointed by the Council rather than by the University. In 1955, 450 acres of land were purchased at Hawkshead, Hertfordshire, to which the departments of Medicine and Surgery were moved in 1958. Successful fundraising by the Animal Care Trust, formed in 1982, enabled the Hawkshead site to be expanded. New facilities included the Sefton Equine Surgery Wing, opened in 1986, the Queen Mother Hospital for Animals, opened in two phases in 1986 and 1991, and a number of purpose built pathology laboratories, which were opened in 1995. Additionally, a major refurbishment of the facilities at Camden Town was carried out during the 1990s.

Anon, *The Royal Veterinary College, London 1791–1991* (London, 1991); Anon, *An Account of the Veterinary College from its Institution in 1791* (London, 1973); Anon, *The Royal Veterinary College and Hospital* (London, 1937); E Cotchin, *The Royal Veterinary College, London: a bicentenary history* (Buckingham, 1990); I Pattison, *John McFadyean, a Great British Veterinarian* (London, 1981); J B Simonds, *The Foundation of the Royal Veterinary College, With Biographical Sketches of St Bel, Edward Coleman, William Sewell and Charles Spooner* (London, 1987).

Records (1): The Library, The Royal Veterinary College, Royal College Street, London NW1 0TU

College foundation letters 1790–93; charters c1874–1979; minute books: College 1790–1877, 1922–31, Council 1948–75, governors 1907, 1932, 1936, examinations 1797–1813, 1819–21, general purposes committee 1890–1921, 1930–39 [w], executive committee 1937, 1943, 1973–83, academic board 1937–82, professorial staff committee 1965–82 [w], general committees 1886–98; minutes and accounts re examinations 1790–1830; Council meeting reports 19th cent; attendance books: governors 1953–80, academic board 1953–73; governors and subscribers election lists 1931–38; lists of governors 1840, 1848, c1878; annual reports 20th cent; annual accounts 1904–26; general accounts 1955–70; ledgers and cash books 19th–20th cent; deposit account books 20th cent; student transfer journal re Hawkshead property 1955–91; subscription ledger 1796–nd; standing orders, nd; stock account book 1819–49; seal books 1947–70; calendars, regulations and reports 19th–20th cent; bicentenary scrolls 1991; lists of veterinary surgeons (former students only) 1794, 1798–1842; pupil registers 1794–1907; student lists 1891–1937; student entry books 1839–1930 [w]; students' lecture notes 19th–20th cent; examination records 1791–1844 [w], 1871–82, 1926–33; record of post-mortem examinations for Board of Agriculture 1890–91; matriculation and college reports c1871–83; matriculation book 1870–93; certificates issued by Royal Veterinary College, Royal College of Veterinary Surgeons and Veterinary Medical Association early 19th–early 20th cent; list of medal and prize winners 1882–91, c1910–36; register of medals presented at centenary 1891; professors' comments on the curriculum 19th cent; register of patients treated 1793–1809; patient treatment records, Hawkshead 1950–74; register of diseased horses treated 1819–80; remedies recipe books c1803, 1836, nd; misc regulations 1875–77; William Moorcroft, *Report on Farcy* 1811; James Beart Simonds, scrapbooks, tracts, volumes and manuscripts compiled as first Chief Inspector and Veterinary Advisor to the Privy Council on cattle plague, pleuro-pneumonia, smallpox, other diseases and personalities within the veterinary profession c1828–1900; W J T Morton: *The Pharmacopoeia of the Royal Veterinary College* 1833, extract from notebook entitled 'A day in the veterinary college at Alfort near Paris' 1834; Frederick Hobday, scrapbooks of press cuttings 20th cent; Ernest Cotchin, notes for book on College history 1990; advertising material incl drug and remedy packaging, leaflets and posters, nd; commemorative brochure re opening of residential college and hospital by George VI 1937; promotional video cassettes 20th cent; films 20th cent; student posters re coursework and student societies 19th–20th cent; scrapbook of press cuttings re fundraising for rebuilding of college c1927–37; misc press cuttings 19th–20th cent; report and papers re Camden Town premises 1937–40; architectural plans and drawings: Hawkshead and Boltons Park Farm, nd, general 19th–20th cent; scrapbook re Nosebag Appeal incl letters, autographs, photographs and animal portraits 1934–35; superannuation records c1929; papers and correspondence re staff appointments 20th cent; misc correspondence and staff records, nd; visitor books c1946–74; library donations book 19th cent; library catalogues 1791, nd; autograph collection re publication of *The Veterinary Record* 19th–20th cent; memoranda book, nd; correspondence: Richard A Powys, Secretary 1879–1909, animal treatment and fundraising for rebuilding 19th–20th cent, Beaumont Animals' Hospital 20th cent, general 19th–20th cent; photographs and drawings of premises, students, societies and sports 19th–20th cent; lists of theatre group productions and cast members 20th cent; William Gilchrist, pre-publication draft of book on practical treatment of diseases of the camel 1841; college medical association: ordinary meetings, minutes 1935–40, Streatley division, minutes 1946–56, Camden Town division, minutes 1946–54, field station sub-division, minutes 1936–49, essays c1942; student union: Council, minute books 1949–66, executive committee, minute books 1942–55, general and divisional, minutes 1945–58, minutes and accounts for various sporting clubs, nd, account books 1965–79, nd, magazines 1891–, general papers 20th cent, visitor book 1969–74; Research Institute in Animal Pathology, committee minutes 1926–37; Beaumont Animals' Hospital: accounts, nd, day books 1933–64, patient treatment records 1952–72, x-ray records 1955–59, patient record forms 1966–68; H & W Brown, printers and publishers, correspondence and ephemera re worldwide delivery of *The Veterinary Record*; W J Hall, war-time postcards with messages and biographical notes 1914–20; Veterinary Students' Association of Great Britain and Eire, executive committee minutes 1955–56; correspondence, accounts and reports re Aberdeenshire Rinderpest Association and cattle plague in Scotland 1865–66. [Ref: A M Johnson Collection]

Records (2): in private ownership of Miss Mary Brancker, 38 Streetly Lane, Sutton Coldfield B74 4TU

Photographs of class D students c1910.

Records (3): in private ownership of Dr C A Spinage, Wickwood House, Stanford Road, Faringdon SN7 8EZ

Questionnaire re cattle plague issued in conjunction with French government 1854.

Records (4): in private ownership of Dr Virginia Hobday, c/o 1 Dolphine Lane, Melbourn, Hertfordshire SG8 6AF

Photographs of staff, students, lecture rooms, etc 1890s.

Records (5): Wellcome Library, Royal College of Veterinary Surgeons, Belgravia House, 62–64 Horseferry Road, London SW1P 2AF

Physiology practical notes 1942; information for prospective students pre 1949; preclinical examination papers 1953–54.

Records (6): in private ownership of Mr R D Locke, 4 Rathmore Road, Cambridge CB1 7AD

Photograph of football team with results and some names 1922.

UNIVERSITY OF BRISTOL, SCHOOL OF VETERINARY SCIENCE

Langford, Bristol

History: The veterinary school at Bristol was established in 1949 following the publication of the second Loveday Report (1944) which recommended the creation of two new veterinary schools in Britain. The new school, with an initial intake of thirty students, was formed within the Faculty of Medicine, largely to encourage the full integration of students within the Faculty and to facilitate joint or closely related research amongst its staff. Three departments were created – Animal Husbandry, Veterinary Medicine and Veterinary Surgery. The preclinical school was set up in Park Row, close to the main university campus, while the clinical school and teaching hospital were located at Langford House near Bristol, which already housed a Ministry of Agriculture, Fisheries and Food veterinary investigation centre. During the 1990s the school underwent substantial reorganisation. The three original departments were merged with research groups from the former Institute of Food Research and the Tsetse Research Laboratory to create a single Clinical Veterinary Science Department with four divisions – Companion Animals, Animal Health and Husbandry, Food Animal Science and Molecular and Cell Biology. The preclinical building in Park Row was replaced by a new building at Southwell Street, while the acquisition of the Institute of Food Research's former Bristol Research Station provided additional teaching, research and administrative facilities at Langford. Two new hospital units were built to provide treatment for small animals and horses and the curriculum was totally revised. During the late 1990s the school featured in the British Broadcasting Corporation television series *Vet School.*

J Webster, 'University of Bristol School of Veterinary Science', *The Veterinary Record*, vol 141, no 9, 30 August 1997.

Records (1): Faculty of Medicine, Senate House, Tyndall Avenue, Clifton, Bristol BS8 1TH

Minutes: faculty of medicine 1988–, board of veterinary studies 1987–, veterinary education committee 1994–, veterinary planning committee 1995–, medical sciences management group 1989–, library committee 1989–; examination records 1950–.

Records (2): Department of Clinical Veterinary Science, Langford House, Langford BS40 5DU

Minutes: board of veterinary studies 1989–, veterinary education committee 1989–, quality management and enhancement committee 1989–, veterinary planning committee 1989–, progress of students committee 1989–, year working groups 1989–, department of anatomy teaching committee and staff/student liaison committee 1989–, department of clinical veterinary science management committee 1989–, department of clinical veterinary science teaching committee 1989–, staff/student liaison committee 1989–, department of pathology and microbiology teaching committee staff/student liaison committee 1989–, department of physiology teaching committee 1989–, preclinical staff/liaison committee 1989–, Langford library users group 1989–, hospital management committee 1989–, farm policy committee 1989–, animal users group 1989–, equine steering group 1989–, space committee 1989–; papers re admission, curriculum, teaching, assessment, examinations, prizes and awards, student support, Royal College of Veterinary Surgeons visitations, extra-mural studies 1990s.

Records (3): University of Bristol, Arts and Social Sciences Library (Special Collections), Tyndall Avenue, Bristol BS8 1TJ

Annual reports 1947–; papers re opening of school 1952; papers, visitor book and brochure re opening of Meat Research Institute by Elizabeth II 1968; pamphlets: inauguration of school at Langford 1948, opening of school at Langford 1952; correspondence re construction of buildings at Park Row 1943–55; notes re school by Professor Charles Bruce Perry c1980; information submitted to group visiting from Royal College of

Veterinary Surgeons 1991; video cassette of British Broadcasting Corporation *Vet School* broadcast 1996. [Ref: DM 485, 538, 651, 873, 1446, 1462/1, 1778, 1831/3/1]

Records (4): University of Bristol, Medical Library, School of Medical Sciences, University Walk, Bristol BS8 1TD

Medical library sub-committee, minutes 1951–91; Langford library users group, minutes 1971–.

Records (5): Wellcome Library, Royal College of Veterinary Surgeons, Belgravia House, 62–64 Horseferry Road, London SW1P 2AF

Prospectuses 1946–47, nd; examination papers 1954–56.

UNIVERSITY OF CAMBRIDGE, SCHOOL OF VETERINARY MEDICINE

Cambridge, Cambridgeshire

History: The origins of the veterinary school at Cambridge can be traced back to 1909 when G Sims Woodhead, Professor of Pathology, purchased a piece of land on Milton Road with a view to establishing a centre for the investigation of large animal diseases. In 1923, following several years of agitation by Sir Clifford Allbutt, Regius Professor of Physic, the Institute of Animal Pathology was established at Milton Road. An endowment from the Agricultural Research Council enabled the university to set up a Chair in Animal Pathology, held initially by Professor J B Buxton. In 1935, after discussions with the Royal College of Veterinary Surgeons, the University set up a preclinical course and postgraduate diploma, the final two years of which were to be spent at one of the four established veterinary colleges. Following the recommendation of the second Loveday Report (1944) that two new veterinary schools be set up in addition to the four already in existence, the veterinary school at Cambridge was established in 1949. Initially there were two departments – Animal Pathology (incorporating the former Institute of Animal Pathology) and Veterinary Clinical Studies. Professor Leslie Pugh was appointed as head of the latter department, which was divided into three divisions, namely Animal Health, Animal Surgery and Veterinary Medicine. The first intake of fifteen students was based at Milton Road and Merton Hall Farm, the latter having invested in a herd of Ayrshire cattle and a flock of Clun Forest sheep. A 'temporary' building provided a lecture room, laboratories, an operating theatre and offices. At first, the two departments were placed in separate faculties. Animal Pathology was part of the Faculty of Biology 'B' while Veterinary Clinical Studies was part of the Faculty of Medicine. Later both became part of the Faculty of Medicine, under the supervision of the Faculty Board of Medicine. With the setting up of the School of Clinical Medicine in 1975, however, the administrative system was changed and a Syndicate of Clinical Veterinary Medicine was formed with a new single Department of Clinical Veterinary Medicine. Full faculty status within the Council of the School of the Biological Sciences was awarded in 1992. Over the years the school has continued to expand both its teaching resources and its research programmes, the latter placing particular emphasis on comparative medicine. Its existence has at times, however, been perilous. The school was threatened with closure in 1972 but the crisis was averted after changes to the entry system and an increased student intake. In 1984, due largely to the efforts of Professor Soulsby, at that time Professor of Animal Pathology, the Cambridge University Veterinary School Trust (CAMVET) was set up to raise funds for new projects. Two years later, funds from the British Veterinary Association Animal Welfare Foundation enabled the school to appoint the world's first Professor of Animal Welfare. The Riley Report of 1988 again brought the threat of closure, but a major campaign, including a petition with more than 200,000 signatures demanding that all six UK veterinary schools remain open, together with the manpower review of 1990, ensured the school's survival. During the 1990s, the school underwent substantial reorganisation, during which its curriculum, staff and infrastructure were all upgraded. Two new Chairs were introduced. The first, in Farm Animal Health, Food Science and Food Safety, was funded by Marks & Spencer, while the second, in Equine Reproduction, was paid for jointly by the Childwick Trust and the Thoroughbred Breeders' Association. In addition, the site at Madingley Road was developed to include a Cancer Therapy Unit, opened in 1992, and a new Small Animal Wing, opened in 1994, containing a lecture theatre as well as a central diagnostic laboratory and experimental facilities.

Anon, *University of Cambridge: the veterinary school 50th anniversary brochure* (Cambridge, 1999); L Jeffcott, 'Department of Clinical Veterinary Medicine, University of Cambridge', *The Veterinary Record*, vol 141, no 9, 30 August 1997.

Records (1): Faculty Office, University of Cambridge, Department of Clinical Veterinary Medicine, Madingley Road, Cambridge CB3 0ES

Council of the School of Veterinary Medicine, minute book 1949–70; Veterinary Syndicate, minutes 1975–91; faculty minutes 1992–; management committee, minutes 1989–; veterinary education committee, minutes 1990–; staff-student committee, minutes 1987–; student record cards 1949–; official programme re opening of school 1955; hospital: client records 1997–, anaesthetic records 1994–, x-ray figures 1987–98, Royal Society for the Prevention of Cruelty to Animals annual returns 1988–98; plans for new dairy unit, stable block and post-mortem room 1990s; papers, leaflets, etc re student support and guidance 1990s; Royal College of Veterinary Surgeons visitation: submission 1993, report 1993, follow-up report 1997.

Records (2): New Merton Hall Farm, University of Cambridge, Department of Clinical Veterinary Medicine, Madingley Road, Cambridge CB3 0ES

Professor Pugh's album incl: copy of statement by Allbutt re establishment of a central institute of comparative pathology 1919, copy of Elizabeth II's speech on school opening 1955, seating plan for official dinner 1955, copy of Pugh's inaugural lecture 1955, programme and photographs re opening of Veterinary Investigation Centre 1959, examination papers 1955, photographs of buildings, staff, students, school opening, clinical procedures, etc 1950–60s; photographs re campaign against closure 1989; photograph album used for teaching large animal classes 1980s.

Records (3): Library, University of Cambridge, Department of Clinical Veterinary Medicine, Madingley Road, Cambridge CB3 0ES

Examination papers 1953–; examination papers re Fitzwygram, Lawson, Walley and Williams prizes 1975–; letters of support, correspondence, press cuttings, etc re Riley Committee and threat of closure 1989.

Records (4): Cambridge University Library, West Road, Cambridge CB3 9DR

Institute of Animal Pathology: committee minutes 1912–27, building committee, minutes 1935, papers re elections of professors 1923–37, 1946, Professor of Animal Pathology guard book 1923–28; registry file 1923–28; plans 1925–30; Animal Morphology: elections 1882, registry file re readership 1882–1914; Biology B, minutes of Faculty Board 1926–74 [w]; Faculty of Medicine, board minutes 1926–74; papers re elections to Department of Veterinary Clinical Studies 1950–63; building plans for veterinary anatomy laboratory 1956; Central Animal Services, committee papers, correspondence, etc 1965–82. [Ref: O.XIV.54A; P.IX.1–44; P.XLI.1–2; PVII 1–3; O.XIV.54,54A; CANS 1–87; CUR 39.36; PREM.VII.15; MIN.VII.70–71; CUR 108*; MIN.V.67–74; BIOL(J)]

Records (5): Archives and Manuscripts, Wellcome Library for the History and Understanding of Medicine, 183 Euston Road, London NW1 2BE

Institute of Animal Pathology, director's report 1932–35.

UNIVERSITY OF GLASGOW, FACULTY OF VETERINARY MEDICINE

Bearsden, East Dunbartonshire

History: In 1859 James McCall, a graduate of the Edinburgh Veterinary College, started giving informal lectures in veterinary medicine at his practice in Hope Street, Glasgow. Following the removal of the practice to 399 Parliamentary Road in 1862, formal classes were introduced under the title Glasgow Veterinary College. Although generally recognised to be Glasgow's first veterinary college, McCall's idea was not entirely original. Back in 1834 John Stewart had been appointed to the University (Andersonian) Medical School and had given lectures in veterinary medicine there until around 1840. A royal warrant granted to the Glasgow Veterinary College in 1863 allowed its students to sit the Royal College of Veterinary Surgeons' examinations and the first three students qualified in 1865. Shortly afterwards the College moved to new premises at 83 Buccleuch Street, Glasgow. In 1909 the College was incorporated as The Glasgow Veterinary College and its governors purchased the buildings on Buccleuch Street from Professor McCall. Following its incorporation, the College was duly recognised by the Scottish Education Department as a Central Institution and for the next decade or so received limited funding. By 1914 there were forty eight students studying at the College. However, the lack of any government grant from 1925 inevitably meant a precarious existence, with the College having to rely entirely on student fees and grants from local authorities and private individuals. The government grant was only reinstated in 1945, following the publication of the second Loveday Report (1944) which recommended the retention of all four existing veterinary colleges as well as the creation of two new ones. In 1949 the College was incorporated into Glasgow University's Faculty of Medicine and the following year work began on a new veterinary hospital on the Garscube Estate, three miles from the main university campus. Further expansion at Garscube during the 1960s led to the closure of the Buccleuch Street premises in 1969. It was in 1969 too that faculty status was finally achieved. Three further teaching and research units were acquired – Cochno Farm, a 185 hectare commercial dairy/hill farm, Netherton Farm, a three hectare farm animal teaching and research centre, and Lanark Veterinary Practice, a commercial mixed veterinary practice and residential unit. The 1990s saw substantial reorganisation. The curriculum was restructured between 1994 and 1996, and the six academic departments reduced to four – Preclinical Studies, Pathology, Parasitology and Clinical Studies. In 1996 the practice at Lanark was incorporated into the Department of Veterinary Clinical Studies as a new academic division called General Practice. Facilities at Garscube were upgraded with the opening of the James Herriot Library, the Weipers Centre for Equine Welfare, a Gene Therapy Laboratory and a Laboratory Animal Centre.

'Centenary of the Foundation of the Glasgow Veterinary College', Professor Weipers's address reprinted from *The Veterinary Record*, vol 75, no 3, 19 January 1963; N Wright, 'University of Glasgow Veterinary School', *The Veterinary Record*, vol 141, no 9, 30 August 1997.

Records (1): Glasgow University Archives & Business Records Centre, 77–87 Dumbarton Road, Glasgow G11 6PW

Governors' general and committee meetings minutes 1909–50; memorandum and articles of association 1910; draft royal charter in favour of the Royal Veterinary College of Scotland 1834; royal warrant 1863; register of governors 1931–49; annual returns 1930–49; Faculty of Medicine minutes, etc 1949–68; Senate papers re Faculty of Veterinary Medicine 1986–92; University Court papers re Faculty of Veterinary Medicine 1976–84, 1988–93; veterinary papers of Secretary of Court 1986–88; General Council papers re veterinary school closure 1989; balance sheets and accounts 1910–49; comparative statement of revenue account 1920–31; dairy cash book 1883–84; committee meetings papers: veterinary education board of studies 1949–68, committee on a masters degree 1966; prospectuses 1918–19, 1945–46; student registers 1866–85, 1919–49; register of abandoned, excluded and withdrawn students in medicine, veterinary medicine and dentistry 1939–c1970; confidential reports on students 1924–41; class register 1947–49; class marks registers 1926–43; student record cards: graduates 1954–72, non-graduates 1949–68; British Veterinary Medicine Society, examination results 1950–69; lists of prize winners 1946–48; student rules and regulations 1866; introductory addresses and lectures 1880–84; statement by governors for continuance of College as a teaching institution 1924; staff teaching papers and correspondence, academic council and board, joint committee of the representatives of Glasgow University, the Agricultural and Veterinary Colleges of Glasgow, the Department of Agriculture and the Royal College of Veterinary Surgeons 1946–48; Glasgow University ordinances re establishment of veterinary education 1949–50; W L Weipers' papers re staff salaries, examination results, appointment of College principal, premises and annual reports 1945–49; examinations and other staff/student statistics 1950–60; press cuttings: College reconstruction 1906, College, staff and veterinary medicine 1915, 1949–74; property papers: staff establishment and quinquennial estimates 1947–66, establishment of veterinary field station 1945–54, copies of inventories and College valuations 1937, 1947, revised supplementary list re veterinary hospital, Garscube 1956, certificate of registration of 38 Buccleuch Street to be used as a stable 1950; departmental reports: Veterinary Medicine and Veterinary Parasitology 1982–83, Veterinary Surgery and Reproduction 1984, Veterinary Pharmacology, Veterinary Clinical Biochemistry, Veterinary Physiology and Veterinary Anatomy 1983–86; departmental reviews by University Grants Committee on veterinary education 1988; papers, correspondence and reports re: Faculty of Veterinary Medicine 1968–84, Royal College of Veterinary Surgeons and University Grants Committee visits 1971–88, quinquennial visit 1991, sexennial reports 1974–86, Nairobi link with Medical Faculty and Department of Political Economy 1971–73; Development Campaign Office, papers and correspondence 1990–93; papers, correspondence and press cuttings re campaign against closure 1989–90; veterinary hospital: ledger 1981–87, day books 1981–93, payment by installment book 1990–94, medicine, drugs and surgery accounts 1992–93, safe deposit book 1984–91, small animal case lists 1951–88, large animal case lists 1974–88, case records from clinical office 1982–89, weekend book 1979–87, samples 1981–87; centenary celebration: list of exhibits and demonstrations in veterinary hospital 1962, dinner dance menu and order of proceedings 1962; silver jubilee programme 1974; invitation and menu re farewell luncheon on transfer of College to Glasgow University 1949; correspondence, papers and notes re brochure written by W L Weipers, nd; photographs: James McCall, nd, Arthur W Whitehouse 1944, Sir William L Weipers, nd, academic board c1930, royal warrant 1863, nd, student rules and regulations with first page of student signatures, nd, staff, students and laboratories c1930, 1960, premises and apparatus c1960, nd; Sir Hector Hetherington: speech to graduates 1954, papers re purchase of Cochno Farm as a veterinary field station 1953–61, general correspondence 1937–61; historical notes and articles 1910, 1941, 1960–62. [Ref: DC144/1–10; GUA 36248–9; GUA 3935; ACC127/4/15,

133/1–3, 157/71, 177/1/8, 194/8/8–10, 194/9/1–2, 202/2/16, 210/3/14, 217/14, 245/7/13, 17, 245/8/9, 16, 19, 22–24, 245/9/11–13, 255/1/66, 286/1/1–6, 286/3/1, 286/4/1, 4, 337/78–79, 356/19; DC8/400, 914–917, 938, 948]

Records (2): Faculty Office, University of Glasgow, Faculty of Veterinary Medicine, Bearsden Road, Glasgow G61 1QH

Senate, minutes 1987–92; Faculty: minutes 1968–, agenda 1990–; board of studies, minutes, etc 1957–62; Garscube committee, minutes 1965–92; academic development committee, minutes 1964–90; faculty development committee: agenda 1978–89, academic correspondence 1980–85, papers re equipment 1980–86; faculty progress committee: minutes 1979–87, agenda 1984–87, regulations c1980; faculty library advisory committee, minutes 1979–92; university court committee on animal houses, minutes 1982–85; Wellcome surgical research committee, minutes 1964–90; Dean's Office, papers and correspondence incl re committees, visitations, relations with other bodies, scholarships and prizes, rationalisation and planning 1970s–; Sub-Dean: faculty development committee, minutes and general correspondence 1978–92, Wellcome surgical institute committee, correspondence 1983–91, University Grants Committee, general correspondence 1974–89, staff/student committee, minutes 1969–92, research support committee, minutes, etc 1984–91, academic committee of review, general correspondence 1970–72, academic development committee, papers 1988, animal house committee, minutes 1980–85, papers re: animal cages 1951–91, equipment 1955–82, brucellosis 1968–75, Animals Scientific Procedures Act 1986–90; correspondence re post-graduate examinations 1976–92; correspondence re Acre Road 1970–88; Clerk of the Faculty: outgoing letter files 1984–96, faculty curriculum review committee, minutes 1983–90, faculty of science committee, minutes 1985–89, faculty board of studies committee, minutes, agenda and correspondence 1991–95, faculty information services committee, minutes, agenda and correspondence 1993–96, correspondence and papers re: roads 1952–80, radioactive waste 1964–72, Senate 1968–92, staff/student ratio 1971–84, supplemental grants group 1971–84, Royal College of Veterinary Surgeons' visits 1978, 1987, Agricultural Research Council fellowships 1983–91, external examiners' expenses and entertaining 1984–89, publications 1985–88, grants 1985–90, elections 1986, students 1986–89, response to Riley Committee 1989, Jarrett report 1980s, post-graduates 1990–95, general correspondence 1973–92; correspondence and papers re Swann Committee: general 1970–74, visit 1972, memorandum submitted by Glasgow University Veterinary Medical Association 1972; student record sheets 1945–75, 1988–90; student record cards 1978–86, 1996; records of students who left 1945–53; graduate cards 1986–93; graduate book 1972–80; transfers, exclusions and withdrawals 1969–73; students no longer on the veterinary course 1951–71; student wastage cards 1978–95; student files higher degrees 1980s–90s; student marks sheets 1969–84; official results sheets (copies) 1951–73; professional examination results 1970–93; papers re examinations and prizes 1980–94; progress of direct entries to second year 1949–76; first year progress 1949–80; class lists 1967–81; staff list 1969–74; curricula 1967–77; general information for students 1972–81; general regulations for veterinary course 1980s; papers re scholarships and bursaries 1970–71; instructions received from medical faculty re record keeping for new veterinary faculty 1968; examination regulations 1980s; papers and plans re building and opening of new small animal hospital 1979–86; Department of Veterinary Surgery/Reproduction submission for Royal College of Veterinary Surgeons visit 1987; papers, etc re professorships 1978–97; plans and sketches of Garscube estate 1990s, nd; new accommodation: plans and papers re microbiology building 1970, first equipping of surgical block 1968–69, new building 1962–72, new surgery building 1970–72; Wellcome Surgical Research Institute (University of Glasgow) report 1960–71; correspondence and papers re Weipers lecture 1976–90; papers re William Weipers silver jubilee celebrations 1974; menu for John Robert's dinner 1990; pamphlets: *Experiment on Brute Animals* 1882, *Introductory Lecture*, Charles Cameron 1883, *Public Health as Affected by Food Supply Obtained from Animals,* James McCall, 1884, *The Veterinary Profession as a Career*, Dr A W Whitehouse 1929, *Studying Veterinary Medicine in the University of Glasgow* 1973, *Glasgow Veterinary School 1862–1962*, 1975, *Introductory Address*, John Cleland, nd; prospectuses 1942, 1947; final year magazines 1990, 1992; *The Veteran*, school magazine, 1948–54, 1956–60, 1962; *Garscube Gazette* 1962–71; photographs: staff and students c1950, Garscube from the air 1990s, operation on a horse 1990s.

Records (3): James Herriot Library, University of Glasgow, Faculty of Veterinary Medicine, Bearsden Road, Glasgow G61 1QH

Sir William Weipers: engagement diaries (mostly blank) 1966–85, correspondence and papers re University Grants Committee veterinary sub-committee incl visits to Royal Veterinary College, London 1960, 1965–66, Glasgow Veterinary College 1965, 1971, Royal (Dick) Veterinary College, Edinburgh 1965, Cambridge 1961, 1965, Liverpool 1961, Bristol 1965, 1971, Bristol quinquennial report 1961, Edinburgh quinquennial estimates 1962–67, Glasgow quinquennial estimates 1962–67, equipment for Edinburgh field station 1960–64, equipment for surgery wing at Bristol 1963–67, meetings 1961–67; Professor N G Wright, day books 1976–95; yearbooks 1947–98 [w]; Glasgow University Veterinary Medical Association: minute book 1949–66, membership roll 1953–54; Joshua Bruce, college notebook for pathology, medicine and surgery lectures given by Professor McCall, nd; biology class registers 1890–1919; copy of letter from Professor McCall to Colonel Frederick Smith 1904; James F Forrest, MRCVS certificate 1892; autograph print of John Gamgee 19th cent; print of Joseph [Lorter?] 19th cent; photographs: staff and students c1930, James McCall c1900, Alf Wight c1990, William Weipers, nd.

Records (4): Wellcome Library, Royal College of Veterinary Surgeons, Belgravia House, 62–64 Horseferry Road, London SW1P 2AF

Prospectus 1945; medicine and surgery examination papers 1950–56.

Records (5): Local History Room, Bearsden Library, Brookwood House, Drymen Road, Bearsden G61 3RJ

Milngavie and Bearsden Herald, photographs re Glasgow Veterinary College, incl Malcolm Rifkind's visit 1989, Provost's visit 1989, commencement of work on Weipers Equine Centre 1993, student's charity rodeo 1994–96, petition to save horses 1995, university success 1997.

Records (6): Glasgow City Archives, Mitchell Library, North Street, Glasgow G3 7DN

Claim for state aid 1907. [Ref: MP35.70]

UNIVERSITY OF LIVERPOOL, FACULTY OF VETERINARY SCIENCE

Liverpool, Merseyside

History: Although the idea of a veterinary college in Liverpool had been put forward as early as 1898, it was 1902 before veterinary education was introduced to the city, with the foundation of the Institute of Comparative Pathology and the establishment of an affiliated farm station at Runcorn, Halton. Although the Institute went into liquidation in 1911 and the research unit at Runcorn was sold to the pharmaceutical company Evans Sons Lescher & Webb Ltd, a lectureship in comparative pathology established at the University's Medical Faculty in 1903 proved more successful. Shortly afterwards the University received an offer of £450 per year for five years towards the provision of veterinary education from various interested parties including shipowners engaged in the transport of cattle. This was followed in 1904 by the transfer to Liverpool of the New Veterinary College, Edinburgh (est 1873), and the appointment of its Principal, William Owen Williams, as Professor of Veterinary Medicine and Surgery. Although based within the Faculty of Medicine, the college operated under an independent Board of Veterinary Medicine, renamed the Board of Veterinary Studies in 1912. Students were initially offered a four year course, although a new five year Bachelor of Veterinary Science degree course was introduced in 1914, followed shortly afterwards by a Master of Veterinary Science and a Doctor of Veterinary Science. However, as the college was a teaching school only, graduates still had to sit the Royal College of Veterinary Surgeons' examinations before being allowed to register and practise as veterinary surgeons. It was only after the Veterinary Surgeons Act of 1948 came into force in 1950 that the university's degree carried with it automatic membership of the Royal College of Veterinary Surgeons. Further changes were made in the period following the First World War. J Share Jones, lecturer in Veterinary Anatomy since 1904, was awarded a Chair in Veterinary Anatomy in 1919, while a Chair in Veterinary Pathology, with the title of Care of Animals: Causation and Prevention of Disease, was established in 1926. Two further Chairs, in Veterinary Surgery and Veterinary Pathology, were introduced in 1941 and 1949 respectively. The school's facilities, too, were improved. In 1929, the school moved from Brownlow Street, its home since 1908, to Bedford Street North, a move made possible largely by the Development Commission's recommendation in 1925 that a grant for new buildings be made on a pound for pound basis up to a limit of £15,000. This increase in funding also allowed a veterinary hospital to be built in Pembroke Gardens, Liverpool, in 1928. It was at Liverpool, too, that the first veterinary field station was established, due largely due to the vision and effort of one man, John George Wright, Professor of Veterinary Surgery from 1941. Recognising that the decline of the city dairies and a sharp fall in the number of heavy horses being employed at the docks would lead to fewer large animals being made available to his students, Wright arranged for the lease and subsequent purchase of land at Leahurst on the Wirral. This allowed his students to gain valuable experience in large animal work in a rural setting and improved the level of training they received in farm animal practice. By 1952, the school had expanded to such an extent that it gained independence from the Faculty of Medicine, becoming the Faculty of Veterinary Science. The duties of the former Board of Veterinary Studies were taken over by a new Board of the Faculty of Veterinary Science. Initially there were four departments within the Faculty: Veterinary Surgery and Veterinary Preventative Medicine, both based at Leahurst, and Veterinary Anatomy and Veterinary Pathology, based at Bedford Street North. In 1960 the latter two relocated to a purpose built building on Brownlow Hill. Between 1967 and 1971 the Leahurst premises was expanded and in 1977 a nearby veterinary practice was acquired for teaching purposes. Also in 1977, the animal hospital in Pembroke Gardens was replaced with a new hospital alongside the main building on Brownlow Hill. The Faculty's structure was reoganised in 1983 into three main departments, Veterinary Preclinical Sciences, Veterinary Pathology and Veterinary Clinical Science & Animal Husbandry, with the last of these split into divisions along species lines. In the early 1990s, the Faculty initiated a vigorous development campaign to improve its clinical, research and teaching facilities, out of which emerged the Philip Leverhulme Large Animal Hospital, opened in 1995, and the Farm Animal Hospital, opened in 1996. By 2000 plans were underway to build a new Small Animal Hospital that would consolidate all the clinical facilities at Leahurst.

C Gaskell, 'University of Liverpool Faculty of Veterinary Science', *The Veterinary Record*, vol 141, no 9, 30 August 1997; S Harrop, *Decade of Change, The University of Liverpool 1981–1991* (Liverpool, 1994); T Kelly, *For Advancement of Learning: the University of Liverpool 1881–1981* (Liverpool, 1981); M Procter (ed), *Education on Merseyside: a guide to the sources* (Liverpool, 1992).

Records (1): Department of Special Collections and Archives, Sydney Jones Library, University of Liverpool, PO Box 123, Liverpool L69 3DA

Royal College of Veterinary Surgeons, minutes and correspondence re establishment of school (p) 1904; royal warrant affiliating veterinary school to Royal College of Veterinary Surgeons 1904; papers re establishment and early development c1904–12; Board of Veterinary Studies (of the Faculty of Medicine), later the Board of the Faculty of Veterinary Science: minute books 1904–68, 1978–93, report books 1908–69, 1984–94; petition to Privy Council re grant of charter to Royal College of Veterinary Surgeons (copy) 1921; trust deeds re William Prescott Chair of the Care of Animals 1924; managing committee of the Board of Veterinary Studies, minute book 1906–13; veterinary building committee, minute book 1950–52; veterinary building sub-committee, minute book 1955–63; committee on progress of students, minute books 1960–68, 1982–91; Leahurst veterinary field station building sub-committee, minute books 1965–69; staff-student committee, minutes

1969–91; Leahurst management committee, minutes 1974–83; research committee, minutes and reports 1983–91; general purposes committee, minutes 1986–96; committee for staff development and appraisal, minutes 1987–91; committee for animal experimentation and usage, minutes 1989–93; faculty review committee, minutes and agenda 1990–95; preclinical core course steering group, minutes and agenda 1991–96; Dean's Leahurst advisory group, minutes, agenda and related papers 1994–97; sub-group of the academic committee of the faculty, minutes, agenda and related papers 1996–99; Faculty Deans and Administrators' meetings, summaries, agenda and notes 1993–96; operational statistics 1985–88; annual review papers 1991–96; correspondence and papers re planning and restructuring 1982–87; faculty handbooks 1982–93; Royal College of Veterinary Surgeons' examinations marks book 1904–35; veterinary anatomy text books (copies) 1978–87; staff research and teaching papers and correspondence: Howel Vaughan Hughes 1905–93, C Wentworth Elam c1910–66, J Share Jones 1913–49, S H Gaiger, G O Davies and Thomas Dalling 1920–32, nd, A C Shuttleworth 1927–62, E J H Ford 1936–43, J G Wright 1941–63, Ronald S Jones 1948–62, R J Fitzpatrick 1950–92, Joan O Joshua 1962–94; papers and photographs re veterinary pathology and school as a whole 1903–90; examination papers 20th cent; student registers 1904–90; James Sumner: notes on lectures given by Professor Simonds at Royal Veterinary College, London 1864–65, letter re outbreak of cattle plague in Altrincham and proposed post-mortem 1865, Lancashire Veterinary Association, names and addresses of members (p) c1866–85; Thomas Weston Woodhead, lecture notes on anatomy and stable management 1921–22, nd; Hawkeshead Seddon Caldwell: notes and lectures on veterinary anatomy possibly given by J Share Jones 1921–22, photograph, nd; Roger B Hornby: veterinary hospital out-patient record sheets and form c1930s, Royal College of Veterinary Surgeons' examination papers and instructions 1936–39, copies of publications by and about J Share Jones 1940s, photograph of staff and students 1939, veterinary hospital opening brochure 1929; John Hoare, lecture, practical and case notes 1960–65; deeds re property at Leahurst, Neston, and university precinct 1942–nd; veterinary hospital, Pembroke Gardens, foundation and floor plans and elevations 1926–27; veterinary field station, Neston, plans 1971, 1974; booklet re proposed field station 1965; copy brochure re new veterinary building 1962; correspondence and related papers re Association of Veterinary Students Annual Conference, particularly the problems which arose from the conference held in Liverpool 1966–68, 1971, 1976; Leahurst students' Christmas revue programmes 1960–62; photographs of staff, students, accommodation, specimens, examination of animals, classes, University Veterinary Society members, Leahurst Veterinary Society and National

Veterinary Association members 1893–1979; transparencies of premises, staff and students 1961–85, nd; University Veterinary Society: *Rumen* magazine c1982–83, photographs of speakers addressing Society at Greenbank 1992. [Ref: A.31, 38/136, 38/522–4, 38/668–81, 59, 68, 73, 109, 115, 133, 135, 173, 184, 213, 246; D.26, 57, 83, 161, 218, 227, 234, 246/22, 284/1–2, 292, 333, 375, 393, 405, 426, 472, 485, 489, 492, 519, 524, 546, 553–4, 577, 605–6, 634, 652, 654, 663, 701, 742, 769; P.90, 8043, 8048; S.165, 175–6, 2950–9, 3424, 3481, 4042–7]

Records (2): Edinburgh Room, Edinburgh Central Library, George IV Bridge, Edinburgh EH1 1EG

New Veterinary College, Edinburgh: photographs of Gayfield House 1912, 1955. [Ref: YSF 9284–5, 9583, 9585]

Records (3): Wellcome Library, Royal College of Veterinary Surgeons, Belgravia House, 62–64 Horseferry Road, London SW1P 2AF

Bachelor of Veterinary Science: 1st examination papers 1951, 1954, 2nd examination papers 1951–56, final examination papers 1952–56.

Records (4): in private ownership of Mr R D Locke, 4 Rathmore Road, Cambridge CB1 7AD

Photographs: football team with names and results 1948–49, rugby team with names and results 1949, final year students and staff at Leahurst 1950.

Records (5): Farm Animal Studies Practice, University of Liverpool, Leahurst, Chester High Road, Neston, Cheshire CH64 7TE

Day books 1976–85, 1988, 1990–; invoices 1977–; client records 1960–; tuberculosis testing records 1963–; brucella testing records 1966–.

UNIVERSITY OF NEWCASTLE, DEPARTMENT OF AGRICULTURE

Newcastle upon Tyne, Tyne & Wear

History: The Department of Agriculture at Newcastle University, established in 1891, is one of the oldest in the country. It forms part of the Faculty of Agriculture and Biological Sciences and in addition to its teaching commitments carries out applied research into crop and animal production and farm business management. The Department is responsible for two farms – a mixed farm of about 250 hectares at Cockle Park, Northumberland, supporting separate pig, sheep, beef and dairy herd research units, and a farm of 300 hectares at Nafferton in the Tyne Valley, home to a dairy herd and a silage beef unit. There is also an extensive agricultural science research unit at Close House, near Nafferton.

Records (1): Registrar's Office, 6 Kensington Terrace, University of Newcastle, Newcastle upon Tyne NE1 7RU

Agricultural committee, minutes 1926–37; Board of the Faculty of Agriculture: minutes 1962–88, other papers 1971–87; committee of Council on agricultural department, minutes 1935; higher degrees committee (agriculture), minutes 1971–82, 1988; faculty planning committee (agriculture), minutes 1975–82; papers re: lectureships in agriculture 1923–35, visit by Minister for Agriculture and Fisheries 1935–37, appointment of veterinary bacteriologist to Department of Agriculture 1942, general board of studies 1975–81; general correspondence 1937–56; University of Durham Board of Faculty of Agriculture, minute books 1953–67.

Records: (2): The Robinson Library, University of Newcastle, Newcastle upon Tyne NE2 4HQ

References to Department of Agriculture in annual reports and university calendars 1890s–.

USK AGRICULTURAL COLLEGE
Usk, Monmouthshire

History: Monmouthshire Institute of Agriculture was established at Usk in 1913, funded partly by an endowment set up under the terms of the will of William Jones of Monmouth, who died in 1614, and partly by a Board of Agriculture and Fisheries grant. With the funds Rhadyr Farm was acquired and new buildings added. After 1923, when administration of the Institute was assumed by Monmouthshire County Council, one year courses in agriculture, horticulture, dairying and poultry keeping were established alongside the existing part time courses and the advisory service offered to farmers and market gardeners. The Institute grew steadily over the next decade and by 1940 was offering five one year courses – in agriculture, dairying, horticulture, poultry husbandry and rural domestic economy. With the creation of the National Agricultural Advisory Service in 1946, the Institute was no longer required to advise farmers, but continued to advise part time food producers including domestic pig and poultry keepers. At the same time, the Government restricted courses in dairying to colleges in Cheshire and Somerset, forcing the Institute to replace its dairying course with one in dairy farming and milk production. In 1961, following recommendations by the Ministry of Education, the number of institutes in England and Wales providing courses in poultry husbandry was reduced to four, of which Usk was one. The poultry department was reorganised and updated at that time. From 1964 the Institute offered students the opportunity to study for the National Diploma in Dairying. Veterinary surgeons are regularly appointed as visiting lecturers.

Records: Gwent Record Office, County Hall, Cwmbran NP44 2XH

Collections books 1914–49; disbursements books 1914–48; cash book 1940–41; ledger 1921–55; farm/dairy sales books 1914–19, 1924–30; livestock books 1913–37; deadstock book 1914–22; student fee book 1916–46; labour account book 1913–16; wages sheets 1918–56 [w]; correspondence files 1944–64; Agricultural Institute's *Journal* 1933–56 [w]; student magazines 1925, 1938–39, 1961–62; press cuttings 1915–33; photographs: aerial view, buildings, students, principal and horses, Horticultural Department, Poultry Department, Dairy Department, cattle management, sheep shearing, piggeries, open day, ducks 20th cent. [Ref: CE.G.I; CE.G.F, P; CPN]

List of records of charities

THE BLUE CROSS
Burford, Oxfordshire

History: Our Dumb Friends' League was established in London in 1897 by a small group of people who were anxious 'to encourage in individuals humanity to dumb animals, by education, co-operation and where desirable, grants of money'. In the first year alone, twenty three local branches were formed across the country, all of which reported to the League's headquarters at 164 Buckingham Palace Road, London. Administration was centred in the Grand Council, although the day to day administrative work was carried out by a committee composed of twenty members which was convened monthly. The annual subscription was set at 2/6-, while membership of the children's branch cost 1d a year. Much of the League's income, however, was derived from legacies, donations and fundraising. By the 1920s, the League was concentrating on six spheres of activity, known as the Special Funds, each of which was run by a committee chosen from the members of the Grand Council. Each Special Fund controlled its own finances but relied on the Grand Council for advances of capital. For the everyday administration of the League's finances, the Grand Council appointed a General Purposes Committee, made up of eight members. The most popular of the Special Funds was the Animal Hospital, opened on Hugh Street, Belgrave Road, London, in 1906. Three consulting veterinary surgeons, William Sewell, Alfred Sewell and F W Cousins, were appointed to the hospital, which provided veterinary treatment to those otherwise unable to afford it. During its first three years the hospital saw over 40,000 animals. The Drivers' and Horsekeepers' Fund provided working horses with waterproofs in winter and oatmeal and water in summer. It also maintained trace horses on several steep hills in and around London. The Blue Cross Fund was set up in 1912 to bring medical help and comforts to horses in the Balkan War, complementing the services already provided by the Red Cross to sick and injured soldiers. During the First World War, the Fund established a number of hospitals in France, which between them treated over 2800 horses in their first year. Similar hospitals were introduced in 1917 to treat the growing number of army dogs being used as messengers and watchers. The Blue Cross Fund also maintained a fleet of ambulances across London and beyond for the removal of injured horses from the roads, and kennels at Charlton which quarantined soldiers' dogs free of charge. Other Special Funds included the North London Dogs' Home, established in 1912 to care for stray dogs, and the Receiving Shelters for Stray Cats. In 1950, Our Dumb Friends' League was renamed The Blue Cross. A new Centre and Head Office was opened at Shilton Road, Burford, in 1991. By 1999, the Blue Cross maintained four veterinary hospitals, three in London and one in Grimsby, North East Lincolnshire, employing 19 veterinary surgeons, 47 veterinary nurses and 27 support staff who between them treated 60,000 animals each year. In addition, eleven adoption centres across England re-homed some 8000 animals each year. The charity also operates a horse ambulance welfare service providing emergency care to injured horses at equestrian events.

C W Forward, *Under the Blue Cross: a story of two horses in the war, etc* (London, 1915); C Smith, *The Blue Cross at War 1914–18 and 1939–45* (London, 1990).

Records (1): The Blue Cross, Shilton Road, Burford OX18 4PF

Annual reports 1898–1998 [w]; Dublin branch, annual report 1981; Receiving Shelters for Stray Cats, annual report 1917; Bournemouth and District Shelter for lost and starving dogs and cats, annual reports 1910–49 [w]; minute books: board of governors 1904–, finance committee 1904–; regulations 1914 amended 1938; in house magazines: *Blue Cross Illustrated* 1927–, *The Blue Cross Journal of Our Dumb Friends' League* 1953–, *Pals* 1972–73, 1976, *Pawprint* 1988–; James Combe, file re public relations activities incl attendance at shows, magazines, talks, etc 1970s; papers re general election co-ordinating committee 1979; misc letters and telegrams re horses in First World War 1915–19; horse records 1950s; North London Dogs' Home, appeal leaflet early 20th cent; photographs 20th cent; 16mm film re Torbay Cats' Hotel c1970; misc press cuttings 1949–71, 1986–; press cuttings re export of Irish horses 1954–57, 1960; leaflets re appeals 1954–55; misc pamphlets, annual reports re other welfare charities 1937, 1950s.

Records (2): Hammersmith & Fulham Archives and Local History Centre, The Lilla Huset, 191 Talgeth Road, London W6 8BJ

Photographs of animal hospital, Argyle Place, London 1972, 1986. [Ref: H619]

Records (3): Durham Record Office, County Hall, Durham DH1 5UL

Duplicate licence from Reverend F A Rainbow to Our Dumb Friends' League for use of 60 Etherley Road, Tottenham, as a veterinary surgery 1950. [Ref: EP/Ke/98]

GREAT BUSTARD TRUST
Porton Down, Wiltshire

History: The great bustard, Europe's largest land bird, was extinct as a breeding species in England by about 1826. Before this date it had been a familiar sight, particularly in Wiltshire and Cambridgeshire. In an attempt to re-introduce the species to England, the Great Bustard Trust was established in 1970 and based at a ten acre pen at Porton Down, Salisbury Plain, Wiltshire, leased from the Ministry of Defence. The first bird acquired by the Trust was a hen that landed on Fair Isle in a starving and exhausted condition. Other birds were provided by Victor Reynolds, who undertook the task of catching and rearing enough young birds at his home in Portugal to build up a breeding stock. By 1975 four cocks and seven hens had been acquired in this way. The Trust was dissolved in c1997.

Records: Estate Office, Whipsnade Wild Animal Park, Dunstable LU6 2LF

Correspondence and papers: negotiations for bustard that landed on Fair Isle 1970–72, Charity Commissioners Charities Aid Fund 1971–75, Spanish contacts 1972–75, transport of birds from Portugal 1972–77, research students 1973–81, visitors, talks and exhibitions 1973–81, publicity 1974–86, grants 1976–90, insurance 1977–89, feeding 1981–84, importation 1986; correspondence of Aylmer D Tryon, chairman with/re: Sir John Mogg 1970–73, Fletcher & Partners, accountants 1970–75, Porton Down 1970–75, publicity 1970–75, Macfarlanes, solicitors 1971–72, W R Royle and Son, printers 1971–75, Victor Reynolds 1971–75, open day 1973, game fair 1974, general 1970–75; veterinary reports 1980–87; scientific reports 1982–86; receipts 1978–79; membership cards, nd; Christmas cards, nd; bank statements 1970–75; lists of names to be targeted in appeal 1971.

PEOPLE'S DISPENSARY FOR SICK ANIMALS
Telford, Telford & Wrekin

History: The People's Dispensary for Sick Animals (PDSA) was established in 1917 by Maria Dickin to provide free treatment for the animals of those too poor to pay for veterinary treatment. Based in a cellar in Whitechapel, London, it initially relied on the assistance of one person with some veterinary knowledge and several volunteers, but by the time the PDSA was incorporated in 1923 fourteen Dispensaries had been set up across London and public subscriptions had reached £8000 a year. Mobile units were introduced in 1922 and continued until 1975. Education was a priority from the outset. From 1934, 500 branches of the 'Busy Bees' club were established in schools, giving demonstrations and teaching children how to look after their pets. The Dickin medal, otherwise known as the Animals' Victoria Cross, was created to reward acts of bravery by animals. In 1928, the PDSA opened its first overseas dispensaries in Ireland and France. Further clinics were established in Romania, Morocco, Egypt, the Dutch East Indies, Greece, South Africa and Palestine, although after 1945 all overseas branches were closed with the exception of those in South Africa, Cairo and Tangiers. During the Second World War, the PDSA organised a rescue service to locate animals buried beneath bomb damaged buildings. After incorporation in 1949 the PDSA employed only qualified veterinary surgeons at its Animal Treatment Centres. By 2000 there were 45 animal hospitals in major towns across the country and 89 PDSA PetAid Services run through private practices, employing over 200 veterinary surgeons and carrying out 1.4 million treatments each year.

Anon, *Maria Dickin: the story of Maria Dickin, founder of the PDSA and pioneer in the field of animal welfare* (private publication, 1990s); Anon, *The PDSA in Wartime: an account of the national humane work of the PDSA 1939–1945* (private publication, c1945); Anon, *The Work of the PDSA in Pictures* (private publication, c1930s); M Dickin, *The Cry of the Animal* (private publication, c1940); M Dickin, *Can Animals Suffer?* (private publication, c1940); F Montague, *Let the Good Work Go On* (London, 1947); C Stone, *Salute to the National Animal Guard* (private publication, 1945); C Stone, *The PDSA* (private publication, c1930s).

Records (1): Head Office, People's Dispensary for Sick Animals, Whitechapel Way, Priorslee, Telford TF2 9PQ

Annual reports 1921–; annual reports for Scottish PDSA 1947–48, 1964, 1968, 1970–71, 1975, 1977; annual report for Johannesburg branch 1961;

balance sheets and accounts 1981–82, 1986, 1989–90; a review of the PDSA 1988–89; handbook 1924; area secretaries' handbook 1968; Cardiff district handbook c1960; assistants' handbook, nd; associates: handbook c1940, cards 1930, newsletter 1946; printed lecture notes c1940; leaflets, cards, etc re fundraising appeals, publicity, Dickin medal, etc c1930–97; memoranda and other papers re funding of veterinary centres 1992; misc papers re National Air Raid Precautions Animals Service 1939–45; Busy Bees: membership cards 1936, nd, collecting box, nd, sheet music for *The Song of the Busy Bees*, nd; transcript of British Broadcasting Corporation interview with Maria Dickin 1950; order of service for Maria Dickin's memorial service with an appreciation by Edward Bridges Webb 1951; poster for Bristol branch Christmas market, nd; press cuttings 1920s–; staff journal (monthly) 1953–54, 1987; *PDSA News* 1941, nd; *The Animal's Magazine* 1947, 1949, 1964; *Busy Bees News* 1959, 1972, 1975; *Guild News* 1969–70; *Animal Forum* 1973; *Southern Region Newsletter* 1984; *North East Region Newsletter* 1984; *North Central Newsletter* 1984; *South Eastern Region Newsletter* 1984; newsletter of the Japanese Society for the Prevention of Cruelty to Animals 1957–59 [w]; misc leaflets on the care of dogs, cats, etc, nd; booklets: *The PDSA Sanitorium Souvenir*, nd, *Common Sense series: The Horse, Poultry, The Donkey, The Rabbit, The Goat*, nd, *Practical Advice on the Management of Household Pets* issued by PDSA Johannesburg c1960s, *The PDSA of the Poor* c1930, *Wartime Aids for All Animal Owners* issued by National Air Raid Precautions animals committee c1939; photographs: patients, veterinary equipment, dispensaries, ambulances, war rescues, hospitals, mobile units, overseas establishments, events and functions, publicity and education, awards and presentations incl Dickin medal, staff, volunteer workers, royal visits, Busy Bees c1930s.

Records (2): Tower Hamlets Local History Library and Archives, 277 Bancroft Road, London E1 4D

Annual reports 1921–23 [w]; Dickin medal incl notes on Rip, a dog who located air raid victims in Poplar, London, in 1940, and Upstart, a police horse involved in a flying bomb explosion in Bethnal Green in 1947, nd. [Ref: 631.3]

Records (3): Lambeth Palace Library, London SE1 7JU

Papers criticising the PDSA 1935–36. [Ref: Lang 145, ff.311–44]

Records (4): Hammersmith & Fulham Archives and Local History Centre, The Lilla Huset, 191 Talgarth Road, London W6 8BJ

Fulham branch, photograph of push cart ambulance c1926. [Ref: F619]

Records (5): West Sussex Record Office, County Hall, Chichester PO19 1RN

Chichester Guild Christmas market: committee minute book 1952–53, statement of account 1952. [Ref: ADD. MSS. 16,090–16,091]

Records (6): PDSA Veterinary Centre, 6 Amersham Vale, New Cross, London SE14 6LD

Minutes of staff meetings and meetings with head office 1992–; cash books 1997–; invoices 1992–; value added tax returns 1992–; client records 1985–; promotional leaflets 1998–; photographs 1992–; general correspondence, mainly thank you letters and complaints 1992–.

RESEARCH DEFENCE SOCIETY
London

History: The Research Defence Society was established in 1908 to protect the interests of those who used animals for medical research purposes. Initial funding was provided by Stephen Paget, secretary of the Association for the Advancement of Medicine by Research, a similar body set up in 1882. Using lectures, debates and publications, the Research Defence Society aims to highlight the importance of research and the necessity of experiments on animals, and to offer advice to members on how to cope with aggressive anti-vivisection activity. The Society also advises the government and Royal Commissions on the legal aspects of medical research on animals. Charitable status was granted in 1980.

Records: Archives and Manuscripts, Wellcome Library for the History and Understanding of Medicine, 183 Euston Road, London NW1 2BE

Committee and Council minutes 1908–81; lists of members, officers and associates c1914–29; list of branch members c1908–19; alphabetical list of members of Hampstead and north west London branch c1913–20; circulation/membership posting lists 1957, 1970; annual reports incl treasurer's report 1910–91 [w]; accounts 1914–69 [w]; attendance books:

general meetings 1914–32, other 1950–90; rules 1980; provisional rules, nd; recruitment poster c1930s; pamphlets, booklets, publicity material, copies of Acts, copies of Stephen Paget memorial lectures 1927–89; papers re Royal Commission on the Practice of Subjecting Live Animals to Experiments for Scientific Purposes and formation of Association for the Advancement of Medicine by Research c1875–83; Gloucestershire Vaccine Association, resolutions for promoting cowpox and discouraging smallpox inoculation 1811. [Ref: SA/RDS A1, A3, C1–12, D1–9, E1–19, F1–11, H8, H16]

ROYAL SOCIETY FOR THE PREVENTION OF CRUELTY TO ANIMALS
Horsham, West Sussex

History: The Society for the Prevention of Cruelty to Animals was established in London in 1824, two years after the Animal Protection Act outlawing cruelty to cattle, horses and sheep made its way onto the statute books. Generally recognised to be the first animal welfare organisation in the world, the Society was responsible for 149 convictions on charges of cruelty to animals in its first year alone. The name 'Royal Society for the Prevention of Cruelty to Animals' was officially 'fixed' by the 1932 Act of Incorporation and in 1840, Queen Victoria granted permission for the Society to use the 'Royal' prefix. Based initially at 15 The Quadrant, Regent Street, London, the Society's headquarters moved several times within London over the next decade or so: to 6 John Street, off Oxford Street, in 1832, 3 Exeter Hall, Strand, in 1833 and Pall Mall in 1842. In 1867 temporary offices were taken at 172 New Bond Street until the move to 105 Jermyn Street was completed in 1869. Jermyn Street remained the Society's headquarters until 1973, when it moved to The Causeway, Horsham, West Sussex. In 2001 another move was made, this time to Oakhurst Business Park, Horsham. By 2000 the Royal Society for the Prevention of Cruelty to Animals employed 328 inspectors who between them were investigating over 100,000 cruelty complaints a year and undertaking thousands of animal rescues, collections and establishment visits. In addition, the Society's clinics and hospitals treat over 270,000 animals each year and support a variety of animal welfare projects including neutering campaigns.

A Brown, *Who Cares for Animals: 150 years of the RSPCA* (London, 1974); A W Moss, *Valiant Crusade: the history of the RSPCA* (London, 1961); A W Moss and E Kirby, *Animals Were There: a record of the work of the RSPCA during the war of 1939–1945* (London, 1947).

Records (1): Library, Royal Society for the Prevention of Cruelty to Animals Headquarters, Wilberforce Way, Oakhurst Business Park, Southwater, Horsham RH13 7WN

Annual reports 1832–; details of proceedings re general meetings 1843–1994 [w]; papers re extraordinary general meetings 1927–80; proceedings of annual conferences of branch and auxiliary secretaries 1916, 1919–23, 1925–26, 1932; minute books: Council 1824–, finance committee (budgetary control committee from 1982) 1911–91, humane slaughter committee 1922–56, branches committee 1930–75, education committee 1935–52, education and publicity committee 1952–70, general purposes committee 1953–70, international and overseas committee 1955–76, homeless animals committee 1966–75, publicity and appeals committee 1970–75, branches and overseas committee 1970–90, farm livestock advisory committee 1971–91, animal welfare establishments committee 1971–92, animal experimentation committee 1972–91, inspectorate committee 1973–90, wild animals advisory committee 1973–91, education and information committee 1975–81, operations committee 1990–92; accounts: animal aid and welfare club 1957–68, animals help branch 1957, 1959–60, 1962, 1965, 1968, animal war memorial dispensary 1957–68, birds fund 1957–68, Mortimer's fund for cats 1957–68, Mayhew home 1957–61, Putney and Roehampton Animals Free Clinic and Convalescent Ward 1957–61, Sir John Partridge Memorial Clinic 1957–68, Wyndham Cottle Home of Rest for Horses 1957–68; general orders to inspectors 1936–95 [w]; rules and instructions for inspectors 1949, 1961, 1972–86 [w]; letters to honorary secretary 1925–90; letters sent to branch secretaries 1957–70, 1977–90; papers, photographs, etc re work of the veterinary unit in Abyssinia 1936; correspondence with Ministry of Defence re retired army horses 1969–90s; British Veterinary Association: agreements 1964, 1973, 1979, 1991, correspondence re administration of voucher system, nd; general correspondence incl: awards 1909–97, death of army horses during First World War 1914–18, rescue of animals and humans by animals 1969–95, establishment and running of clinics 20th cent; correspondence, reports and related papers re legislation, campaigns, etc 20th cent; notes re branch histories 20th cent; papers re junior membership (Animal Defenders) 1934–92; press cuttings, leaflets, articles, photographs 19th–20th cent.

Records (2): Lambeth Palace Library, London SE1 7JU

Question paper for prize awarded to pupils of London School Board late 19th cent. [Ref: MS.1387, f.145]

Records (3): Horsham Museum, 9 The Causeway, Horsham RH12 1HE

Band of Mercy: newsletter 1897, melody leaflet c1900. [Ref: 1987.165–166]

Records (4): Cumbria Record Office, 140 Duke Street, Barrow in Furness LA14 1XW

Poster entitled 'Directions for using humane killers,' nd.

Records (5): Tower Hamlets Local History Library and Archives, 277 Bancroft Road, London E1 4DQ

Poplar Free Clinic for Sick Animals of the Poor: annual reports 1936–39, photograph of clinic in Grundy Street, nd. [Ref: 631.3]

Records (6): Warrington Library, Museum Street, Warrington WA1 1JB

Warrington branch, annual reports 1928–42. [Ref: PS26]

Records (7): Hammersmith & Fulham Archives and Local History Centre, The Lilla Huset, 191 Talgarth Road, London W6 8BJ

Sir John Partridge Memorial Clinic, Chelsea & Fulham Districts, annual reports 1968, 1973; Mayhew Home, photograph of premises 1972. [Ref: F619; H619]

Records (8): Hampshire Record Office, Sussex Street, Winchester SO23 8TH

Henry John George Herbert, 3rd Earl of Carnarvon, letters and papers as president incl correspondence re establishment of a similar society in France 1835–42; Fareham, Hampshire branch: executive minute book 1929–39, plans for buildings to house dogs and cats c1950. [Ref: 65M78/G1; 210M85/252; 75M91/E41]

Records (9): Dorset Record Office, Bridport Road, Dorchester DT1 1RP

Lyme Regis and Charmouth branch: minute book 1892–1981, secretary's reports 1964–66, summary of income 1914–46, statement of accounts 1954, receipt from Montague Club Home Committee 1981, press cutting re establishment of new committee following resignation of previous committee 1977. [Ref: D/LRM/G1/1–6]

Records (10): Gloucestershire Record Office, Clarence Row, Alvin Street, Gloucester GL1 3DW

Gloucester & West Gloucestershire branch: copy of trust deeds and related papers 1889–1922, applications for post of part time inspector 1916, licence for humane killers and ammunition 1918–20. [Ref: D4115/19–21]

Records (11): Liverpool Record Office, William Brown Street, Liverpool L3 8EW

Liverpool branch: annual reports 1872–1960, branch committee, minute books 1871–1963, ladies' committee, minute books 1873–78, 1885–97, 1914–39, Irish cattle traffic sub-committee, minute books 1895, dogs' home committee, minute books 1923–53, Birkenhead sub-committee, minute books 1930–47, horse purchase board, minute books 1932–50, Wallasey sub-committee, minute books 1938–60, general sub-committee and joint sub-committee, minute books 1918–28; Liverpool Dogs' Home, annual reports 1884–1904. [Ref: 179 ANI 1–9]

Records (12): Glasgow City Archives, Mitchell Library, North Street, Glasgow G3 7DN

Reports 1904–14 [w]. [Ref: T–PAR 1]

SCOTTISH SOCIETY FOR THE PREVENTION OF CRUELTY TO ANIMALS

Edinburgh

History: The Scottish Society for the Prevention of Cruelty to Animals (SSPCA) was established in Edinburgh in 1839. Widespread concern raised both by the cruel treatment being suffered by animals, particularly horses, and the lack of sufficient protective legislation within Scotland prompted the forming of a committee which would investigate the whole issue of cruelty and press for any legislation deemed necessary. Additionally, an endowment by its patroness, Mrs Gibson, enabled the SSPCA to award prizes for the best essays written on animal cruelty at the Universities of Edinburgh, Glasgow and Aberdeen. Having taken these steps, the Society then appeared to fall into abeyance until 5 July 1840, when a paragraph in *The Scotsman* announced its resumption. This was followed on 5 August by an advertisement calling upon members of the public to report cases of cruelty to the Superintendent of Police. By 1850 the SSPCA had helped secure the passing of the Cruelty to Animals (Scotland) Act, which imposed penalties for the ill-treatment and over-driving of animals and outlawed 'fighting or baiting [of] any bull, bear, badger, dog, cock or other kind of animal, whether of domestic or wild nature'. Although broadly similar to an Act passed in England the previous year, the Scottish Act contained one important difference, namely that the Society's inspectors were to be given the same powers as police constables with regard to the Protection of Animals Acts and the Slaughter of Animals Act. Consequently they were obliged to take an oath before a Justice of the Peace. By 1890, inspectors (known as Officers until 1928) were visiting the whole of Scotland except the counties of Argyll & Bute, Dumbarton, Renfrewshire and Lanark, which were visited by the Glasgow and West of Scotland Society, set up in 1856. William Mitchell became the first SSPCA inspector to be stationed outside Edinburgh when he was posted to Perth in 1890. A second inspector was based in Perth from 1892, while others were appointed to Dumfries (1891), Inverness (1893), Kirkcaldy (1894), Moray and Roxburghshire (1897) and Dingwall (1899). Their caseload grew rapidly too, from 197 cases in 1873 to 985 by 1893. Bicycles were first issued in 1898, followed by motorcycles in 1913, while in 1902 the Society acquired its first ambulance. As the SSPCA grew, a number of branch committees were established, at Galashiels and Peebles (1867), Dunfermline and Kirkcudbright (1869), Inverness and Melrose (1873), Falkirk (1874), Nairn (1888), Brechin (1889) and Montrose (1890). In 1884, the Perthshire SPCA became a branch of the SSPCA, followed later in the same year by the Dumfries & Galloway SPCA. Representatives from all branches were invited to attend the directors' quarterly meetings from 1885. The Society's activities gradually became more wide-ranging. In 1873, for example, the SSPCA commissioned two veterinary surgeons, Charles S Romanis, Inspecting Veterinary Surgeon to the Privy Council, and Thomas Walley, Professor of Cattle Pathology at Edinburgh Veterinary College, to investigate the plight of the horses used to draw city tramcars in Edinburgh. Their report revealed that 25 per cent of all the horses being used were unfit to work and prompted the introduction of various practical measures such as the provision of drinking troughs and periodic inspection programmes. In 1907, a large-scale inspection programme was carried out at a number of collieries, with prizes being distributed to pit ponies' drivers and stablemen. Overall, education was believed to be one of the most effective ways of improving the working conditions of animals and reducing ill-treatment. Essay prizes continued to be awarded to university students while an annual essay competition aimed at children, set up in Edinburgh in 1891, was extended to include schools across Scotland in 1895. In 1920, a series of lantern lectures was instituted in Edinburgh schools and a course of lectures on the care and management of horses and ponies was given by a veterinary surgeon, with an average attendance of sixty. Films were introduced as part of the Society's humane education programme in 1927. Nor was the education of inspectors neglected. From 1900, the Edinburgh inspectors were obliged to attend a course of veterinary classes at Heriot-Watt College. The SSPCA also continued to press for legislation on such issues as the humane slaughter of animals, the licensing of drovers, the keeping of wild animals in captivity, the monitoring of greyhound tracks and the importation and exportation of animals. Following the introduction of the Exportation of Horses Order of 1921, which limited the number of ports across the UK from which horses could be exported to seven, an SSPCA inspector regularly attended the presentation and inspection of horses at Leith. Funding for all the Society's activities was largely derived from donations and membership schemes. From the late 1860s, it benefited from an annual subscription by the Highland and Agricultural Society of Scotland, while the first substantial bequest, from the estate of Dr Fraser of Hampstead, London, was received in 1883. In 1928 the SSPCA's directors purchased a small farm at Balerno, Edinburgh, which opened as a rest farm and dog boarding kennels in 1930. Also in 1928, as part of a major reorganisation, a General Council was formed, made up of SSPCA directors and branch delegates. The junior membership was reorganised in 1935, resulting in the amalgamation of the Animal Defender Corps and the Band of Mercy under the title of the SSPCA Junior Division. By 1939 the Junior Division had over 10,000 members. In 1936, a Free Veterinary Scheme, by which inspectors were able to issue vouchers allowing those unable to afford veterinary fees to secure free treatment for their sick animals, was introduced. Further reorganisation was necessary in 1987 after the Glasgow and West of Scotland Society (est 1856) agreed to merge with the SSPCA. This was followed by the absorption of two further previously autonomous bodies, the Society for the Prevention of Cruelty to Animals, Dundee, in 1994, and the Aberdeen Association for the Prevention of Cruelty to Animals in 1996. By the time the SSPCA was incorporated in 1999, it had been divided into 4 administrative areas, had 89 branches, and employed approximately 55 inspectors. Although the Society ceased to appoint its own veterinary surgeon after 1896, believing that this would encourage better co-operation from the profession in general, two veterinary surgeons continued to sit on the Board of Directors. In 1995 the Society's headquarters moved from 19 Melville Street, Edinburgh, to Braehead Mains, Queensferry Road, Edinburgh. The new offices included a call centre covering Edinburgh, Glasgow, East, West and Central Scotland and the Scottish Borders which by 1999 was handling over 600 calls a day. In addition, the Society operates the Middlebank Wildlife Centre, near Inverkeithing, where children can learn how to care for their pets. Inspectors monitor a range of establishments, including farms, intensive units, markets, ports, pet shops, kennels and catteries in addition to responding to emergency calls. A new Animal Welfare Centre was opened at Bothwell Bridge, South Lanarkshire, in 1999, complementing those at Milton, West Dunbartonshire, and Glasgow. All three centres offer refuge to injured, abused or abandoned animals and have fully-equipped veterinary rooms and services contracted out to the University of Glasgow's Faculty of Veterinary Medicine. Services provided by the centres include neutering programmes, micro-chipping of dogs and cats and re-homing. The Society's commitment to education is reflected by the work of its Education Officers, who give talks across the country, arrange visits to the Animal Welfare Centres and are responsible for the production of the Society's magazines.

Records (1): Scottish Society for the Prevention of Cruelty to Animals, Braehead Mains, 603 Queensferry Road, Edinburgh EH4 6EA

Annual reports 1867–; minutes of directors' meetings, general meetings, finance committee, other committees and sub-committees 1906–; staff book re inspectors c1870–1980, incl rules and regulations 1909, 1932; papers re administration of estate of Mrs Sarah Macadam 1902–29; weekly contributions registers 1946; photographs incl staff, royal visits, horse ambulances, etc 19th–20th cent; Glasgow Dog and Cat Home, board minutes 1993–95; various papers (unlisted) 19th–20th cent.

Glasgow and West of Scotland Society for the Prevention of Cruelty to Animals
Annual reports 1857–79; board minutes 1952–87; executive committee, minutes 1976–87; finance committee, minutes 1952–76; accounts 1966–75; official collecting book 1961–68; Greenock branch, secretary's outgoing letter books 1907–29; merger agreement with Scottish Society for the Prevention of Cruelty to Animals 1987; misc papers incl agenda for board and executive meetings, financial statements, reports from homes, inspectors, etc 1982.

Records (2): Glasgow City Archives, Mitchell Library, North Street, Glasgow G3 7DN

Scottish Society for the Prevention of Cruelty to Animals, abstract of Act for the Prevention of Cruelty to Animals with suggestions for guidance c1850. [Ref: D–TC6/94]

Records (3): Dundee City Archives, 21 City Square, Dundee DD1 3BY

Dundee branch (Society for the Prevention of Cruelty to Animals, Dundee, until 1994): annual reports 1865–1973 [w], minute book 1896–1918, constitution and rules 1899, 1971, photographs of animals helped 1970–72. [Ref: GD/AY/10]

Records (4): Aberdeen City Archives, Town House, Broad Street, Aberdeen AB10 1AQ

Aberdeen branch (Aberdeen Association for the Prevention of Cruelty to Animals until 1996): directors' and committee meetings, minute books 1870–1978, draft minutes 1889–1927 [w], 1968–71, annual reports 1872–1994, draft annual reports 1889–1978, annual accounts and supporting papers 1882–1980 [w], capital ledgers 1891–1977, draft ledgers 1889–92, cash books 1889–91, 1923–44, 1963–67, pension fund book 1938–71, petty cash book 1894–95, revenue account books 1907–30, current account passbooks 1877–95, vouchers 1889–96, 1933, 1946–47, cheque book stubs 1890–1941, returned cheques 1915–33, taxation papers 1896–1927, insurance papers 1895, wage books 1894–95, 1908–11, wage receipts 1889–94, 1920–33, Association secretary's wage receipts 1908–23, collection books 1889–92, 1949–51, 1969–70, subscription lists and papers 1889–1900, 1913–17, legal papers and correspondence re bequest from Frederick Chalmers Lumsden 1877–94, papers re bequests 1890–1927, sundry legal papers 1891–92, 1906–21, prosecutions register 1896–1912, complaints books 1887–91, record of telephone complaints 1976–79, inspectors' reports 1888–1969, inspectors' diaries 1882–89, 1974, 1979, general papers re inspectors 1888–1910, reports and by-laws 1887–1908, 1948–71, papers re Acts of Parliament 1876–1933, papers re cross-group anti-vivisection lobby 1892–95, applications for post of sub-inspector 1891, 1969, copy of award of merit certificate 1950–60, registration certificates for motorcycles purchased for use by inspectors 1915, property papers re Union Grove 1891–1951, Osborne Place, Blenheim Place and 107 Hamilton Place 1909, 67 Charlotte Street 1922, general property papers 1893–1917, 1922, mortgage papers 1924, 1933, architectural plans for 44 Union Grove c1890–1900 and Seaton animal sanctuary 1972, press cuttings 1892–1932, 1987, posters 1920–77, information and educational leaflets c1921–92, general administrative papers 1967–80, general office papers, reports and correspondence 1950–86, outgoing letterbooks 1886–1928, 1934–76, incoming letters and letterbooks 1888–1933, 1938–57, general correspondence 1888–1924, photographs of inspectors 1960–80, film of inspectors and animals 1960–70, film re association history 1960–70, centenary dinner ticket and incomplete copy of after dinner speech 1970, association publication c1880, annual reports of various animal protection societies 1885–1971. [Ref: AAPCA]

VETERINARY BENEVOLENT FUND

London

History: In 1897 George Upton of the Central Veterinary Society called for the establishment of a national society which would offer financial relief to the widows and orphans of veterinary surgeons. Like many others, Upton was concerned that the National Veterinary Benevolent & Mutual Defence Society (NVBMDS), based in Manchester since its establishment in 1865, was concerning itself too much with legal defence work and doing little to compensate those affected by death or injury. Shortly afterwards, a committee was set up to examine the possibility of founding a national society devoted to benevolence, a move which led to the inauguration of the Victoria Veterinary Benevolent Fund on 30 December 1897. From the outset, the Fund was a charitable organisation, collecting donations and subscriptions from local veterinary societies and making grants to needy veterinary surgeons and their families. At first there was considerable rivalry with the NVBMDS, but this gradually subsided during the course of the twentieth century, and the two organisations eventually came to work alongside each other. In 1976, the NVBMDS, which had by this time become known as the Veterinary Defence & Benevolent Society, invited the Victoria Veterinary Benevolent Fund to adopt its benevolent functions, which it did from 1978. At the same time, the Victoria Veterinary Benevolent Fund was renamed the Veterinary Benevolent Fund. It continues to operate from the offices of the British Veterinary Association.

R D Locke, 'The Origins of Benevolence in the Veterinary Profession', *The Veterinary Record*, 27 Sept 1997.

Records: in private ownership of Mr R D Locke, 4 Rathmore Road, Cambridge CB1 7AD

Memorandum and articles of association 1919; annual reports and accounts 1914, 1916–99; appeal letters 1935, 1938.

List of records of zoos

BRISTOL ZOO GARDENS
Clifton, Bristol

History: Although the establishment of the Bristol, Clifton and West of England Zoological Society was first proposed in 1823 by members of the Bristol Institution, it was not until 1835 that the Society finally came into being. Its aim from the outset was 'the diffusion of useful knowledge by facilitating observation of the habits, form and structure of the animal kingdom as well as affording rational amusement and recreation to the visitors of the neighbourhood'. The original 220 subscribers included many famous Bristol names but the initial driving force was the Society's first Secretary, Dr Henry Riley (1797–1848), a lecturer at the School of Anatomy. It was largely through Riley's efforts that land was purchased, at a cost of £3500, and the buildings and gardens created, costing a further £3500. During the First World War, many of the animals were disposed of and the zoo suffered considerable financial difficulties in the period immediately following the war. Only the combined efforts of Dr Richard Clarke, President of the Society from 1928 to 1929, his cousin Sefton Clarke, the Superintendent Mr Greed and a businessman called Freddie Burgess stopped the dissolution of the Society and the sale of its land to Clifton College. A period of sustained growth followed this crisis, with new buildings and research projects being developed. Following the establishment of the University of Bristol's School of Veterinary Science in 1949, an association was formed with the Society, which led eventually to its funding various posts at the school. The zoo appointed its first full time veterinary surgeon in 1999.

R P Warin, 'Medicine and Bristol Zoo', *Bristol Medico-Chirurgical Journal*, Jul/Oct 1982.

Records (1): Bristol Zoo Gardens, Clifton, Bristol BS8 3HA

Annual reports 1836–; general meetings, minutes 1871–; Council, minutes 1944–83; general committee: minutes 1836–48, 1866–80, 1893–1911, 1931–44, rough minute book 1925–28, agenda 1891–93, 1908–25, proceedings of general meetings 1835–54; general and special committee, minutes 1861–66; executive committee, minutes 1970–; finance and general committee, minutes 1880–93; finance committee: minutes 1897–1971, rough minute book 1918–28, agenda 1894–1907; animal committee (from 1988 part of zoo gardens committee), minutes 1928–; medical and veterinary committee (est 1960 as a sub-committee), minutes 1967–81, 1990–93; scientific committee, minutes 1981–86; education, research, conservation and scientific committee, minutes 1988–90; committee of management, financial reports 1941–49; Hollywood Tower estate committee, minutes 1966–84; sub-committees, minutes 1836–56, 1949–66; various committees: minutes 1856–61, 1873–96, agenda 1891–94; committee meetings' attendance books 1907–93; science advisory panel meetings, minutes 1993–; cash payment book 1929–32; cash book 1932–46; valuation 1932; audited accounts 1937–44; financial statements 1960–66; papers re shares 19th–20th cent; deeds 19th–20th cent; deed of regulations 1837; animal reports 1923–51, 1969–77; post-mortem sheets 20th cent; summary veterinary report 1998–99; photographs 20th cent.

Records (2): Bristol Record Office, B Bond Warehouse, Smeaton Road, Bristol BS1 6XN

Subscription book 1845–48.

CHESTER ZOO

Chester, Cheshire

History: Chester Zoo was established by George Saul Mottershead in 1930 and opened to the public the following year. Inspired by his childhood visits to a Manchester zoo, Mottershead set about creating a 'zoo without bars' at his home, Oakfield House, Chester, using the animals from an earlier zoo at Shavington, Cheshire. In doing so he succeeded in creating the country's first large-scale garden zoo which moved away from the out-moded urban menagerie-style zoos. The zoo continued to develop, helped in part by the establishment in 1934 of the North of England Zoological Society Ltd. One of its most notable successes was the birth in 1977 of Jubilee, the first elephant to be born and raised in Britain. The veterinary laboratory was completed in 1965, at which time the first full time veterinary officer was appointed. From 1967 veterinary services have been contracted out to a local veterinary practice.

Records (1): Director's Office, North of England Zoological Society, Chester Zoo, Caughill Road, Upton, Chester CH2 1LH

Memorandum and articles of association 1932; annual reports and balance sheets 1935– [w]; balance sheet and income/expenditure accounts 1948–81 [w]; general meeting reports 1935–55 [w]; veterinary laboratory annual reports 1969–77 [w]; observations and preliminary pathology report re birth of an African/Asian elephant 1978; pathology reports on two baby rhinos 1993–94; animal management species policies 1989; animal management notes 1990s; Mr Mottershead's correspondence re elephants 1941; lectures to keepers from: Mr Mottershead 1963, W J Jordan, veterinary surgeon, on parasites 1963 and diets 1964; Directors of the Zoological Societies of Great Britain and Ireland: minutes, programmes, etc re annual conferences 1956, 1961, 1966, 1988, report by W J Jordan, veterinary surgeon 1961; International Union of Directors of Zoological Gardens Conference: minutes, programme, proceedings 1963; copy of paper by Derek G Lyon, veterinary surgeon, 'A Survey of Parasitic Problems, Treatment and Control at Chester Zoo' 1971; *Chester Zoo News* 1937–; clinical case summaries 1969–89; clinical case full records 1990–; post-mortem report summaries 1969–89; post-mortem register 1969–; full post-mortem reports 1990–; laboratory analysis reports 1969–; veterinary day book/annual diary 1993–; controlled drugs/poisons register 1969–.

GLASGOW ZOOPARK
Calderpark, South Lanarkshire

History: The Zoological Society of Glasgow (later the Zoological Society of Glasgow and West of Scotland) was formed in 1936 with the purpose of founding a zoo for Glasgow. To this end a 93 acre estate at Calderpark was purchased in 1939 and the first plans drawn up. Shortly after the end of the Second World War, 30 acres of land were enclosed by a team of ex-servicemen and a number of animals donated to the Society. By the time the zoo opened in 1947 there were 160 specimens on show. Veterinary services are provided by J Taylor and Partners, Rutherglen, and by Glasgow University's Faculty of Veterinary Medicine.

Records: Glasgow Zoopark, Calderpark, Glasgow G71 7RZ

Annual reports 1947–; committee minutes and reports 1980–.

ROYAL ZOOLOGICAL SOCIETY OF SCOTLAND
Edinburgh

History: The Royal Zoological Society of Scotland was established in 1909 but it was 1913 before its founder, Thomas Gillespie, was able to open his 'Zoo for Scotland' in Edinburgh. Veterinary support from the outset was provided by the Royal (Dick) Veterinary College, Edinburgh.

Records (1): National Register of Archives (Scotland), HM General Register House, Edinburgh EH1 3YY

Minutes 1913–53, 1967–73; correspondence and accounting records 1913–69; animal committee reports 1926–33; veterinary post-mortem reports 1928–34; wage sheets 1919–42; daily occurrence sheets 1913–46; gate returns 1923–26. [Ref: NRA(S) 2587]

Records (2): The Registry, Edinburgh Zoo, Murrayfield, Edinburgh EH12 6TS

Annual reports 1910–; animal health and management advisory committee, minutes 1973–92; records of births 1914–57; registers of arrivals 1913–72; registers of departures 1933–72; registers of deaths 1915–52; notebook giving names, habitats, etc of animals, birds, reptiles and fish c1970; diary of events 1970–74; daily occurences book 1990–94; daily occurrences book for ape house 1961–66; post-mortems and test results 1959–; record cards for animals no longer at the zoo, incl post-mortems where appropriate c1960–; correspondence and papers re sales of animals 1987–90, 1994–; correspondence and papers re purchase of animals 1995–; notebook re sales of specimens 1985–87; summaries of visits by veterinary surgeons 1967–84; veterinary surgeons' notes 1983–; anaesthesia records 1988; register of incubations 1982; order books 1978–90; curators' diaries 1985–91; notes kept of a period of observation on red pandas 1986; notebook of repairs 1985–86; petty cash book 1985–89; address book, possibly McBone's, nd; slides and photographs 1914–.

Records (3): National Archives, Ruskin Avenue, Kew, Richmond TW9 4DU

Charter 1913. [Ref: PC 8/761]

THE ZOOLOGICAL SOCIETY OF LONDON
London

History: The Zoological Society of London was established in 1826 by a group of scientifically minded men including Sir Stamford Raffles and Sir Humphry Davy. Their aim was to gather together a zoological collection that would not only be of interest to the Society's members but would also provide them with unrivalled opportunities for scientific research. The Zoological Gardens, based in Regent's Park, were opened to Fellows of the Zoological Society in 1828 and to the public in 1847. Additionally, regular scientific meetings were inaugurated and a dissecting room set up in the Society's offices. In 1829, the Society was granted a royal charter. The first veterinary attendant, Charles Spooner, appointed by the Society's Council in 1829, was required to 'attend three times in each week, and oftener when necessary, to prescribe for and examine all the animals and to keep a record of his observations and practice'. Spooner was replaced in 1833 by William Youatt, who, in addition to attending the Gardens twice a week, was also expected to carry out post-mortems. After Youatt's death in 1847, responsibility for animal care was entirely assumed by the Superintendent, with occasional advice from the Royal Veterinary College, London. In 1865, however, the Society, anxious to reintroduce the systematic post-mortem of animals that had ended with Youatt's death, set up a Zootomical Committee which appointed a prosector and provided him with a dissecting room. This was followed in 1903 by the appointment of a pathologist who reported to the Prosectorial Committee and the Council. From that time, every animal was examined after death and the exact cause of death recorded. A further development, in 1907, was the opening of a sanatorium, complete with isolation rooms, for the treatment of sick animals. Although the day to day running of the sanatorium was placed in the hands of the keepers, Messrs Sewell & Cousens MsRCVS were appointed Consulting Veterinary Surgeons to the Society in 1909. Within a year, though, Sewell & Cousens had resigned, claiming that they were unable to devote enough time to the zoo. The Society then entered into an arrangement with the Royal Veterinary College, London, by which Professors McQueen and Wooldridge were appointed Honorary Veterinary Surgeons and B Gorton Veterinary Surgeon to the Society. Gorton was given overall charge of the sanatorium and required to visit the Gardens each day. When he left to join up during the First World War, however, the Society did not appoint a replacement, but once again transferred responsibility for the sanatorium to the Superintendent and continued to rely on the Royal Veterinary College, London, for advice. This system continued until 1951 when a new resident Veterinary Officer was appointed. Shortly afterwards a new sanatorium was built, complete with pathological and research facilities. Various studies were then developed, relating to such issues as breeding and diet. By the 1970s, the zoo was employing two full time veterinary surgeons and twelve lay staff. Clinical and pathological records were kept relating to all the animals and summaries published in the Society's scientific reports. In 1927, the Society purchased 480 acres of land near Dunstable, Bedfordshire, which it aimed to turn into the first 'open' zoo in the world. It was generally recognised by this time that some animals could more easily be kept in large groups and it was hoped that those animals which struggled to survive in the restrictive conditions of Regent's Park would flourish in the more spacious surroundings at Dunstable. The new park, known as Whipsnade Wild Animal Park, opened in 1931, also afforded increased opportunities to develop breeding programmes for rare species at a time when the general research emphasis had shifted from anatomy and the classification of species to conservation. Notable early successes have included Pere David's deer and cheetahs.

P C Mitchell, *Centenary History of the Zoological Society of London* (London, 1929); O Graham-Jones, *First Catch Your Tiger* (London, 1970); Lord Zuckerman et al, *The Zoological Society of London 1826–1976 and Beyond* (London, 1976).

Records (1): Archivist, The Library, Zoological Society of London, Regent's Park, London NW1 4RY

Council minutes 1826–; committee minutes 1826–; annual reports 1826–; daily occurrences books 1826–; Medical Superintendent's journal 1830–[w]; post-mortem and veterinary reports, press cuttings, scrap albums, lantern slides and photographs 1864–.

Records (2): Department of Veterinary Science, Whipsnade Wild Animal Park, Dunstable LU6 2LF

Post-mortem and laboratory results for animals in the collection 1962–; veterinary correspondence 1962–.

Records (3): Archives and Manuscripts, Wellcome Library for the History and Understanding of Medicine, 183 Euston Road, London NW1 2BE

Scientific reports 1972–73, 1979–81.

Guide to minor collections

This section lists archives held mainly by record offices and libraries. Entries are arranged by county and the material within each is in chronological order.

ENGLAND

BATH & NORTH EAST SOMERSET

BATH & NORTH EAST SOMERSET RECORD OFFICE
Guildhall, High Street, Bath BA1 5AW

Bath and West of England Agricultural Society, secretary's correspondence re veterinary arrangements 1937–39, 1963. [Ref: 0038/6/24, 56]

BEDFORDSHIRE

BEDFORDSHIRE AND LUTON ARCHIVES AND RECORD SERVICE
County Hall, Cauldwell Street, Bedford MK42 9AP

Churchwardens' accounts, Edworth, containing medicine recipes for horses and cattle c1725–99 [Ref: P110/5/1]; veterinary recipes c1780s [Ref: PM2996]; recipe book incl some for animals late 18th cent [Ref: SM/E49]; Peter Kempson, cow doctor and cutter, title deeds re property in Flitwick 1807–09 [Ref: WE89; X168/98]; Gibbard family, Sharnbrook, veterinary surgeons' bills 1815, 1847 [Ref: GA.78.2528]; G Turner, 63 High Street, Biggleswade, chemist, recipe books incl recipes for worms in horses and animal diseases c1821–33, early 20th cent [Ref: X346/109, 111]; Josh Powell, farrier, bill 1831 [Ref: BO1267]; letter re sheep rot losses on Bedford estates 1831 [Ref: R3/3690]; apprenticeship indenture, Robert Goddard to Charles Gown Goddard, farrier c1840 [Ref: DDX171/62/23]; William Wontor, Ampthill, veterinary surgeon: trade card 1841 [Ref: CRT130/CRAN13], papers re application for position as clerk or overseer 1849 [Ref: R4/927]; John Saunders, Stotfold, cattle doctor, bond 1855 [Ref: X108/11]; press cutting re sheep scab and sheep sent to Little Staughton 1881 [Ref: *Bedfordshire Mercury* 26 Mar 1881];

K Leggett, Luton, veterinary surgeon, party to deed 1883 [Ref: CCE/3865/16/6]; William Withington, Dunstable Road, Luton, veterinary surgeon, party to deed 1895 [Ref: CCE5309/3]; F J Powell, veterinary surgeon, bill to Alfred Ginn, Potton 1896 [Ref: Z723/101/13]; Benjamin Harrison, Duck Mill, Bedford, veterinary surgeon's bill late 19th cent [Ref: X128/7]; William Hill, veterinary surgeon, Bedfordshire Yeomanry, photograph c1901 [Ref: X468/1]; information re foot-and-mouth disease 1906–28 [Ref: LHE438]; papers re distemper among hounds 1908–18 [Ref: LHE505]; E A Wilshaw, Biggleswade, veterinary surgeon, bill for treatment of horses 1914 [Ref: X758/4/2(12)]; papers re anthrax 1914 [Ref: LHE437]; Veterinary Camp, London Road and Trapps Lane, Luton, papers re sale with site plan 1923–25 [Ref: LHE/451]; Speed Farm, Chicksands, record book re movement of animals 1926–31 [Ref: X752/3]; papers re sheep dipping and quarantine 1933–35 [Ref: LHE465]; J Macarthur, Leighton Buzzard, bill for treating cow 1939 [Ref: Z849/13/7]; report on myxomatosis, first noticed in Ridgmont 1954 [Ref: Z916/2/9]; Kingswood Chemists, 19 Market Square, Potton: animal prescription book 1973–76 [Ref: Z585/12], general prescription books incl veterinary prescriptions 1950–70 [Ref: Z585/8, 10, 13]; sketches by Bernard West of 7 De Parys Avenue, Bedford, showing proposed conversion of first and second floors of veterinary practice to form two self-contained flats 1973 [Ref: Z 284/217]; veterinary surgery, Shotmead Street, Biggleswade, photographs 1976. [Ref: X758/1/4 (97–101)]

BRISTOL

BRISTOL RECORD OFFICE

B Bond Warehouse, Smeaton Road, Bristol BS1 6XN

Andrew Jordan of Bristol, farrier, party to deeds re property in North Street, Bedminster 1656, 1663 [Ref: P/St.Jbed/D/1/5; P/St.Jbed/D/1/7]; Robert Goning of Barton Regis, farrier, party to lease re the King's Head and the White Hart, Lawford's Gate 1682 [Ref: P/St.P and J/D/13(I)]; William Goding, farrier, party to deeds 1753, 1754, 1758 [Ref: P/Xch/D/25(a) i–ii; P/Xch/D/25(b) i–ii; P/Xch/D/25(c)]; William House, veterinary surgeon, party to lease 1826 [Ref: P/AS/D/L/57]; Samuel Hicks Withers of College Green, veterinary surgeon, party to deed 1850. [Ref: P/St.Aug/D/10/1]

BUCKINGHAMSHIRE

BUCKINGHAMSHIRE RECORDS AND LOCAL STUDIES SERVICE
County Hall, Aylesbury HP20 1UU

Gilbert Pickering of Broughton, farrier, party to mortgage 1715 [Ref: D 117/27]; Richard Stratton of Coleman Street, London, farrier, party to mortgage re land in Hartwell 1731 [Ref: D/LE/1/527]; Earl of Buckinghamshire, veterinary bills and receipts 1754–73 [Ref: D/MH/32/3]; Robert Ewers of Blendon, Bexley, Kent, farrier, party to assignment 1772 [Ref: D/D/8/50]; John Nash of Sunninghill, Berkshire, farrier, party to deeds re Rockall End Farm and land in Hambleden 1781, 1786 [Ref: D 62/8/12, 13, 33, 34]; insolvency papers re Joseph Mobbs, formerly of Fenny Stratford, farrier 1809 [Ref: Q/SD/15]; Thomas Mobbs of Fenny Stratford, farrier, party to deed 1817 [Ref: D/DU/3/79]; letter to 11th Duke of Somerset from Professor [Edward] Coleman of the Veterinary College, London 1818 [Ref: D/RA/4/44]; William Weedon of Church Street, Blackfriars Road, Surrey, veterinary surgeon, party to deed re land in Chesham 1832 [Ref: D/CH/A/220]; Anne Allnutt, widow of Henry Allnutt of Windsor, veterinary surgeon, party to conveyance of land in Chesham Bois 1866 [Ref: D/CH/A/465]; Joseph Reynolds, notification of registration of trade mark for embrocations for human use and veterinary purposes 1890. [Ref: D 52/4/12]

CAMBRIDGESHIRE

CAMBRIDGE UNIVERSITY LIBRARY
West Road, Cambridge CB3 9DR

'The True Briton's Answer to a Farmer's Letter', being a treatise on communion, with recipes and accounts, incl some for animals 1752 [Ref: Add. MS 4124]; letter from Richard A Powys, secretary of Royal Veterinary College, London, to Lord Crewe 1911 [Ref: CREWE C.43.1.272]; Joseph Stanley Mitchell, correspondence with G W Osbaldiston, research student at the Cambridge University School of Veterinary Medicine 1963–67, 1970–71 [Ref: NCUACS 36.4.92/H.295, H.296]; Sir Peter Markham Scott: speech given at International Veterinary Congress 1969 [Ref: NCUACS 87.8.99/G.23], correspondence and papers re Scott's support for plans by Royal Veterinary College, London, to build Cedric Price Aviary c1984 [Ref: NCUACS 87.8.99/M.2477], correspondence with British Veterinary Association re

Scott's acceptance and subsequent resignation of vice presidency 1988–89 [Ref: NCUACS 87.8.99/C.321]; Vickers plc, photographs of animal health products in use at Royal Veterinary College, London, and veterinary college, Weybridge, Surrey 1971–73 [Ref: Vickers negatives 6951 41, 6958 26–32, 6981 13–19; C 088 1–4, 38–39; C 093 18–21]; Buxton papers, veterinary recipes, nd.

CAMBRIDGE UNIVERSITY, TRINITY COLLEGE LIBRARY
Cambridge CB1 1TQ

Richard Laurence Millington Synge, biochemist: letters from K Halse of physiology department of Veterinary College of Oslo, Norway 1951–61, 1965, letters from P E Jakobsen, Royal Veterinary and Agricultural College, Copenhagen, Denmark, and Rowett Research Institute, Aberdeen 1954–56, papers re annual conference of New Zealand Veterinary Association 1959, invitation to address central branch of New Zealand Veterinary Association 1959. [Ref: Synge]

CAMBRIDGESHIRE COUNTY RECORD OFFICE
Shire Hall, Castle Hill, Cambridge CB3 0AP

Correspondence and copies of articles re John Shipp [army veterinary surgeon from 1796] 1936, 1984–88 [Ref: R98/18]; William Taylor, Cottenham, extracts from account book with memoranda and veterinary recipes, nd. [Ref: R81/142]

IN PRIVATE OWNERSHIP, MR S HALL
14 Huntingdon Road, Cambridge CB3 0HH

George Banham's national survey on shoeing forges and veterinary practices: circular notice 1883, individual replies 1883, nd, booklet summarising replies [1883?]; cassette recorded interviews: Leslie Pugh 1978, Sir William Weipers 1979, Sir William Henderson 1980, Geoffrey Spicer Muir 1982, T A R Chipperfield 1984, Ruth D'Arcy Thompson, daughter of D'Arcy Wentworth Thompson 1984.

CORNWALL

CORNWALL RECORD OFFICE
County Hall, Truro TR1 3AY

Antony house: small printed volume, unbound, entitled *A Very Perfect Discourse and Order How to Know the Age of a Horse, and the Diseases that Bred in Him*, by T W C 1624, grooms' inventories, veterinary remedies, etc 1708–10 [Ref: CE/E/19, 20]; misc household and veterinary recipes c1750–70 [Ref: X355/66]; Tom family, St Ervin, recipes for sheep diseases 1840, copied by Mary Martyn [Ref: AD/915/46]; medicinal herbal remedies for animals 1840–70 [Ref: X223/6]; William Bolitho junior, Ponsandale, Gulval, notebook of papers and regulations re contagious diseases in animals, especially foot-and-mouth disease 1869–74 [Ref: X/576]; veterinary remedies early 19th cent [Ref: DD/AM/64]; recipe for horse powders 19th cent [Ref: X347/8]; cures for mad dogs, fleas, etc 19th cent [Ref: WH/5085]; Royal Cornwall Show dog committee, minutes 1930–31 [Ref: DDX/584/32]; Werrington parish technical education committee, minutes and press cuttings incl re poultry keeping, dairying, sheepshearing and veterinary hygiene. [Ref: P251/28/1]

COURTNEY LIBRARY AND CORNISH HISTORY RESEARCH CENTRE
Royal Institution of Cornwall, River Street, Truro TR1 2SJ

Photographs: Edward George Pearce Arnall, veterinary surgeon, Camelford and Bodmin 19th cent [Ref: Arnall], C Crowhurst, veterinary surgeon 20th cent. [Ref: Crowhurst]

CUMBRIA

CUMBRIA RECORD OFFICE
140 Duke Street, Barrow in Furness LA14 1XW

Press cutting re Urswick Animal Surgery 1907 [Ref: BDX 123]; Hannah Hall McKinlay, wife of Patrick of Stranraer, veterinary surgeon, party to deeds 1911–12. [Ref: BDSo/41/63, 66]

CUMBRIA RECORD OFFICE
The Castle, Carlisle CA3 8UR

Grainger family, Holm Cultram, notes on various subjects incl veterinary and medical recipes c1786–95 [Ref: DX/74/2]; Thomas Brockbank Veterinary Establishment, posting and livery stables, Albert Square and Blackfriars Street, Carlisle: veterinary and shoeing ledger 1854–60 [Ref: DB/29/1], hack ledger for horses and carriages, etc 1859–60 [Ref: DB/29/2]; Papes, Keswick, chemists: prescription books 1906–55, veterinary cures c1910. [Ref: DB 102/1–57]

CUMBRIA RECORD OFFICE
County Offices, Kendal LA9 4RQ

Veterinary recipes late 17th cent [Ref: WD/Ry/Box34/Miscellaneous papers]; Thomas Harrison, horse doctor, Crosthwaite, account book 1769–1803 [Ref: WDX 188/1]; Thomas Thompson, Middleshaw, Old Hutton, book of animal cures 1793 [Ref: WDX 161]; recipes for cure of farm animals c1930 [Ref: WDX 454/16]; J W Youdell, Grasmere, lecture notes re veterinary science 1939–40. [Ref: WDX 728/4]

DERBYSHIRE

DERBYSHIRE RECORD OFFICE
County Hall, Matlock DE4 3AG

Illustration re horses' ailments 18th cent [Ref: D331/26/7]; Mr Boyle, veterinary surgeon, correspondence and papers c1888–1920s [Ref: D3017]; Buxton Cattle Breeding Centre (formerly Buxton Artificial Insemination Centre), records 1946–74 [Ref: D5069]; Pan's [Zoological] Garden, Ashover, records c1960–75. [Ref: D5295]

DEVON

DEVON RECORD OFFICE
Castle Street, Exeter EX4 3PU

Peter de Troubrygge, Exeter, farrier, party to lease 1347 [Ref: 51/1/3/2]; J White, veterinary surgeon, Exeter, bill 1804 [Ref: 2741 M/FV 25]; apprenticeship indenture, William Woodford Hayman, Exmouth, to John Tosswell, farrier 1817 [Ref: 2932 A/PO 105/4/46]; [-] Clarke, veterinary surgeon at St Helena, application to Henry Addington, 1st Viscount Sidmouth 1815 [Ref: 152M]; apprenticeship indenture, John Cann, Cheriton Bishop, to John Haydon, farrier 1833 [Ref: 132A/PO 692–694]; farming ledger with cures for animal ailments 1869–71 [Ref: 181 M/E 6]; unidentified veterinary surgeon's account book 1898–1904 [Ref: 74 B/Z 42]; Veterinary Infirmary, Musbury, sale particulars 1916 [Ref: 547 B/P 1465]; Dispensary for Sick Animals, Exmouth, accounts 1924–55. [Ref: 3761 R/Accounts/Exmouth]

NORTH DEVON RECORD OFFICE
Tuly Street, Barnstaple EX31 1EL

William Ascot of Bideford, veterinary surgeon, declaration of trust as trustee of church institute 1912. [Ref: 799A–1/PW 52]

DORSET

DORSET RECORD OFFICE
Bridport Road, Dorchester DT1 1RP

[J B and Robert Nineham], farmers, account book incl veterinary recipes and remedies for horses, sheep and cows 1812–30 [Ref: D.1428/1]; veterinary, farming and iron-founding recipes 1839. [Ref: D.1428/2]

CO DURHAM

DURHAM RECORD OFFICE
County Hall, Durham DH1 5UL

Misc recipes and prescriptions, animal and human 17th–19th cent [Ref: D/Sa/X 165–179]; Thomas Atkinson, Newton Cap and Merrington, farrier, deeds mentioning him 1729–31 [Ref: D/Br/D 928, 934]; Jane Bowes, bill received for veterinary expenses 1760–65 [Ref: D/St/C1/2/121]; William Story, Willington, blacksmith and farrier, deeds mentioning him 1780 [Ref: D/Br/D 1846–1847]; Veterinary Doctor Marshall, verse appeal to creditors 1837 [Ref: D/X 202/1]; Francis Henry Salvin, diary incl references to treatment of animal diseases 1839–1949 [Ref: D/X 871/1]; papers re Peele family, Durham City, veterinary surgeons 1849–1953 [Ref: D/X 820]; Ralph George Wheatley, Colepike Hill, farrier, deed mentioning him 1850 [Ref: D/X 610/2–3]; veterinary surgeon's bills 1857 [Ref: D/Lo/E 834]; Fred R Stevens, veterinary surgeon, bills and receipts 1865–1906 [Ref: D/Ad 2]; Robert Brydon, veterinary surgeon and land agent, Seaham, correspondence with Marquess of Londonderry's secretary 1874–82 [Ref: D/Lo/C 288]; King & Gillespie's Veterinary, Shoeing and Livery Establishment, letter re suitable brougham horse 1880 [Ref: D/CG 14/133]; Cuthbert Joseph Hubbick, New Elvet, Durham City, veterinary surgeon, deeds 1881, 1890 [Ref: EP/DuSO 248–249]; Charles Hunting, South Hetton, veterinary surgeon, deeds mentioning him 1882, 1886 [Ref: D/X 668/19, D/Sh.H 393]; J E Hodgson, chemist, prescription book incl recipes for animal medicines 1882–98 [Ref: D/Hg 55]; Thomas Foreman, Leadgate, veterinary surgeon, deeds mentioning him 1886 [Ref: D/CG 7/1400–1]; James Furniss, notebooks probably of lectures at Glasgow Veterinary College 1890s [Ref: D/XD 92/16/1–7]; correspondence between J W Rider and N Nesbit re conditions of appointment as veterinary surgeon for J Joicey and Co Ltd 1914 [Ref: NCB 7/4/11]; National Master Farriers' and Blacksmiths' Association: price lists and general account 1915–31, *The Farrier's Journal* 1946 [Ref: D/X 1018/35–42]; notebook containing cures for animal and human ailments 1916–19 [Ref: D/X 700/138]; veterinary surgeon's invoices for attending cows 1921–48 [Ref: D/X 1021/21]; report by veterinary surgeon on illness and death of several horses (copy) c1940 [Ref: D/Ed 17/475]; Wallis family, Darlington, correspondence re government veterinary scheme 1942 [Ref: D/Wa 5/1/1591–2]; T W Dowson, Tow Law, agricultural engineer and farrier, letter 1952 [Ref: D/X 1041/25]; negatives of veterinary surgeons at work in Newton Aycliffe c1975 [Ref: NT/Ay 7/5/3/96]; Waters the Chemists, veterinary recipe books, nd. [Ref: D/XD 38]

EAST RIDING OF YORKSHIRE

EAST RIDING RECORD OFFICE

County Hall, Beverley HU17 9BA

Misc letters incl references to dogs, horses and cattle plague 1740s–50s [Ref: DDGR 41]; notebook incl recipes for horse and beast drenches' 1756 [Ref: DDSA 1065]; Robert Mawson, account book incl recipes for human and animal ailments 1758–70 [Ref: DDSA 1051/1]; notebook incl animal prescriptions 1775–1818 [Ref: DDX 128/15]; recipes incl treatments for disorders in horses 18th cent [Ref: DDGR 38/94]; notebook incl recipe for 'green salve for any green wound in horse or beast' c1818 [Ref: DDX 128/17]; estate vouchers incl payment for remedies and veterinary work 18th–19th cent [Ref: DDCC]; notebook mainly re animals incl recipes for ailments c1890s [Ref: DDSD 649]; J Read, 35

Regent Circus, Piccadilly, London, illustrated advertisement for veterinary instruments, nd. [Ref: DDBD 91/44]

EAST SUSSEX

EAST SUSSEX RECORD OFFICE

The Maltings, Castle Precincts, Lewes BN7 1YT

John Lovell, citizen and farrier of London, assignment of land in Selmeston 1673 [Ref: SAS/G33/12]; Samuel Waghorn of Goudhurst, farrier, party to leases 1756–57 [Ref: DAN/1688, 1689]; veterinary house, Framfield, title deeds 1774–1935 [Ref: ACC 5637]; Simon Grover, farrier and veterinary surgeon, The Cliffe, receipted bills 1795–1815 [Ref: AMS 634]; John Vinall of Fletching, farrier, party to deeds 1804, 1806 [Ref: SRL 2/7/8; SRL 2/17/6]; William Leaver, Wrotham Heath, Kent, veterinary surgeon, letter to Thomas Frewen, Northiam 1844 [Ref: FRE/4090]; Schiffner estate, accounts incl for veterinary services 1850–52 [Ref: SHR/3610]; Harold Leeney, veterinary surgeon, Forest Row, attendance book 1891–93. [Ref: AMS 5780]

ESSEX

ESSEX RECORD OFFICE

Wharf Road, Chelmsford CM2 6YT

Philip Howard, volume containing recipes for equine and human complaints c1725 [Ref: D/DP/Z39]; John Grayling, farmer, Theydon Garnon, accounts incl drinks and ointments for sick horses and cows 1748–51 [Ref: D/DB/A1]; Nicholas Pearse, recipes for animal and plant diseases 1810–24 [Ref: D/DHt/A1/1/1]; Martin Gatward, farmer, Finchingfield, account book incl note re treatment of foot-and-mouth disease 1824–73 [Ref: D/DU/845]; recipes for human and animal diseases 1834–73 [Ref: D/Dse/35]; George Drought Warburton, Henley House, Frant, Sussex, receipted bills incl some for services of veterinary surgeon and blacksmith 1847–52 [Ref: D/DU/572/5–7]; Robert Andrews, farm accounts incl recipe for 'drink for the plague disease in cattle' 1865–66 [Ref: D/DU/441/62]; Charles DuCane, Coldstream Guards, receipted bills incl veterinary expenses and saddlers' bills 1882–84 [Ref: D/DBs/F58]; notebook containing formulae for medicines for horses and humans c1889 [Ref: D/DU/892]; George Rayment, Gardners Farm, Burnham on Crouch, notebook of veterinary remedies 19th cent [Ref: D/DU/275]; Peter Gard and Andy Taylor, veterinary surgeons, Frinton, cassette recorded interview 20th cent [Ref: SA 29]; unidentified chemist and druggist, Dunmow, recipe book incl several veterinary recipes, nd. [Ref: D/DU/260/15]

GLOUCESTERSHIRE

GLOUCESTERSHIRE RECORD OFFICE

Clarence Row, Alvin Street, Gloucester GL1 3DW

Recipes for animal and human medicines 1653–99 [Ref: D2026 A1]; recipe for medicine for horse colic c1663 [Ref: P307 IN 3/1]; recipe to prevent crows coming upon new sown corn c1700 [Ref: D1833 Z3]; cures for horse ailments 1724–60 [Ref: D3566/1]; horse ailments and remedies 1746–1800 [Ref: D6798/1]; misc bill for ointments 1775 [Ref: D2857/2/20/42]; recipes, charms and spells 1770–96 [Ref: P218 MI 1]; recipes for sick farm animals 1777–84 [Ref: D3596/1]; veterinary recipes and remedies 18th cent [Ref: P251 IN 3/1], recipes for a horse drench 18th–19th cent [Ref: D5024 Z1]; cures for animal illnesses 18th–19th cent [Ref: D2929/1]; recipes for human and animal ailments c1804–38 [Ref: D5136]; recipes for cattle and sheep cures 1816–33 [Ref: P63 CW 2/2]; recipe for rat poison c1820 [Ref: D4194]; cures for animal ailments c1830–37 [Ref: D4764/4/8]; treatment for farm animals c1830–85 [Ref: D5792/1]; John Paradise, veterinary surgeon, Dursley, ledger 1851–59 [Ref: D1578, Acc 2364]; cure for foot-rot c1860 [Ref: D1358/4]; veterinary recipes and remedies c1865 [Ref: D3724/2]; R B Sellors, Tewkesbury, agricultural and dispensing chemist, notebook of medical recipes, many accompanied by appropriate pill box or bottle label c1870–85 [Ref: D5792/1]; cures for human and animal sickness 19th cent [Ref: P244a MI 8/1]; veterinary recipes and remedies c1903–09 [Ref: D2426/A7]; remedies for human and animal ailments c1910 [Ref: D7681/2]; remedy for 'grease in a horse' c1914 [Ref: D6843/2/3]; veterinary recipes and remedies 1918–46 [Ref: D4128/1]; file re improvement works incl plan of St George's Road showing Pyatt's Hotel and James Brain's veterinary forge 1920 [Ref: CBR/C5/4/1/19]; William Barton, farrier, Slimbridge, accounts 1921–35 [Ref: D3751]; recipes for trapping vermin, making oil of worm, 'quicking' a horse and decoying a dog, nd [Ref: D3471/389]; cure for 'shab' on sheep, nd. [Ref: D6297/5/1]

GREATER LONDON

DEPARTMENT OF MANUSCRIPTS, BRITISH LIBRARY
96 Euston Road, London NW1 2DB

De veterinaria medicina libri duo ex operibus auctorum plurimorum collecti 14th cent [Ref: Sloane 745]; miscellaneous veterinary directions and recipes 15–17th cent [Ref: Sloane 333 ff. 44, 50b–61b, Sloane 393 ff. 204–238b, Sloane 680 ff. 49–68b, Sloane 3465 ff. 5b–23, passim, Sloane 3991 ff. 71–93b, passim]; Anne Glydd, recipe book incl veterinary recipes 1656–1700 [Ref: Add Ms 45196]; John Jebbe, farrier, Wormleighton, bill 1666 [Ref: Add Ms 61490 f. 184]; Henry Hunston, farrier, receipted bill 1676 [Ref: Add Ms 61490 f. 197]; Richard Wattes, farrier, London, receipts 1684–85 [Ref: Add Ms 61346 ff. 88, 98, 116, 128]; Andrew Snape, Serjeant-Farrier to Charles II, extracts from *The Anatomy of the Horse* 1687 [Ref: Sloane 256 ff. 9b–15b]; Pasquale Caracciolo, *On The Veterinary Art* 17th cent Italian [Ref: Sloane 2757 ff. 80–237]; John Warde, veterinary prescriptions 17th cent [Ref: Sloane 2562 ff. 66–81]; miscellaneous veterinary recipes 17th–18th cent [Ref: Add Ms 39289]; Edward Manning, veterinarian, receipted bill 1714 [Ref: Add Ms 61656 f. 98]; John Buriand, farrier, agreement with H Morice 1718 [Ref: Add Ms 48590 f. 26]; Edward Stamp, farrier, receipted bills 1730–31 [Ref: Add Ms 61678 ff. 40, 43]; John Drake, citizen and farrier of London: assignment by of a legacy to his creditors 1732 [Ref: Add Ch 70576], general quitclaim 1736 [Ref: Add Ms 42607 f. 63]; medical, household and veterinary recipes c1750 [Ref: Add Ms 29740]; J Huntingford, Secretary to the Veterinary College, London, letters to A Young 1785, 1792 [Ref: Add Ms 35126 f. 287, Add Ms 35127 f. 141]; P M A Broussonet, letter to Sir Joseph Banks introducing de St Bel 1790 [Ref: Add Ms 8097 f. 277]; Bracy Clark, veterinary surgeon, letters to J L Phillips 1790–92 [Ref: Add Ms 29533 ff. 106–122]; Charles Benôit Vial de St Bel, Professor at the Veterinary College, London, letter to Sir Joseph Banks 1793 [Ref: Add Ms 33979 f. 202]; Edward Brown, farrier, receipted bill 1798 [Ref: Add Ms 49186 f. 33]; Robert Johnson, horse doctor, petition to the Duke of Marlborough 18th cent [Ref: Add Ms 61290 ff. 34–35b]; William Sewell, assistant at the Veterinary College, London, prescription for W Windham's horse 1803 [Ref: Add Ms 37870 f. 9]; J White, veterinary surgeon, Exeter, letter to W Sharman [1810] [Ref: Add Ms 71594 ff. 56–57v]; William Stockley, veterinary surgeon, Royal Artillery, report to Sir R Peel 1817 [Ref: Add Ms 40269 f. 49]; William Youatt, veterinary surgeon, letters to J C Hobhouse 1825 [Ref: Add Ms 36461 ff. 132, 135]; Thomas Burrell of Great Windmill Street, Soho, veterinary surgeon, bill and receipt for work carried out by his uncle and predecessor, Charles Newsham 1831 [Ref: Add Ms 74648 ff. 115–116]; John Field, veterinary surgeon, London, certificate of examination of a bay gelding for Prince Lieven 1833 [Ref: Add Ms 47296 f. 113]; Ann Mason, wife of J Mason, veterinary surgeon, London, letters to Lady Peel 1845 [Ref: Add Ms 40580 ff. 80–83b]; John Mason, veterinary surgeon, London: letter to W H Stephenson 1845 [Ref: Add Ms 40561 f. 358], letters to Lady Peel 1845 [Ref: Add Ms 40561 ff. 352, 354, 360]; John Poyntz, 5th Earl Spencer: letters and official papers re foot-and-mouth disease 1865–78, nd [Ref: Add Mss 77374, 77375], letters and horse examination certificates from John Merrick, veterinary surgeon 1866–88 [Ref: Add Ms 77209]; Alexander Williams, Secretary to the Privy Council Office Veterinary Department, letter to Sir B Seton 1869 [Ref: Add Ms 43513 f. 275]; Francis Savage Reilly, barrister, legal advisor to the Veterinary Department, copy of letter to Sir A Helps 1869 [Ref: Add Ms 43539 f. 84]; Alexander Mavor, veterinary surgeon, certificate 1872 [Ref: Add Ms 49330 f. 67]; William Hunting, veterinary surgeon, letter to Sir C Dilke 1906 [Ref: Add Ms 43919 f. 80]; Charles Rowland Chadwick, Director, Civil Veterinary Department, Baghdad: correspondence with Sir A T Wilson 1920 [Ref: Add Ms 52458A ff. 130, 225, Add Ms 52459B f. 55], letter from his staff 1920 [Ref: Add Ms 52458A f. 131]; J K Gupta, Head Clerk, Civil Veterinary Department, Baghdad, letter on behalf of Indian personnel to Sir A T Wilson 1920 [Ref: Add Ms 52459B f. 56]; Francis Albert Eley Crew, Director, Animal Breeding Research Department, Edinburgh University, correspondence with Marie Stopes 1927–28 [Ref: Add Ms 58483 f. 138, Add Ms 58570 ff. 3, 4, 6]; Mrs Dickin, Honorary Director, People's Dispensary for Sick Animals, letter to Marie Stopes 1936 [Ref: Add Ms 58718 f. 86]; Arabic treatise on the veterinary art, nd [Ref: Add Ms 19448]; Arabic treatise on veterinary medicine, nd. [Ref: Add Ms 14056]

ORIENTAL AND INDIA OFFICE COLLECTIONS, BRITISH LIBRARY
96 Euston Road, London NW1 2DB

Mary Fitzgibbon (1813–62) and Sarah Ann Fitzgibbon (c1836–94), second and third wives of Richmond Allen Fitzgibbon (c1805–71), veterinary surgeon, Madras Army, diaries 1831–76 [Ref: B205]; William Gilchrist, Madras Medical Service, manuscript entitled 'A Practical Memoir on the History and Treatment of the Diseases of the Elephant' 1848 [Ref: K503]; Sir Roger Thomas, agriculturalist and government advisor, India and Pakistan, papers re agriculture and development planning, incl veterinary subjects 1913–60. [Ref: F235]

SCIENCE AND TECHNOLOGY SERVICE, BRITISH LIBRARY

96 Euston Road, London NW1 2DB

Patents: purging and diuretic balls for the cure of several diseases incident to horses 1769 [Ref: 941], Thomas Johnson, preparation for staining horses and other animals so as to make them match in colour, also for preserving cattle from flies and other insects, and for making such marks on animals as cannot be effaced without injury to the said animals 1774 [Ref: 1060], Thomas Watson, purging paste for horses and dogs 1783 [Ref: 1387], Thomas Fleet, medicine to prevent the rot in sheep, and to check its progress in those already affected 1794 [Ref: 2014], Edward Coleman, artificial frogs to be applied to horses' feet, for prevention of contracted hoofs, thrushes and canker 1800, construction and application of horseshoes to prevent diseases to which the feet of horses are subject, especially contraction of the hoof 1808, 1820 [Ref: 2370, 3128, 4446], Bracy Clark, horseshoes 1806 [Ref: 2923], John Lewis, horseshoes 1812 [Ref: 3605], Francis Purden, horse boots for the preservation of sound hoofs and the restoration of contracted hoofs 1812 [Ref: 3542], Joseph Manton, shoeing horses 1816 [Ref: 3985], Benjamin Rotch, flexible elastic horse shoe 1816, guards or protections for horses' feet and legs 1830 [Ref: 4025, 5922], Henry Goldfinch, formation of horseshoes 1821 [Ref: 4548], Thomas Barnard Williamson Dudley, making malleable cast metal shoes for draught and riding horses and other animals 1822 [Ref: 4735], James Harris, manufacture of shoes for horses and other cattle 1822 [Ref: 4635], Robert Dickinson, shoeing, stopping and treatment of horses' feet 1823 [Ref: 4827], William Woodman, horseshoe denominated 'Bevilled Heeled Expanding Shoe' 1823 [Ref: 4841], John James Hodgson, construction and manufacture of shoes, or substitutes for shoes, for horses and other cattle, applying the same to the feet 1824 [Ref: 5014], William Percivall, construction and application of shoes, without nails, to the feet of horses and other animals 1828 [Ref: 5610], John Weiss, instruments for bleeding horses and other animals 1828 [Ref: 5612], John James Watt, application of a certain chemical agent for destroying animal poison, and for preventing the disease consequent thereon 1828 [Ref: 5643], Alexander Stocker, machinery for manufacturing horseshoes and certain other articles 1835 [Ref: 6816], Miles Berry, machinery for making horseshoes 1837 [Ref: 7354], John Springall, shoes for horses and other animals 1837 [Ref: 7293], Whitmore Baker, truss applicable to the nicking of horses' tails 1837 [Ref: 7403, h], Alexander Francis Campbell, horseshoes 1839 [Ref: 8108], Charles White, horseshoes 1839 [Ref: 8108], Jules Alphonse Simon Degourney, manufacture of horseshoes 1840 [Ref: 8358], Thomas Harris, horseshoes 1841 [Ref: 8782], Thomas Vaux, horseshoes 1841, 1846 [Ref: 8789,

11131], Henry Barron Rodway, manufacture of horseshoes 1842 [Ref: 9286], James Home, manufacture of horseshoes 1843 [Ref: 9861], James Neville, form and manufacture of horseshoes 1843 [Ref: 9818], Thomas Clarendon, shoeing horses 1843 [Ref: 9933], Stephen Bencraft, making and fitting up harness for prevention and cure of galled shoulders in draught horses 1844 [Ref: 10246], Laurence Hill, machinery for manufacturing shoes for horses and other animals 1844 [Ref: 10007], Dennis Woodin, forms of shoes for horses or other animals, and process of accomplishing same 1845 [Ref: 10581], Alfred Watney, manufacture of horseshoes, and applying shoes to horses and other animals 1845 [Ref: 10917], Charles Powell, construction of horseshoes 1845 [Ref: 10605], Charles Black, manufacture of horseshoes 1845 [Ref: 10620], Richard Hobson, manufacture of horseshoes, apparatus for measuring horses' shoes or hoofs 1849 [Ref: 12900], William Parry, horseshoes 1849 [Ref: 12560], James Smith, treating the fleeces of sheep when on the animals 1849 [Ref: 12902], Alexander Mein, treating the fleeces of sheep when on the animals 1849 [Ref: 13391], Thomas Huckvale, instruments for administrating medicine to horses and other animals 1852 [Ref: 35], Joseph Major, removing spavins, ringbones, curbs, splents and other unnatural ossifications and humours from horses, *Major's Celebrated British Remedy* 1852 [Ref: 387], George Stuart, treating the fleeces or natural coverings of sheep and other animals when on the animals 1852 [Ref: 195], William Edward Newton, horseshoes 1853 [Ref: 1847], William George Reeve, an appendage to horseshoes to supersede the necessity of roughing 1853 [Ref: 2844], Auguste Castels, composition for curing diseases in the feet of animals 1853 [Ref: 2689], John Baily, cure of the roup and other diseases in fowls and poultry 1853 [Ref: 2442], trocars or cannulas for teats, vaccine appliances [Ref: A61D/1/02], cropping devices for tails or ears [Ref: A61D/1/04], castrating appliances [Ref: A61/D/1/06], obstetrical instruments or devices [Ref: A61D/1/08], embryotomic instruments [Ref: A61D/1/10], instruments for removing foreign bodies from animals' throats, oesophagus or stomachs [Ref: A61D/1/12], devices for degrassing animals' stomachs [Ref: A61D/1/14], magnets for the stomach [Ref: A61D/1/16], appliances for supporting or fettering animals for operative purposes [Ref: A61D/3/00], instruments for treating animals' teeth [Ref: A61D/5/00], devices or methods for introducing solid, liquid or gaseous remedies or other materials into or onto the bodies of animals [Ref: A61D/7/00], devices for artificial insemination [Ref: A61D/7/02], devices for anaesthetising animals by gases or vapours, inhaling devices [Ref: A61D/7/04], bandages, poultices, compresses specially adapted to veterinary purposes [Ref: A61D/9/00], prolapsus appliances [Ref: A61D/9/02], washing devices or gaseous curative baths specially adapted to veterinary purposes [Ref:

A61D/11/00], thermometer holders specially adapted to veterinary purposes [Ref: A61D/13/00], mouth openers [Ref: A61/15/00], devices for indicating trouble during labour of animals [Ref: A61D/17/00], veterinary preparations. [Ref: A61K]

HACKNEY ARCHIVES DEPARTMENT
43 De Beauvoir Road, London N1 5SQ

Farrier, Sandford Lane, London, sale catalogue 1846. [Ref: HAD M3987]

HAMMERSMITH & FULHAM ARCHIVES AND LOCAL HISTORY CENTRE
The Lilla Huset, 191 Talgarth Road, London W6 8BJ

J Woodger & Broad, The Veterinary Infirmary, 39b Goldhawk Road, London, receipted invoices 1912, 1936 [Ref: DD/491 Box 8]; Animals' Help Society, 281 Goldhawk Road, London, programme of entertainment 1937. [Ref: H619]

INSTITUTE OF EDUCATION
20 Bedford Way, London WC1H 0AL

Animal Defence Society, verbatim report of proceedings of a conference on humane and inhumane methods of destroying animals 1933.

KINGS COLLEGE ARCHIVES
Strand, London WC2R 2LS

Chelsea College Nuffield archives, correspondence with veterinary colleges re acceptability of Schools Council Integrated Science Project qualification in admissions policy 1978–79. [Ref: C/SCISP10/F48, F51]

KINGSTON MUSEUM AND HERITAGE SERVICE
North Kingston Centre, Richmond Road, Kingston upon Thames KT2 5PE

William Harding of Kingston, farrier, party to lease and release 1832 [Ref: KT55/34a–b]; Louis Charles Welfare of 24 Gardiners Place, Dublin, Ireland, veterinary surgeon, party to conveyance 1895 [Ref: KT24/5]; plan showing land leased to Mr Edwards, veterinary surgeon, nd. [Ref: KT1044/4/133]

LAMBETH PALACE LIBRARY
Lambeth, London SE1 7JU

A medycyne for a syck ox 15th cent [Ref: MS.241, f. 263]; apprenticeship of Henry Gloster as a surgeon, incl training in curing distempers in cows, horses, etc 1673 [Ref: VX 1A/10/208]; prayers for animals 1942 [Ref: W Temple 1, ff. 329–336]; letters and papers re prayers for animals 1966. [Ref: Ramsey 91, ff. 39–40]

THE LINNEAN SOCIETY OF LONDON
Burlington House, Piccadilly, London W1V 0LQ

Carolus Linnaeus, diagnosis of animals incl some made during his visit to England 18th cent.

LONDON METROPOLITAN ARCHIVES
40 Northampton Road, London EC1R 0HB

Robert Hassell, citizen and farrier of London, party to deeds 1589, 1590 [Ref: E/HOD/041, 048]; Edward Salisbury, citizen and farrier of London, party to deeds re meadow commonly called Two Acres 1659 [Ref: ACC/0401/050/051, 052]; Joseph Comfort senior of Clapham, farrier, party to lease 1697 [Ref: E/DCA/141]; William Benskin, St Mary Newington Butts, Surrey, farrier, party to lease 1714 [Ref: O/027/020]; Thomas Stanton of Limehouse, farrier, probate of will 1726 [Ref: ACC/1045/138]; William Bowers of St Martin in the Fields, farrier, and Elizabeth, wife of John Palmer, farrier, parties to assignment of interest to Mary Stanton 1728 [Ref: ACC/1045/139]; Nathaniel Preston of St James, Westminster, farrier, party to deeds re 43 and 45 Beak Street 1729, 1735 [Ref: ACC/1871/037–039]; deeds re The King of Prussia's Head [public house], farrier's shop, tenement and messuage in Stratford Langthorne, Westham, Essex 1729, 1770 [Ref: H01/ST/Y/343/001, 005]; William Beck of Twickenham, farrier, party to deeds 1714, 1731 [Ref: ACC/1246/024; ACC/1087/038]; John Palmer and Robert Franklin of St James, Westminster, farriers, parties to deeds re property in Rupert Street, Westminster 1736, 1743 [Ref: ACC/1045/116, 117]; bill for attention to, and medicines for, horses with burns 1771 [Ref: Acc. 446/H23/85]; James Jarvis of Enfield, farrier, party to deeds re land in Enfield 1779, 1786, 1787 [Ref: ACC/0371/060–063]; George Pepper: receipts from William Kingston of Harden, Hertfordshire, for veterinary treatment 1788 [Ref: Q/STB/091], receipts from Thomas Hickson for veterinary treatment 1791 [Ref: Q/STB/092], bills and receipts from Robert Rogers, blacksmith, for veterinary attendance 1815–16 [Ref: Q/STB/125], bills and receipts from Alexander Henderson of 8 Park Lane, London, veterinary surgeon 1825–26 [Ref: Q/STB/130]; William Newport of Grays Inn Lane, St Andrew Holborn, farrier, party to release and assignment 1793 [Ref: ACC/0015/008]; Read family, account book containing veterinary recipes 1823–30 [Ref: ACC/1093/031]; James Beart Simonds of Twickenham, veterinary surgeon, party to conveyance by bargain and sale 1838 [Ref: ACC/638/410]; James Pepper, High Street, Bow, farrier, party to counterpart lease 1840 [Ref: M/093/344]; Joseph Mead, 41 Old Street, St Luke, Middlesex, farrier, party to lease 1845 [Ref: O/065/002]; recipe for curing warts on cow's teats mid 19th cent [Ref: Acc. 1040/79]; Thomas Taylor of Charlton, farrier, party to lease 1857 [Ref: E/MW/C/839]; James Frederick Hall of Twickenham, veterinary surgeon, party to leases re premises in Twickenham and Old Brentford 1882, 1888, 1889 [Ref: ACC/1269/002–004]; Francis Walker of Meerut, India, inspecting veterinary surgeon, party to reconveyance 1892 [Ref: ACC/1013/073]; particulars of sale re property incl Harringay Arms beer house, stabling, farrier's premises, house and garden at corner of Crouch Hill and Crouch Hill End 1894 [Ref: ACC/1289/004]; photograph of workers and dogs at Battersea Dogs' Home c1900 [Ref: 47.4 BAT]; Sidney Villar of Greenhill, Harrow, veterinary surgeon, party to conveyance 1901 [Ref: ACC/0076/0998]; London County Council, education officer's department, papers re Royal Veterinary College, London 1913–36 [Ref: LCC/EO/HFE/5/145]; Metropolitan Drinking Fountain and Cattle Trough Association, papers re appeal to rebuild Royal Veterinary College, London 1922–27 [Ref: ACC/3168/251]; Board of Deputies of British Jews, presidents and secretaries papers: veterinary congress papers on Shechita 1930 [Ref: ACC/3121/B/04/V007], correspondence with Sir Frederick Hobday re Shechita 1931–38 [Ref: ACC/3121/B/04/H0A001], reports re attitude of Dutch veterinary surgeons towards Shechita as represented by the Sophia Society 1933 [Ref: ACC/3121/B/04/H0A004], correspondence with British Veterinary Association 1963–69 [Ref: ACC/3121/C/16/039]; Greater London Council, Legal Department, file re parliamentary bills concerning veterinary surgeons, nd. [Ref: LRB/LD/P/081/044]

LIBRARY OF THE RELIGIOUS SOCIETY OF FRIENDS
Religious Society of Friends in Britain, Friends House, 173–177 Euston Road, London NW1 2BJ

Bracy Clark, veterinarian: letter to William Phillips 1813 [Ref: MS VOL 337/27], signature, nd [Ref: MS PORT 27/48]; John Barlow, veterinarian: manuscript entitled 'A Few Expressions of our Beloved John Barlow' 1856 [Ref: TRACT BOX 234], letter M Nicholson to P Green re John

Barlow 1856 [Ref: MS PORT/B/83], published memoir re John Barlow 1858 [Ref: TRACT VOL 542/4], signature, nd [Ref: MS VOL 338/87]; S Hoare, letter to 'Wombwell' advising him not to proceed with a fight between a lion and six dogs, nd. [Ref: MS PORT 42/10]

NATIONAL ARCHIVES
Ruskin Avenue, Kew, Richmond TW9 4DU

Board of Customs and Excise
Consideration of principles of exemption of certain medical, dental and veterinary instruments and drugs from purchase tax 1940–43 [Ref: CUST49/2636]; Northern Ireland land boundary, use of unapproved roads by veterinary surgeons 1942–47. [Ref: CUST49/2764]

British Council
Inter-University Council for Higher Education Overseas, correspondence and papers re Kenya Veterinary School and other schools 1946–80. [Ref: BW90]

British Transport Commission
Commercial committee veterinary sub-committee, minutes 1954–58. [Ref: AN97/41]

Cabinet Office
Files re: medical and veterinary supplies 1924–26 [Ref: CAB60/19], veterinary service in Italy 1946 [Ref: CAB106/453], adjournment debate on veterinary services 1954 [Ref: CAB124/2956], British Veterinary Association representations about field trials 1954–55 [Ref: CAB124/2955], future organisation of veterinary research 1954–57 [Ref: CAB124/2954], use of radioactive materials and x-rays in veterinary practice 1964 [Ref: CAB124/2569], preparation of code of practice for the protection of persons exposed to ionising radiation in veterinary practice 1964–65. [Ref: CAB124/3043]

Central Criminal Court
Depositions re food offences against Shaw's Veterinary Products Limited and others 1942. [Ref: CRIM1/1450]

Chancery
Men and tenants of Shipdham and East Dereham v John de Wesenham, alleged extortion of the King's farrier of the temporalities of the bishopric of Ely County 1358/59 [Ref: C44/2/30]; John Bell of London, draper, v John Hornbye, churchwarden, of St Dunstan's Fleet St and others, shop in

the said parish bequeathed to a chantry in the said church by Robert Hay citizen and farrier of London 1413 [Ref: C1/1289/20–23]; lease, Thomas Hatton of London, grocer, to Edward Salisbury of London, farrier, of property on Broad Street, All Hallows, London Wall, and assignment of lease to Nicholas Grice of Grays Inn, Middlesex, of the same property 1664 and 1670 [Ref: C104/269 Bundle 48]; assignment of Edward Salisbury of London, farrier, to Thomas Harkett of Cheshunt, Hertfordshire, doctor of divinity, of property on Broad Street, All Hallows, London Wall 1667 [Ref: C104/267 Bundle 44]; Munn & Tinnewell, veterinary and horse fodder receipts 1839–41 [Ref: C171/49]; Robert Browne of London, carter, v the Sheriffs of London, detention of complainant under an alderman's commandment pending an action of debt brought by Richard Watson of London, farrier, petition for a writ of *corpus cum causa*, nd [Ref: C1/31/517]; Richard Watson of London, farrier, v the Sheriffs of London and Walter Bewfild, arrest for debt arising out of a dispute as to the repair of a forge in the parish of St Peter, Cornhill, nd [Ref: C1/176/18]; William Harbery, citizen and farrier of London v William Tomlynson of Stanton, messuage and land at Langley in Hever, Kent, nd [Ref: C1/703/30]; William Randall, citizen and farrier of London v the Mayor and Sheriffs of London and Joan Mongham, action on a bond for rent of a tenement in Fenchurch Street, held of the masters of the Bridge-house, nd [Ref: C1/883/6]; Robert Watson of London, minstral, v the Mayor, Aldermen and Sheriffs of London, John Bradley of Southwark, farrier, Roger Sankee of London, shoemaker, and Thomas his brother, action on a bond given on behalf of the said Roger in error, nd [Ref: C1/919/1]; John Wylson v the Sheriffs of London, Thomas Dyxon, farrier, action of debt in breach of an arbitral award by Thomas Wyngfield, knight, nd [Ref: C1/927/43]; William Bodyley of London, farrier, v Richard Laplowe and Agnes his wife, cattle and goods sold to William Porter of Fradsowe, nd [Ref: C1/1288/46]; William Bodeley of London, farrier, v Thomas Momford the elder and Thomas Momford the younger, meadow in Norton granted on a nine year lease by Hugh Balle, nd. [Ref: C1/1331/38]

Civil Service Commission

Tables of examination marks and results 1907–08, 1921 [Ref: CSC10]; regulations, rules and memoranda re open and limited competitions re veterinary officers 1907–08, 1926, 1933, 1966–73 [Ref: CSC6]; revised recruiting arrangements for veterinary officers, research officers, assistant veterinary investigation officers 1962 [Ref: CSC5/960]; papers re recruitment problems 1969–70. [Ref: CSC5/1746]

Civil Service Pay Research Unit
Veterinary grades survey no 55 1961. [Ref: CSPR1/64]

Copies of captured records of German, Italian and Japanese governments
German delegation to Moscow Conference 1924–25, veterinary agreement 1925. [Ref: GFM33/3783]

Court of Bankruptcy
J Home, veterinary surgeon 1845. [Ref: B9/70]

Crown Estate Commissioners
Appointment of veterinary surgeons to Windsor Establishment 1864–1935. [Ref: CRES4/78]

Defunct temporary bodies
Evidence from British Veterinary Association and Royal College of Veterinary Surgeons to Royal Commission on Gambling 1976. [Ref: BS3/29, 117, 346, 362]

Department of Education and Science
Royal College of Veterinary Surgeons, file re Clement Stephenson scholarship 1919 [Ref: ED39/740]; Royal Veterinary College, London, file re Ewin scholarship 1937–38 [Ref: ED39/1250]; standard inventories of basic scientific equipment, part III geology, agriculture, veterinary science 1945 [Ref: ED42/30]; G White, approval given to payment of additional grant to veterinary student in respect of six months 'seeing practice' necessitating residence in lodgings during two vacation periods 1948–55 [Ref: ED94/234]; M K Snow, additional grant of £3 paid to veterinary student 1951–55 [Ref: ED94/260]; request for veterinary school in Wales, file re facilities and manpower problems 1964–72 [Ref: ED188/175]; follow-up to Pilkington Report, papers on Veterinary Surgeons Act 1966 [Ref: ED46/803]; department's comments on draft training regulations of Royal College of Veterinary Surgeons 1966–68. [Ref: ED188/185]

Department of the Environment
British Veterinary Association, evidence submitted to committee of enquiry into local government finance 1974. [Ref: AT10/464]

Department responsible for labour and employment matters and related bodies
General policy for veterinary surgeons 1939–41 [Ref: LAB6/132]; allocation of veterinary students on graduation in 1947 and 1948 [Ref: LAB8/1413]; publications re careers 1948, 1968, 1975 [Ref: LAB44/19, 68; LAB52/93]; National Service Acts, veterinary students completing full time studies in 1951. [Ref: LAB8/1828]

Department of Scientific and Industrial Research
Committee for analytical methods to determine residues of pesticides and veterinary products in foodstuffs, terms of reference 1967–70. [Ref: DSIR26/1034]

Department of Technical Co-Operation and of successive Overseas Development Bodies
File re secondment of veterinary surgeons 1964–66 [Ref: OD8/251]; correspondence with British Veterinary Association 1964–66 [Ref: OD25/27, 28]; papers re veterinary staff recruitment, incl animal husbandry experts for Kenya 1964–66 [Ref: OD8/252, 253]; papers re assistance towards expansion of Veterinary School of Edinburgh University 1964–67 [Ref: OD25/24, 25]; proposal to establish a training institution on tropical veterinary medicine 1964–67 [Ref: OD25/27]; papers re veterinary clinician for Iran 1965 [Ref: OD34/119]; papers re veterinary studentship scheme 1967–69 [Ref: OD8/387]; file re establishment of Centre for Tropical Veterinary Medicine and Applied Protozoology Research Department at Edinburgh 1967–69 [Ref: OD11/237–39]; papers re links between Glasgow and East African veterinary schools 1968–69. [Ref: OD17/311]

Deposits, gifts, etc
Deeds re a messuage, The Boar's Head, near Clements Inn 'foregate' from Gilbert, Earl of Clare, to Thomas Halfepenny, farrier, of St Martin in the Fields parish 1669 [Ref: PRO30/26, 74/7; PRO30/26, 74/8]; letter from Kitchener to Brodrick with information on field veterinary hospitals 1901. [Ref: PRO30/57/22]

Exchequer and related bodies
Expenses of the king's horses at Chester in the keeping of Richard Farrier 1308/09 [Ref: E101/97/2]; accounts of William the Farrier, keeper of horses south of Trent 1344–46 [Ref: E101/102/35, 36]; leases of messuages in Long Lane, Great St Bartholomews, London, to Thomas Younge, farrier 1647, 1656 [Ref: E214/86; E214/758; E214/759]; Robert Young, farrier, lease of a house called The Spotted Dog, etc 1727 [Ref:

E367/6747]; William Spynke, farrier, will 1427 [Ref: E210/4982]; John Lovich of Pirton, Worcestershire, farrier, to Margery late the wife of William Ravel and Richard her son, Pershore, deed, nd. [Ref: E210/1874]

Foreign and Commonwealth Office
Discussion on possible appointment of veterinary attaché to embassy in Uruguay 1969. [Ref: FCO7/315]

General Nursing Council for England and Wales
Medical, Nursing, Dental and Veterinary Qualifications (European Economic Community Recognition) Order SI1982/1076. [Ref: DT1/10]

General Register Office
Notification of deaths to Royal College of Veterinary Surgeons, Veterinary Surgeons Act 1948 [Ref: RG48/2312]; leaflets issued on death of veterinary surgeons 1974. [Ref: RG41/70]

Government Actuary Department
Forecast of future number of veterinary surgeons 1963. [Ref: ACT1/1435]

High Court of Delegates
Memorandum by John Fisher and Anne Mather on nuncupative will of William Nicholls, farrier, of Islington 1672 [Ref: DEL10/57]; Samuel Palfrey, veterinary surgeon, Worcester, signed will made 1824 proved 1829. [Ref: DEL10/157]

Higher Education Funding Council for England
File re possible move of Royal Veterinary College, London, from Camden Town to Potters Bar 1971–76. [Ref: UGC7/1095]

Inland Revenue
Royal College of Veterinary Surgeons: allowance of subscriptions 1924–25 [Ref: IR40/2832], corporation duty files 1916–18, 1939–52. [Ref: IR41/134]

Keeper of Privy Purse
Correspondence with Royal College of Veterinary Surgeons, nd. [Ref: PP1/102, 504]

Law Officer's Department
Validity of Veterinary Surgeons (Agreement with Republic of Ireland) Order 1954, opinion 1956. [Ref: LO2/841]

Lord Chancellor's Office
Royal College of Veterinary Surgeons, files re charters and supplementary charters 1932, 1960, 1963, 1965, 1967 [Ref: LCO6/271, 2476, 2505, 2476, 2602]; Royal Veterinary College, London, files re charters of incorporation and supplementary charters 1936, 1946, 1956 [Ref: LCO6/333, 1695, 2029]; Veterinary Surgeons Act 1948, rules of court to provide for hearing of appeals 1948–49 [Ref: LCO2/4109]; Royal Commission of Civil Liability and Compensation for Personal Injury, evidence from British Veterinary Association 1974–75. [Ref: LCO 20/815]

Metropolitan Police Office
Police Order, payment of veterinary surgeons' fees in cruelty cases 1895–1933 [Ref: MEPO2/5701]; wrongful diagnosis by a veterinary surgeon 1905 [Ref: MEPO2/796]; Injured Animals Act 1907, recovery of veterinary fees 1908 [Ref: MEPO2/1210]; animals injured in street accidents, arrangements by Royal Society for the Prevention of Cruelty to Animals to pay veterinary surgeons' fees and provide a twenty four hour service for injuries and complaints of cruelty, conveyance of injured animals in police utility vans 1924–29, 1936 [Ref: MEPO2/5883]; notification of convictions to Royal College of Veterinary Surgeons 1929 [Ref: MEPO2/2012]; horses for police service purchased at provincial sales, examination by local veterinary surgeons 1931–46 [Ref: MEPO2/7479]; instruction of Chelsea Barracks farrier by police in the rubber shoeing of horses 1934 [Ref: MEPO2/3985]; Home Office authority, payment of veterinary surgeon's fee when called out at night 1934–35 [Ref: MEPO2/5733]; file re Royal Veterinary College, London, Miniature Rifle Club 1938–44 [Ref: MEPO2/4398]; veterinary officer attested as a Special Constable 1939 [Ref: MEPO2/4018]; fees payable to veterinary surgeons 1946–60. [Ref: MEPO2/7898]

Ministry of Housing and Local Government
National Veterinary Medical Association Annual Congress 1950, delegates' expenses 1938–53. [Ref: HLG52/1541]

Ministry of Munitions
Plant for disposing of carcasses of dead animals at field veterinary hospitals in France 1918–19. [Ref: MUN4/5272]

Ministry of National Service
Request by Royal College of Veterinary Surgeons for demobilisation of students under certain conditions to address shortage of veterinary surgeons 1917–18. [Ref: NATS1/1059]

Ministry of Pensions and National Insurance
Royal Army Veterinary Corps, effect of increased rates of service retired pay on regular officers' retired pay 1920–29 [Ref: PIN15/139]; assistant to sales representative of firm of veterinary chemists 1949–50 [Ref: PIN48/45]; correspondence, statistics, personal cases and extracts from Hansard re resolutions by Trades Union Congress, British Veterinary Association and others on brucellosis 1951–70 [Ref: PIN20/79]; Royal Society for the Prevention of Cruelty to Animals, honorary veterinary surgeons 1955 [Ref: PIN49/28]; papers re veterinary inspector (employed earner) 1976–78. [Ref: PIN48/336]

Ministry of Power
Coal Mines Act 1911, appointment of consulting veterinary surgeons, payment of fees, travelling and subsistence allowances 1912–23 [Ref: POWE10/284]; accident prevention, contravention of section 35(1) by inspecting veterinary surgeon taking matches into mine 1913. [Ref: POWE8/40]

Ministry of Supply, Ordnance Board and related bodies
Civil requirements of foodstuffs, medical and veterinary supplies 1925–1930s [Ref: SUPP14/622, 623]; suggested enquiry into foodstuffs, medical and veterinary supplies 1928. [Ref: SUPP3/70]

National Coal Board
East Midlands division, veterinary reports re pit ponies at area collieries 1947–67 [Ref: COAL75/4563, 4564]; veterinary reports re ponies 1964–66. [Ref: COAL50/672]

National Incomes Commission
Memorandum on salaries at Royal Veterinary College, London 1963. [Ref: NICO1/5]

National Savings Committee, Post Office Savings Department and Department for National Savings
Campaign posters re girls in veterinary surgery 1960. [Ref: NSC25/280]

Pre-nationalised railway companies, etc
Memoranda book with details of agencies, boat horse stations, wagon stations, distance tables and statistics re provender purchased, veterinary prescriptions for horses, etc 1829–1935 [Ref: RAIL1133/129]; accounts paid, incl blacksmith and veterinary surgeon 1838–45 [Ref: RAIL371/36]; agreement between Great Western Railway Company and Joseph Claymouth, veterinary surgeon, Birmingham, for appointment as

veterinary surgeon at Hockley, Warwickshire 1871 [Ref: RAIL252/425]; agreement between Thomas Greaves, veterinary surgeon, Manchester, and Lancashire & Yorkshire Railway for attending their horses at Manchester and Salford goods stations three times per week and in cases of emergency 1871 [Ref: RAIL795/558]; agreement between John Scholfield and William George Scholfield, veterinary surgeons, Pontefract, for attending Lancashire & Yorkshire Railway's horses at all stations in Yorkshire except Todmorden 1871 [Ref: 795/559]; correspondence re resignations of W Allen, traffic manager, and W Martin, veterinary surgeon 1888–1900 [Ref: RAIL1130/81]; alleged lime burning of pigs by chemists and veterinary surgeons 1910 [Ref: RAIL1080/363]; Southern Area cartage committee, closing of Lodge Road Veterinary Hospital, Marylebone 1926–27. [Ref: RAIL390/589]

Prerogative Court of Canterbury

Roger King, citizen and farrier of London, will 1663 [Ref: PROB4/20626]; John Toombes, citizen and farrier of London, will 1664 [Ref: PROB4/1169]; John Griffin of St Andrew in the Wardrobe, London, farrier, will 1665 [Ref: PROB4/11538]; William Nicholls of Islington, farrier, will 1672 [Ref: PROB5/2392]; George Pittman of Petworth, West Sussex, farrier, will 1675 [Ref: PROB4/10/109]; John Lovell of St Sephulchre, Middlesex, farrier, will 1676/77 [Ref: PROB4/1678]; Henry Price of Eldersfield alias Elsfield, Worcestershire, farrier, will 1677 [Ref: PROB4/7146]; Thomas Waller, citizen and farrier, London, will 1679 [Ref: PROB4/10179]; William Smith of Twickenham, Middlesex, farrier, will 1688 [Ref: PROB4/7730]; Thomas Ambrose of Rugby, Warwickshire, farrier, will 1690 [Ref: PROB4/2406]; Francis Flower, London, farrier, will 1714 [Ref: PROB20/947]; John Motteram, Uttoxeter, Staffordshire, farrier, will 1783 [Ref: PROB3/37/1244]; Palfrey and Palfrey v Price and others testator or intestate, Samuel Palfrey of Worcester, veterinary surgeon 1825–28 [Ref: PROB37/606]; Smith and others v Smith testator or intestate, James Smith, late of Prospect Cottages, Thornhill Road, Islington, veterinary surgeon and farrier 1847–48. [Ref: PROB37/1438]

Prison Commission and Home Office Prison Department

Veterinary attendance, issue of tenders discounted, veterinary surgeons appointed 1927–28. [Ref: PCOM7/74]

State Paper Office

Account of Haniball Zynzan, marshal farrier of the royal stable, for medicines and ointments for the King's horses for one year ending 25 March 1547 [Ref: SP46/1/fo9]; William Golightlye, the Queen's serjeant farrier, to the township of Stratford Langthorne 1572. [Ref: SP46/15/fo55]

Supreme Court of Judicature
Counterpart of lease of house of farrier and veterinary surgeon in Datchet Road, New Windsor, Berkshire, belonging to infant John Newlands 1862 [Ref: J90/1076]; medical, surgical and veterinary instruments, appliances and pharmaceutical products mainly for hospital or professional use 1967. [Ref: J90/1076]

Transport Department
Provision of veterinary stores on transports 1905. [Ref: MT23/187]

Treasury Solicitor and HM Procurator Fiscal Department
W H Turner, veterinary surgeon, an insolvent in the county court, Hereford, Herefordshire 1870 [Ref: TS25/1671]; Veterinary Department Ireland, file re establishment, appointment of officers, salaries 1872 [Ref: TS 25/1747]; Development and Road Improvement Funds Acts 1909 and 1910, Central Veterinary Laboratory, Weybridge, Surrey, whether land can be compulsorily acquired 1935. [Ref: TS27/1087]

Various research institutes
Kenya Veterinary Department: papers re Dr Furlong's East Africa visit 1953–55, report by Dr Mann on survey of Nigerian hides, skins and animal by-products 1955, report by Dr Mann on improvement of slaughter and meat handling facilities and development of animal by-products industry in the British Caribbean 1956–57, sample of wild game meat for vitamin analysis 1962–65 [Ref: AY4/927, 976, 1021, 1526, 2795]; Tropical Products Institute, comments on pyrethrum extract monograph being prepared for *British Veterinary Codex* 1952. [Ref: AY4/1889]

Welsh Office
Agricultural panel re veterinary college in Wales, papers 1958–64. [Ref: BD23/36]

NATIONAL FILM AND TELEVISION ARCHIVE
21 Stephen Street, London W1P 1PL

Between 100 and 200 films on veterinary medicine and animal husbandry c1940–.

ROYAL BOROUGH OF KENSINGTON AND CHELSEA
Local Studies Library, Central Library, Phillimore Walk, London W8 7RX

Wharves and plant committee, minutes incl references to purchase, care and treatment of horses 1877–1900; wharves and plant committee, horse sub-committee appointed to consider present arrangements for purchase, care and treatment of horses and stable management 1892–93; veterinary surgeons' receipts and letters re care of horses belonging to Edward Linley Sambourne, artist, Kensington 1881, 1889–90 [Ref: ST/1/6/123]; J Stonebridge, Veterinary Shoeing Forge, Earl's Court Road, receipted bills issued to Edward Linley Sambourne, artist, Kensington 1889–97. [Ref: ST/1/6/122]

ROYAL BOTANIC GARDENS
Library and Archives, Kew, Richmond TW9 3AB

Research correspondence with universities, botanical gardens and individuals re medicinal uses and toxicity of plants incl some veterinary, nd.

ROYAL COLLEGE OF VETERINARY SURGEONS
Wellcome Library, Belgravia House, 62–64 Horseferry Road, London SW1P 2AF

Day book for unidentified practice in Thornhill, Dumfries & Galloway 1914–18.

UNIVERSITY COLLEGE LONDON
Manuscripts Room, The Library, Gower Street, London WC1E 6BT

Society for Diffusion of Useful Knowledge, correspondence: Sir Charles Bell re animal mechanics 1827, 1829 and animal physiology 1829, Thomas Southwood Smith re animal mechanics 1828, Peter Mark Roget re animal physiology 1828–30, William Youatt, veterinary surgeon, re veterinary, agricultural and farriery matters 1828–45, David Jardine re animal physiology 1829, Henry Bellenden Ker re animal mechanics 1829 and animal physiology c1829, Robert Baldwin re animal mechanics 1829 and animal physiology 1829–32, John Connolly re animal physiology 1829–30, G Layton re animal physiology 1830, Stephen Sly re animal physiology 1830, John Parratt re animal physiology 1830, William Coulson re animal motion 1833.

WALTHAM FOREST ARCHIVES
Vestry House Museum, London Borough of Waltham Forest, Vestry Road, Walthamstow, London E17 9NH

Jones' Forge, Station Road, Chingford, deeds and associated papers 1784–1956 [Ref: V67.1–53]; Permanent Amalgamated Farriers' Protection Society, Walthamstow branch, out of work book 1902–40. [Ref: W 29.2 PAF1]

ARCHIVES AND MANUSCRIPTS, WELLCOME LIBRARY FOR THE HISTORY AND UNDERSTANDING OF MEDICINE
183 Euston Road, London NW1 2BE

Medical compendium comprising 'the boke of marschalse', a treatise on medicine and horse breeding 15th cent [Ref: MS 5650]; Robert Barret, 'The Buds of Experience', a treatise on horse medicine and farriery c1660 [Ref: MS 1070]; medicines, human and animal, supplied to Lord Leigh, Mrs Monks, Mrs Browne and a nurse by J Bett 1687, medicines supplied to 'Old Gascoyn' (probably a horse) by J Yardley, to be paid for by Lord Leigh 1738 [Ref: MS 7526]; Eusebius Ashby, *The First Book of Horses* and *The Second Book of Horses* 1705–40 [Ref: MS 993, 994]; correspondence from veterinary surgeons and veterinary manufacturers 1796–1913 [Ref: MS 7568]; recipes for cure of horses, cattle, etc mid 18th cent [Ref: MS 4124]; Repps family, Norfolk, recipe book incl veterinary recipes 18th cent [Ref: 7788]; James Clark, observations upon the shoeing of horses late 18th cent [Ref: MS 1658]; unidentified apothecary, recipe book incl veterinary preparations c1800 [Ref: MS 5712]; veterinary surgeons, misc bills and receipts 1808–1933 [Ref: MS 7562]; farriers and blacksmiths, misc bills and receipts 1815–1916 [Ref: MS 7563]; Edward Coleman, Guy's Hospital, London, lectures on the veterinary art 1817, 1822 [Ref: MS 1709, MS 7794]; Edward Barrett Curteis, commonplace book containing notes on veterinary medicine and other subjects 1823–26 [Ref: MS 1981]; Charles Wallwork, chemist and druggist, recipe book containing veterinary preparations c1829 [Ref: MS 5728]; veterinary medicine manufacturers and animal feedstuffs merchants, misc bills and one recipe 1829–1926 [Ref: MS 7564]; apprenticeship agreement binding George South to William Mavor, veterinary surgeon 1833 [Ref: MS 7569]; James Brocklehurst, Hyde, Manchester, chemist and druggist, prescription book incl veterinary prescriptions 1844–73 [Ref: MS 5946]; Thomas Dunlop, Thorn, papers re purchase of horse subsequently found to be unsound from James Newall, Newton Stewart, incl certificate from examining veterinary surgeon, John Simpson, Kilmarnock, East Ayrshire 1854–55 [Ref: MS 7567];

photograph of delegates at 1st International Veterinary Congress 1863; Thomas Hodgkin, physician and philanthropist, letterbook containing letter to Lord Granville with a memorandum on the Brown Trust (later the Brown Animal Sanatory Institution) 1865–66 [Ref: MS 5683]; certificates re veterinary examination of animals, chiefly horses 1876–99 [Ref: MS 7565]; George Fleming, commission of appointment to post of veterinary surgeon, Army Second Life Guards 1877 [Ref: MS 5777]; Louis Pasteur, correspondence re inoculation against swine fever 1883 [Ref: MS 5127]; J Blench, announcement of his acquisition of the late William Stephenson's veterinary practice, Pickering, North Yorkshire, 1884 [Ref: MS 7569]; papers re purchase of animals and feedstuffs 1887–1901 [Ref: MS 7566]; Frederick Parkes Weber, papers re animals and their disorders and diseases, mostly those communicable to humans 1890s–1940s [Ref: FPW]; veterinary receipts mid 19th cent [Ref: MS 4125]; James Henry Bennett, notes of lectures at Royal Veterinary College, London 19th cent [Ref: MS 7652]; W R Brumet, veterinary recipe book 19th cent [Ref: MS 7653]; Thomas Brigstocke Humphreys, chemist, veterinary recipes 19th cent [Ref: MS 7702]; chemist's notebook 19th cent [Ref: 7791]; Edward and May Mellanby, papers re experiments into diet, vitamins, teeth and dentition using dogs c1910–60 [Ref: MEL]; Thomas Lewis, correspondence re animal supply 1920–35 [Ref: LEW]; William Arthur Pool, army veterinarian, notes taken at Institut Pasteur, Paris, while following a course on animal disease c1921 [Ref: GC/111]; film of delegates at 11th International Veterinary Congress 1930 [Ref: GC/129]; Honor Bridget Fell, notebooks re experiments on animals 1930s–40s [Ref: HBF]; Alexander Haddow, research notebooks re grafting, operations, injections, etc using animals 1940s–50s [Ref: HAD]; Dr Geoffrey Clough Ainsworth, mycologist, University of Exeter: report on Agricultural Research Council survey of animal mycosis 1952–53, history of medical mycology committee, nd [Ref: GC/1/2–3]; J Hugh Baron, articles, correspondence and photographs re the Brown Dog of University College [London] 1955–56, 1985–86 [Ref: GC/199]; Henry Foy and Athena Kondi, papers re use of a colony of baboons in Kenya for study of vitamin B deficiency 1950s–70s [Ref: FAK]; Alan Sterling Parkes: papers re poultry science and British Egg Marketing Board 1960–70, correspondence and reports from Nuffield Unit of Tropical Animal Ecology, Uganda 1968–82 [Ref: ASP]; Robert J Hetherington, subject file on animals re work on oral contraceptives 1960s–80s [Ref: RJH]; Martin Folkes, President, Royal Society, correspondence re several matters incl veterinary medicine, nd [Ref: MS 5403]; Sydney Galvayne, lecture notes re horse dentition, nd [Ref: MS 3579]; Guy's Hospital, London, notebook containing veterinary remedies, nd [Ref: MS 5267]; R Elkington, announcement of acquisition of John Gunn's shoeing forge, Coventry, nd

[Ref: MS 7569]; annual reports: Natal Government Bacteriologist and Director of the Veterinary Department horse-sickness investigation 1903, Natal Government Bacteriologist 1903–05, Nigeria (southern region) veterinary reports 1908–09, South Africa Department of Agriculture, Government Veterinary Bacteriologist 1909–10, South Africa Department of Agriculture, Director of Veterinary Education and Research 1912, 1915, 1918, 1929, Ministry of Agriculture Veterinary Service, Egypt 1913–36, Burma Civil Veterinary Department 1914–41, Nigeria (Northern region) veterinary reports 1921–25, 1927–37, 1942–44, 1946–53, Tanganyika Ministry of Agriculture Department of Veterinary Service 1921–60, National Institute for Research in Dairying 1923, 1925, 1930–54, 1957–72, Madras Civil Veterinary Department 1929–30, South Africa Department of Agriculture, Director of Veterinary Services and Animal Industry 1930–32, Agricultural Research Council 1931–81, Veterinary Director General, Department of Agriculture, Canada 1935–36, 1955, Foot-and-Mouth Disease Research Institute 1937–53, Sind Civil Veterinary Department 1941–46, Department of Animal Health, Gold Coast 1954–55, Institute of Animal Genetics, University of Edinburgh 1955–57, National Association of Poultry Packers Ltd, technical year book 1955, 1958–62, Ditton Laboratory 1956–68, Institute of Animal Physiology, Cambridge 1960–61, 1972–73, Poultry Research Centre 1963–65, 1984, Houghton Poultry Research Station 1981–82.

GREATER MANCHESTER

BURY ARCHIVE SERVICE

First Floor, Derby Hall Annexe, Edwin Street, Bury BL9 0AS

Thomas Briggs, veterinary surgeon, Castle Buildings, Bury, building regulation plans c1874, 1920s. [Ref: ABU/T no.476]

JOHN RYLANDS UNIVERSITY LIBRARY

University of Manchester, 150 Deansgate, Manchester M3 3EH

Grey family, Earls of Stamford, Dunham Massey: blacksmiths' accounts 1772–1840, 1859–1939 [Ref: EGR 7/3, 7/12/1–4, 7–8, 12, 7/14/1, 11/2/2/13–30, 11/3/5/1–10, 14/1/33, 14/18/5/575–1091, 7–11, 14/20, 23, 53/11, 54–55, 59/30, 74/3–4], papers re treatment of horses 1806–07, 1814–16, 1822, 1858–1939 [Ref: EGR 4/1/6/2/7–8, 4/1/6/21/69, 4/1/6/23/72, 4/1/6/25/48, 7/12/3–4, 8, 14/20, 14/23, 14/53/11, 14/54–55, 14/59/30], veterinary surgeons' accounts 1822, 1858–1939. [Ref: EGR 7/12/3–4, 8, 14/20, 14/23, 14/53/11, 14/54–55, 14/59/30]

MANCHESTER CENTRAL LIBRARY, LOCAL STUDIES UNIT
St Peter's Square, Manchester M2 5PD

Recipe for horse medicine 1688 [Ref: L1/48/10/9]; recipe, 'a good purge for a horse' c1730 [Ref: L1/46/6]; Robert Midgley, accounts for medicaments incl some for horses 1751–56 [Ref: L1/4/1/2]; Cuthbert Simpson, veterinary surgeon, Store Street, London Road, Manchester, bills with engraved headings showing premises incl infirmary for sick horses 1857–63 [Ref: M35/9/62/4–12]; William Coates, veterinary surgeon, Longsight, bills 1862, 1865 [Ref: M35/9/62/1–3]; bills issued by the Veterinary Infirmary 1869–70 [Ref: M35/9/62/18–22]; unnamed veterinary surgeon, bill 1864 [Ref: M35/9/62/23]; cards advertising horses, cure for swollen fetlock 1880–1905. [Ref: M173/1/2/1–15]

SALFORD ARCHIVES CENTRE
658–662 Liverpool Road, Irlam, Manchester M44 5AD

Joseph Faulkner, chemist and general provisions retailer, recipe book incl some for treatment of cattle 1859–1915 [Ref: U311/B1]; unnamed chemist, recipe book incl some for treatment of cattle, nd. [Ref: U311/B2]

WIGAN ARCHIVES SERVICE
Leigh Town Hall, Leigh WN7 2DY

Mr McNish, Wigan, registers of veterinary practice 1969–94. [Ref: D/DY/Acc]

HAMPSHIRE

HAMPSHIRE RECORD OFFICE
Sussex Street, Winchester SO23 8TH

Recipes to cure colds and strained back in horses late 17th–early 18th cent [Ref: 63M84/235]; Jervoise family of Herriard: medical and veterinary recipes incl cures for horses and sheep 17th–18th cent [Ref: 44M69/M2/4 items 6,8,20,21,23,26], recipe for cure for horse cough sent to Richard Jervoise 18th cent [Ref: 44M69/F7/14/67], Reverend G H P Jervoise, bills for veterinary care 1797, 1801 [Ref: 44M69/E12/13&24], G P Jervoise, bills for veterinary care of horses 1814 [Ref: 44M69/E13/6/7]; John Reeves of Poulner, farrier, party to leases 1751, 1756 [Ref: 6M80/E/B465, 517]; Broughton overseers' account book incl recipe for curing horses with tack 18th cent [Ref: 137M71/PO1]; Dogmersfield parish register, incl recipe to cure sick horse 18th cent [Ref: 59M72/PR2]; veterinary prescriptions 18th cent [Ref: 3M51/607]; recipes for cures of animal diseases 18th cent [Ref: 5M50/2243–2245]; Hall family of Preston Candover, recipe for horse ointment late 18th cent or early 19th cent [Ref: 44M69/E18/1/217]; Winchester butcher's veterinary bills c1850 [Ref: 88M89W/7]; bills for treatment of horses by Jeffrey Dawtrey of Chichester 1868 [Ref: 129/M90/A44]; posters re swine fever 1887–92 [Ref: W/B3/21, 24–26]; printed volume of biographies of notable Hampshire persons incl veterinary surgeons 1905. [Ref: 62M91/1]

HEREFORDSHIRE

HEREFORDSHIRE RECORD OFFICE
Old Barracks, Harold Street, Hereford HR1 2QX

James Staunton of Much Cowarne, farrier, party to deed 1740 [Ref: Q/RD/8/2]; John Stevens of Oldford, St Mary of Stratford Bow, farrier, party to deed 1751 [Ref: AL40/885]; deeds and copies of wills giving the title and descent of property at one time belonging to James Enoe of Leominster, farrier 1763–1820 [Ref: C94/109]; Pybus family, farm account books incl veterinary recipes 1808–50 [Ref: AH75/1–2]; James Griffiths, Weobley, 'The Waggoner's Friend', notebook containing remedies for sick horses 1852 [Ref: C74/1]; Arkwright family, Hampton Court Estate, Hope under Dinmore: stable account for farriery medicines supplied by Davis, chemist 1858–68 [Ref: E41/328], certificate of veterinary examination for a bay harness mare 1888 [Ref: A63/IV/22/13], request for photograph of bull 'Prince Bulbo' from Robert Holding, veterinary lecturer 1890 [Ref: A63/IV/22/13/1–30], printed circular re visiting lecturers on fruit culture and veterinary science, with covering letter from H Colley 1898 [Ref: A63/IV/49/8]; Chave & Jackson, 6–7 Broad Street, Hereford, chemists, veterinary book 1890 [Ref: BR13/1]; misc receipts for livestock, veterinary surgeons and slaughterhouses c1920–60 [Ref: BE94/4]; William Stewart Wood, Whitehouse Estate, Vowchurch, notebook containing remedies for illnesses in humans and animals, nd. [Ref: F37/192]

HERTFORDSHIRE

HERTFORDSHIRE ARCHIVES AND LOCAL STUDIES
County Hall, Hertford SG13 8EJ

Apprenticeship indenture, John Lawford junior to John Lawford, his father, grocer and [farrier?] 1708 [Ref: HB/4]; report re distemper in cattle at Islington 1714 [Ref: D/EP F125]; Isaac Bulsingh, London, letter to Ralph Radcliffe, Hitchin, offering remedies for distemper in hounds 1729 [Ref: D/ER/C41/10]; recipes incl some for treating farcy in horses c1730–50 [Ref: D/EP/F279]; Jane Radcliffe, Hitchin, letter re sickness amongst cows and attempted remedies 1746 [Ref: D/ER/C169/6]; John Radcliffe, recipe for cold in horses on flyleaf of 'London Account Book' 1771–76 [Ref: D/ER/F190]; John Duncombe, Northchurch, recipe for bruise on horse's back 1781 [Ref: 29686]; Randall Lawrence of Bromley St Leonard, Middlesex, farrier, party to deeds re property at Welham Green, Roestock, North Mimms and Hatfield 1795, 1800, 1808 [Ref: 34070–34071, 34247, 34260–34261, 34264–34265, 34267–34268]; notebook re care of horses and dogs c1800 [Ref: 25921]; George Lines & Co, chemist, Hertford, prescription books, incl occasional veterinary scripts c1817–1922, 1925–87 [Ref: D/Eli]; George Spalding, advertisement for *Bovinospedica*, a foot-and-mouth disease remedy c1872 [Ref: D/EHe/C33/14]; Stevenage development corporation, architect's department, file re veterinary surgeries 1963–72. [Ref: CNT/ST/5/1/AP/V1 Vol 1]

IN PRIVATE OWNERSHIP, MR NORMAN COMBEN
Gillams, Cross Oak Road, Berkhamsted HP4 3NA

Captain O'Kelly and Edmund Bond, receipts for covering mares by Eclipse and Volunteer 1787, 1792; four prints lampooning work of Veterinary College, London, and its professors 1792; print of Mr Taplin, author of *The Gentleman's Stable Directory* and *New Compendium of Farriery*, etc 1796; Thomas Brookes, farrier and cow leech, advertisement 1818; wallchart re care of horses, taken from J White (French) 1825; Thomas Spires, farrier and cow leech, advertisement c1840; James Ward, late coachman to Alexander Campbell of Gatcomb House, now farrier understanding 'the Veterinary Art in no mean degree', advertisement c1850; William Dick, veterinary surgeon, bill for treatment 1856; John Gamgee, veterinary surgeon, letter to Bracy Clark re purchase of skeleton of racehorse Eclipse 1860; advertisement for cures for cattle diseases c1860; *Long's Non-Poisonous Specific* for scab in sheep, advertisement c1880; certificate for life membership of Sydney Galvayne's school for horse taming and training 1886; Thomas Walley, veterinary surgeon, letter re non-payment of bill 1889; advertisement for *Stevens' Ointment*, the substitute for firing horses c1890s; R Long, veterinary instrument maker, advertisement early 19th cent; advertisements for cow keepers, horse slaughterers, etc 19th cent; labels for chemists' remedies 19th–20th cent; Royal Veterinary College, London, certificate 1910; postcards of colleges, animal hospitals, etc c1900–20; Bracy Clark, veterinary surgeon, printed wallchart of recommendations to farriers and shoeing smiths in respect to the injurious practice of slicing and cutting away the horn from the frogs of horses' feet, nd; directions for using instrument for relieving cattle that are hoven, nd; W Fowke and Son, druggists, advertisement for remedy for colds, etc in cattle, nd; J Wilkinson, druggist, York, advertisements for various horse and dog medicines, nd; J W Sill, agricultural chemist, Beaminster, Dorset, advertisement for *Pine's Devonshire Oils* for horses, cattle and sheep, nd.

ISLE OF WIGHT

ISLE OF WIGHT COUNTY RECORD OFFICE
26 Hillside, Newport PO30 2EB

James White, farmer, Briddlesford, veterinary recipe book 1845 [Ref: WHT/13]; letter from A V Sewell, veterinary surgeon, veterinary infirmary, 55 Elizabeth Street, Eaton Square, London, to John H G Oglander, Nunwell, Brading 1899. [Ref: OG/CC/2014A]

KENT

CENTRE FOR KENTISH STUDIES
County Hall, Maidstone ME14 1XQ

William Maylesden, veterinary surgeon, Tunbridge Wells, account books 1824–31 [Ref: Q/CI/86]; Brett & Ransley family, veterinary recipes 19th cent. [Ref: U1957 Z12]

EAST KENT ARCHIVES CENTRE
The Enterprise Business Park, Honeywood Road, Whitfield, Dover CT16 3EH

J Pilcher, Littlebourne, veterinary surgeon, request to be appointed to the regiment as a veterinary surgeon following service as a farrier 1820. [Ref: U1231 O65]

KINGSTON UPON HULL

BRYNMORE JONES LIBRARY, UNIVERSITY OF HULL

Brynmor Jones Library, Cottingham Road, Kingston upon Hull HU6 7RX

Edward Pilkington of Mitton, Staffordshire, farrier, bond 1652 [Ref: DDEV/69/17]; overseers of the poor account book, South Frodingham, Lincolnshire, incl prescriptions for diseases of animals 1742–1811 [Ref: PR/6]; overseers of the poor account book, Sproatley, East Riding, incl prescriptions for diseases of animals 1771–1812 [Ref: PR/7]; letters to Sir Carnaby Haggerston re cattle, horse and sheep plague 18th cent [Ref: DDEV/60–61]; Countess of Stradbroke's cookery, medicinal, veterinary and household recipes c1820 [Ref: DDHO/19/5]; lease and release, Thomas Duesbery, etc to John Lythe, veterinary surgeon 1825 [Ref: DDCV/15/474]; John Walker of Seaton Ross, East Riding, farrier, will 1856 [Ref: DDCV/207/92]; Diseases of Animals Amendment Act 1866 [Ref: DDEV/63/16]; cattle plague rate receipt book 1866 [Ref: DDLG/30/895]; valuation of cattle lost to plague in Holme Beacon Division 1866 [Ref: DDEV/68/213]; letters by William Constable Maxwell, 10th Lord Herries, re cattle plague in Escrick, North Yorkshire and Lincolnshire 1860s [Ref: DDEV/60/31xiv]; letters to William Mortimer Baines re cattle plague in Naburn area 1860s [Ref: DDBH/26/11]; Jonathan Douthwaite of Leven, East Riding, farrier, will 1878 [Ref: DDCV2/86/266]; memorandum on veterinary work by J F D Tutt 1947 [Ref: DSM/6/18]; misc societies, file re animals 1968–72; British Small Animal Veterinary Association, file 1974 [Ref: DBV/22/15]; Alan Plater, playwright, papers re screenplay *It Shouldn't Happen to a Vet* by James Herriot 1976 [Ref: DPR/5/4, 5]; All Party Pharmaceutical Group and the Association of the British Pharmaceutical Industry, file re veterinary matters 1981–83 [Ref: DMC/1618]; press cuttings re animal experiments 1983–84 [Ref: DBV/30/76]; British Union for the Abolition of Vivisection, factsheet re veterinary research 1989. [Ref: DBV(2)/21/61]

HULL CITY ARCHIVES
79 Lowgate, Kingston upon Hull HU1 1HN

Papers re partnership between John Freeman and Richard Philip, both of Hull, veterinary surgeons 1884 [Ref: DBX9]; London Midland & Scottish Railway, Goole, East Riding, file re land for veterinary surgeon's office incl agreement with Aire and Calder Navigation 1920 and payment sheet 1925–50. [Ref: DPD/3/1/1971]

LANCASHIRE

LANCASHIRE RECORD OFFICE
Bow Lane, Preston PR1 2RE

Henry Crook of Preston, farrier, admittance to a premises and land in Haslingden 1736 [Ref: PUH/6/2]; Lonsdale cattle plague watch assessment 1747 [Ref: DP]; charm for curing cows 1773 [Ref: DDX 611/4/8]; James Bradley of Poulton-le-Fylde, innkeeper and farrier, insolvency papers 1774–75 [Ref: QJB/41/41]; recipe book for human and animal sickness 1840 [Ref: DDX 235/1]; Lancaster canal horse sickness book 1932–48. [Ref: DDX 1052/2/1]

LEICESTERSHIRE

RECORD OFFICE FOR LEICESTERSHIRE, LEICESTER AND RUTLAND
Long Street, Wigston Magna, Leicester LE18 2AH

Archibald Palmer, Wanlip, recipe book containing recipes of a medicinal and veterinary nature c1658–72 [Ref: DE 2918]; Curzon family, Breedon on the Hill and Lockington Hall: pedigree of horse named 'Moses' and receipt for a cure for rheumatism and bruises c1770 [Ref: DE 1536/385A], recipe entitled 'a drink for a cow that has a bad alder at calving' c1770 [Ref: DE 1536/389]; Joseph Lucas, veterinary surgeon, Lutterworth: cash accounts re rents received 1834–36 [Ref: DE 783/44], visiting books 1857–59 [Ref: DE 783/41–43]; recipes for horse medicines with envelope addressed to Mr Simons, groom at the vicarage, Weedon, Northamptonshire c1845–93 [Ref: DE 3376/6]; unidentified veterinary practitioner: notebooks 1853–56 [Ref: 18 D 67/417–421], day book 1856 [Ref: 18 D 67/416]; J Wiggins: notice of acquisition of veterinary practice from Samuel Banks, Market Harborough and district 1861 [Ref: DE

513/36], card, nd [Ref: DE 513/33]; John Harvey, South Croxton, farrier, party to deed re The Anchor, Woodhouse 1863 [Ref: DG 9/966]; Quorn Hunt: minute and account books, bills and receipts, incl from chemists for medicines and liniments and from veterinary surgeons for treatments 1886–1980 [Ref: DE 3030/1–511]; W Cooper, Woodboy Street, Leicester, shoeing smith, books containing recipes for horse and pig ailments 1894–1903 [Ref: MISC 342]; George James Baldwin, chemist, Loughborough: customer ledger for animal prescriptions incl cows, horses, pigs, poultry and sheep c1900–29 [Ref: DE 3711/10], papers re mixture for fish bait and lotion for foul in cattle c1900–29 [Ref: DE 3711/11/1, 2]; Belvoir Hunt, bills of G E Gibson & Sons, veterinary surgeons, Oakham and Grantham, Lincolnshire 1928–34 [Ref: DE 4797/57]; North Atherstone Hunt: assorted bills and receipts incl veterinary expenses 1937–39 [Ref: DE 3031/1–53, 55–141], veterinary surgeon's 'hunter account' detailing injuries to horses and hounds, treatments given and cost 1938 [Ref: DE 3031/142/142–143]; Littler & Sons, Melton Mowbray and Long Clawson, blotter advertising remedy for tapeworm and scour in lambs c1950 [Ref: MISC 1017]; Francis Baxter, veterinary surgeon, Whitwick, trade card, nd. [Ref: MISC 226]

LINCOLNSHIRE

LINCOLNSHIRE ARCHIVES

St Rumbold Street, Lincoln LN1 3AB

Farming memoranda incl veterinary remedies c1690–1725 [Ref: EXLEY 27/3]; John Strey, farmer, account book incl memoranda on animal medicines 1783–90 [Ref: FIELD 2/7/1]; T Rose, West Deeping, advertisement for horse and beast medical remedies c1790 [Ref: DIXON 21/5/6/13]; poor rate book, incl remedies for horse and cattle diseases late 18th cent [Ref: BRACE 23/5]; farming account book, incl veterinary remedies late 18th–early 19th cent [Ref: MISC DEP 150]; George Wallis, veterinary surgeon, Stamford, additional mortgage to George Edward Watts, Langton Grange, near Darlington 1830 [Ref: BRA 766]; recipe book of animal medicines 1845 [Ref: SCORER FARM 3/6]; Warters Richardson, veterinary surgeon, Lincoln, conveyance of property in parish of St Peter at Gowts, Lincoln 1849 [Ref: BS 21/7/1]; John William Dixon of Caistor, bills incl from George Capes, Snitterby, blacksmith, and Richard Wilson, Caistor, veterinary surgeon 1855 [Ref: 1 DIXON 12/9/2]; Robert Wilson, Caistor, veterinary surgeon, party to deeds re Wold Farm, Nettleton 1869 [Ref: 1 DIXON 1/C/14/65]; Thomas Brightman Sharman, veterinary surgeon, Leake, North Yorkshire, will

1869 [Ref: LCC WILLS 1869/599]; Joseph Clarke, veterinary surgeon, Horncastle, will 1870 [Ref: LCC WILLS 1870/752]; William Lovitt, blacksmith and farrier, Hayton, Nottinghamshire, account book 1871–78; Robert Dyball, veterinary surgeon, Moulton, will 1872 [Ref: LCC WILLS 1872/1]; Charles Nowell, veterinary practitioner, Bassingham, ledger 1875–94 [Ref: MISC DEP 620]; Battles, chemists, horse and cattle prescription books 1876–1936 [Ref: BATTLES IB/1–3]; John Holmes, veterinary surgeon, Bourne: bill of professional charges 1880–90, papers re account with Robert Mills, chemist, nd [Ref: WHIT 4/1/57]; two horse remedies, nd. [Ref: MONSON 16/2/1/5]

MUSEUM OF LINCOLNSHIRE LIFE
Burton Road, Lincoln LN1 3LY

William Chapman, recipe book for horses 1826; Robert Hardy, photograph following veterinary qualification 1837; J W Dawson, Alford, apprenticeship indenture binding him to C Smith 1872; cures, ailments and recipes from Mrs Cobb 1872–74; unnamed veterinary surgeon, Grimsby, ledger 1899–1902; Fiskerton Pig Club, ledger 1901–40; recipe book for livestock from Old Hall, Hagworthingham 1912; Henry [Sawyer?], veterinary surgeon, notebooks 1918; Thomas Rands, veterinary surgeon, recipe book, nd; Joseph Skayman, remedies for sick livestock, nd.

NORTH EAST LINCOLNSHIRE ARCHIVES
Town Hall, Town Hall Square, Grimsby DN31 1HY

Papers of W H Eliot-Boyden of Massachusetts, US, studying veterinary science in London 1853–60. [Ref: 233]

MEDWAY

MEDWAY ARCHIVES & LOCAL STUDIES CENTRE
Civic Centre, Strood, Rochester ME2 4AU

Vestry minutes, Swanscombe, mentioning collections for cattle losses sustained by London cow keepers 1715 [Ref: P362/8/1]; churchwarden's accounts, Southfleet, mentioning Act of Parliament and prayer re distemper amongst horned cattle 1746–47 [Ref: P343/5/19]; recipes to cure mange in dogs 1763, to stop scouring of hogs 1763 and outlining method of fattening poultry 1781 [Ref: U480/B875]; Thomas Law, veterinary bill issued to Mr Everist for medicines for farm animals and culling 1821 [Ref: U/245–21]; Best family, Chatham, recipes for diseases in dogs and horses c1850–64 [Ref: U480/F92]; Harveyland alias Harbourland Farm: copy inventory and valuation 1880, detailed pedigree of Sussex herd 1881–89, account of livestock and feeding materials 1892 [Ref: U480/E35]; file of complaints re noisy animals at veterinary premises, 99 High Street, Rochester 1959–61. [Ref: RCA Box 001]

NORFOLK

HISTORY OF ADVERTISING TRUST

History of Advertising House, 12 Raveningham Centre, Raveningham, Norwich NR14 6NU

Imperial Chemical Industries Ltd, proofs, advertisements and press cuttings re animal health products incl cattle and game bird wormers, sheep dips, artificial insemination treatments, etc 1956–57, 1960–71 [Ref: OM(L) 01, 06, 11, 14–17, 20, 29, 32, 43]; British Oxygen Company, advertisements and proofs for products incl some re artificial insemination 1969–70. [Ref: OM(L) 35]

NORFOLK RECORD OFFICE

Gildengate House, Anglia Square, Upper Green Lane, Norwich NR3 1AX

Richard [Grand?], Hackford and Reepham, farrier, accounts 1780–84 [Ref: BR 167/1]; letters from Horace Hamond to his cousin Anthony Hamond incl re resiting of Veterinary College, London 1800–04 [Ref: HMN 4/]; Isaac Lansdell, Winfarthing, farrier: customer accounts 1813–17, 1824–32, cash journals 1848–51 [Ref: BR 41/1–8]; Meade of Earsham, farrier's bills 1831 [Ref: MEA3/141, 654 x 4]; Johnson Wallis, New Buckenham, farrier, customer accounts 1858–63 [Ref: MC 22/15]; Freebridge Lynn cattle plague committee, correspondence and papers 1863–66 [Ref: HMN 5/154–164]; Woodrow family, Blofield, blacksmiths and farriers: ledgers 1869–1933, day books 1917–43 [Ref: BR 120/1–13]; Henry Cleveland, Brooke, veterinary surgeon, accounts with William Chapman junior 1894–96 [Ref: BR242/1]; Henry [Chapman?], Mundford, veterinary surgeon, notebook of veterinary recipes late 19th cent [Ref: MC 302/9]; agreement between Docking rural district council and Celia M Bray re room in The Manor Cottage, Docking, formerly used as a veterinary surgery 1952. [Ref: DC 17/7/14]

UNIVERSITY OF EAST ANGLIA
Library, University of East Anglia, Norwich NR4 7TJ

Correspondence and papers between Royal College of Veterinary Surgeons, Ministry of Agriculture, Fisheries and Food, Department of Education and Science and liaison committee of Veterinarians of the European Economic Community re harmonisation of professional qualifications and Veterinary Surgeons Act 1965–74 [Ref: AR/JH/POL/PARL/13]; European parliament standing veterinary committee: papers and correspondence from UK veterinary organisations incl liaison committee of Veterinarians of European Economic Community, British Veterinary Association and Royal College of Veterinary Surgeons re better liaison between European Parliament, British veterinary surgeons and state veterinary service, list of existing draft directives and proposed amendments on veterinary issues, etc 1973–74, papers on procedures and powers, briefing notes and extracts from official journal, correspondence with H R Nord and P Minoprio, notes 1970s. [Ref: AF/JH/POL/EUR/13/1–2]

NORTH YORKSHIRE

NORTH YORKSHIRE COUNTY RECORD OFFICE
Malpas Road, Northallerton DL7 8TB

Farrier's accounts 1811–37, 1868 [Ref: ZV 4, MIC 1855]; Mrs Ibbotson's book incl veterinary remedies c1829–32 [Ref: TD 129, MIC 3868]; John Lacy, farrier and blacksmith, papers 1897-1921. [Ref: ZW III5, MIC 3377]

THE WORLD OF JAMES HERRIOT
23 Kirkgate, Thirsk YO7 1PL

Manuscript for *It Shouldn't Happen to a Vet* by James Herriot c1970; George Frederick Fox, Sheffield, student notes of lectures given by Professors Simonds and Spooner at Royal Veterinary College, London, nd; recipes for purging balls, nd.

NORTHAMPTONSHIRE

NORTHAMPTONSHIRE RECORD OFFICE
Wootton Hall Park, Northampton NN4 8BQ

Clement Darlow of Kingsthorpe, farrier, party to deed 1663 [Ref: Th 1958]; Italian commentaries on the veterinary arts 17th cent [Ref: Fitzwilliam Misc Vol 791, 192]; recipe for a poultice for horses' heels 1701 [Ref: Fitzwilliam Misc Vol 260]; George Osborn of Northampton, farrier, probate of will 1774 [Ref: O(N)/1]; veterinary recipe book c1800 [Ref: YZ 2585]; account due for veterinary services 1808–28 [Ref: BK (0) 1]; Robert Elliott, farrier, billhead c1825 [Ref: O(N)/51]; accounts for horse medicines 1826–32 [Ref: G 3933]; Mrs John Winns Abbott, veterinary bill from William Blunson of Daventry, blacksmith 1829 [Ref: B(HH)/558]; bill for bleeding a mare 1833 [Ref: ZA 7617]; supplies bill 1835 [Ref: NPL 2452, 2455]; accounts for cattle medicines 1835, 1840–59 [Ref: G 2006, ML 1276]; Thomas Garlick, Greens Norton, account book 1842–55 [Ref: ML 1274]; kennels account book 1862–83 [Ref: G 3934]; misc veterinary bill 1864 [Ref: YZ 4796]; Towcester Cattle Plague Association for Mutual Insurance Against Cattle Plague, minutes 1865–75 [Ref: ZB 30]; bills for cattle plague tax from Duke of Grafton's estate 1866 [Ref: G 2043, 2047–2081]; papers re cattle plague 1866–68 [Ref: X 296–298]; Henry Joseph Cartwright, veterinary surgeon, mortgage transfer 1876 [Ref: ZB 516/4]; Northamptonshire Association for Insuring Against Cattle Plague, list of officers and rules 1877 [Ref: CAM 477]; veterinary accounts, Potterspury 1878 [Ref: G 1832]; farm accounts 1882–83 [Ref: G 2086]; Thomas Pettifer, Eydon, dealer in cattle medicines, conveyance 1896 [Ref: X 6187 bundle 2]; C W Crofts, St Giles Street, Northampton, account book and bank statements 1931–50 [Ref: X 6168]; J R Fisher, article entitled 'Not Quite a Profession: the aspirations of veterinary surgeons in England in the mid 19th century', nd. [Ref: ROP 1376 vol 66 and 161]

NOTTINGHAMSHIRE

NOTTINGHAMSHIRE ARCHIVES
County House, Castle Meadow Road, Nottingham NG2 1AG

John Stevens of Milthorpe, Cuckney, farrier, party to leases re property in Norton, Northamptonshire 1689, 1743 [Ref: 157 DD/2P/28/361, 366]; Nathaniel Hurst of Mansfield, farrier, party to leases 1734/35, 1741 [Ref: 157 DD/2P/28/312, 314]; William Henry Cavendish Bentinck, 4th Duke of Portland: bills and receipts from local tradesmen incl veterinary surgeon and farrier 1801–28, 1833–34, 1839–54 [Ref: DD/P/6/7/10], bills and receipts from London tradesmen incl veterinary surgeons and farriers 1821–54 [Ref: DD/P/6/8/2], Richard Prince's bills incl one for veterinary work at Newmarket 1836–41 [Ref: DD/P/6/8/7/2]; Lord Henry Bentinck, papers re his responsibilities for stables and kennels at Welbeck and Burton near Lincoln incl bills and receipts for veterinary care 1827–58 [Ref: DD/P/6/9/49–65]; 5th Duke of Portland: letters from W T Stanley, veterinary surgeon of Leamington Spa, Warwickshire, incl reports on horses to buy and care of horses sent to him 1860–75 [Ref: DD/4P/62/94/1–27], letters to Charles Neale re veterinary treatment for the Duke's horses, incl use of Turkish baths 1869 [Ref: DD/P/6/13/15/99–101, 109–123], letter from John Barker, veterinary surgeon, of Sheffield, Yorkshire, applying to be stud groom 1872 [Ref: DD/4P/62/106/38]; Izaac Timms, commission as veterinary surgeon in the Clumber Troop of Yeomanry Cavalry 1820 [Ref: C/QALT/6/1/4]; Savile of Rufford, stable accounts incl for veterinary attention 1837–45. [Ref: DD/SR/235/1]

OXFORDSHIRE

OXFORDSHIRE RECORD OFFICE
St Luke's Church, Temple Road, Cowley, Oxford OX4 2EX

Will of farrier, bequeathing his veterinary books, recipes and instruments to William Hawkins Arding 1838–47. [Ref: Ost/V/ii/1]

RHODES HOUSE LIBRARY
South Parks Road, Oxford OX1 3RG

William Walker Henderson, Chief Veterinary Officer, Nigeria: memoir of his work in setting up the Laboratory Service 1924–27, staff addresses 1940s [Ref: MSS.Afr.s.1082]; Edward Finch Peck, Director of Agricultural and Veterinary Services, Somalia: veterinary history of Somaliland Protectorate 1924–60, paper re organisation of government services 1946 [Ref: MSS.Afr.s.141, ff. 108–120]; Wilfrid Frank Poulton, Director of Veterinary Services, Uganda, report on results of clearing and burning programme in South Ankole incl maps and photographs 1937 [Ref: MSS.Afr.s.784]; K D S Macowan, memoranda re livestock industry in Kenya and experiences in Veterinary Service there 1937–63 [Ref: MSS Afr. s. 1717/104]; Adam Fulton, Senior Veterinary Officer, Ghana, and Director of Veterinary Services, Sierra Leone and Gambia, reports on meat supply in Gambia and other papers 1930s–50s [Ref:

MSS.Afr.s.365]; R W E Lewis, memorandum on work in Kenya Veterinary Service, with related report 1941–65 [Ref: MSS Afr. s. 1717/96]; Ernest Beaumont, Director of Veterinary Services, Kenya, papers re dispute between East African High Commission and Kenya government re responsibility for and control over Veterinary Laboratory services in Kenya 1949–51 [Ref: MSS.Afr.s.1344]; Robert M Gambles, Senior Veterinary Officer, circular letters from Nigeria 1949–62 [Ref: MSS Afr. s. 1311]; R L Wooldridge, transcript of interviews on work in Kenya Veterinary Service 1949–65 [Ref: MSS Afr. s. 1717/179]; Robert Joseph Simmons, Director of Veterinary Services, Uganda 1938–45, account of experiences 1940s [Ref: MSS.Afr.s.1674, ff.35–41]; John MacDonald, memorandum on service as Veterinary Officer in Kenya 1950–63, with transcript [MSS Afr. s. 1717/102]; Edgar Yates, transcripts of interviews on work as Veterinary Officer in Kenya 1951–64 [Ref: MSS Afr. s. 1717/183]; William John Herbert, Senior Veterinary Officer, Nigeria, personal account book 1953–54 [Ref: MSS.Afr.s.1780]; Michael C Butler, memorandum on service as Veterinary Officer in Kenya 1953–63 [Ref: MSS Afr. s. 1717/21]; Marcus P E Durand, memorandum on work in Kenya Veterinary Service 1954–59, with related text of lecture and notes [Ref: MSS Afr. s. 1717/44]; Domasi, Nyasaland: Domasi community development scheme 1949–54, memorandum on hides and skins industry 1957, beef production 1959, policy and future development of Department of Veterinary Services and Animal Industry 1960, analysis of cattle population trends, nd [Ref: MSS Afr. s. 939]; Ian G Gibson, memorandum on work in Kenya Veterinary Service 1958–71 [Ref: MSS Afr. s. 1717/58]; B W Sellwood, description of training programme for African students and staff and of research in virology, bacteriology and animal reproduction c1960 [Ref: MSS.Afr.s.983]; J Smith, memorandum on work in Kenya Veterinary Service c1960s [Ref: MSS Afr. s. 1717/141]; David Shannon, memorandum on teaching veterinary science in Uganda and Nigeria 1972–78 [Ref: MSS Afr. s. 1825/104]; R W Crowther and Robert M Gambles, *The History of the Veterinary Service in Cyprus, 1905–76*, account by Crowther and Gambles, typescript c1980 [Ref: MSS Medit. s. 24]; W G G Pevie, memoirs of Colonial Veterinary Service, Tanganyika and Nigeria, nd [Ref: MSS Afr. s. 2075]; Patrick Desmond Langford Guilbride, Veterinary Officer, Zambia, account of service in Zambia entitled 'Pawpaw Picnic', nd [Ref: MSS.Afr.s.1315]; R G Syme, papers on rinderpest, Gold Coast and Togoland, nd. [Ref: MSS Afr. s. 512]

IN PRIVATE OWNERSHIP, DR C A SPINAGE
Wickwood House, Stanford Road, Faringdon SN7 8EZ

Acts of Parliament, orders in Council, government reports and returns re rinderpest 1741–68, 1848–75; advice circular re 'infection raging amongst horned cattle' 1748–49; John Giblett, chair of committee appointed to respond to Cattle Diseases Prevention Bill, circular 1864; resolutions of meeting of importers and salesmen of foreign cattle and meat re Cattle & Meat Importation Act 1864; County of Glamorgan Mutual Association for Protection Against Loss by the Cattle Plague, rules and draft rules 1865; Leek and Moorlands Association for Protection Against Loss by the Cattle Plague, letter and proposed rules 1865; Newark Cattle Plague Mutual Compensation Association, membership receipt 1865; North Staffordshire Mutual Cattle Insurance Co: prospectus 1865, circular to stockholders 1865; prayer for relief from cattle plague and cholera 1865–66; press cuttings re cattle plague c1865, 1868–69; Central Committee of the Commissioners of Supply, Argyllshire, circular re cattle plague 1866; County of Dumfries Fifth Division Rinderpest Stamping Out Fund, invoice for rates 1866; Daniel Stone, Professor of Chemistry, Royal Manchester School of Medicine, report to Committee of Justices on suppression of cattle plague re fumigation and disinfection 1866; hymn on the cattle plague, Warwick c1866; Mrs Duckett, Oswestry, Shropshire, receipt for payment of local cattle plague rate 1867; notebook re cattle plague with suggested cures and recipes c1860s; instructions for using crude carbolic acid as a disinfectant for cow sheds, nd.

READING

BERKSHIRE RECORD OFFICE
Shire Hall, Shinfield Park, Reading RG2 9XD

Recipes for medicines for animal ailments c1705–10 [Ref: D/ELV A1]; attorney-general, opinion re effect of order in council for slaughter of distempered cattle 1750 [Ref: D/ED O29]; veterinary surgeons' recipes c1775, 1780, 1785, 1851 [Ref: D/Els Z1–3, 11, D/Esv (M) F54, F59]; Buscot Park, Oxfordshire: stable and kennel accounts 1786–1822 [Ref: D/ELV E38–41], details of grain supplied to fowl 1788–1807 [Ref: D/ELV E81]; recipes for worms and mange in dogs 1812–15 [Ref: E/ELV E133]; veterinary surgeon's bills 1821–33 [Ref: D/Ecb F6/1–3]; advertisement for horse blister ointment c1865 [Ref: D/EX284/542]; note on treatment of disease in cattle and sheep 19th cent [Ref: D/Eby E 139];

Forest Petty Sessional Division: court document re swine fever 1953 [Ref: PS/FT 1A/14], claims re exemption from payment of dog licence duty 1956. [Ref: PS/FT 1A/15]

BRITISH BROADCASTING CORPORATION WRITTEN ARCHIVES CENTRE

Caversham Park, Reading RG4 8TZ

Central agricultural broadcasting advisory committee, minutes 1944–54 [Ref: R6/12, 13]; correspondence and papers re radio broadcasts: farming programmes 1932–64 [Ref: R51/165/1–18, 819], *Farming Today* series 1944–46, 1960–74 [Ref: R51/168–170, 823, 824, 1125], programmes re pets 1947–48 [Ref: R19/901], proposed series *Can't We Do Better Than This?* re veterinary services 1954 [Ref: T32/11], British Veterinary Association 1954–67 [Ref: RCONT/1,12], *On Your Farm* series 1958–63 [Ref: R51/827], *Farm Bulletin* series 1961–64 [Ref: R51/823], Ministry of Agriculture, Fisheries and Food 1965–76 [Ref: R19/1120]; papers and correspondence re television broadcasts: agricultural programmes 1951–57 [Ref: T32/11], Ministry of Agriculture, Fisheries and Food 1953–57 [Ref: T32/12], farming programmes 1957–64 [Ref: T32/902–903]; radio scripts re veterinary matters: *Careers – veterinary work* 1930 [Ref: B/C 7.3.30], Dr P J Du Toit, *Empire Exchange – veterinary work in the British Empire* 1938 [Ref: B/C23/24.6.46], H J Bedford, *Dispensary for Sick Animals* 1940 [Ref:B/C 23.2.40], Sir Robert Gower, *Appeal for veterinary supplies for Russian army horses* 1942 [Ref: B/C 1.2.42], T J Margarson, *The Countryman's Part – veterinary surgeon* 1942 [Ref: B/C 6.9.42], H E Harbour, *Veterinary Research Work* 1943 [Ref: B/C 3.11.43], John Spellman, veterinary surgeon, interviewed on *Country Magazine* 1943 [Ref: B/C 16.1.43], H R Jude, *A Country Calendar*, re veterinary work 1944 [Ref: B/C 24.3.44], Dr J Carmichael, *Calling Southern Rhodesia: some recent advances in veterinary research, particularly in dairy cattle* 1946 [Ref: B/C 4.10.46], Major R C G Hancock, *Farming Today: the vet and your herd* 1946 [Ref: B/C 18.4.46], *A Veterinary Surgeon Talks About His Job* 1946 [Ref: B/C 5.2.46], *Outwit the Vet* 1946 [Ref: B/C 21.2.46], *Pets as a Profession* 1947 [Ref: B/C 14.7.47 (hp)], S L Hignett, *A British View of Argentine Veterinary Problems* 1948 [Ref: B/C HS 15.2.50], T K Ewer, *Positive Stock Health* 1948 [Ref: B/C HS 15.7.48], Thomas Dalling, *Agriculture no 8 – animal health* 1948 [Ref: B/C 21.2.48], *Animal Diseases – agriculture and the veterinary scientist*, for farmers in Northern Ireland 1948, 1949 [Ref: 26.4.48–49], *Protecting Our Cattle* 1949 [Ref: B/C HS 27.10.49], *A Veterinary Surgeon* 1949 [Ref: B/C SHS 31/10, 49], Dr Mark L Morris and Dr Edwin Lattimer, *The American Attitude Towards Domestic Pets* (Inter-Veterinary Congress,

London) 1949 [Ref: B/C LP 12.8.49], *The Veterinary Surgeon* 1950, 1952, 1953 [Ref: B/C HS 15.2.50, 52, 53], *Science and the Larder – the veterinary surgeon* 1952, 1953 [Ref: B/C HS 7.2.52, B/C HS 19.11.53], Brian Branston, *Visit to Central Veterinary Laboratory, Weybridge* 1953 [Ref: B/C HS 19.2.53], Iain Pattison, *Work of a Veterinary Officer* 1953 [Ref: B/C HS 12.12.53], Alistair Dannett, *Working with Animals – interviews with Royal Society for the Prevention of Cruelty to Animals workers* 1953 [Ref: B/C GOS 10.7.52], Roger Massey, *The Causes of Mastitis* 1953 [Ref: B/C HS 7.10.53], Noreen Twyman, *Starting a Veterinary Practice in Ireland* 1953 [Ref: B/C LP 24.4.53], *Science and Your Food – the veterinary surgeon* 1958, 1961 [Ref: HS 26.6.58, HS 26.6.61], Tyler Whittle, *Veterinary Vagaries* 1959 [Ref: LP 20.5.59], W R Wooldridge, R S T Bowden and W B Singleton, *Veterinary Medicine and Surgery* 1959 [Ref: NIII 31.8.59], Sydney Jennings, President of the British Veterinary Association, interviewed on *Guest of the Week* 1960 [Ref: LP 7.12.60], Percy Edwards, interview with Mrs Phillips and Captain Phillips on veterinary work 1965 [Ref: HS 6.1.65], Alasdair Steele-Bodger, President, British Veterinary Association, interviewed on *Guest of the Week* 1965 [Ref: LP 29.9.65], E C Straiton, *The Effect on the Housewife of Recent Advances in Veterinary Science* 1967 [Ref: B/C LP 4.9.67], Jameson Clark interview with R Naismith, author of *Highland Vet* on his work 1968 [Ref: R2 26.4.68], David Hammond, *Woman Veterinary Surgeon* 1968 [Ref: R4.7.5.68], *Tony Van Den Bergh spends a day with a veterinary surgeon* 1970. [Ref: R4 17.4.70]

RURAL HISTORY CENTRE
University of Reading, Whiteknights, PO Box 229, Reading RG6 6AG

William Johnson, notebook of veterinary recipes 1780 [Ref: D69/32]; veterinary recipe book 1802–06 [Ref: D66/11]; Khrone & Sesemann, catalogue c1901 [Ref: TR CXL P2/A1]; Holborn Surgical Instrument Co Ltd, catalogue 1957 [Ref: TR MRL P2/B78]; Alfred Cox (Surgical) Ltd, catalogues 1966, 1968. [Ref: TR HSE, TR CXL P2/A2]

UNIVERSITY OF READING
The Library, Whiteknights, PO Box 223, Reading RG6 6AE

John Standen of St George, Southwark, farrier, party to lease re property in Turnmill Street, St James, Clerkenwell 1678 [Ref: MS 145/EN1/2/228]; recipe book, incl human and animal remedies for such conditions as bad heels in horses, rabies, bog spavin, fowl water in cows, wound swellings and sprains and making hair grow on a horse or cow c1790–1830 [Ref: MS 4455]; farm diary for Little Somborne farm,

King's Somborne, Hampshire, incl brief veterinary recipes 1815–67 [Ref: HAN 11/2/1]; farm account book kept by Thomas Ream of Newton, Cambridgeshire, incl veterinary recipes 1848–56 [Ref: CAM 4/1/1]; Easingwold, Yorkshire, notebook containing veterinary and other remedies 1850 [Ref: YOR 2/1/1]; account book for Eyton farm, Eyton on the Weald Moors, Salop, and Wappenshall farm, Wellington, Salop, incl veterinary recipes 1871–93 [Ref: SAL 6/1/1]; photograph of Mr Bickford, veterinary surgeon at Kingsclere, Devon c1890 [Ref: DEV 3A/8/26]; Sidehead farm, Westgate in Weardale, Durham, veterinary notebook c1900. [Ref: DUR 1/3/2]

SHROPSHIRE

SHROPSHIRE RECORDS AND RESEARCH CENTRE

Castle Gates, Shrewsbury SY1 2AQ

Edward Nicholas of Prees Henlley p Whittington, farrier, party to deed 1728 [Ref: SRO 2847/5/145–146]; Attingham collection, bills and vouchers incl for veterinary treatment 1729–1815 [Ref: 112/6/Box 34/4, Box 36/92–93, Box 39/636, 670, 762, 859, 915, Box 48/259, 342, Box 53/242]; Richard Hughes of Leebotwood, farrier, party to lease 1743/44 [Ref: 2922/14/1/11]; William Feriday, notebook incl recipes for cure of sheep scab, etc 1777–90 [Ref: 1681/32/2]; letter re veterinary treatment given to Mr Hill's horse c18th cent [Ref: 112/12/Box 28/58]; Richard Williams of Pitchford, farrier, party to lease 1809 [Ref: 2922/14/1/18/1–3]; H Reginald Corbet, account of cattle plague at Adderley Farm 1865 [Ref: 1096/37]; letter from H J Cartwright, veterinary infirmary, Wolverhampton, to M R B re a hunter for William Clive Bridgeman 1884 [Ref: 4629/1/1884/177]; cattle charm, Llanyblodwell c1900 [Ref: MI 371/1]; Roberts & Carter, veterinary surgeons, Ludlow, papers re bankruptcy 1903–04 [Ref: 4924/9/2/5]; recipe to prevent flies troubling cattle, nd [Ref: MI 1448/1]; *The Pocket Farrier, or Approved Receipts Collected From Different Authors with an Intent to Cure or Assist any Immediate Accident that may Happen to a Horse Till Further Help Can Be Got*, nd. [Ref: 549/548]

SOMERSET

SOMERSET ARCHIVE AND RECORD SERVICE
Obridge Road, Taunton TA2 7PU

The Gentleman's Pocket Farrier With Large Additions and Remarks by Dr Henry Bracken of Lancaster 1735 [Ref: DD\SF/3850]; bills incl for farrier's work 1762–63 [Ref: DD\SAS\C/909/2]; letter from William Calla of Broadway, Worcestershire, to William Gore of Barrow, soliciting a loan of £30–£40 to set him up as a farrier 1763 [Ref: DD/GB/149/143]; William Stillman of Bath, farrier: account book 1773–79, day books 1774–79, receipt book 1777–78, misc papers 1770s [Ref: DD\WLM/4]; notice of intended publication of veterinary work early 19th cent [Ref: DD/SAS 5X 101]; Samuel Vallis Gregory of Yeovil, veterinary surgeon, assignment of his personal estate and effects in trust for his creditors 1837 [Ref: DD/NP/1/28/2]; John Pope, farrier, party to deed re cottage etc adjoining turnpike road 1838 [Ref: DD\CM/88]; Joseph Gibbs of Bishop's Lydeard, veterinary surgeon, party to draft mortgage of shares in Bristol & Essex Railway 1846 [Ref: DD\DP/75/6]; unnamed veterinary surgeon, accounts 1867 [Ref: DD/WY 151]; H Leeney, veterinary surgeon, Banwell, day book 1896–97 [Ref: DD/X/BYN 1]; Taunton rural district council, planning department, plans re veterinary surgery, Westerkirk, Staplegrove 1963 [Ref: D\R\ta/24/1/845]; S R Bunyan, veterinary surgeon, Sandford, Winscombe, day book 1972–73. [Ref: DD/X/BYN 2]

SOUTH YORKSHIRE

ROTHERHAM METROPOLITAN BOROUGH ARCHIVES AND LOCAL STUDIES SECTION
Brian O'Malley Central Library, Walker Place, Rotherham S65 1JH

Humphry Davy, chemist and druggist, recipe book incl veterinary remedies 19th cent. [Ref: 85/B]

SHEFFIELD ARCHIVES
52 Shoreham Street, Sheffield S1 4SP

Samuel Peech, letter to Mr Schofield re treatment for a horse 1834. [Ref: MD 3613]

STAFFORDSHIRE

STAFFORDSHIRE RECORD OFFICE
Eastgate Street, Stafford ST16 2LZ

Earls of Stafford, Jerningham papers, bills and receipts incl for farriery work 1794–1801, 1818 [Ref: D641/3/H/2/4]; formulae for remedies for diseases of cows and sheep c18th cent [Ref: D661/21/6/1e]; Knight family, Milwich, recipe books, mainly for treatment of cattle and sheep 1824 [Ref: D864/3/3/6a, b]; Victor Cartwright, dispensing chemist, High Street, Uttoxeter: prescription books 1871–1920, accounts, 1893–1915 [Ref: D1349]; Anson family of Shugborough, Alrewas estate, papers re deaths of sheep at Hilliards Cross Farm and alleged pollution of water, incl veterinary report and analysis of samples 1896 [Ref: D615/ES/1/11]; recipes for diseases in horses late 19th cent [Ref: D110/M1]; Green family, High House Farm, Great Wyrley, notebooks containing veterinary recipes c19th cent [Ref: D3632/2/17]; Forebridge Shoeing Forge Ltd, Bridge Street, Stafford: directors' minutes 1917–23, accounts 1917–30 [Ref: D4338/A/23/1–2]; P Dodd, farrier, Bradley, accounts 1930–38. [Ref: D 4338/A/17]

IN PRIVATE OWNERSHIP, MR E C STRAITON
Darlaston Hall, Darlaston Park, Stone ST15 0ND

Photographs of veterinary instruments, practices, surgical procedures, veterinary staff at work, etc 20th cent.

STOKE ON TRENT

IN PRIVATE OWNERSHIP, MR J CLEWLOW
Ferndale, 5 Grange Road, Biddulph, Stoke on Trent ST8 7SB

Charles Seal, farrier, receipt book 1772; North Staffordshire Mutual Cattle Insurance Co: prospectus 1865, notice re premiums 1865, letter re desirability of insurance 1865, letter from Clerk of the Peace's office to Clerk to the Leek Board of Guardians re insurance 1865; Staffordshire County Association for Protection against Loss by the Cattle Plague, proposals for formation and draft rules 1865; Lichfield Union Aid Association, notice of proposal to form association c1865; letter from Secretary of National Association for the Prevention of Cattle Diseases to Clerk to Leek Board of Guardians re difficulty of alerting farmers to the dangers of cattle plague 1865; circulars and correspondence re cattle plague insurance 1865; County of Stafford Mutual Insurance Society against the Cattle Plague, application form for registration and insurance c1865; Staffordshire farmers' declarations that their cattle are free from plague 1866; licences to move cattle 1866; cattle plague enquiry reports, Staffordshire 1866; Joseph Edge, veterinary surgeon, 43 Stockwell Street, Leek: receipts 1866–68, 1875, authorisation to Uriah Hudson to give receipt for money owed 1868; foot-and-mouth disease orders and regulations 1875–83; Dr R Hill, veterinary surgeon, Veterinary Infirmary and Shoeing Forge, Shoebridge Street, Leek, receipt 1887; farrier's recipe book, nd.

SUFFOLK

IN PRIVATE OWNERSHIP, JOHN RUSSELL GIBBS
Longlands, Nettlestead, Ipswich IP8 4QL

Uganda Veterinary Service, annual reports incl staff lists 1920–30; staff lists (p) 1914, 1938.

SUFFOLK RECORD OFFICE, BURY ST EDMUNDS BRANCH
Raingate Street, Bury St Edmunds IP33 2AR

Abraham Garrad of Colchester, Essex, veterinary surgeon, party to assignment of mortgage re cottages on North Street, Sudbury 1851 [Ref: EE 501/11/210]; Newmarket urban district council, surveyor's department, plans re veterinary infirmary establishment near Jubilee Clock Tower, Exeter Road, for E H Leach 1894 [Ref: EF 506/6/1/H79]; photograph of Turner house and members of family, High Street, Ixworth, with P Turner's veterinary surgery c1905 [Ref: K 797/9]; photograph of farrier's trademark of a stallion's tail on a house in Kersey 1956 [Ref: K 562/3/18]; unnamed veterinary surgeon, Bury St Edmunds, day book 1962–63. [Ref: HC 540]

SUFFOLK RECORD OFFICE, IPSWICH BRANCH
Gatacre Road, Ipswich IP1 2LQ

Apprenticeship indenture, John Pallant to James Durrant of Ipswich, farrier 1777 [Ref: C/2/9/1/1/1/118]; Robert Smith, veterinary surgeon, 3 Great Colman Street, Ipswich, account books 1831–39, incl notes of lectures by Professor Coleman at Royal Veterinary College, London 1828–29 [Ref: C/2/9/1/1/7/23/1–2]; Thomas Goodburgh, veterinary medicine agent, advertisement 1833–34 [Ref: HA 34:50/21/6.1(e)];

papers re estate of late Alfred John Shorten, veterinary surgeon in Ipswich, Stratford St Mary and Rushmere St Andrew and the family settlement 1861–1907 [Ref: HB 54/E48/1]; *East Anglian Magazine*, photograph of farrier's trademark of a stallion's tail on a veterinary surgeon's house in Kersey, nd. [Ref: K 626/1/122/21]

SUFFOLK RECORD OFFICE, LOWESTOFT BRANCH
Central Library, Clapham Road, Lowestoft NR32 1DR

James Beart Simonds, late of Bungay and now of Twickenham, Middlesex, veterinary surgeon, party to deed re 26 Bridge Street, Bungay 1840. [Ref: 870/1]

SURREY

SURREY HISTORY CENTRE
130 Goldsworth Road, Woking GU21 1ND

Richard Binn of Whitwell, Derbyshire, farrier, copy of will 1704 [Ref: LM/2011/9]; letters of administration with will of Thomas Streete of Shere, farrier 1735 [Ref: G85/13/468]; John Leadbetter of Stoke, farrier, party to deeds re The Ship, Guildford 1766 [Ref: G97/17/7]; letters and papers re outbreak of cattle disease in south west Surrey and Hampshire 1770–71 [Ref: G85/2/4/1/75]; Bray family of Shere, account book and veterinary recipes 1811–45 [Ref: 1589]; Howard family, Elford Hall, remedy for sheep sickness 1824 [Ref: 203/29/49]; Elliott family of Bramley and Cranleigh, notebook chiefly containing remedies for livestock ailments (p) c1840–43 [Ref: Z323/2/4]; John Roalfe Cox of Berkeley Square, London, veterinary surgeon, party to mortgage 1893 [Ref: K61/11/159]; plan of The Duke's Head Inn and adjacent premises of H H Roberts, veterinary surgeon 1913. [Ref: 6145/7/7]

TELFORD & WREKIN

PEOPLE'S DISPENSARY FOR SICK ANIMALS
Head Office, Whitechapel Way, Priorslee, Telford TE2 9PQ

Mr Crawford of Edinburgh, veterinary surgeon, dosage book 1930s.

TYNE & WEAR

TYNE AND WEAR ARCHIVES SERVICE

Blandford House, Blandford Square, Newcastle upon Tyne NE1 4JA

John Tyzack of Newcastle upon Tyne, veterinary surgeon, party to deeds re 17–20 High Claremont Place 1817–63. [Ref: DT.SC/348/1–13]

WARRINGTON

WARRINGTON LIBRARY

Museum Street, Warrington WA1 1JB

Robert Dandy of Rixton, Warrington, farmer, farriers' bills for veterinary work c1910–30. [Ref: MS2822]

WARWICKSHIRE

SHAKESPEARE BIRTHPLACE TRUST RECORDS OFFICE

Henley Street, Stratford upon Avon CV37 6QW

John Ingram of Stratford upon Avon, farrier, party to lease in Bridge Street 1612 [Ref: ER 2/33]; Symon Godwyn senior and Symon Godwyn junior of Stratford upon Avon, farriers, parties to deeds 1615, 1619, 1646 [Ref: ER 2/38, 45; ER 3/4]; Lord Robert Russell, farrier's bill 1695 [Ref: DR 37/3/20]; Christopher Wareing of Stratford upon Avon, farrier, and John Wareing his brother, farrier, parties to deeds re a messuage in Bridge Street known as The Old Swann 1699/1700 [Ref: ER 3/53–55]; Sir William Lemon, recipe to cure bite of a mad dog 17th cent [Ref: BRU15/16/38]; misc veterinary remedies late 17th cent [Ref: DR10/2113]; recipe to cure bite of a mad dog 1726 [Ref: BRU15/15/28]; Nathaniel Earnall [Arnold] of Stratford upon Avon, blacksmith and farrier, probate copy of will 1729 [Ref: ER 3/89]; Elizabeth Smith, bill to [William] Peyto for farrier's work 1729–1733 [Ref: DR 98/1654/48]; John Treen, Great Kington, farrier, party to deeds re cottage in Old Stratford 1761, 1762 [Ref: DR 469/462/2–3]; commonplace book incl veterinary prescriptions c1770 [Ref: DR73]; William Benton, farrier, veterinary bills 1771–91 [Ref: DR165/298/6]; John Marshall of Rose Ash, Devon, farrier, party to lease of messuage called Honey Cliff 1789 [Ref: DR5/741, 742]; Thomas Bones, veterinary prescriptions for cow with 'the body gargle' and for 'stick lice upon sheep' 1796 [Ref: DR68]; William

Goff of Halford, farrier, will (copy) 1803 [Ref: DR 165/267]; Thomas Fisher of Childswickham, Worcestershire, farmer and farrier, party to agreement re rent of premises in Bartholomew Street, Birmingham 1823 [Ref: ER 3/1296]; draft agreements between William Umbers of Alveston, gentleman, and William Lucas of Atherstone, veterinary surgeon, referring certain disputes concerning a horserace at Warwick to arbitration 1830 [Ref: ER 3/816, 990]; Thomas Rose of Stratford upon Avon, farrier and innkeeper, party to lease of The King's Arms, Wood Street 1836 [Ref: DR 165/301/1]; Edward Stanley of Banbury, Oxfordshire, veterinary surgeon, party to conveyances 1849 [Ref: DR 18/10/69/25]; Leigh of Stoneleigh, veterinary bills from William Amos Packwood of Coventry c1850 [Ref: DR 18/17/21/22]; Thomas Rose the elder of Stratford upon Avon, farrier and innkeeper, probate and testamentary papers, correspondence, draft deed re land on College Lane 1852–73 [Ref: DR325/2017]; Shipston on Stour Cattle Plague Assurance Association, minute book 1865–67 [Ref: ER145/448]; W E Evans, veterinary surgeon: papers re case brought by Lloyds Bank to recover overdraft deficit 1880–1904 [Ref: DR325/1659], papers re prosecution by Lloyds Bank for debt 1902 [Ref: DR325/2661]; [Frank] Sharp of Stratford upon Avon, veterinary surgeon, party to tenancy agreement re 14 Guild Street 1883 [Ref: DR574/141]; papers re executorship of John Rose, Henley Street, Stratford upon Avon, veterinary surgeon, incl rent books re garden property in College Lane, Stratford upon Avon, and houses in Evesham street, Alcester 1883–94 [Ref: DR 469/365]; accounts of executors with residuary legatees of John Rose of Stratford upon Avon, veterinary surgeon, with legacy duty receipts and bank pay in book 1887–93 [Ref: DR 469/364]; draft apprenticeship indenture, Harry Jewell Verney, son of Richard Grange Verney of Stratford upon Avon, veterinary surgeon, to Sydney Petter, ironmonger and house furnisher 1889 [Ref: DR 153/272]; John James Crowhurst, veterinary surgeon: apprenticeship agreement with W H Barlow 1890 [Ref: DR325/2723], tenancy agreement 1906 [Ref: DR574/144]; Charles Winter of Kilburn, London, farrier, party to draft conveyance re house in Loxley 1903 [Ref: DR 149/154/234]; veterinary inspection of horses on Leigh estates 1904–08 [Ref: DR962/31–32]; Francis Seeney, 11 John Street, Stratford upon Avon, blacksmith and farrier, died intestate, administration accounts 1948 [Ref: DR 469/382]; Needham & Newey, veterinary practice, dissolution papers 1964. [Ref: DR885/4/14]

WARWICKSHIRE COUNTY RECORD OFFICE
Priory Park, Cape Road, Warwick CV34 4JS

John Lovell, citizen and farrier of London, party to assignment of land in Croft, Winthorpe and Theddlethorpe St Hellin 1668 [Ref: CR 611/791/1–36]; William Butler of Birmingham, farrier and blacksmith, party to deeds re mill and land in Studley 1760, 1790 [Ref: CR 3097/108, 109, 111, 112]; Newdegate of Arbury, household, animal husbandry, medical and veterinary recipes 17th–18th cent [Ref: CR 136/B/2411–2515]; Shipston on Stour Cattle Plague Insurance Co, policy ledger 1866–67 [Ref: CR 609/box 25]; J Rose & Son, veterinary practice, Stratford upon Avon and Alcester: ledgers 1876–92, residuary papers of William Rose and John Rose, nd [Ref: CR 1596/box 133]; apprenticeship indenture, William Edward Baldwin of Warwick to Henry Rose Perrins of 45 Foregate Street, Worcester, veterinary surgeon 1879 [Ref: CR 611/38/5]; W P Stokes, D R Lane & P W Franks, veterinary practice, Leamington Spa, day books 1961–62. [Ref: CR 1609]

WEST MIDLANDS

BIRMINGHAM CITY ARCHIVES
Central Library, Chamberlain Square, Birmingham B3 3HQ

William Weaver of Over Hanley, Worcestershire, farrier, will 1685 [Ref: MS 3312/394784]; misc receipts and vouchers re treatment and care of horses 1732–1823 [Ref: Gough 260–314]; recipe for curing sheep of the scab 1733 [Ref: Gough 304/6]; recipe to treat a lame bullock 1757 [Ref: Gough 287/32]; Thomas Malie, Paymaster of King's Dragoon-guards, Holland, account book incl entries re payments to farrier for transportation of horses from England 1758–59 [Ref: DV 912 [607392]]; J Hawkesford, horse doctor, daily journals 1759–60 [Ref: MS 367864–5]; papers re bulling of eight cows 1769 [Ref: Gough 300/6]; papers re lime, lambs, ducks and bulling cows 1773 [Ref: Gough 303/52, 75]; William Fisher of Childswickham, farrier, party to deeds re land in Childswickham 1792 [Ref: MS 3192/Acc1928–015/361363, 361364]; Thomas Fisher of Childswickham, farrier, party to deeds re land in Childswickham and Evesham, Worcestershire, and Winchcomb, Gloucestershire 1792–93 [Ref: MS 3192/Acc1928–015/361364, 362413, 362141]; William Perks, Coleshill Street, farrier, handbill 1797 [Ref: MS 690/90/96]; King family, Gospel Farm, Hall Green, farm diary and account book incl cure for 'horse belley hake' and list of 'blistering oils' 1800–66 [Ref: MS 2091/1]; indenture between Thomas Miller and his son John Miller, both farriers of

Epping, Essex, being a settlement of the former's household goods and implements of his trade together with land in Hockerill, Hertfordshire 1804 [Ref: MS 3733/Acc 1940–055/581522]; Joseph Rawlins of Wigginton, Tamworth, Staffordshire, farrier, will 1823 [Ref: MS 3375/1782]; James Aston of Studley, veterinary surgeon, party to deed re land in Feckenham, Worcestershire 1825 [Ref: MS 3292/Acc 1926–027/329219]; Thomas Fisher of Childswickham, farmer and veterinary surgeon, party to deeds re premises in Duddeston Row and Bartholomew Street, Birmingham 1828 [Ref: MS 3192/Acc1928–41/360368, 360369]; Joseph Parker of Edgbaston, veterinary surgeon, copy probated will [1832] [Ref: MS 3/Box10/bdll 8]; Rupert Holmes of Birmingham, veterinary surgeon, party to assignment of mortgage 1850 [Ref: MS 58/52]; William Joseph Godwin of Birmingham, veterinary surgeon, party to assignment of land and premises in Great Charles Street, Birmingham 1851 [Ref: MS 3375/409971]; Robert Lewis Hunt of Birmingham, veterinary surgeon and smith: articles of partnership with Joseph Marston Parker 1856 [Ref: MS 3/Box5/bdl 21], party to mortgage of interest in estate of Abraham Hopkins deceased 1866 [Ref: MS 3/Box 4/bdl 19]; papers re transfer of George Bodington's veterinary infirmary and shoeing forge, Stephenson Place, New Street, Birmingham, to E Stanley 1858 [Ref: MS 1342/31]; Edward Stanley of Birmingham, veterinary surgeon, party to lease re a dwelling house in Broad Street 1859 [Ref: MS 3375/411187]; Henry Margetts Stanley of Birmingham, veterinary surgeon, party to deeds re land adjoining Broad Street and Sheepcote Street 1877, 1884, 1898 [Ref: MS 3375/409971, 411184, 411190–411192]; guarantee by Francis Blakeway to Joseph Clayworth of Birmingham, veterinary surgeon, of payments by his son John under a partnership agreement 1886 [Ref: MS 3/Box6/bdl 6]; Lawrence Clarke Tipper, veterinary inspector and local politician, correspondence re local Conservative activities 1886–1921 [Ref: MS 709]; Birch family, Curdworth, Warwickshire, papers incl blacksmiths' accounts c1890–1950. [Ref: MS 1957]

COVENTRY ARCHIVES
Mandela House, Bayley Lane, Coventry CV1 5RG

Edward Jackson Palfrey of Chapelfield, Coventry, veterinary surgeon, party to deeds 1812 1814 [Ref: PA/101/1/309–310; PA/202/3/4–5, PA/101/8/654–655]; William Amos Packwood of Coventry, veterinary surgeon, party to deeds 1837, 1848. [Ref: PA/101/8/689, 691]

IN PRIVATE OWNERSHIP, MR F C HAMMOND
5 Bracken Wood, off Skip Lane, Walsall WS5 3LH

Misc prescriptions 19th–20th cent; cine film of animal infections, testing and surgery 20th cent.

WALSALL LOCAL HISTORY CENTRE
Essex Street, Walsall WS2 7AS

Edward George Jarrett, horse keeper at co-operative dairy: book of horse medicines c1930s–50s [Ref: Acc 542/1], press cuttings c1930s–50s [Ref: 542/2]; F C Hammond, veterinary surgeon, Walsall: typescript of reminiscences re veterinary surgery and his practice early 1990s [Ref: P636.089], cassette recorded interview re his professional life 1990s. [Ref: Acc 426/216, 217]

WOLVERHAMPTON ARCHIVES AND LOCAL STUDIES
42–50 Snow Hill, Wolverhampton WV2 4AG

William Wallace of Wolverhampton, veterinary surgeon, party to deeds re land in Bradley and Bilston 1865, 1867, 1874. [Ref: D/JSR/26/2, 3; D/JSR/44/349/3; D/JSR/44/411/5]

WEST SUSSEX

HORSHAM MUSEUM
9 The Causeway, Horsham RH12 1HE

John Meginnis, veterinary surgeon, bills and receipts to Medwin family 1813–37 [Ref: MS 596]; Gumbrill, blacksmith, account book 1872–74 [Ref: MS 4537]; misc livestock accounts c1895–1907. [Ref: MS 4567.1–3]

WEST SUSSEX RECORD OFFICE
County Hall, Chichester PO19 1RN

Petworth House: receipted bills, letters etc of London tradesmen for goods and services supplied to Thomas Elder incl Thomas Allen, Edward Palmer, William Warden, John Lambert, George Shaw, farriers 1744–49, 1753–55 [Ref: PHA/7356, 7357, 7455, 8435], tradesmens' bills paid for George, 3rd Earl of Egremont, incl Peter Hay, Henry Boulton, Edward Snape, James Hay, Jane Hay, Charles Adams, William Layton, farriers

1753–55, 1774–98 [Ref: PHA/6608, 6611, 6635, 6640, 7528, 7530, 7531, 7536, 7539, 7541, 7543, 7545, 7548–50, 7555, 8051, 8052, 8079, 8101, 8435], abstracts of bills from London and Petworth tradesmen paid by Countess of Egremont as executrix to Charles, 2nd Earl of Egremont, incl Elizabeth Allen and Alexander Hay, farriers 1763 [Ref: PHA/6626, 6613], bills re case for debt brought by executors of George Heald, farrier, against William Frederick Wyndham 1782–88 [Ref: PHA/8315], bills for goods and services supplied to William Frederick Wyndham by local tradesmen incl John Etherton, farrier 1794 [Ref: PHA/8306], bills paid by George, 3rd Earl of Egremont, incl to Veterinary College, London, for keeping a horse 1796 [Ref: PHA/8058]; commonplace book of John Sergent with veterinary and other recipes on reverse 18th cent [Ref: Wilberforce/291]; William Woods of Arundel, farrier, party to mortgage 1812 [Ref: Holmes, Campbell & Co Mss/604]; Cobden of Heyshott, accounts incl for veterinary services 1836–63 [Ref: COBDEN/176. 177]; Dr Robert Druitt, letters on medical matters incl from James Beart Simonds, Royal Veterinary College, London, with Druitt's comments on reverse 1854 [Ref: Druitt Mss/67]; Charles Henry Gordon-Lennox, 6th Duke of Richmond, correspondence incl re Royal Agricultural Commission and Contagious Diseases (Animals) Acts 1882–86 [Ref: GOODWOOD/871]; deeds, plans etc re house and stable in Church Street, Steyning, leased to Thomas Bolton, veterinary surgeon 1893–1909. [Ref: Wiston/2860–2865]

IN PRIVATE OWNERSHIP, MR OLIVER GRAHAM-JONES
The Drey, 16 Park Lane, Selsey, Chichester PO20 0HD

Videos: colostomy on a python late 1960s, correction of an elephant's abnormal tusk 1960s, operations on a chimpanzee and a wolf 1960s, episode of British Broadcasting Corporation's *Animal Magic* showing new animal hospital at London Zoo c1960; photographs taken at London Zoo: apparatus, cages, anaesthetic procedures, toucan's artificial beak, VIP visits, etc c1950–66.

IN PRIVATE OWNERSHIP, DR A G WARREN
6 Meadow Way, Aldwick Bay Estate, Aldwick, Bognor Regis PO21 4HS

Board of Studies, Khartoum, Sudan: minutes, Home Office Inspectors' reports, employment contracts, case histories 20th cent.

WEST YORKSHIRE

BRADFORD DISTRICT ARCHIVES
15 Canal Road, Bradford BD1 4AT

Joseph Wright, Horsforth, Keighley, medical recipe book incl some for animal medicines 1787–1842. [Ref: 23D97]

BROTHERTON LIBRARY, LEEDS UNIVERSITY
Department of Special Collections, Brotherton Library, Leeds University, Leeds LS2 9JT

Thomas Escricke, recipe book for man and beast c1710–c1748 [Ref: MS 422]; Thomas Scattergood, surgeon and lecturer in chemistry at Leeds School of Medicine, case notes re his analyses in cases of suspected poisonings incl animals, also his analysis of *Priest's Condition Powder* for horses 1846–97. [Ref: MS 534/1–3]

YORKSHIRE ARCHAEOLOGICAL SOCIETY
Claremont, 23 Clarendon Road, Leeds LS2 9NZ

Stud book containing veterinary prescriptions 18th cent. [Ref: MD 290/box 11]

WILTSHIRE

WILTSHIRE & SWINDON RECORD OFFICE
County Hall, Trowbridge BA14 8JG

James Kite of Salisbury, veterinary surgeon, account books 1845–47 [Ref: 776/930]; memorandum of agreement between William Peahale of Barnstaple, Devon, veterinary surgeon, and Great Western Railway Company re provision of veterinary services at Barnstaple and Ilfracombe 1881 [Ref: 2515 210 Box 37/7]; correspondence between Walter Hume Long, President of Board of Agriculture, R W Hanbury, MP, and A C Cope, Chief Veterinary Officer to Board of Agriculture and Fisheries, re negotiations for increases in salaries of certain Board officials etc 1897–98 [Ref: 947/46]; agreement between Great Western Railway Company and Joseph Harry of Llwynhendy, Monmouthshire, veterinary surgeon, and others re sidings near Llanelly with subsequent agreements and plans 1903–16. [Ref: 2515 210 Box 121/6]

WORCESTERSHIRE

WORCESTERSHIRE RECORD OFFICE
County Hall, Spetchley Road, Worcester WR5 2NP

Michael Fisher of Childswickham, farrier, party to lease and release 1772 [Ref: 705:962/8965/5/i/1-2]; marriage settlement of Richard Lawrence, veterinary surgeon 1804 [Ref: 889:749/8782/21/D45/2]; commission appointing Joseph Berrington as veterinary surgeon to the Corps of Herefordshire Yeomanry Cavalry 1805 [Ref: 705:24/1472]; partnership agreement re Guise, Lea & Co, chemists and druggists, mentioning Charles Guise of Stoke Prior, veterinary surgeon 1812 [Ref: 899:749/8782/8/B8/12]; James Berrington: commission as veterinary surgeon to the Staff Corps of Cavalry 1813 [Ref: 705:24/1473], party to lease and release re land in Leominster and Hope under Dinmore, Herefordshire 1821 [Ref: 705:24/1326, 1327], draft copy of the specification of his invention known as the Berrington knapsack 1838 [Ref: 705:24/1474], petition to House of Commons re the Berrington knapsack c1850 [Ref: 705:24/1476]; Charles Guise of Stoke Prior, veterinary surgeon, party to marriage settlement 1817 [Ref: 899:749/8782/21/D45/8]; *Horses, Their Food and Treatment Considered in Relation to Henri's Patent Arabian Meal* 1855 [Ref: 705:414 BA 8779/14 (ii)]; catalogue of Hindlip herd of purebred Shorthorns 1878 [Ref: 899:233) BA 4371]; hymn on cattle plague 19th cent [Ref: 850 Besford (in Defford cum Besford) BA 8522/5 (vi)]; letters and papers re case of N Gold, veterinary surgeon, v R V Adams concerning disturbance caused by dogs on premises at 7 Church Green East, Redditch 1939 [Ref: 705:399/8008/42/x]; British Needle Co Ltd, correspondence incl letter re veterinary tattoo pins 1967. [Ref: 705:1321/11235/10i]

IRELAND

PUBLIC RECORD OFFICE OF NORTHERN IRELAND
66 Balmoral Avenue, Belfast BT9 6NY

Letter re 'cattle dying by the thousands' 1744 [Ref: 2092/1/16]; description of epidemic among black cattle in Co Leitrim 1748 [Ref: T/3019/1096]; letters re cattle plague 1750 [Ref: T/3019/1628–29, 1632]; recipe for distemper in horses 1760 [Ref: D/1950/29]; notebook re service of cattle, etc, Co Down 1768–1880 [Ref: T1296]; letter re distemper in cattle, Co Waterford 1769 [Ref: D/572/1/48]; Robert and William Best, Ballycairn, Co Antrim, misc accounts and receipts including veterinary fees c1800–95 [Ref: D/2838/C1/39]; George Linden, deposition as to houghing a cow 1829 [Ref: D/353/3]; J Riley, veterinary surgeon, certificate giving result of examination of a horse 1837 [Ref: D/2838/G/3]; W Youatt, textbook on cattle c1840 [Ref: D/693]; prayer to be read in all churches and chapels in Ireland during prevalence of cholera and cattle plague 1866 [Ref: D/1124/5/32]; W A Moore, letter to J R Moore re disease in his cattle 1872 [Ref: D/2309/3/2/97]; letters and papers re licence to perform experiments on animals 1877–78 [Ref: D/3819]; Walter Ferguson, Bowhouse Bog, Lanarkshire, letter to Thomas [Forserves?], Ballavaine, Co Tyrone, advising him on the treatment for 'magots on the sheep' 1880 [Ref: D/2712/1/89]; papers re livestock exports, etc in records of Larne Harbour Ltd, Co Antrim 1886–1985 [Ref: D/3947]; Robert F Blake, public analyst for Northern Ireland, medical analysis books, notebooks, papers incl some re animals 1887–1944 [Ref: D/2682]; Edward Watson, veterinary surgeon, Killyleagh, Co Down, account book 1892–1909 [Ref: D/3749]; J B Moore, veterinary surgeon, Londonderry, ledger 1895–1916 [Ref: D/4060/7]; Dr John Adair Crawford, diplomas, certificates and testimonials re medical training and career incl diploma as veterinary surgeon granted by French government in 1812 19th cent [Ref: D/1913/2/1–56]; prayer for cow late 19th cent [Ref: D/2312]; Lisahoppen, Co Tyrone, personal account book incl references to veterinary expenses 1904–14 [Ref: D/3578]; government papers re aid to new industries, incl references to veterinary products 1937–39 [Ref: COM17/1]; F T Finney, veterinary surgeon, Newcastle upon Tyne, Tyne & Wear, obituary, nd. [Ref: D/1900/27]

SCOTLAND

ARYLL & BUTE

ARGYLL AND BUTE COUNCIL ARCHIVES

Area Office, Manse Brae, Lochgilphead PA31 8QU

A MacNair, farrier and blacksmith, Campbeltown: general ledgers 1844–47, ledgers re cartwright work 1845–46. [Ref: DR4/4/6–7]

DUMFRIES & GALLOWAY

DUMFRIES & GALLOWAY ARCHIVE CENTRE

33 Burns Street, Dumfries DG1 2PS

Gelston Castle estate, invoice from Robert McAdam, veterinary surgeon 1887 [Ref: GGD 78/1/6/20]; K S Dobie & Son Ltd, seed merchants and pet shop owners, Dumfries: order and customer delivery books 1960s–70s, trade catalogues and magazines 1970s. [Ref: GGC 322]

EDINBURGH

NATIONAL ARCHIVES OF SCOTLAND

HM General Register House, Edinburgh EH1 3YY

Mar and Kellie estate: account by Thomas Downie, smith in Stirling, for shoeing horses 1648 [Ref: GD124/17/11], letters to Lord Grange from George Erskine at Alloa re an injured horse, with related papers 1708 [Ref: GD124/15/762/14]; Airlie estate: papers re treatment of horses 17th cent [Ref: GD16/58/49], papers re cattle plague in Forfarshire 1865 [Ref: GD16/27/432], papers re cattle diseases 1865–68 [Ref GD16/57/84], petition by University of Dublin against Bill confirming bequest by Thomas Brown for advancement of veterinary studies 1867 [Ref: GD16/57/87]; Rosslyn estate: surgeon-apothecary's accounts for 'drugges to the horses' 1722–23 [Ref: GD164/554], vouchers for horses 1734–59 [Ref: GD164/600–739 passim], misc papers re horses 1755–1926 [Ref: GD164/2110–2124], notebook on care and veterinary treatment of horses and dogs mid 19th cent [Ref: GD164/2119]; Clerk of Penicuik estate: accounts of stablers, farriers and veterinary surgeons 1655–1891 [Ref: GD18/2174], correspondence with James Clerk, farrier 1764–82 [Ref: GD18/5753], several improvements for feeding of horses, black cattle, sheep and fowls 18th cent [Ref: GD18/1706]; Robertson of Lude estate: discharged account by Hugh Livingstone, Perth, to Captain John Robertson for shoeing horses 1767 [Ref: GD132/637], account for shoeing horses 18th cent [Ref: GD132/653]; Huntly estate, letter from John Low, blacksmith, to Lord Aboyne, binding himself as smith and farrier in Charlestown 1770 [Ref: GD312/11]; MacKintosh of MacKintosh: discharged accounts for smith work, incl agreement by William Falconer to attend The MacKintosh's sick horses, not accepting payment until horses are cured 1791 [Ref: GD176/1675], Duncan Thompson, report on condition of horses 1874 [Ref: GD176/2324], letter from Messrs Sedgwick, Turner & Oddie, solicitors, requesting payment of an account owed to F Jarvis, South Kensington, for shoeing horses 1890 [Ref: GD176/2484]; Cunninghame estate, Thornton, letter to medical board giving rates of pay for assistant and veterinary surgeons 1797 [Ref: GD21/642]; Warrand of Bught estate: letter from Thomas Gillespie to James Grant prescribing treatment for foot-rot in sheep 1829 [Ref: GD23/6/625], receipted account, Duncan Grant to Archibald Young, surgical instrument maker, Edinburgh, for cattle syringe 1834 [Ref: GD23/5/395]; [Veterinary Hospital, Princes Street, Perth], architectural plans and elevations c1830 [Ref: RHP83345–46]; Seaforth estate, account from Keith Stewart Mackenzie to Duncan MacDonald, smith and farrier, Dingwall, Highland 1850 [Ref: GD46/1/520]; Strathern and Blair estate, specifications for 'Preserving Animal and Vegetable Substances' and 'Slaughtering Animals', the former being US patent no 71,377 in the names of John Gamgee and Arthur Gamgee, with related papers 1861–67 [Ref: GD314/481]; letters to William Smythe of Methven re cattle plague 1865–66 [Ref: GD190/3/377]; King's and Lord Treasurer's Remembrancer (Exchequer): Veterinary Medical Inspector, proposed purchase of camera for use in inspection of slaughterhouses, dairies, etc 1913 [Ref: E 824/31], papers re requests for grants from Glasgow and Edinburgh colleges in respect of loss of income caused by war 1917 [Ref: E 824/240], papers re veterinary college estimates 1923–25 [Ref: E 824/334, 340, 349]; Broughton and Cally estate: correspondence with veterinary surgeons 1945–67 [Ref: GD10/1587], papers re Jersey Cattle herd incl correspondence with agricultural consultants 1942–69, calf registers and cattle record cards 1947–65, general file on herd 1952–66, insemination certificates 1957–66, correspondence re staff 1958–69 [GD10/1605], details of cast cows c1958–c1965, queried accounts with suppliers 1959–69, correspondence with suppliers and customers 1960–65, details of goods for sale 1961–67, furnishings and fittings in shop 1961–67, correspondence and papers re export of Galloway cattle models and Galloway Cattle Society ties 1961–62 [Ref: GD10/1665], correspondence with Scottish Jersey Cattle Club 1967–69 [GD10/1590]; J W Keddie, programmes of Royal (Dick) Veterinary College Athletic Club annual sports meetings 1950–55 [Ref: GD445/1/146]; George Matheson, postmaster, Edinburgh, sederunt book noting that William Dick, veterinary surgeon, is a trustee, nd. [Ref: CS96/4270–71]

NATIONAL LIBRARY OF SCOTLAND
George IV Bridge, Edinburgh EH1 1EW

Prescription for scabbed horses 1689 [Ref: MS 2208 f.15v]; Sir Joseph Banks' prescription for sheep scab 1788 [Ref: MS 3593 f.10]; recipes to cure coughs and diseases in cattle 1790, nd [Ref: MS 8114 ff.66, 67];

misc medical, domestic and veterinary recipes 18th–19th cent [Ref: MS 10693 ff. 153–180]; receipt issued to William Rae McPhun, publisher, by John Stewart, veterinary surgeon 1834 [Ref: MS 30005 f. 66]; copy of letter to John Stewart, veterinary surgeon, with Stewart's reply 1840 [Ref: MS 30007 ff. 125, 126]; assignation of copyright of *Stable Economy* by John Stewart, veterinary surgeon, to Robert Blackwood and Sons, with a letter from James Brash, bookseller, to Robert Blackwood 1840 [Ref: MS 30007 ff. 127–131]; letters re teaching of veterinary surgery in Edinburgh 1844 [Ref: MS 12139 ff. 34–38]; William Dick, Edinburgh Veterinary College: letter and petition 1844 [Ref: 12139 ff. 34–38], letter to [-] 1850 [Ref: MS 7307 f. 55], letter to Spottiswood and Robertson, London, concerning the teaching of his subject 1851 [Ref: 9597]; correspondence and papers of 3rd Earl Minto re various political issues incl cattle plague and Contagious Diseases (Animals) Acts 1858–89 [Ref: MS 12357 ff. 162–191, 202]; receipt issued to John Blackwood by Colin C Baird of Edinburgh, veterinary surgeon 1875 [Ref: MS 30031 ff. 133, 134]; letter and notes re vivisection 1881 [Ref: MS 6077 ff. 29–36]; letter from Florence Nightingale to Sir John J Burden Sanderson re work of veterinary surgeons 1884 [Ref: MS 6103 f. 120]; letters to William Blackwood from: Thomas Walley, Principal, Edinburgh Veterinary College 1887 [Ref: MS 30052 ff. 283, 312, 313, MS 30053 f. 387], W D Connochie and Sons of Selkirk, Scottish Borders, veterinary surgeons 1892 [Ref: MS 30061 f. 11]; certificate of soundness for horses issued by George Williams, veterinary surgeon, Pimlico, to Earl of Minto 1890 [Ref: MS 13228 ff. 152, 153]; misc memoranda re tuberculin testing of milk 1934–35 [Ref: Acc. 6688, box 12 folder 1]; letter from Alasdair Alpin MacGregor to Gerald Curtler re anti-vivisection movement with a draft reply 1966 [Ref: Acc. 7846]; notebook, incl sketches, re animal anatomy, nd. [Ref: Dep. 199]

MISCELLANEOUS REFERENCES WITHIN COLLECTIONS IN PRIVATE OWNERSHIP IN SCOTLAND

National Register of Archives (Scotland), HM General Register House, Edinburgh EH1 3YY

Lauderdale estate: accounts for maintenance of horses 1670 [Ref: NRA(S)832/61/65], Henry Home, factor, contract with Andrew Brabander, smith in Largo, Fife, for shoeing horses, etc 1670, accounts 1672–74 [Ref: NRA(S)832/159]; Hopetoun estate: notes by Charles, 1st Earl of Hopetoun, on horses bred by him, how they were disposed of, medical recipes for a variety of illnesses, etc 1695–1736 [Ref: NRA(S)888/v306], correspondence of 2nd Marquess of Linlithgow re purchase and maintenance of horses 1929–36 [Ref: NRA(S) 888/1019];

Hamilton estate: accounts of money expended on shoes for coach and saddle horses 1723–24 [Ref: NRA(S) 2177/471], letters to 5th Duke of Hamilton and others re care of horses, etc 1731 [Ref: NRA(S)2177/898], misc letters re horses 1734–35 [Ref: NRA(S) 2177/938–939], letters and other papers of Alexander Inglis, Master of Horse, re management of stables, health of horses and dogs, etc 1735–40 [Ref: NRA(S)2177/2808, 2809, 1051, 1052, 1058], bills and receipts, incl farrier 1764–68, 1775 [Ref: NRA(S) 2177/3388, 3391, 3397], accounts re racehorses 1767–78, 1811, 1817 [Ref: NRA(S) 2177/3851, 3768, 3742], accounts for payments to named servants and tradesmen incl James Purdie, smith and farrier at Motherwell, North Lanarkshire, for medicine given to a cow that died 1786 [Ref: NRA(S) 2177/5345], accounts of expenses for individual racehorses 1789 [Ref: NRA(S) 2177/3841], receipted bills from James Gibbs, cutler, New Bond St, London, for a machine for docking horses 1791, and John Norborn, dog doctor, for medicines and bleeding of dogs 1791 [Ref: NRA(S) 2177/5388], receipted bills from John Hume for a variety of medicines for horses and dogs 1791 [Ref: NRA(S) 2177/5393], accounts kept by John Mangle for Duke of Hamilton re horseracing 1793–94 [Ref: NRA(S) 2177/3520], bills from William Purkins, farrier, to Earl of Rochford for shoeing horses and supplying ointment 1795 [Ref: NRA(S)2177/5323], bills from Mr Whitehead, surgeon, for treating horses 1798 [Ref: NRA(S) 2177/6168], letters from Frank Collinson to 9th Duke of Hamilton re health of stables, etc 1807 [Ref: NRA(S)2177/2799], correspondence of Robert Brown, factor, incl veterinary expenses to be paid 1817 [Ref: NRA(S) 2177/1679], notebook with details of expenditure on racehorses 1817 [Ref: NRA(S) 2177/3769], pedigrees, receipts, etc re racehorses 19th cent [Ref: NRA(S) 2177/3849]; Grant of Ballindalloch: account due to David Brodie, physician in Elgin, Moray, incl medicines for horses 1742–43 [Ref: NRA(S)771/1164], account due to George Mitchal in Slack, Aberdeenshire, for shoeing horses 1769 [Ref: NRA(S)771/1149], account due to James Rioch, smith, for shoeing and other work re horses 1806 [Ref: NRA(S) 771/1190]; Mercer of Aldie, account from Patrick Soutar, Meikleour, smith 1775–76 [Ref: NRA(S)3698/653]; Earl of Haddington (Tyninghame), notebook of treatments for illness in horses and dogs 1787 [Ref: NRA(S) 3503/1/72]; memoranda and papers re proposals to establish a stud in India for cavalry horses c1802–12 [Ref: NRA(S)276/1/3, 2/3]; Stuart-Menteth of Closeburn and Mansfield: letter (with drawings) from T Hill, Downton Vale, London, describing method he has perfected for shoeing horses 1848 [Ref: NRA(S)3256/77], John Douglas, veterinary surgeon, Cumnock, East Ayrshire, receipted bills for treatment of cow 1857–58 [Ref: NRA(S)3256/30], letter from William Dick re cattle plague 1866 [Ref: NRA(S) 3256/88], William Turnbull, blacksmith, New Cumnock,

East Ayrshire, receipted bills for shoeing horses, etc 1889 [Ref: NRA(S) 3256/16]; Claude Bowes Lyon, misc papers incl recipes for veterinary medicaments c1850 [Ref: NRA(S)885/193/1]; MacLean of Ardgour, letter from Reverend Archibald Clerk to Alexander MacLean re Campbell's suitability as a tenant 1861 [Ref: NRA(S)3583/42/4]; Forbes of Callendar, accounts and receipts re horses 19th cent [Ref: NRA(S)3626]; Earl of Strathmore, accounts for medical and dental treatment and veterinary surgeons' bills 1940–51 [Ref: NRA(S)3526/384, 386]; Kilkerran family, Ayrshire, collection of receipts and curiosities on different subjects incl notes on veterinary and agricultural procedures, nd [Ref: NRA(S) 3572/1/15]; J Wortley, Professor of Pathology, Royal Veterinary College, London, paper re bovine contagious abortion, its causes, prevention and treatment, nd [Ref: NRA(S)771/646]; Cawdor estate, recipe for curing horses of botts, nd [Ref: NRA(S)1400/495]; proposed draft of *Orders re Care of Horses*, apparently corrected by Sir Horatio Herbert Kitchener, nd. [Ref: NRA(S) 1054/26/2]

SCOTTISH LIFE ARCHIVE
Royal Museum of Scotland, Chambers Street, Edinburgh EH1 1JF

Colonel Alexander Houston of Haddington, East Lothian, recipes for arsenical soap 1839 [Ref: MS.Archives 1980/41]; Thomas Harley, veterinary chemist, Perth, advertising leaflets c1900 [Ref: W.MS.1997.466/20–24]; photograph of veterinary surgeon injecting a lamb c1920 [Ref: C5231]; Royal (Dick) Veterinary College, receipt for veterinary services 1933 [Ref: W.MS.1997.111/35]; Colin C Baird & Son, Edinburgh, receipt for veterinary services 1934 [Ref: W.MS.1997/111/36]; *The Little Red Book Diary* (blank) published by Cooper McDougall & Robertson Ltd to advertise their veterinary products 1939 [Ref: W.MS.1997.722/57]; cure for an ailing cow 1959 [Ref: MS 1986–38]; letter from M L Ryder to Robert Dascotte re castration methods 1966; *Cooper's Sheep Dipping Powder*, advertisement early 20th cent; Edinburgh School of Agriculture, slides re cattle, horses, pigs, dogs, poultry diseases, sheep, nd [Ref: C20929–20932, C20954–21301]; postcards: tilting table for calf, calf on tilting table, collecting vaccine lymph from calf, nd [Ref: P2679–2681]; description of outbreak of foot-and-mouth disease by Mr Geddes of South Powrie, nd [Ref: MS 1977/19]; photographs of fleams, castrating clamps and other veterinary instruments, nd. [Ref: PM26(ii), PM27, PM1969, C12268, PM24]

FALKIRK

FALKIRK COUNCIL ARCHIVES

Falkirk Museums History Research Centre, Callendar House, Callendar Park, Falkirk FK1 1YR

Forbes of Callendar: receipts incl veterinary accounts with sketches of unidentified implements on reverse 1795–96 [Ref: GD171/2418/7–8], account due to veterinary surgeon 1832–33 [Ref: GD171/3118], account due to Arthur Herriot, veterinary surgeon 1842. [Ref: GD171/3170]

GLASGOW

GLASGOW CITY ARCHIVES

Mitchell Library, North Street, Glasgow G3 7DN

Harvie family, Halfway House, Cardonald, blacksmiths: ledgers 1839–47, 1849–60, notebook on veterinary lectures, nd [Ref: TD285/1–3]; Veterinary Association, report of annual meeting 1892 [Ref: MP23, 425]; Purple Cross Service for Wounded and Sick Animals, papers, nd. [Ref: T–PM1/28, p561]

MITCHELL LIBRARY

Arts Department, North Street, Glasgow 7DN

Notebook of veterinary recipes 1730–20 [Ref: D115521]; Veterinary Department of Privy Council Office, report 1878–82 [Ref: L40401]; James McCall, introductory lecture, Glasgow 1884 [Ref: D81744]; regulations for admission to Army Veterinary Corps 1906 [Ref: D23434]; East Kilbride and District Milk Record Society, minute book 1919–50; Scottish Milk Records Association, constitution and rules, nd.

WALES

CARDIFF

MUSEUM OF WELSH LIFE

St Fagans, Cardiff CF5 6XB

Llewellyn Miles, farrier, Wenvoe, testimonials in his favour as a skilled farrier 1870s [Ref: 3590]; David Davies, farrier, Prys Mawr, Gwynedd, veterinary recipe books c1920s [Ref: 2720/1–3]; Eisteddfod essays describing a family of farriers from Llanuwchllyn, Gwynedd (p) c1840–1934, 1966 [Ref: Photocopies 1389–90]; W O Jones, pharmacist and veterinary surgeon, Betws-y-Coed, reminiscences (p) 1978 [Ref: Photocopy 2673]; T G Thomas, Caernarfon, list of Welsh-English veterinary terms (p) 1978. [Ref: Photocopy 3482]

REGIMENTAL MUSEUM, 1ST THE QUEEN'S DRAGOON GUARDS
Cardiff Castle, Cardiff CF10 3RB

Lieutenant Colonel H A Hankey, diary re men and horses 1838–51.

CEREDIGION

NATIONAL LIBRARY OF WALES
Department of Manuscripts and Records, Aberystwyth SY23 3BU

Mary Edwards, Great Ness, Shropshire, notebook containing culinary, medical and veterinary recipes 1716–67 [Ref: NLW MS 23472C]; account book incl veterinary recipes 1752–1844 [Ref: Burchinshaw Deeds and Documents no 15]; Charles Hassall, East Wood, Narberth, Pembrokeshire, recipes for sheep scab 1798 [Ref: Poyston Deeds, no 336]; farmer's accounts incl veterinary recipes 1799 [Ref: Cwmeiddig (Rhayader) Documents, no 20]; Cadwaladr Davies, Gwyddelwern, Denbighshire, *Ail biser Sioned*, collection of poems, medical and veterinary recipes 18th cent [Ref: NLW MS 9047A]; recipe for 'balls for a horse cough' c18th cent [Ref: Wigfair Deeds and Documents no 2294]; veterinary and medical recipes 18th–19th cent [Ref: NLW MS 19662B, Cwrtmawr 514B section X]; John Jones, petty constable, Pencoed, Llanwyddelan, Powys, notebook re his office incl veterinary recipes 1809–21 [Ref: Henblas (Llanwnnog) Papers, no 1]; Morgan Rice James and Mary Ann James, Haverfordwest, notebook containing veterinary, household and culinary recipes c1825–81 [Ref: NLW MS 23216B]; William Crawshay, letter to John Powell recommending a veterinary surgeon 1828 [Ref: Maybery Collection, no 2625]; Richard Jones, Worcester, book of veterinary and other prescriptions 1836 [Ref: D Teifigar Davies MSS (p 1 of schedule)]; John Jones, Llangernyw, Denbighshire, pocket ledger containing medical and veterinary recipes 1840–83 [Ref: NLW MS 22747A]; Thomas Jones, Brynmeheryn, Ystrad Meurig, Ceredigion, weaver's account book containing customer accounts and a few veterinary recipes 1869–1905 [Ref: NLW MS 22835B]; letter re cattle plague in County Montgomery 1883 [Ref: NLW 19460C]; William Simon, Cwm-dwr-Forge, Llansadwrn, Carmarthenshire, account books with notes of veterinary interest 1883–98 [Ref: NLW Misc Vols 360–362]; Hugh Davies & Co, chemist, The Pharmacy, Machynlleth, Gwynedd, prescription books containing veterinary recipes 1885–1930 [Ref: NLW Minor Deposits 1414–17B]; notebooks containing medical and veterinary prescriptions c1895–1951 [Ref: NLW Misc Vols 269, 314–315]; Lieutenant Colonel Knox, letter to Sir Charles Morgan re letting a veterinary surgeon examine a bay horse early 19th cent [Ref: Tredegar Park Muniments 45/1528]; veterinary recipes 19th cent [Ref: Nanteos Papers]; notebooks of medical and veterinary recipes 19th cent [Ref: Maesnewydd Deeds and Documents, nos 383–384]; notebook incl a few medical and veterinary recipes 19th cent [Ref: Cwrtmawr 538B]; notebook incl veterinary recipes 19th cent [Ref: Cwrtmawr 618A]; notebook containing veterinary recipes mid 19th–20th cent [Ref: Henblas (Llanwnnog) Papers, no 2]; University College Wales, Aberystwyth, extension course on agriculture, land surveying, entomology, law, mineralogy and veterinary science, lecture notes 1908–09 [Ref: T J Jenkin Papers 2–19]; University of Wales, papers re veterinary science 1939–57 [Ref: Association of Welsh Local Authorities X85]; papers re Welsh veterinary training and education 1942–46 [Ref: W A O S Archives L3]; Lord Cledwyn, correspondence with British Veterinary Association 1989–92 [Ref: Lord Cledwyn Papers (October 1992 Donation) B24]; notebook containing veterinary and other recipes, nd [Ref: NLW MS 20584B]; research papers re horses and veterinary work, nd [Ref: Ffransis G Payne Papers 818]; Moses Griffith: papers and correspondence re establishment of agricultural and veterinary colleges in Wales, nd, notebook of veterinary and other recipes, nd. [Ref: Moses Griffith Papers]

FLINTSHIRE

FLINTSHIRE COUNTY RECORD OFFICE

The Old Rectory, Hawarden CH5 3NR

Recipe for a cure for rabies c1700 [Ref: D/E/856]; leaflet re homeopathic treatment of cattle plague 1856–60 [Ref: D/E/2747]; correspondence re outbreak of cattle plague 1866–67 [Ref: D/IP/189]; recipe for sheep rot cure 1930s [Ref: D/DM/1107/186]; prescription register and register of poisons, Rhyl and Colwyn Bay areas 1949–73. [Ref: D/DM/1130/1–2]

GWYNEDD

UNIVERSITY OF WALES, BANGOR
Department of Manuscripts, Bangor LL57 2DG

Farriery recipes contained in *The Art of Farriery*, Wrexham 1795 [Ref: Bangor MS.3590]; misc farriery recipes c1800–25. [Ref: MS.1B]

ISLE OF ANGLESEY

ANGLESEY RECORD OFFICE
Shire Hall, Llangefni LL7 7TW

Recipe for curing the bite of a mad dog 1741 [Ref: WM/932/1]; book 'giving an illustration of the diseases met by animals and directions to make them better' pre 1842 [Ref: WDAJ/2]; William and Robert Edwards, Glangorsddu, Gwlachmai, dictionary of daily wants incl horse and calf remedies 1858 [Ref: WM/1640]; cassette recording containing reference to treatment of horses and hounds injured during hunting, nd. [Ref: WM T/69/2]

SWANSEA

UNIVERSITY OF WALES, SWANSEA
Collections Access Officer, Swansea Museum, Victoria Road, Swansea SA1 1SN

Receipt for 'the murren' c1680 [Ref: Swansea Museum Service miscellanea no 2]; medical prescriptions: mange c1730, collick c1730, misc 1812. [Ref: Whitney collection nos 29–31]

WEST GLAMORGAN ARCHIVE SERVICE
County Hall, Oystermouth Road, Swansea SA1 3SN

Ystradgynlais, Powys, notebook with accounts, medical and husbandry advice and legal document formulae incl folk remedies for diseases of farm livestock 1726–68. [Ref: D/D Z 123/1]

TORFAEN

GWENT RECORD OFFICE
County Hall, Cwmbran NP44 2XH

John Gwin and others, Llangwm, commonplace book incl herbal remedies for various ailments 1630–1720 [Ref: D43.4216]; Thomas Phillpotts, Brelston, Herefordshire, farrier, covenant of indenture with Edward Hemond, Brelston, husbandman 1635 [Ref: D917.601 (Davis, Lloyd & Wilson MSS)]; Edmund Davies, Newchurch, farrier, lease of messuages and tenements, Llanvaches and Newchurch 1757 [Ref: D43.431 (M424.6)]; parish register, Llandenny, Monmouthshire, incl recipe for cure of mange c1769 [Ref: D/Pa 37.1]; Moses Daniel, Lanvihangel, Pontymoyle, farrier, lease of messuage, blacksmith's shop, pigstye and gardens 1791 [Ref: D43.1780 (M350)]; misc recipes for human and animal diseases and killing of vermin 18th cent [Ref: Misc.MSS.1443]; Mary Long, recipe book 1828 [Ref: D361.F1.E9]; Edward Harris, Rockfield, farrier, contract for sale of farm and lands called Penny Veddow in Llangattock Vibon Avel 1840 [Ref: D361.32–44]; Catherine Peirce, Abergavenny, recipe book 1848 [Ref: Misc.MSS.1771]; David Whitty, Havod, Brecknock, Powys, veterinary surgeon, counterpart lease 1855 [Ref: D397.822 (Nantyglo and Blaina Estate MSS)]; G Lewis, Monmouth, veterinary surgeon, receipt for veterinary services from Mr Long, Llanthewy 1866 [Ref: D.586.12]; William Sheap, Newport, veterinary surgeon, purchase of farmhouse from Edmund Davies Williams 1890 [Ref: D43.4344 (M428)]; Frederick Tucker, 5 Whitecross Street, Monmouth, veterinary surgeon, conveyance of land and messuages at 5 and 7 St Mary Street, Monmouth 1901 [Ref: D1524.77]; Sidney Smith, Usk, veterinary surgeon, notice to quit premises at Gwehelog, Usk 1910. [Ref: D968.2 (Adams-Williams Estate MSS)]

Index of names

Index of places

Index of subjects

Index of archive repositories